Atlas of

Pediatric Otolaryngology

Illustrators

Jon P. Coulter, M.A., A.M.I.
Carol Coulter, B.A.
Caitlin Hughes, M.A.
Erik Dolnack

CHARLES D. BLUESTONE, M.D.
Professor of Otolaryngology
University of Pittsburgh School of Medicine
Director, Department of Otolaryngology
Children's Hospital of Pittsburgh
Pittsburgh, Pennsylvania

SYLVAN E. STOOL, M.D.
Professor of Otolaryngology and Pediatrics
University of Pittsburgh School of Medicine
Director of Education, Department of Otolaryngology
Children's Hospital of Pittsburgh
Pittsburgh, Pennsylvania

Atlas of Pediatric Otolaryngology

W.B. SAUNDERS COMPANY
A Division of Harcourt Brace & Company
Philadelphia London Toronto Montreal Sydney Tokyo

W.B. SAUNDERS COMPANY
A Division of Harcourt Brace & Company

The Curtis Center
Independence Square West
Philadelphia, Pennsylvania 19106

Library of Congress Cataloging-in-Publication Data

Atlas of pediatric otolaryngology / [edited by] Charles D. Bluestone, Sylvan E. Stool.
p. cm.
ISBN 0-7216-3711-6
1. Pediatric otolaryngology—Atlases. 2. Otolaryngology, Operative—Atlases.
I. Bluestone, Charles D. II. Stool, Sylvan E.
[DNLM: 1. Otorhinolaryngologic Diseases—in infancy & childhood—atlases. WV 17 A8816 1994]

RF47.C4A85 1995
618.92'09751—dc20
DNLM/DLC 93-40737

Atlas of Pediatric Otolaryngology ISBN 0-7216-3711-6

Printed in the United States of America.

Last digit is the print number: 9 8 7 6 5 4 3 2 1

contributors

CHARLES D. BLUESTONE, M.D.
Professor of Otolaryngology
University of Pittsburgh School of Medicine
Director, Department of Otolaryngology
Children's Hospital of Pittsburgh
Pittsburgh, Pennsylvania
Chapter 3: Otologic Surgical Procedures

LINDA BRODSKY, M.D.
Associate Professor of Otolaryngology and Pediatrics
State University of New York at Buffalo
School of Medicine and Biomedical Sciences
Co-Director, Department of Pediatric Otolaryngology
Children's Hospital of Buffalo
Buffalo, New York
Chapter 15: Tonsillectomy and Adenoidectomy
Chapter 16: Uvulopalatopharyngoplasty

MARGARETHA L. CASSELBRANT, M.D., PH.D.
Associate Professor of Otolaryngology
University of Pittsburgh School of Medicine
Director of Clinical Research
Department of Pediatric Otolaryngology
Children's Hospital of Pittsburgh
Pittsburgh, Pennsylvania
Chapter 21: Tracheostomy

KENNY H. CHAN, M.D.
Associate Professor of Otolaryngology
University of Colorado Health Sciences Center
Chairman, Department of Pediatric Otolaryngology
The Children's Hospital
Denver, Colorado
Chapter 20: Endoscopic Surgery of the Upper Aerodigestive Tract

NOEL L. COHEN, M.D.
Chairman, Department of Otolaryngology
New York University School of Medicine
Director of Otolaryngology
Tisch Hospital and Bellevue Hospital Center
Consultant, Veterans Administration Medical Center
New York, New York
Chapter 8: Cochlear Implants

WILLIAM S. CRYSDALE, M.D.
Professor, Department of Otolaryngology
University of Toronto
Otolaryngologist-in-Chief
Hospital for Sick Children
Toronto, Ontario, Canada
Chapter 18: Diseases of the Salivary Glands

MICHAEL J. CUNNINGHAM, M.D.
Assistant Professor of Otology and Laryngology
Harvard Medical School
Associate Surgeon in Otolaryngology
Massachusetts Eye and Ear Infirmary
Boston, Massachusetts
Chapter 25: Tumors of the Head and Neck

ROLAND D. EAVEY, M.D.
Associate Professor, Department of Otology and Laryngology
Harvard Medical School
Director, ENT Pediatric Services
The Massachusetts Eye and Ear Infirmary
Boston, Massachusetts
Chapter 2: Surgical Repair of the Auricle for Microtia

CARLOS GONZALEZ, M.D.
Associate Professor of Surgery (Otolaryngology)
University of Puerto Rico School of Medicine
Chief of Otolaryngology
San Jorge Children's Hospital
Santurce, Puerto Rico
Chapter 19: Tumors of the Mouth and Pharynx

CHARLES W. GROSS, M.D.
Professor, Otolaryngology–Head and Neck Surgery
Professor, Pediatrics
University of Virginia Health Science Center
Charlottesville, Virginia
Chapter 10: Plastic and Reconstructive Surgery

GERALD B. HEALY, M.D.
Professor of Otology and Laryngology
Harvard Medical School
Otolaryngologist-in-Chief
The Children's Hospital
Boston, Massachusetts
Chapter 22: Surgery of the Larynx and Trachea

RAYMOND L. HILSINGER, JR., M.D.
Director, Otolaryngology–Head and Neck Surgery
Residency Training Program
Chief, Department of Head and Neck Surgery
Kaiser Permanente Medical Center
Oakland, California
Consultant Staff, Department of Otolaryngology
Veterans Affairs Medical Center
Martinez, California
Chapter 4: The Facial Nerve

ANDREW J. HOTALING, M.D.
Assistant Professor of Otolaryngology–Head and Neck Surgery
Loyola University Medical Center
Children's Memorial Hospital
Maywood, Illinois
Chapter 14: Inflammation of the Nose and Paranasal Sinuses

DENNIS J. HURWITZ, M.D.
Clinical Associate Professor of Surgery (Plastic)
University of Pittsburgh School of Medicine
Hospitals of the University of Pittsburgh Medical Center
Children's Hospital of Pittsburgh
Pittsburgh, Pennsylvania
Chapter 1: Craniofacial Surgery

GLENN C. ISAACSON, M.D.
Associate Professor and Deputy Chairman, Department of Otorhinolaryngology/Broncho-esophagology
Temple University School of Medicine
Director, Department of Pediatric Otolaryngology
St. Christopher's Hospital for Children
Philadelphia, Pennsylvania
Chapter 7: Endoscopy of the Nose and Nasopharynx

MARGARET A. KENNA, M.D.
Associate Professor of Otolaryngology
University of Pittsburgh School of Medicine
Co-director, Department of Pediatric Otolaryngology
Children's Hospital of Pittsburgh
Associate Attending Physician
Eye and Ear Hospital of Pittsburgh
Pittsburgh, Pennsylvania
Chapter 11: Congenital Malformations of the Nose and Paranasal Sinuses

CHARLES F. KOOPMANN, JR., M.D.
Professor and Associate Chairman and Chief, Pediatric Otolaryngology
Department of Otolaryngology
C.S. Mott Children's Hospital
University of Michigan Medical Center
Ann Arbor, Michigan
Staff, Chelsea Community Hospital
Chelsea, Michigan
Saline Community Hospital
Saline, Michigan
Consultant
Veteran's Administration Medical Center
Ann Arbor, Michigan
Chapter 17: Deep Neck Infections

RODNEY P. LUSK, M.D.
Associate Professor
Washington University School of Medicine
Director, Pediatric Otolaryngology
St. Louis Children's Hospital
Associate Professor of Pediatrics
St. Louis Children's Hospital
St. Louis, Missouri
Chapter 13: Pediatric Endoscopic Ethmoidectomy

SCOTT C. MANNING, M.D.
Associate Professor, Department of Otolaryngology
University of Texas Southwestern Medical Center
Attending Otolaryngologist
Children's Medical Center
Parkland Memorial Hospital
Zale Lipshy University Hospital
Dallas, Texas
Chapter 9: Epistaxis

BRADLEY MARPLE, M.D.
Assistant Professor, Department of Otolaryngology
University of Texas Southwestern Medical Center
Dallas, Texas
Chapter 9: Epistaxis

FRANCIS X. McGOWAN, M.D.
Assistant Professor
Department of Anesthesiology
University of Pittsburgh School of Medicine
Staff Anesthesiologist
Children's Hospital of Pittsburgh
Pittsburgh, Pennsylvania
Chapter 20: Endoscopic Surgery of the Upper Aerodigestive Tract

SIMON C. PARISIER, M.D.
Chairman, Department of Otolaryngology–Head and Neck Surgery
Manhattan Eye, Ear and Throat Hospital
Attending Physician
New York Hospital
Mount Sinai Hospital
New York, New York
Chapter 5: Surgery of the Ear Canal: Split-Thickness Skin Grafts and Surgical Correction of Atresia

JAMES S. REILLY, M.D.
Professor, Otolaryngology and Pediatrics
Jefferson Medical College of Thomas Jefferson University
Philadelphia, Pennsylvania
Chief, Pediatric Otolaryngology
Alfred I. DuPont Institute Children's Hospital
Wilmington, Delaware
Chapter 6: Perilymphatic Fistula

MARK A. RICHARDSON, M.D.
Professor of Otolaryngology–Head and Neck Surgery
University of Washington School of Medicine
Chief, Division of Pediatric Otolaryngology
Children's Hospital and Medical Center
Seattle, Washington
Chapter 24: Congenital Malformations of the Neck

KEITH H. RIDING, M.D.
Clinical Associate Professor
University of British Columbia
Head, Division of Otolaryngology
British Columbia Children's Hospital
Vancouver, British Columbia
Chapter 20: Endoscopic Surgery of the Upper Aerodigestive Tract

ROBERT W. SEIBERT, M.D.
Professor, Department of Otolaryngology–Head and Neck Surgery
University of Arkansas for Medical Sciences
Chief, Pediatric Otolaryngology
Arkansas Children's Hospital
Little Rock, Arkansas
Chapter 12: Cleft Lip and Palate

DAVID A. SEIDMAN, M.D.
Resident Coordinator
Manhattan Eye, Ear and Throat Hospital
Director of Ambulatory Otolaryngology
The Jamaica Hospital
Assistant Clinical Professor
Cornell University Medical Center
New York, New York
Chapter 5: Surgery of the Ear Canal: Split-Thickness Skin Grafts and Surgical Correction of Atresia

SYLVAN E. STOOL, M.D.
Professor of Otolaryngology and Pediatrics
University of Pittsburgh School of Medicine
Director of Education, Department of Otolaryngology
Children's Hospital of Pittsburgh
Pittsburgh, Pennsylvania
Chapter 20: Endoscopic Surgery of the Upper Aerodigestive Tract

PAUL J. WALKER, M.B.B.S.
Otolaryngologist
New Lambton, Australia
Chapter 18: Diseases of the Salivary Glands

JAY C. WERKHAVEN, M.D.
Assistant Professor, Department of Otolaryngology
Vanderbilt University Medical Center
Nashville, Tennessee
Chapter 23: Laryngotracheal Laser Surgery

preface

In the first edition of *Pediatric Otolaryngology*, which was published in 1983, we stated in the Preface that we had made "no attempt to provide extensive details of surgical techniques that have been covered adequately in texts and atlases," and the emphasis of that edition was on the "concepts of surgical management rather than on explicit descriptions of technique." We thought that the atlases available at that time were sufficient, even though the surgical procedures described were for all age groups. This format was continued in the second edition, which was published in 1990.

However, during the past several years we have become increasingly aware that our assumption was incorrect. There was no atlas available that adequately and comprehensively described the surgical procedures that were recommended in *Pediatric Otolaryngology*. In addition, new surgical procedures developed during this period have been specifically modified and designed for pediatric patients, who frequently require specially designed instruments; one such procedure is functional endoscopic sinus surgery (Chapter 16). Also, some complex surgical procedures, such as craniofacial surgery (see Chapter 1), were not included in the standard atlases because they were performed more in children than in adults. As the success of skull-base surgery (Chapter 3) rapidly improved over the years, more and more children became candidates, and information on the procedure was lacking. In addition, cochlear implantation (Chapter 8) was extended to the pediatric age group in recent years.

To meet the needs of the surgeon, this unique *Atlas of Pediatric Otolaryngology* brings together for the first time in one text the otolaryngologic surgical procedures that are performed in infants and children. We have been fortunate in recruiting the leading experts in the field to describe in detail how they have been able to achieve successful surgical outcomes. We have included not only the most commonly performed procedures, such as tympanostomy tube insertion (Chapter 4) and tonsillectomy and adenoidectomy (Chapter 15), but also those operations less frequently performed, such as surgical repair of the injured facial nerve (Chapter 4) and of the auricle for microtia (Chapter 2). The wide scope of the chapters' content reflects the diversity of pediatric otolaryngologic surgery today.

This surgical atlas is also unique in that, unlike others that are currently available, diseases and disorders that affect infants and children are comprehensively addressed. For example, in the chapters that describe surgery for tumors of the temporal bone (Chapter 7), nose, paranasal sinuses, and nasopharynx (Chapter 18), mouth and pharynx (Chapter 19), and neck (Chapter 25), the most common cell types differ in children as compared to adults, and therefore the emphasis is on eradicating these tumors in this specific age group. Likewise, congenital malformations of the ears, nose, throat, head, and neck are extensively covered in many of the chapters, because these abnormalities are commonly encountered in children.

Because otitis media, with its complications and sequelae, is the most common disease requiring surgery in the pediatric age group, the chapter on the middle ear and mastoid (Chapter 4) is comprehensive, describing the many surgical procedures needed to manage these problems.

Another notable justification for this atlas compared with those that include all age groups is that for many of the surgical procedures, the anesthetic considerations, preparation, and postoperative care are different in infants and children as compared with adults. An understanding of these differences can improve the outcome of surgery in this age group, because children have special needs related to changes in anatomy, physiology, and psychosocial adjustment during growth and development.

We are pleased to have had Jon Coulter, who is not only our artist but also a colleague and friend, prepare the artwork that describes in detail the surgical techniques. His expertise has added consistency and clarity to the text. We are also indebted to our excellent editorial assistants, Mary D. Scheetz and Suzanne K. Stewart, who integrated the entire text into a highly readable form. We also want to thank Lawrence J. McGrew, our editor at Saunders, for his special interest in this project.

We hope the reader will benefit from the fine contributions made by the authors of this text, each of whom is an authority in this area, and that this atlas will enhance the health care of infants and children who require otolaryngologic surgery.

CHARLES D. BLUESTONE, M.D.
SYLVAN E. STOOL, M.D.
Pittsburgh, Pennsylvania

contents

chapter

1

Craniofacial Surgery

DENNIS J. HURWITZ, M.D.

The surgery of craniofacial malformations is an evolving discipline. Each anomaly must be analyzed thoroughly with examination by state-of-the-art imaging techniques and may require extensive surgical exposure. It is important for the surgeon to understand the dynamics of growth in order to plan the timing and execution of these procedures. Three procedures that are typical of the spectrum of correctable anomalies are presented in this chapter.

TREATMENT OF PLAGIOCEPHALY

Indications (Fig. 1–1*A* and *B*)

- Unilateral cranial and orbital retrusion and distortion associated with craniosynostosis. A contralateral frontal bone bulge is variably present.
- The ideal age of the patient is 6 months, because bone is malleable enough for recontouring but is strong enough to maintain an advanced position. In addition, the calvarial bone donor site will reossify readily.
- Surgery within the first 3 years of life takes advantage of normal brain expansion unrestricted by the sutural synostosis.
- Associated major malformations such as midface deficiency or, in the case presented here, hypertelorism are probably best treated later when the facial structures are more firmly developed.

Anesthetic considerations

The procedure is performed with the patient under general anesthesia and using an oral endotracheal tube. A neuroanesthesia technique is used.

Preparation

Analysis of head CT scans with 3-D reformatting for planning of osteotomies and grafts and to rule out intracranial pathology.

The patient is in the supine position unless subtotal calvarial correction is necessary, and then the prone position with the head extended is used.

Procedure (Fig. 1–1*C* and *D*)

A coronal scalp incision is made over the vertex, followed by a subperiosteal dissection of a forehead flap.

The flattened forehead is compared with the opposite side, which may have a compensatory bulge. A wire template of the frontal deformity is made and is compared with the ideal shape.

The coronal suture is resected by formal craniotomy. The temporal bone osteotomies are extended along the lateral orbital walls, releasing the orbits from the temporal bone. Superiorly, the bone cuts traverse the orbital roof and come to lie in front of the crista galli. A horizontal osteotomy through the nasal extension of the frontal bone is done, thus releasing a frontal bar extending from each pteryon.

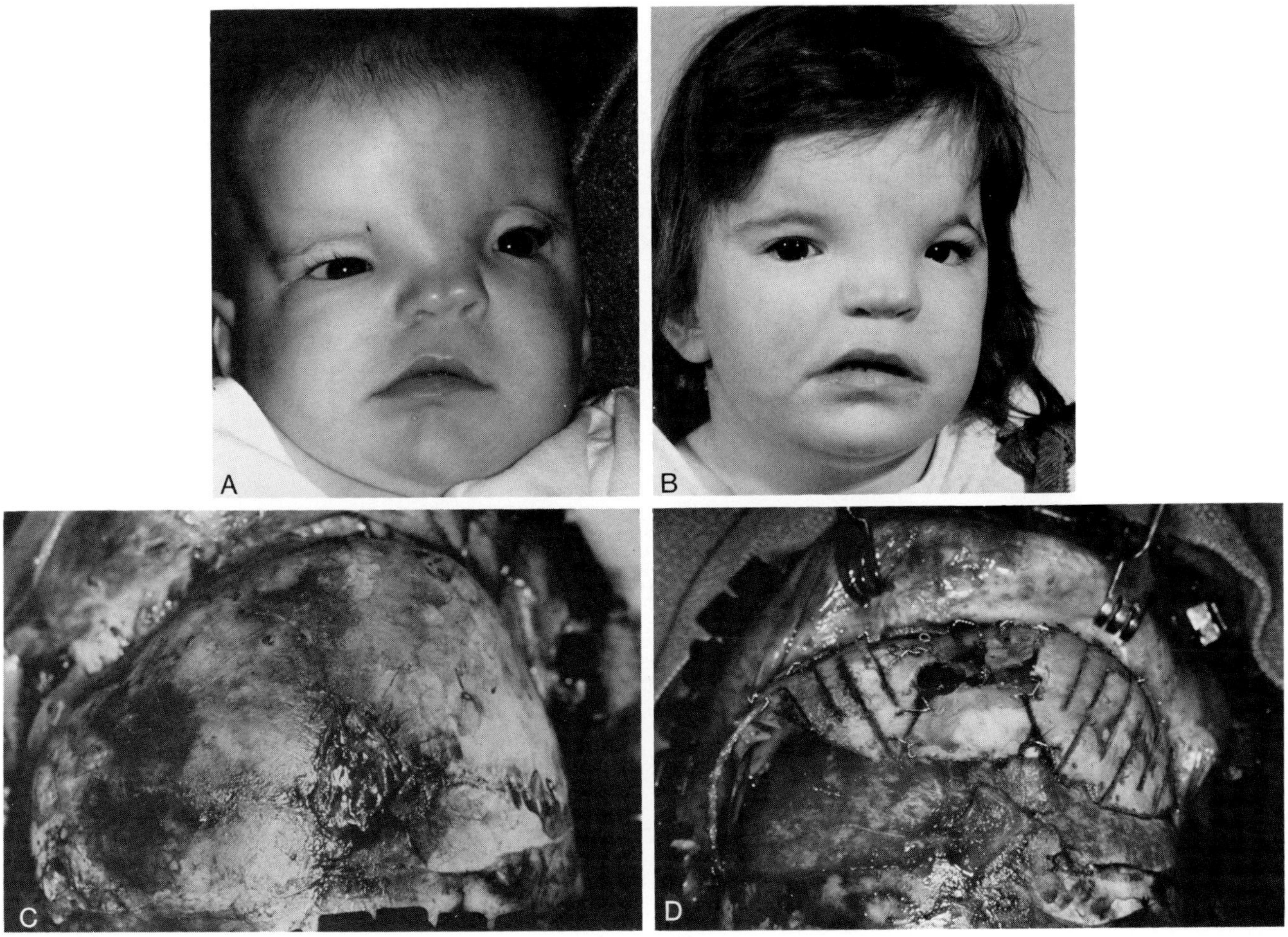

• **FIGURE 1-1.**

A, Preoperative photographs of a 6-month-old female with frontonasal dysplasia and hypertelorism and retrusion of the left brow and left orbit associated with left unilateral coronal synostosis. *B*, The results 2 years later showing good bilateral and symmetric orbital contour and position. The hypertelorism was not corrected because recurrence is likely if the deformity is treated before 3 years of age. *C*, Intraoperative photographs of the early deformity. *D*, Intraoperative photograph of the alternating osteotomies and repositioning of the bone with fixation using wires.

The vertical plate of the frontal bone extending to the coronal suture osteotomy is divided into several pieces. Cross-cuts are made in the bone to reshape the dome. The frontal bar with its lateral orbital extensions is curved to the desired shape and is advanced 14 mm to an overcorrected position. It is fixed with steel wires laterally. Miniplates and screws are used for additional rigidity. Cranial bone grafts are frequently necessary in the cranial base midline to support the frontal bar advancement. Finally, the frontal bones are reoriented for their best position on the superior margin of the advanced frontal bar. There will be a substantial gap between the dura on the side of the plagiocephaly and the advanced frontal bone and frontal bar. The scalp is closed over the reconstruction and is repaired in two layers. Drains are not used. A light head dressing is applied.

Postoperative care

The patient is immediately transferred to the intensive care unit with the endotracheal tube in place. The tube is left in place until the next morning, and ventilation is assisted as necessary. Fluid balance is carefully monitored, because on rare occasions an inappropriate antidiuretic response may occur. The neurologic signs are monitored carefully, as for all craniotomies, and particular attention is paid to the mental status, eye signs, and frontoscopic examination. No drains are placed when craniotomies are done in conjunction with skull reshaping, and dressings are placed carefully so that they are not restricting. Small hematomas and rather marked periorbital swelling are anticipated. A liquid diet is initiated upon extubation, and the patient is transferred to the neurosurgical postoperative care area. Within 5 days, when the swelling has satisfactorily reduced, it is customary for the patient to be measured for a protective plastic helmet that will be available at the time of discharge several days later. This helmet is worn until bone healing is complete in 3 months.

CORRECTION OF HYPERTELORISM CAUSED BY FRONTONASAL DYSPLASIA AND RIGHT HEMIFACIAL MICROSOMIA AS PART OF GOLDENHAR SYNDROME

(Fig. 1–2*A*, *D*, *E*, *F*)

Indications

- Grade III orbital hypertelorism (38-mm bony intraorbital distance — normal is 22 mm for a 4-year-old)
- Dermoid of the nasal bridge
- Tessier No. 1 cleft through the right nasal ala
- Right macrostomia
- Grade III right hemicraniofacial microsomia with absence of the ascending ramus of the mandible and the zygomatic arch. The entire right orbit is depressed by 5 mm.
- Anteriorly displaced right auricle
- Prior operations for middle ear effusion, preauricular skin paddles, epibulbar dermoids, and cleft palate

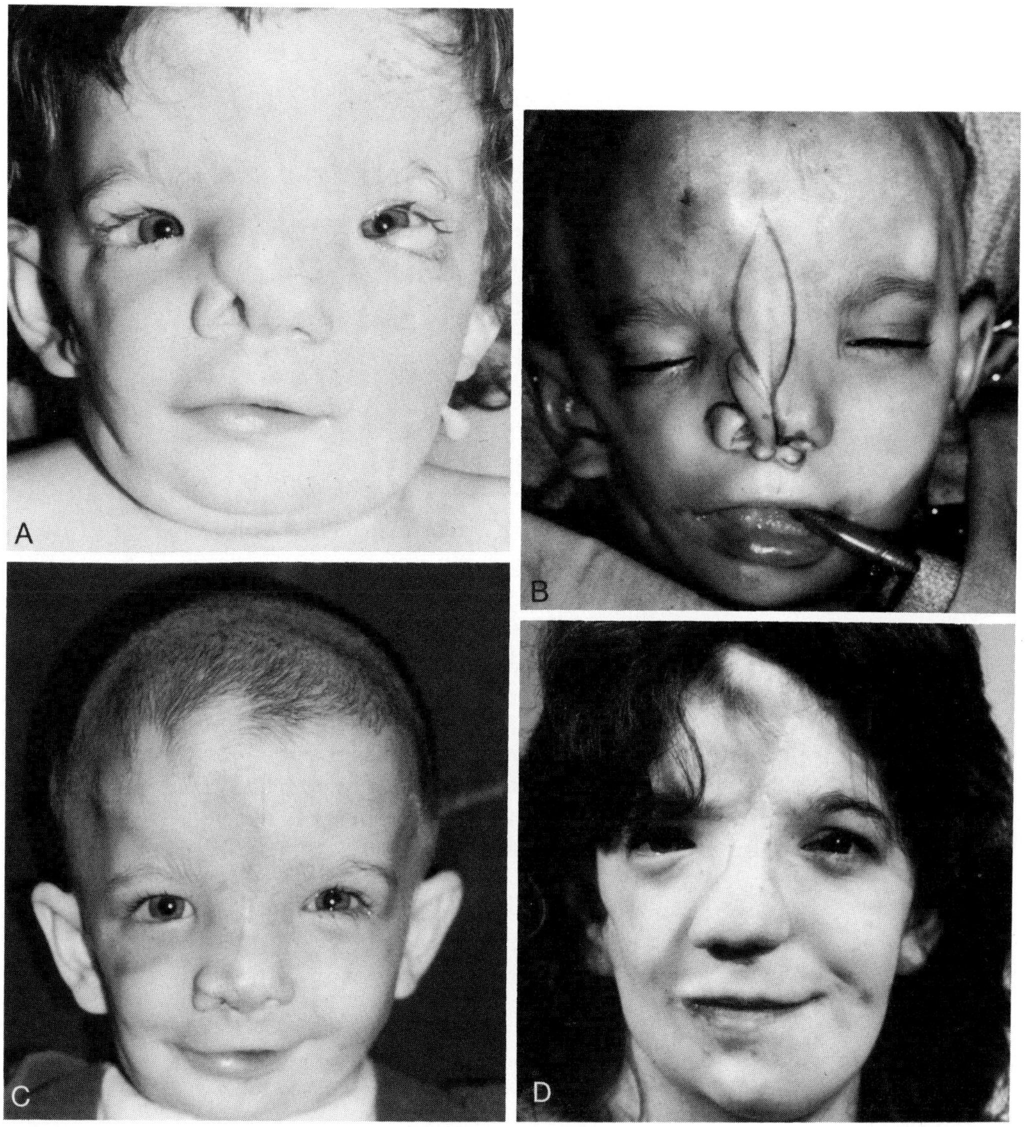

• FIGURE 1-2.

A, Goldenhar syndrome with frontonasal dysplasia. For a description, see under Indications. *B*, An intraoperative photograph of the nasal incision. *C*, The results are shown 6 weeks later. *D*, Photograph 12 years later after forehead flap and mandibular bone graft reconstruction of the nose and augmentation of the right angle of the mandible with Proplast.

Illustration continued on page 7

Anesthetic considerations

General oral endotracheal anesthesia is given using a neuroanesthesia technique.

Preparation

Analysis of head CT scans with 3-D reformatting for planning of osteotomies and grafts.

Intermaxillary fixation is not necessary despite the use of a costochondral bone graft reconstruction of the mandible in young patients.

Procedure (Fig. 1–2*B* and *C*)

Correction of the hypertelorism is a medial translocation of the "useful" orbits, orbital bone that surrounds the equators of the globes. A forehead flap exposes the frontal bone and orbits, and a midline nasal incision includes the removal of an anticipated ellipse of excess skin at the root of the nose caused by the orbital movement. An inferiorly based right nasal transposition skin flap corrects the right alar notch, and a 3-cm right upper neck incision helps to place and stabilize the costochondral bone graft to the right mandibular body.

A broad frontal craniotomy is made over the intact supraorbital bar. A rectangular segment of right frontal bone is removed to raise that orbit. Circumferential orbital osteotomies are made, and care is taken to place the inferior cut just below the infraorbital nerve foramen to avoid injury to developing maxillary teeth. The "eyeglass frame" orbital osteotomies are made with a power saw. A radical nasal bone and ethmoid sinus resection creates a midline space for the orbit. Because of soft tissue memory, a 50% bony overresection is done.

Free rib grafts reconstruct the right zygomatic arch and ascending ramus of the mandible.

Postoperative care

Immediate postoperative care focuses on airway management and fluid balance. The patient is transferred to the intensive care unit from the operating room with the oral endotracheal tube and a central intravenous (IV) line in place. The child is monitored carefully for neurologic changes, including a frontoscopic examination on a regular basis. Oral endotracheal intubation lasts for 48 to 72 hours and is stopped only when the child is fully alert and able to cooperate. A chest x-ray is taken soon after the operation to determine if a pneumothorax has occurred inadvertently owing to the harvesting of rib grafts. If a pneumothorax is present, a chest tube is placed at the bedside. Transfusions are occasionally required if the hematocrit drops below 24%. Active mandibular exercises are begun 2 weeks after surgery to minimize a tendency toward ankylosis of the reconstructed temporomandibular joint.

The patient is discharged between 1 week and 10 days from the time of surgery, with careful observation for possible cerebrospinal fluid (CSF) leakage. If any suggestion of leakage occurs, care is taken to avoid forced inspiration or positive end-expiratory expiration that may cause air to travel up the cranial base. An indwelling spinal catheter is placed for drainage of CSF up to 50 ml daily for 1 week. If the CSF leak is not controlled, intracranial repair is necessary.

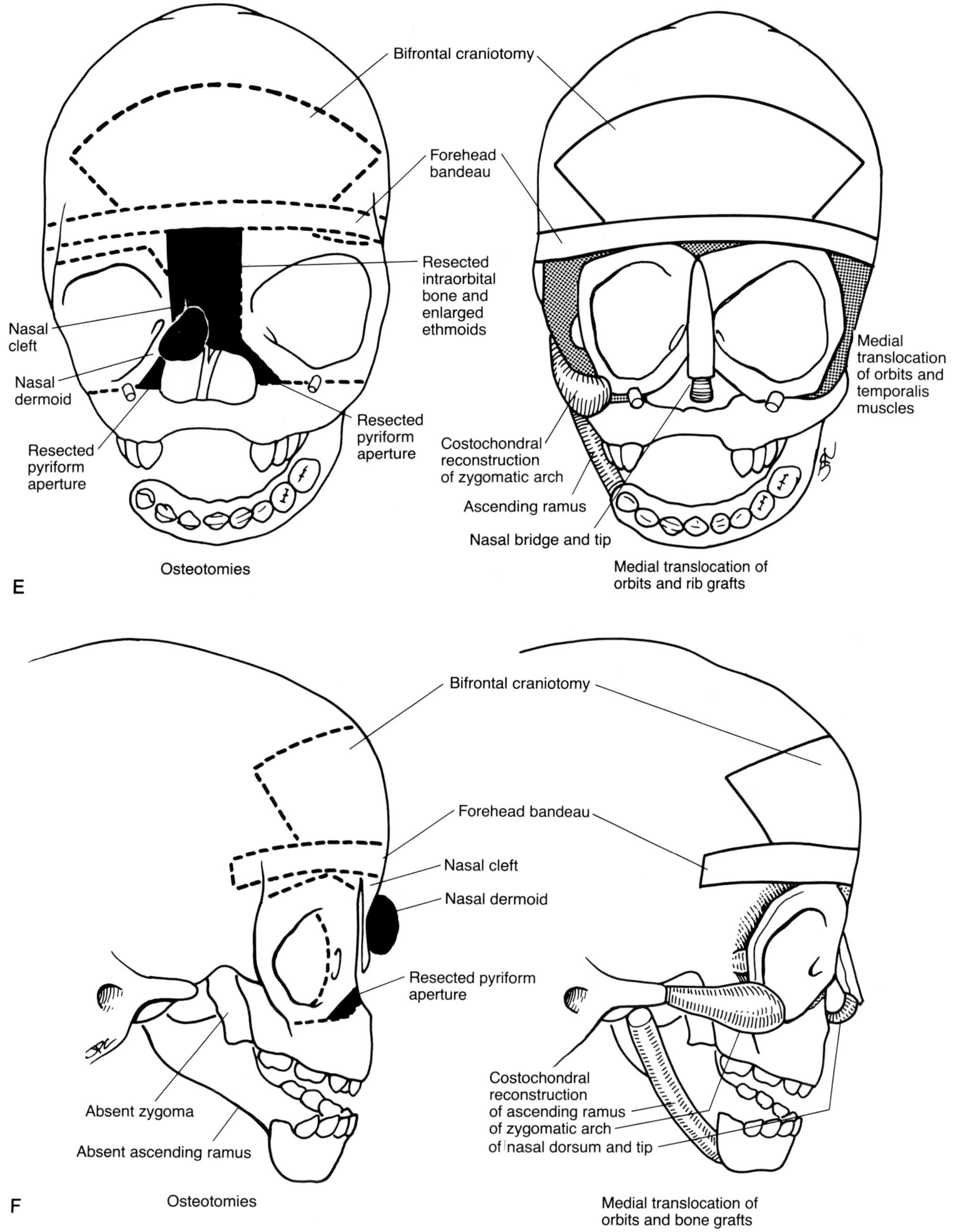

• **FIGURE 1-2.** *(continued)*

E and *F*, Diagrams of the frontal and lateral views of the skull deformity and its reconstruction. The osteotomies are described under Procedure.

CORRECTION OF CROUZON'S DEFORMITY

Indications (Fig. 1–3A_1–C_2)

- Prominent exorbitism
- Midface deficiency
- Patient self-awareness of facial deformity
- Tracheostomy is considered but is rarely necessary
- Middle ear disease is controlled
- Fronto-orbital facial advancement is performed in one or two stages. To avoid base of the skull communication between the nasal and intracranial cavities, a fronto-orbital advancement is staged about 6 months before a Le Fort III type of facial advancement.

Anesthetic considerations

General oral endotracheal anesthesia with neurosurgical anesthesia technique is used. Cervicofacial deformities may require a presurgical tracheostomy. Nasal endotracheal intubation may be elected if intermaxillary fixation is planned; however, the intranasal tube is vulnerable to midline nasofacial osteotomies. With advancement of more than 1 cm, an intraoral tube placement can be accommodated owing to the additional space behind the advanced maxillary tuberosities. Postsurgical intubation is indicated for 1 to 2 days.

Preparation

The fronto-orbital advancement is preceded by a head CT scan with 3-D reformatting to document the deformity and to reveal any cerebral malformation. Type-specific blood may be donated and cross-matched.

The second-stage facial advancement is preceded by a thorough orthodontic dentofacial work-up. Lateral cephalometric x-rays and dental models permit construction of a postoperative dental splint that will support the new position of the maxilla. Dental hygiene and condition are optimized.

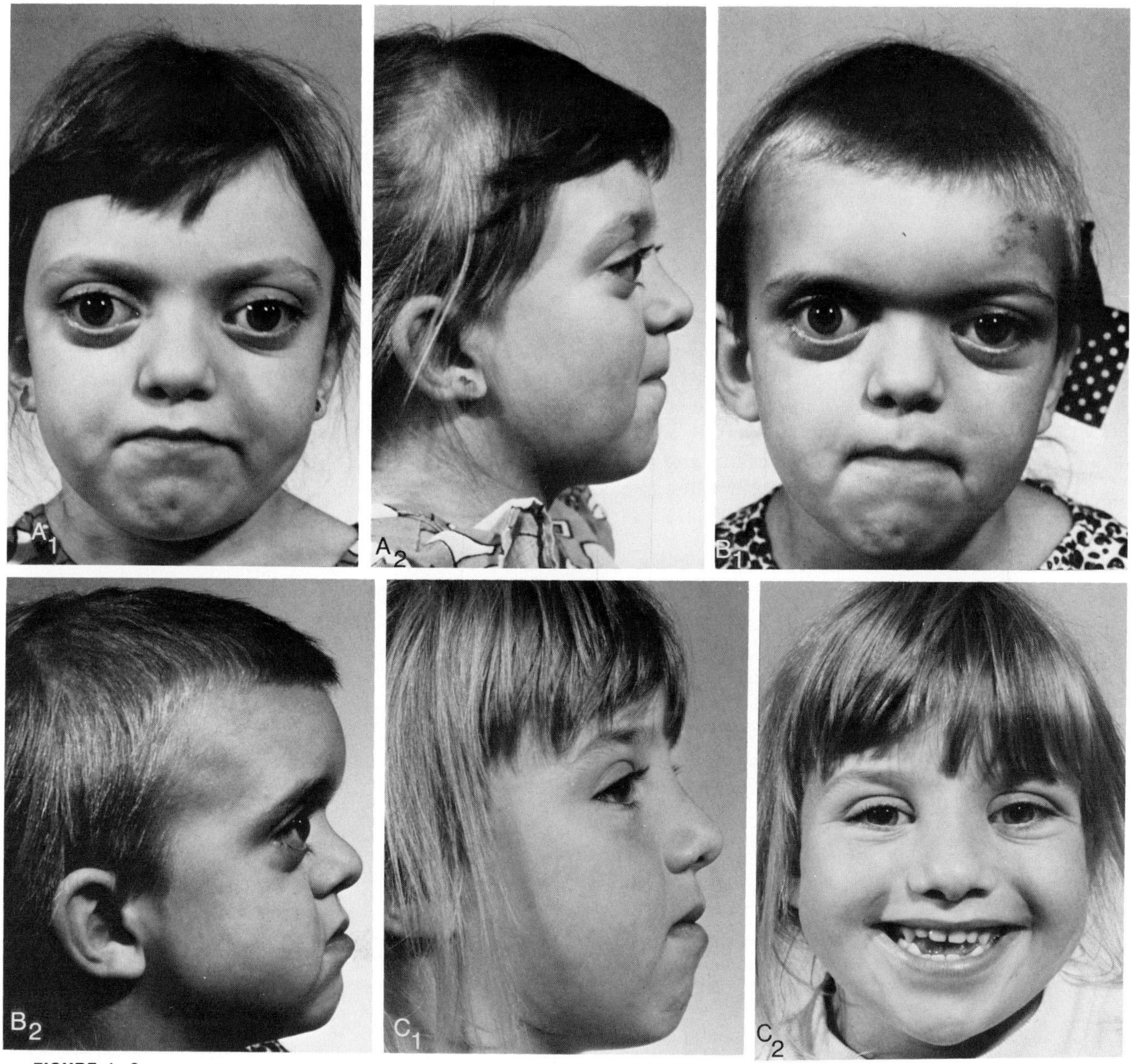

• FIGURE 1–3.

A_1 and A_2, Preoperative frontal and lateral views. B_1 and B_2, Two months after first-stage reconstruction. Notice what appears to be an overly advanced forehead with very deep frontonasal grooving and correction of the upper portion of the exorbitism. *C*, Two years after a Le Fort III osteotomy, orbital bony relationships are normal. There is mild but improving ptosis of the right upper eyelid. Facial convexity and dental occlusion are appropriate.

Illustration continued on following page

Procedure (Fig. 1–3*D–J*)

The first procedure requires a bicoronal scalp incision and a forehead flap for access to the frontal bone and orbits. The supraorbital bar with lateral orbital extensions is advanced far enough to correct the exorbitism, using osteotomies previously described for the treatment of plagiocephaly. When the forehead deformity is symmetric, the entire vertical portion of the frontal bone is advanced and is sometimes turned 180 degrees for better contour. Split cranial bone grafts support the frontal bone advancement. Microplates and screws as well as surgical-steel wires are used.

Eight months later, a 15-mm lower orbital and facial advancement is performed through the bicoronal scar on the scalp. The new facial position completes the correction of the exorbitism and establishes a normal dental occlusion.

The procedure is started with an intercartilaginous and caudal septal transfixion incision to allow for dissection of the soft tissues surrounding the bony and cartilaginous dorsum of the nose, and a submucous dissection of the mucoperichondrium and periosteum of the septum. The periosteum of the nasal bones is dissected to the medial canthal ligaments. Following elevation of the frontal scalp, soft tissues are elevated in the subperiosteal plane about the orbit and midface.

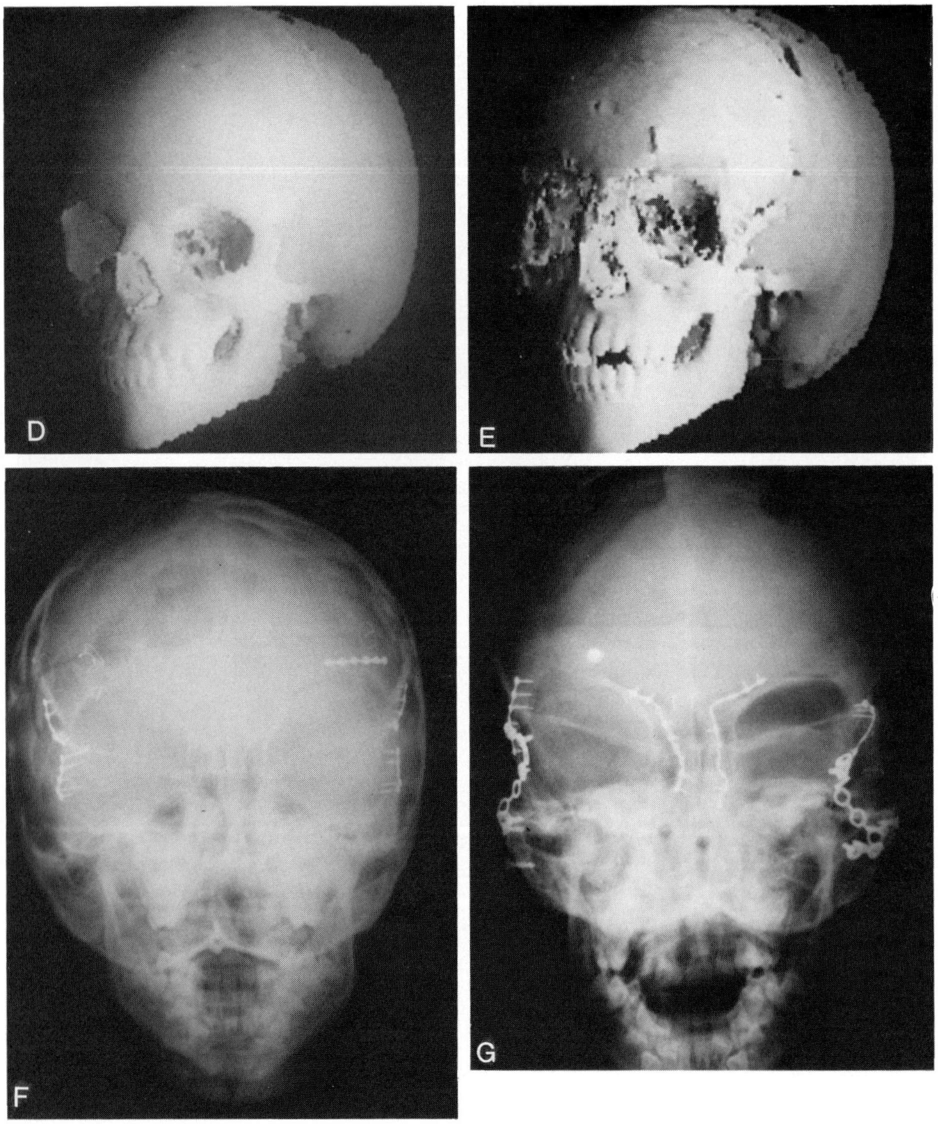

• **FIGURE 1–3.** *(continued)*

D, Initial 3-D reformatting of the oblique view of the craniofacial bones of a CT scan shows forehead, orbital, and maxillary retrusion. *E*, Postoperative 3-D reformatting of the same oblique view shows the cumulative craniofacial advancement of the midface with a small open bite. Metal fixation plates obscure the lateral orbital and zygomatic arch osteotomy. *F*, Frontal plane facial x-ray after fronto-orbital advancement shows the position of wires and microplates that secure the advancement. When the frontal bone was advanced it was curved further, and in order to maintain that curvature, wires were used on the patient's right side and microplates on the left side. *G*, A plane frontal x-ray of the face following the Le Fort III advancement. A combination of miniplates and microplates secures the midface and orbits in an advanced position. A single right frontal lag screw secures an onlay bone graft.

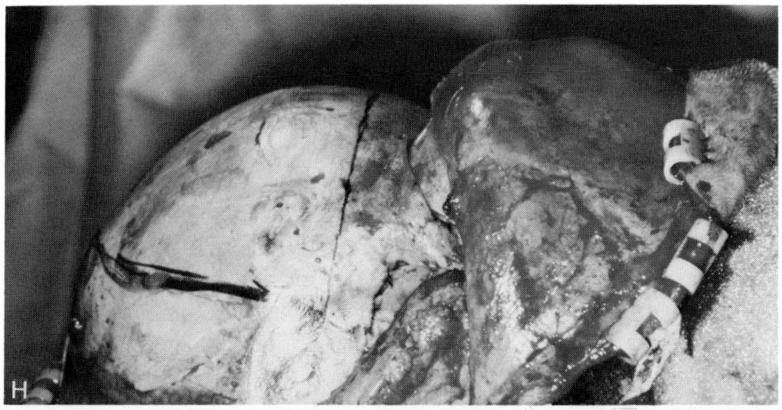

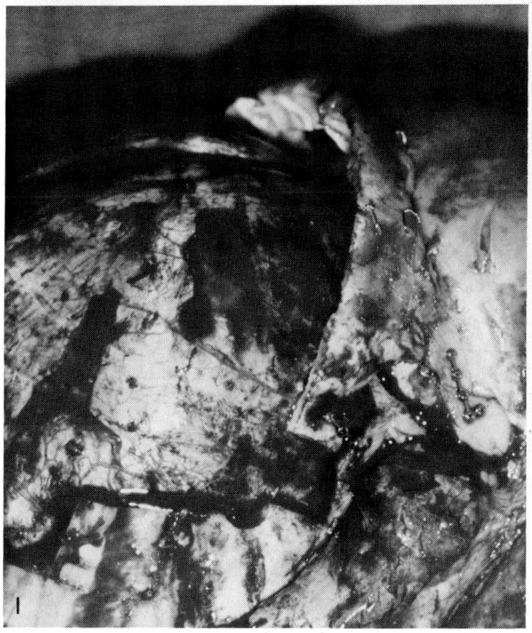

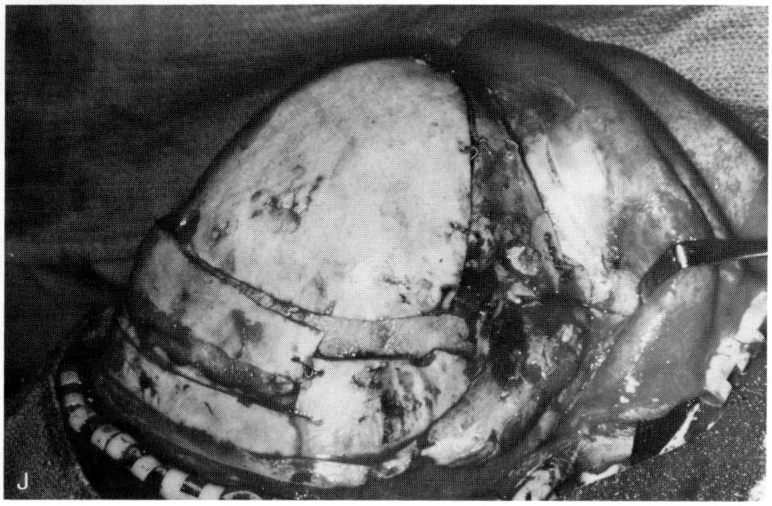

• FIGURE 1-3. *(continued)*

H, Intraoperative photographs during the first stage demonstrate the proposed osteotomies for the forehead and frontal bone advancement. *I*, The frontal bone and supraorbital bar have been advanced, leaving a 2-cm gap of the dura. *J*, This final intraoperative photograph shows the frontal bone advanced and wired in position with the gap filled with 2 split cranial bone grafts.

The temporalis muscle is dissected from the orbits and zygomatic arch, and the periorbit is freed circumferentially, except at the level of the medial canthal ligament and lacrimal sac. The masseteric muscle is dissected from the zygomatic arch and maxilla.

A Le Fort III subcranial osteotomy is made transversely immediately inferior to the first-stage fronto-orbital advancement. It extends along the lateral orbital wall across the floor of the orbit just posterior to the rims and lacrimal fossa. The osteotomy then crosses the nasion at the level of the prior frontonasal advancement. A 5-mm osteotome is then angled in the midline through the nasal osteotomy and the bony septum with a slight posterior direction. Previously dissected mucoperiosteum of the septum allows for disjunction without mucosal lacerations and allows for unimpeded advancement. A maxillary tuberosity disjunction from the pterygoid plates is performed through the coronal incision, with the assistance of a finger behind the soft palate. Using Rowe's disimpaction forceps, the posterior maxillary wall is fractured, and the maxilla is slowly but forcefully advanced forward.

Split cranial bone grafts are harvested from the parietal skull for interposition behind the advanced orbits and nasal bones. Microplates and screws fix the medial orbits and nose, and miniplates and screws hold the lateral orbits and maxilla forward.

Postoperative care

The patient is transferred from the operating room to the intensive care unit with an oral endotracheal tube in place, which is removed within 24 hours when the patient is alert and cooperative. The neurologic status is monitored carefully by the nursing and physician personnel and includes an intermittent frontoscopic examination. The eyelids are not bandaged closed. Extensive periorbital eyelid swelling occurs, but generally the patient can see beneath the swollen eyelids. Careful monitoring and maintenance of fluid balance are performed. The patient is allowed to leave the intensive care unit as soon as airway and fluid management is under control, and the patient is generally discharged from the hospital within 1 week of surgery. Care is simplified because intermaxillary splints are no longer necessary for craniofacial procedures.

BIBLIOGRAPHY

Bluestone CD and Stool SE: Pediatric Otolaryngology, Vol 1, 2nd ed. Philadelphia, WB Saunders, 1990, pp 62, 68, 72.

Hurwitz DJ, Pang D, and Albright L: Creation of a dome in the surgery of craniosynostosis: Six cases of plagiocephaly. *In* Caronni E (ed): Craniofacial Surgery. Proceedings of The Second International Society of Craniomaxillofacial Surgery. Bologna, Italy: Mondazzi: Editore, 1991.

chapter

2

Surgical Repair of the Auricle for Microtia

ROLAND D. EAVEY, M.D.

Anxious parents of a newborn with severe microtia should be counseled that successful surgical correction of a severely malformed auricle is possible.[1-4] The repair requires augmentation with cartilaginous rib, and definitive correction should be postponed until 6 to 7 years of age. Until then, hearing assessment and monitoring for otitis media in both ears is necessary.

The repair involves at least three stages, which are illustrated. A fourth stage, to add a tragus or to perform a contralateral "otoplasty" of the normal auricle, is needed occasionally. If surgical correction of hearing for aural atresia is contemplated, auricular reconstruction for microtia should always precede it so that the regional skin coverage is not violated.

The discomfort from this surgery is surprisingly well tolerated; the most painful first stage is caused by the rib harvest. The patient requires a 2- to 3-night hospital stay for that stage owing to discomfort and drainage requirements; all other hospital stays are shorter.

The alternatives to surgery are to cover the ear with long hair or to use a prosthesis. The trade-off for an improved auricular appearance is a linear scar over the contralateral lower chest and a donor skin graft site on the ipsilateral buttock.

The goal of surgery is to provide the patient with an auricular appearance that is sufficiently close to normal that no attention will be called to the ear. The results of surgery are sufficiently consistent and reliable that this goal can be achieved, and children need no longer be deprived of the surgical option of auricular correction.

Indications

Correction of a severe auricular congenital malformation that will require augmentation by an autogenous rib.

Anesthetic considerations

General anesthesia is given for all surgical stages.

Preparation

- Measure the normal contralateral ear: vertical height, distance from the lateral canthus of the eye to the anterior insertion helix and to the lobule; note the axis of the auricle (nearly parallel with the nasal dorsum); note the position of each lobule viewed en face. The microtic lobule lies more superiorly (Figs. 2–1 to 2–3).

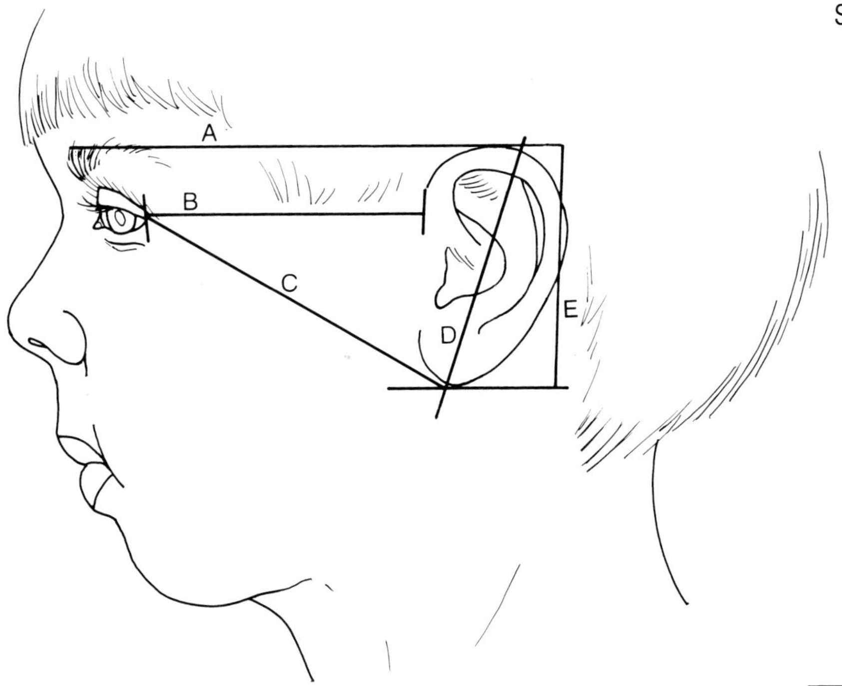

• FIGURE 2-1.

Preoperative measurements of a normal contralateral ear. *A*, Relationship of the superior auricle to the brow. *B*, Distance from the lateral canthus to the auricle. *C*, Distance from the lateral canthus to the lobule. *D*, Axis of the auricle relative to the nasal dorsum. *E*, Vertical height of the auricle.

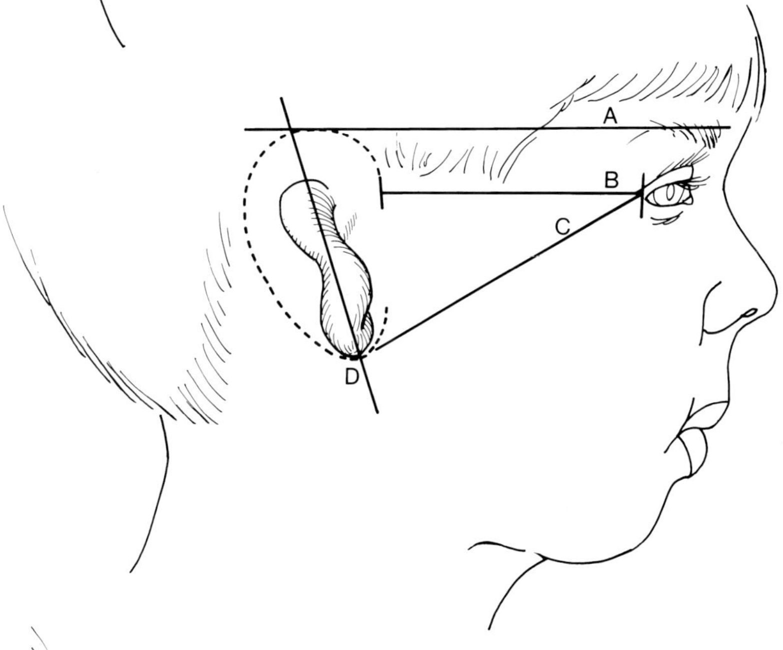

• FIGURE 2-2.

Measurements for the malformed ear are taken from the normal ear.

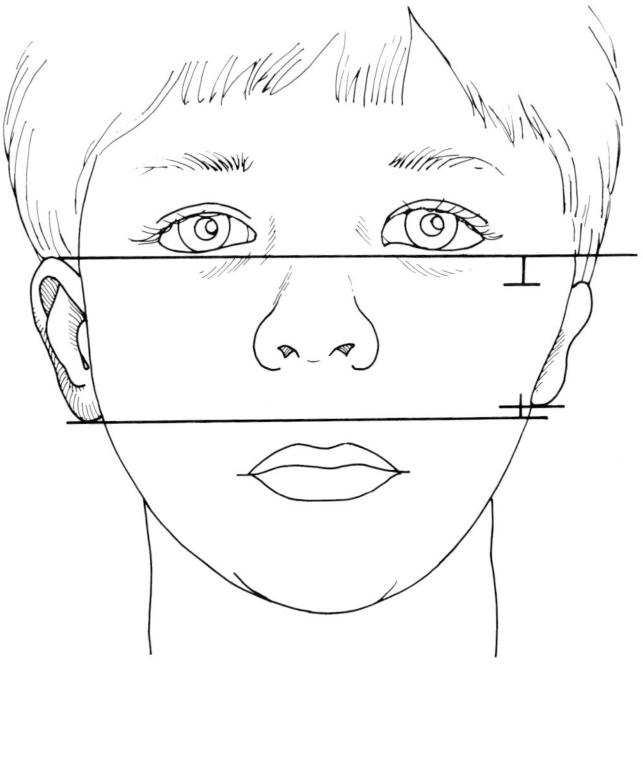

• FIGURE 2-3.

An en face view reveals a difference in vertical height and relationships of the superior and inferior aspects of the auricle.

- Create a template from the normal ear using an x-ray film and a marker (Fig. 2–4).
- Examine for other potential facial asymmetry and facial nerve malfunction.
- Evaluate the child's overall size (the child should be at least 6 years of age and preferably older). Evaluate the size of the contralateral cartilaginous ribs by palpation. Check for possible trauma to the ribs or a congenital malformation that could create the need to use an ipsilateral rib.

STAGE 1: RIB HARVEST

Preparation

The contralateral chest is prepared with an iodine solution. Those ribs have a curvature that is favorable for reconstruction. Towels are placed with a square window sufficiently generous to harvest several cartilaginous ribs from the lower costal margin. Injection of local anesthesia and epinephrine is optional.

Procedure

HARVEST OF THE RIB

- A linear incision is made over the lower contralateral ribs.
- Isolate three lower cartilaginous ribs. Use a film template, and place it over two ribs connected at the synchondrosis to select for the base of the framework. The third rib is to be used for the helix. Cut the ribs cleanly at the costochondral junction. Remove with the perichondrium (Fig. 2–5).
- Repair the pleura if entered with a pursestring suture, which is tightened as a suction tube is removed. Close the incision without a drain. Use a nonpermanent subcutaneous suture. Place a sterile dressing.

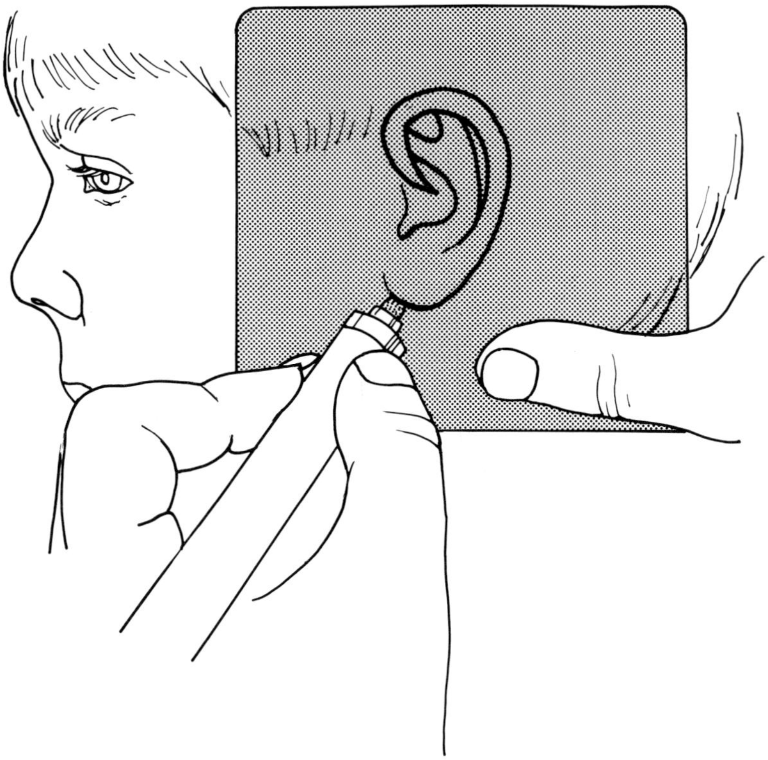

• FIGURE 2-4.

An x-ray film template is created from the normal ear.

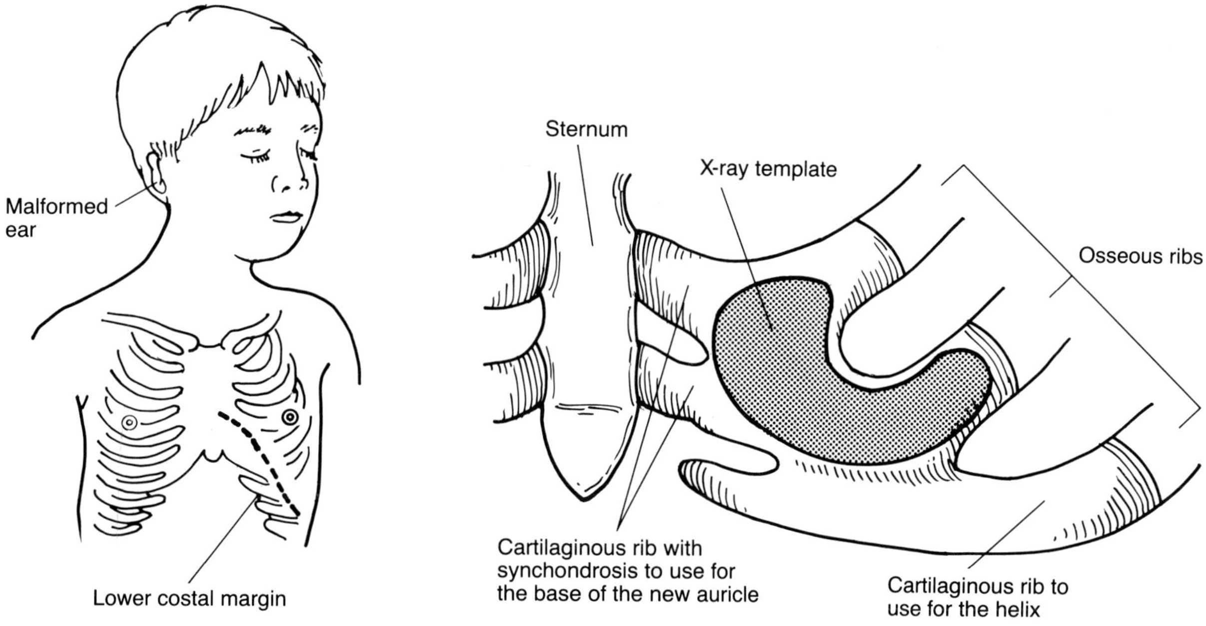

• FIGURE 2-5.

Rib harvest procedure.

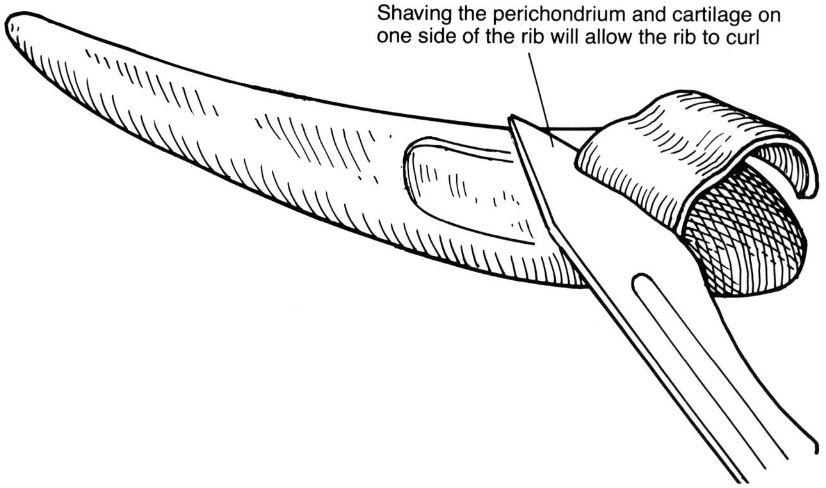

• FIGURE 2–6.

Creation of a helix. Shaving the perichondrium and cartilage on one side of the rib allows the rib to curl.

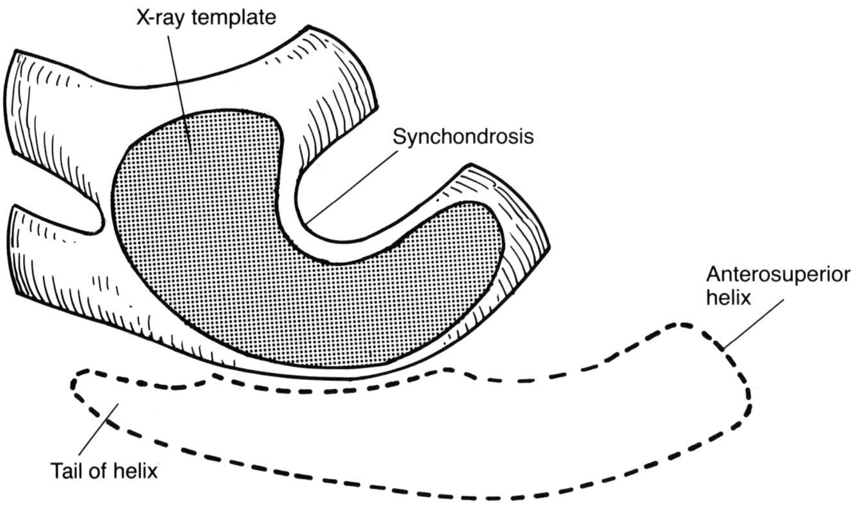

• FIGURE 2–7.

Shaping of the auricle. A solid block is carved as a base using the x-ray template.

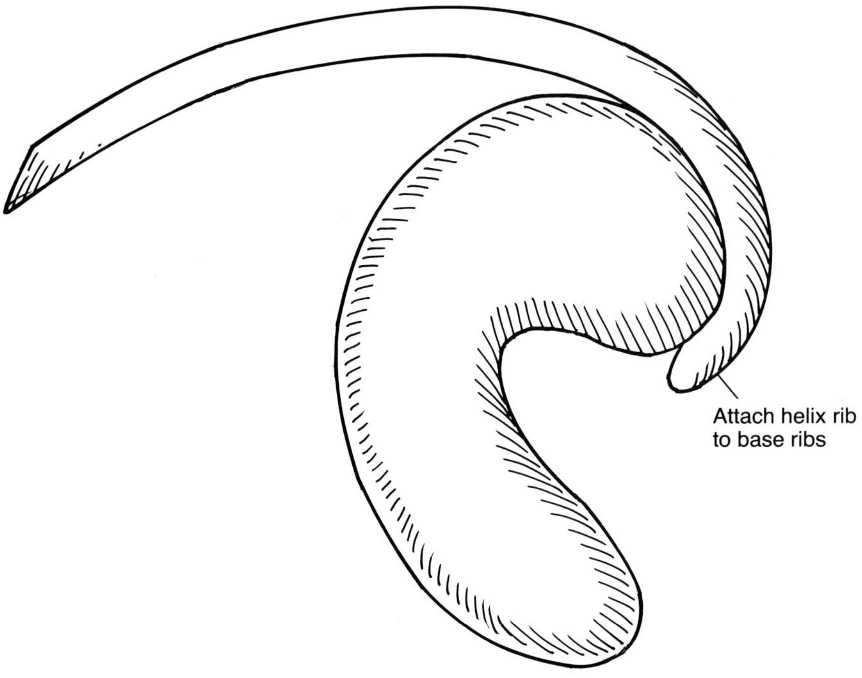

• FIGURE 2–8.

A helix is attached to the base ribs.

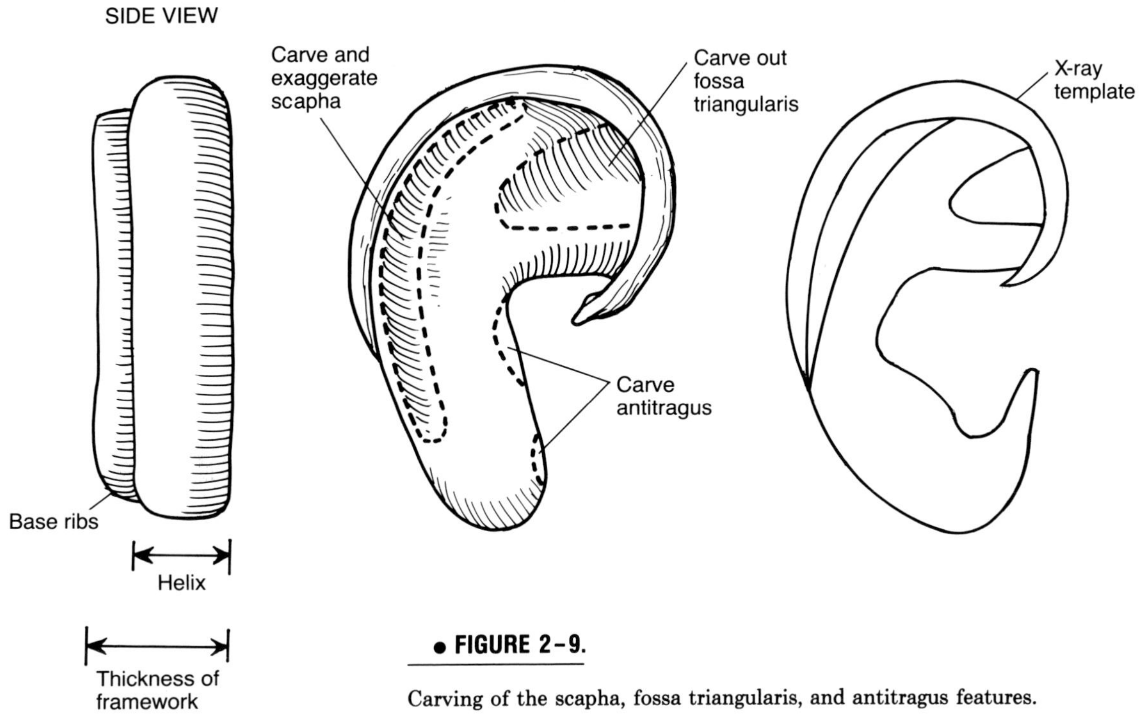

• FIGURE 2-9.

Carving of the scapha, fossa triangularis, and antitragus features.

CREATION OF THE FRAMEWORK

- Clean the adherent muscle attachments.
- Use a No. 10 blade to shave lower, and free the rib to create a helix (Fig. 2–6). Preserve the perichondrium on the inner curve.
- Place the film template on the upper two ribs with the synchondrosis, and carve around the template to create the shape of the auricle (Fig. 2–7).
- Suture the helix (lower free rib) to the base (upper two ribs of the synchondrosis) using a 5-0 wire and clear nylon (Fig. 2–8). Sutures must purchase the perichondrium for strength.
- Draw the outline of the fossa triangularis and the scaphoid fossa. Use a septal gouge to carve these areas to create realistic contours (Fig. 2–9).
- Keep the cartilage moist.

Preparation of a skin pocket

- Place the template over the malformed ear. Using preoperative measurements, locate and outline the correct position.
- Create a 2- to 3-cm vertical incision preauricularly (Fig. 2–10).
- Remove the malformed cartilage of the auricle. Do not remove the fatty tissue or the skin.
- Elevate the skin pocket. The plane is an extension of the skin depth already achieved over the malformed cartilage. During dissection, the scissor tips should be slightly visible tenting the skin (Fig. 2–11).
- Apply pressure for hemostasis; the pocket dissection is bloody.
- Insert the framework, and check the measurements.
- Use a suction drain (Fig. 2–12).
- Close the incision with a running Prolene suture. Tiny skin fenestrations are closed with a 6-0 mild chromic suture.
- Apply a mastoid dressing.

Postoperative care

- Manage rib area pain as necessary with patient-controlled anesthesia.
- The suction drain requires an hourly change of red-topped vacuum tubes that are displayed in a test tube rack to monitor drainage.
- The mastoid dressing is changed daily or at the surgeon's discretion when the patient is discharged from the hospital.
- Discharge the patient on postoperative day 2 or 3, depending on the amount of drainage and pain.
- Suture removal is done in the ear area at 7 to 10 days. No new dressings are necessary.

• FIGURE 2-10.

A template is placed over the malformed ear to outline the correct position for the incision.

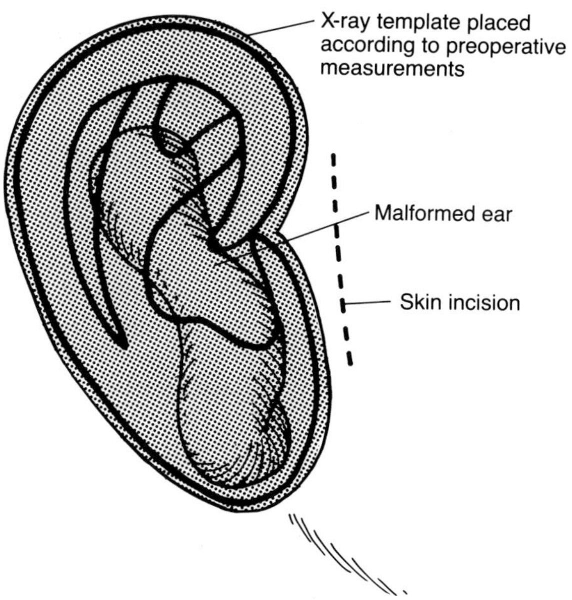

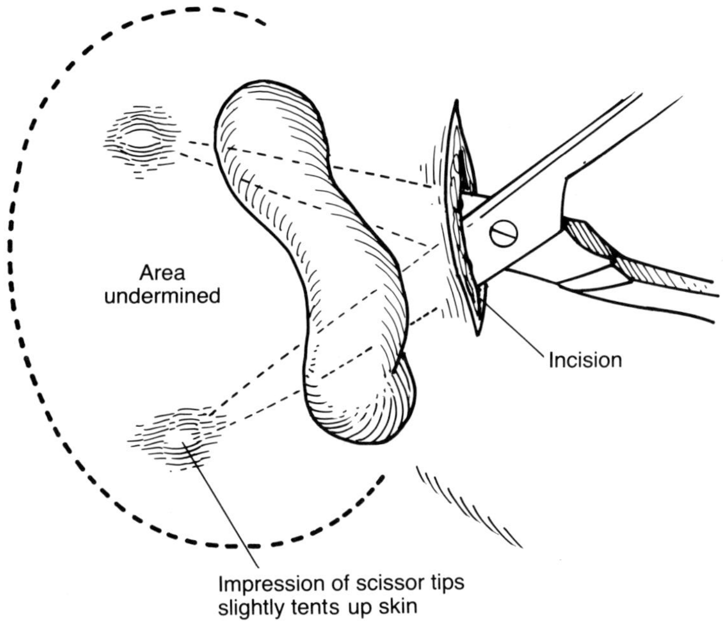

• FIGURE 2-11.

Elevation of the skin pocket.

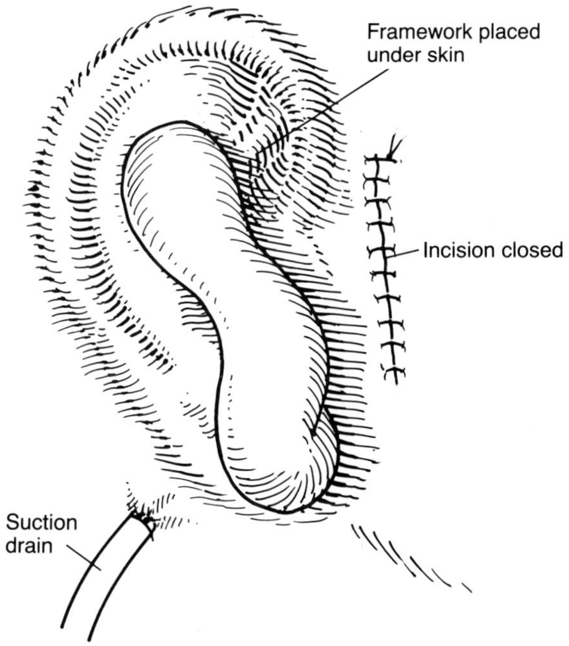

• FIGURE 2-12.

The framework is inserted, and the incision is closed.

STAGE II: LOBULE TRANSPOSITION (Fig. 2–13)

Preparation

The malformed ear is prepared with an iodine solution. An adherent, transparent plastic drape is applied anteriorly in the towel window to permit a view of the eyebrow and the nasal dorsum to assist with later placement of the framework. Use of vasoconstriction is prohibited because skin blanching will confuse the surgeon in his or her determination of skin tension once the framework has been placed in the subcutaneous pocket.

Procedure

- The microtic ear usually has a lobule-like appendage located anterior to where it should be located.
- Mark the area of excision as well as the area for transfer over the lower area of the framework.
- Remove the skin over the framework. Preserve the subcutaneous connective tissue over the framework.
- Elevate the lobule-like remnant, retaining the inferior pedicle.
- Rotate the remnant posteriorly to the lower framework.
- Trim the skin and fat until a realistic lobule contour is achieved.
- Close the sites without drains. The donor site may be closed with a small graft of skin obtained from the recipient site. Prolene sutures are used. A sterile mastoid dressing is applied.

Postoperative care

- Pain is managed with acetaminophen.
- The mastoid dressing and the sutures are removed after 1 week.

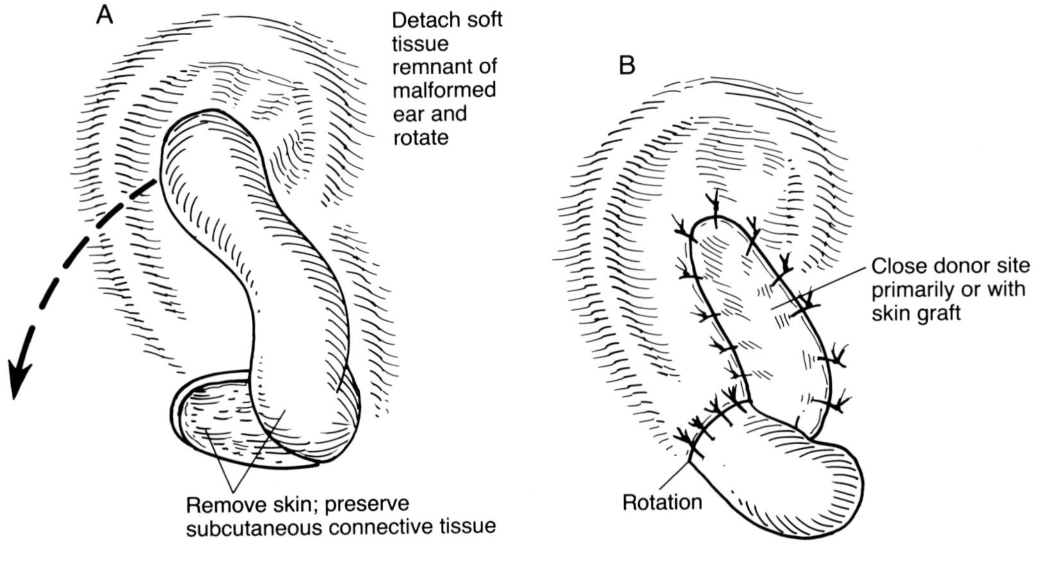

• FIGURE 2–13.

A, The soft tissue remnant of the malformed ear is detached and rotated. The skin is removed, and subcutaneous connective tissue is preserved. *B*, The donor site is closed either primarily or with a skin graft.

STAGE III: SEPARATION FROM THE SIDE OF THE HEAD

(Fig. 2–14)

Procedure

- Obtain a skin graft (18/1000-inch thickness) from the right buttock. Place a sterile plastic dressing on the donor site.
- Incise the skin along the helical rim to the depth preserving connective tissue over the cartilage. The incision placement depends on the zone of hair-bearing skin.
- Elevate the framework and preserve the thin layer of subcutaneous connective tissue over the cartilage.
- Create a sulcus under approximately one half of the framework; do not undermine the entire framework.
- Advance the scalp skin behind the framework.
- Attach the split-thickness skin graft to the superior edge of the skin, covering the framework with a mild chromic suture. Tuck the skin medially under the framework to create a rounded helical contour.
- Apply a bolster with long nylon sutures and apply a mastoid dressing.

Postoperative care

- Provide pain management with acetaminophen and perhaps codeine.
- A plastic dressing is left on the buttock donor site.
- A sterile mastoid dressing and sutured bolster are left in place for 1 week.

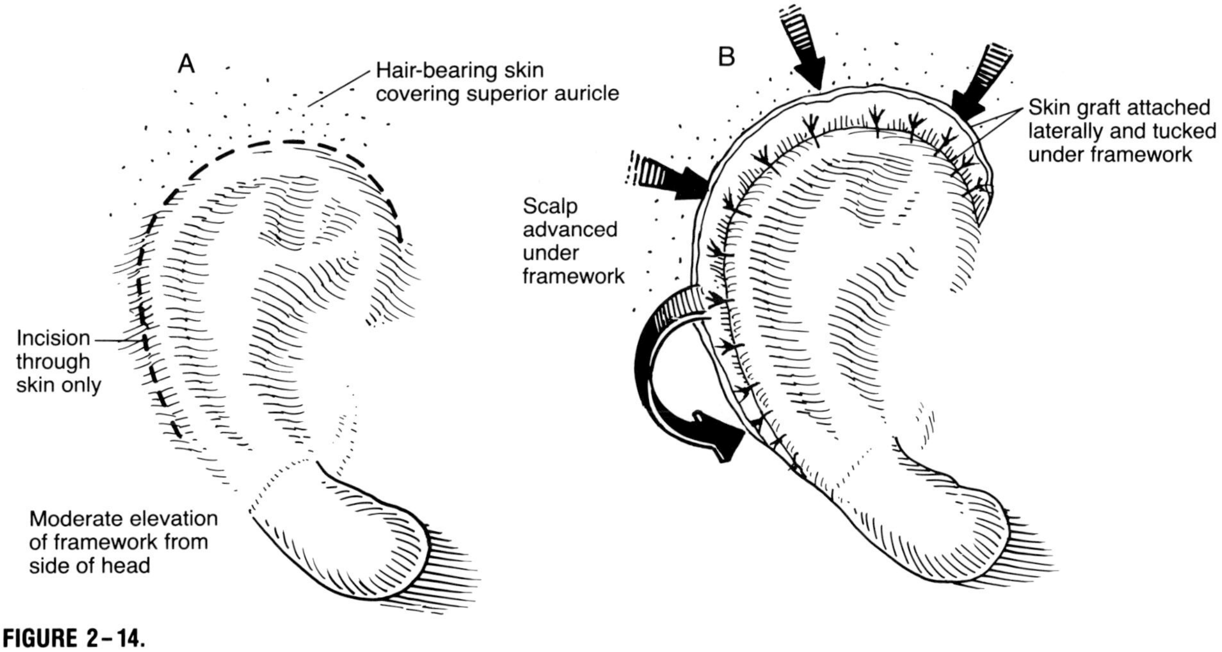

• FIGURE 2–14.

A, An incision is made through the skin only. Placement is determined by the area of hair-bearing skin. *B*, The scalp is advanced under the framework. The skin graft is then attached laterally and is tucked under the framework.

STAGE IV: OPTIONAL CREATION OF THE TRAGUS OR CONTRALATERAL OTOPLASTY

Procedure

- Crescent-shaped cartilage is harvested from the contralateral ear. This provides a further opportunity to complete the symmetry by tailoring the normal ear.
- A J-shaped incision is created in the reconstructed ear.
- A cartilage is inserted with skin still attached on one side.
- A small skin graft with a bolster is applied to the raw surface to create a conchal bowl appearance (Fig. 2–15).

Postoperative care/complications

- Use perioperative antibiotics for wound infection. If an infection occurs, an incision and drainage should be performed if the skin envelope is fluctuant. Antibiotics should be continued until the soft tissue is normal.
- Skin breakdown occurs usually over the helix anterosuperiorly. Observe for this, and allow to demarcate. The skin may re-epithelialize if the area is small; therefore, use antibacterial ointment for several weeks and débride the underlying cartilage to fresh white substance if cartilage sloughs; otherwise, one will need a soft tissue cover of either a bilobed scalp flap or a temporalis fascia flap to cover the cartilage and to provide a bed for a skin graft.
- A hypertrophic scar may occur.

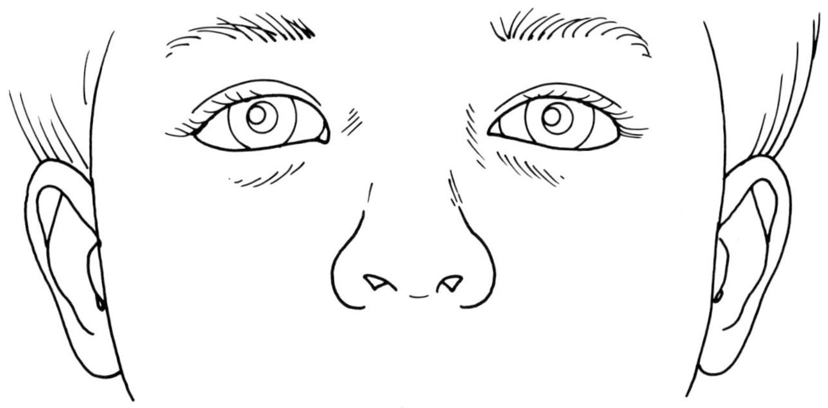

• FIGURE 2–15.

Postoperative appearance following the removal of the suture.

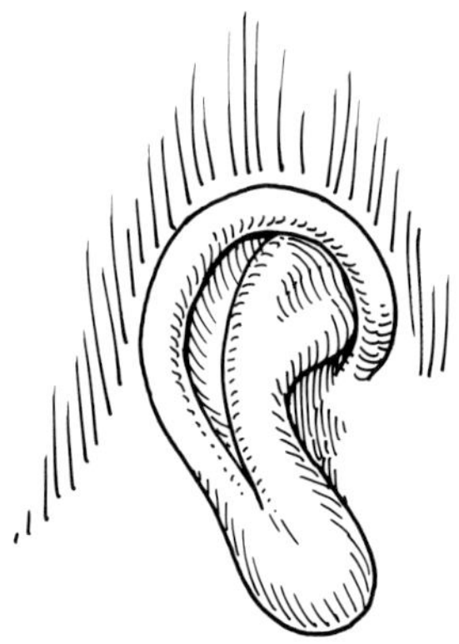

BIBLIOGRAPHY

Brent B: The correction of microtia with autogenous cartilage graft. I: The classic deformity. Plast Reconstr Surg 66:1–12, 1980.

Brent B: Total auricular construction with sculpted costal cartilage: Case No. 15. *In* Brent B (ed): The Artistry of Reconstructive Surgery. St. Louis, CV Mosby, 1987.

Eavey RD: Management strategies for congenital ear malformations. Pediatr Clin North Am 36:1521–1534, 1989.

Eavey RD and Cheney ML: Reconstruction of congenital auricular malformation. *In* Nadol JB and Schuknecht HF (eds): Surgery of the Ear and Temporal Bone. New York, Raven Press, 1992, pp 435–447.

chapter

3

Otologic Surgical Procedures

CHARLES D. BLUESTONE, M.D.

This chapter contains the most common otologic procedures performed on children, but I have also included some of the operations that we have developed, such as the techniques for closing the eustachian tube (see later) and operations for which the technique was described in the past but that have not been included in other currently available texts. The procedure for correction of lop ears is an example of the latter. The otoplasty technique used for the last 30 years is one that was described originally by Becker.[1] I have added a few modifications that have resulted in a more pleasing and longer-lasting cosmetic outcome. The common otologic procedures described are ones that are not unique to me or to my colleagues, but most are techniques that we have modified specifically for children and that have stood the test of time.

Numerous methods are described in the literature on how to repair a perforation of the tympanic membrane, but almost all are designed with the adult patient in mind. We have used most of these procedures in children during the last 3 decades, but we have had only a few successes when children have been followed for a long time. In general, when the child has a large central perforation, the lateral graft tympanoplasty has been more successful than have procedures that employ the medial graft technique.[2, 3]

The section on cholesteatoma is designed to follow the course of the operation in the child. Each step in the procedure and the final operation chosen depend on the anatomic site and on the extent of the cholesteatoma. One procedure is not advocated for all cholesteatomas. On the contrary, we select the external incision and approach, as well as the decision for or against removal of the posterior canal wall, based on the individual child's cholesteatoma. We have published the outcome of these methods.[4]

In this chapter, I do not describe in detail indications for many of the surgical procedures, because the indications are included in *Pediatric Otolaryngology*;[5] for example, my indications for performing a tympanoplasty. However, for procedures not covered in those chapters, I have provided the reader with a more detailed discussion of those indications (e.g., in the section on otoplasty).

Finally, I did not wish to completely cover every aspect of every otologic procedure that is currently advocated and employed, but I have attempted to provide information on the methods that we use routinely. Other texts that I recommend to supplement this chapter are those by Glasscock and Shambaugh,[6] Goycoolea and associates,[7] and Nadol and Schuknecht.[8] These surgeons provide the reader with extensive descriptions of procedures that are not included in this chapter, such as those that are used for otosclerosis (a disease that is infrequently encountered in children). When indicated in the adolescent, the techniques described by these surgeons are ones that I perform. Furthermore, I have not included a section on the otologic surgical procedures that are indicated for children who have a suppurative complication of otitis media or middle cranial fossa surgery, because they have been adequately described by the aforementioned authors.

TYMPANOCENTESIS, MYRINGOTOMY, AND TYMPANOSTOMY TUBE INSERTION

An extensive description of my indications and technique for tympanocentesis, myringotomy, and tympanostomy tube insertion can be found in *Pediatric Otolaryngology*.[5]

Tympanocentesis is a needle aspiration of the middle ear and is indicated to identify the causative organism when a middle ear effusion is present. Myringotomy is performed when drainage of the middle ear cleft is required. Insertion of a tympanostomy tube into a myringotomy incision is indicated when long-term ventilation, drainage, or both is desired.

TYMPANOCENTESIS

Indications

- Otitis media in children who are seriously ill or have toxic signs or symptoms[9]
- Unsatisfactory response to antimicrobial therapy
- Onset of otitis media in a patient who is receiving antimicrobial agents
- Presence or suspicion of suppurative complications
- Otitis media in the newborn, the very young infant, or the immunologically deficient patient, in each of whom an unusual organism may be suspected

Anesthetic considerations

- The procedure can usually be performed without general anesthesia.
- In certain cases, premedication with a combination of a short-acting barbiturate and either morphine or meperidine, or even a general anesthetic, is advisable.

Preparation

- For older children and adolescents, a small amount of phenol can be used on the tympanic membrane before the needle is inserted.

Procedure

- Aspiration can be carried out using an otoscope with a surgical head or with the otomicroscope. Adequate immobilization of the patient is essential when a general anesthetic is not used.[5]

- The needle is inserted through the inferior portion of the tympanic membrane, using an 18-gauge spinal needle that is attached to a syringe or collection trap.[5]

- The following method is recommended for tympanocentesis and aspiration of a middle ear effusion for microbiologic assessment:

  A culture of the external auditory canal can be obtained with a Calgiswab that is moistened with trypticase soy broth. The external canal is then filled with 70% ethyl alcohol for 1 minute (Fig. 3–1).

  Alcohol is removed from the ear canal by aspiration. Tympanocentesis is performed in the inferior portion of the tympanic membrane with an Alden-Senturia trap with a needle attached (Fig. 3–2). Care is taken not to close the suction hole in the trap before entering the middle ear. A tuberculin syringe with an 18-gauge needle attached is an alternative. (Note that a myringotomy can be performed after tympanocentesis to provide adequate drainage.)

Postoperative care

- The middle ear aspirate should be sent to the microbiology laboratory for Gram stain, culture, and susceptibility studies.

MYRINGOTOMY

Indications

- Presence or suspicion of suppurative complications of otitis media, such as facial paralysis or mastoiditis

- Relief of severe otalgia at the onset of the illness, or persistent signs and symptoms of acute middle ear (mastoid) infection

Note that myringotomy is useful primarily to provide drainage of the middle ear and frequently the mastoid. Tympanocentesis with needle aspiration should precede the myringotomy when microbiologic assessment is indicated (see earlier). Myringotomy as a *routine* adjunct to antimicrobial therapy is not required; however, the procedure is helpful for relief of otalgia.[10] Furthermore, in selected cases, a tympanostomy tube may be indicated to provide adequate drainage, such as when a suppurative complication is present or when the child has had recurrent otitis media in the recent past.

Anesthetic considerations

- The anesthetic considerations and immobilization of the child are similar to those described under tympanocentesis.

● FIGURE 3–1.

Ethyl alcohol (70%) is instilled in the external canal for 1 minute.

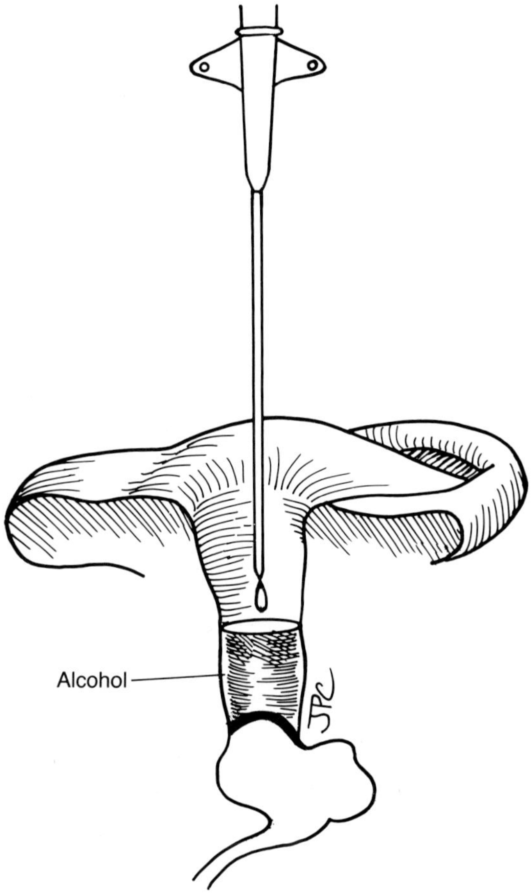

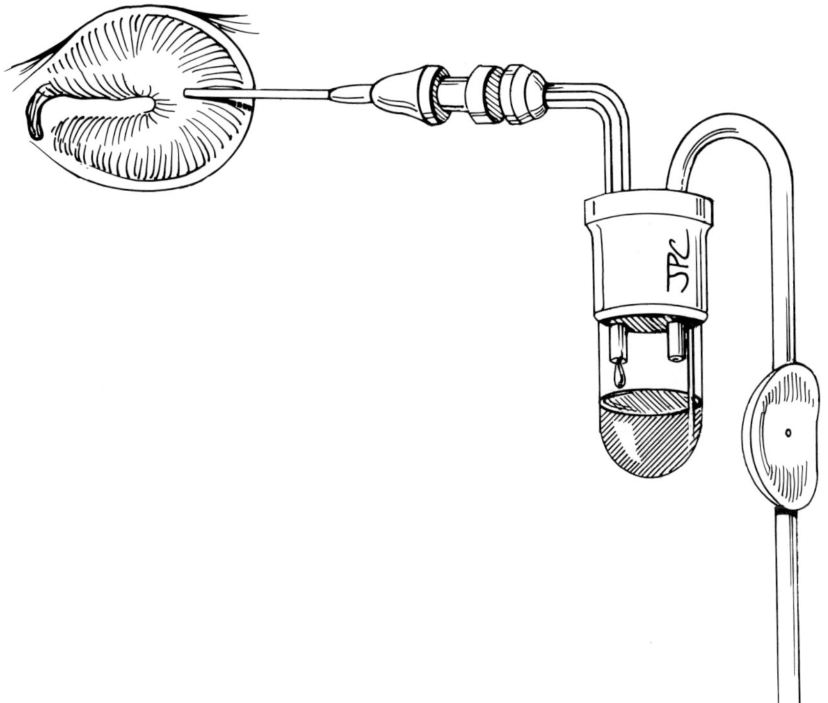

● FIGURE 3–2.

Alcohol is removed from the ear canal by aspiration, and tympanocentesis is performed with an Alden-Senturia trap (Storz Instrument Co., St. Louis, MO) with a needle attached.

Procedure

- A wide-field incision is made in the inferior portion of the pars tensa (instillation of 70% alcohol for 1 minute precedes the procedure) (Fig. 3–3*A*).

- A radial incision is made in the anterosuperior quadrant of the pars tensa, if a tympanostomy tube is to be inserted (Fig. 3–3*B*). (An incision in the anteroinferior quadrant is a reasonable alternative.)

- Middle ear effusion is aspirated with a small Baron or Fraser aspirator (Fig. 3–4*A*).

- When a wide-field inferiorly placed myringotomy is indicated, a larger aspirator is used (Fig. 3–4*B*). Also, if during myringotomy, the effusion is too viscid to be aspirated through the anterosuperior radial myringotomy, a "counter incision" myringotomy can also be performed and the thick effusion aspirated through the inferiorly placed incision.

Postoperative care

- The patient (or family member) should be warned that otorrhea may become a problem.

- When otorrhea is profuse, infectious eczematoid dermatitis may develop. Cotton should be placed in the external auditory canal, and ototopical cortisone-antibiotic drops are usually helpful in preventing dermatitis and chronic suppurative otitis media that could result from bacterial organisms from the external canal entering and contaminating the middle ear through the myringotomy incision. The cotton should be changed whenever it becomes wet, or at least once a day.

TYMPANOSTOMY TUBE INSERTION

Of the many types of tubes currently available, the Armstrong-type biflanged tube is preferred for routine placement. Our studies have shown that it remains functional for approximately 1 year.[11–13]

Indications

- For chronic middle ear effusion that is relatively asymptomatic and does not respond to medical management (and is not improving), and has persisted for at least 3 months when bilateral or 6 months when unilateral. Insertion at an earlier time would be reasonable when there is significant hearing loss (e.g., >25 dB), speech or language delay, a severe retraction pocket, or disequilibrium/vertigo, or when tinnitus is present.

- For recurrent acute otitis media, especially when antimicrobial prophylaxis fails to prevent frequent, severe, and long-lasting disease. Minimum frequency for considering tympanostomy tube insertion would be three or more episodes during the previous 6 months or four or more attacks during the previous year, with one being recent.

  Also, recurrent episodes of otitis media with effusion in which the duration of each episode does not meet the criteria for chronic disease, but the cumulative duration is considered to be excessive (e.g., 6 to 12 months).

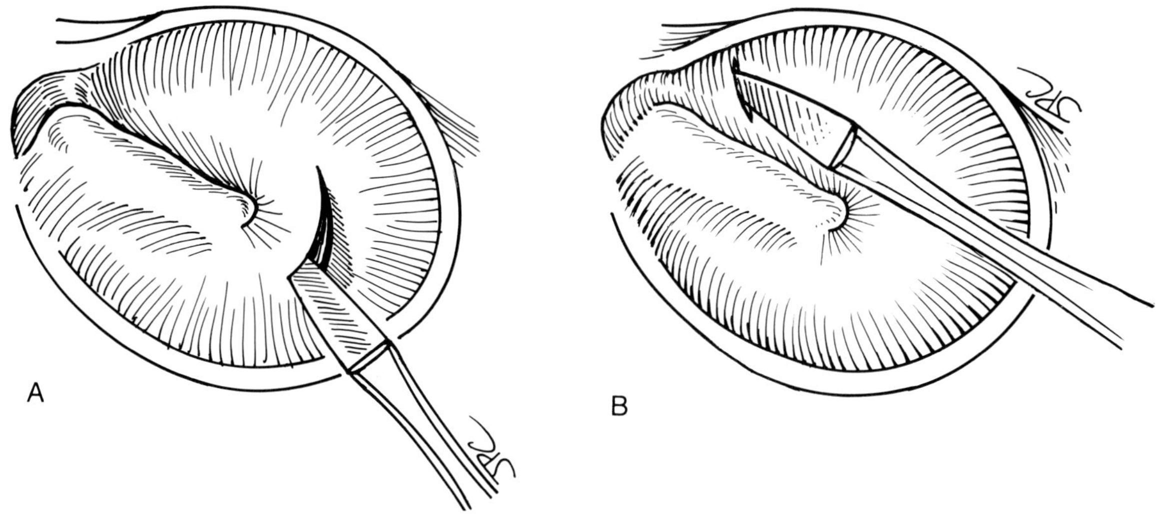

• FIGURE 3-3.

A, A wide-field incision is made in the inferior portion of the pars tensa. *B*, A radial incision is made in the anteroposterior (or anteroinferior) quadrant of the pars tensa.

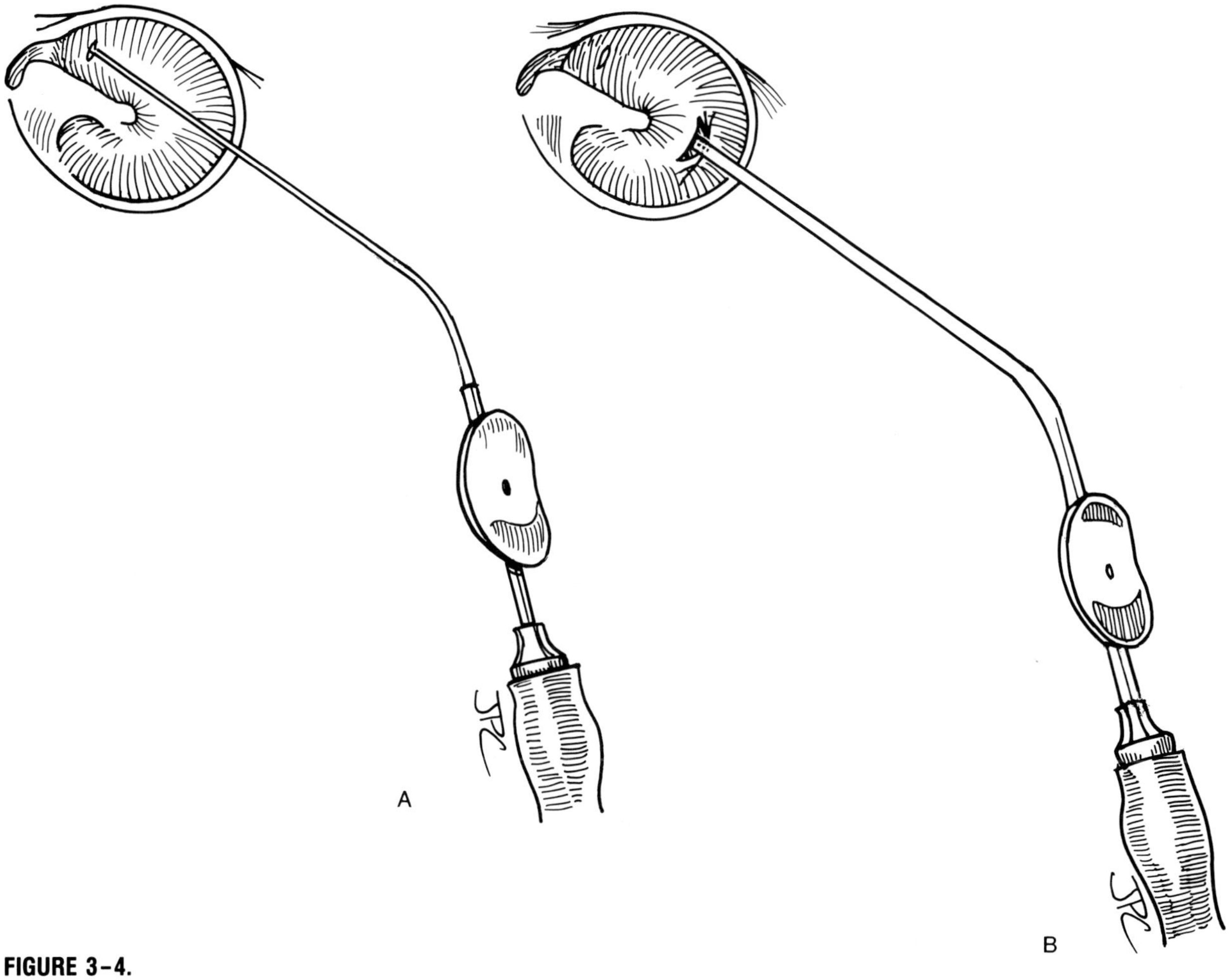

• FIGURE 3-4.

A, A small Baron or Fraser aspirator is used for aspiration of middle ear effusion. *B*, When a wide-field inferiorly placed myringotomy is indicated, a larger aspirator is used.

- When a suppurative complication is suspected or is present. Insertion of a tympanostomy tube at the time of tympanocentesis/myringotomy can provide more prolonged drainage and aeration of the middle ear cleft. A wide-field myringotomy should also be performed in the inferior portion of the tympanic membrane to provide adequate drainage; the tympanostomy tube is inserted through a radial incision in the anterosuperior quadrant. A Gram stain, culture, and susceptibility study are done, as described later.

- For eustachian tube dysfunction, even in the absence of middle ear effusion, when the patient has persistent or recurrent signs and symptoms that are not relieved by medical treatment. Signs and symptoms would include hearing loss (usually fluctuating), disequilibrium/vertigo, tinnitus, or a severe retraction pocket (see *Pediatric Otolaryngology*).[5]

- When a tympanoplasty (with or without a mastoidectomy) is performed and when eustachian tube function is thought to be poor, such as when an acquired cholesteatoma is present in an infant or young child (see Figs. 3–104 and 3–116). (Eustachian tube function testing is usually not feasible prior to surgery for cholesteatoma, unless a tympanostomy tube is in place or a perforation is present. If a tube or perforation is present, the middle ear should not be infected.) Tympanostomy tube insertion at the time of the surgery for the cholesteatoma can be helpful in preventing a recurrence of the disease, by preventing a recurrence of middle ear atelectasis and, more important, development of another retraction pocket (see *Pediatric Otolaryngology*).[5]

Anesthetic considerations

- In children, the procedure is performed under general anesthesia. In some older, cooperative teenagers, local infiltrative anesthesia (1% xylocaine with 1:100,000 epinephrine) can be used successfully (see Fig. 3–15 for injection sites), or a small amount of topical phenol can be applied to the myringotomy site, or both methods of local anesthesia can be used.

Procedure

- Alligator forceps are used to insert the tympanostomy tube into the previously performed myringotomy in the anterosuperior quadrant of the pars tensa (Fig. 3–5). An Armstrong-type tube is preferred, because it usually lasts for about 1 year (range of 6 to 18 months).[3, 12, 13]

- A tube is placed in the anterosuperior quadrant (Fig. 3–6). A radial incision is made that is small enough to prevent premature extrusion but is long enough to permit the tube to be inserted easily. When purulent or mucopurulent fluid is aspirated, a culture of middle ear effusion is helpful, especially if the child develops persistent postoperative otorrhea; a Quik-Cath (Baxter Healthcare Corporation, Deerfield, IL) attached to an Alden-Senturia trap is used to aspirate the effusion. Ototopical drops are instilled into the external auditory canal when a middle ear effusion is aspirated, and instillation is continued if otorrhea occurs.

Postoperative care

- Otorrhea that occurs after surgery is usually treated effectively with ototopical medication. A culture and susceptibility testing of the effusion at the time of the

• FIGURE 3–5.

An alligator forceps is used to insert the tympanostomy tube into the previously performed myringotomy in the anterosuperior quadrant of the pars tensa.

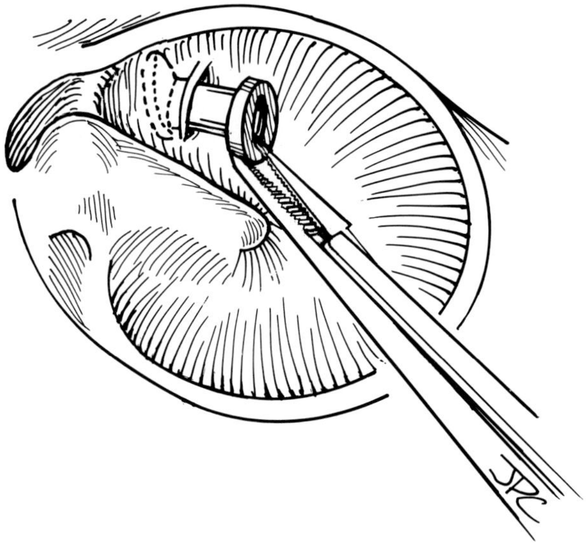

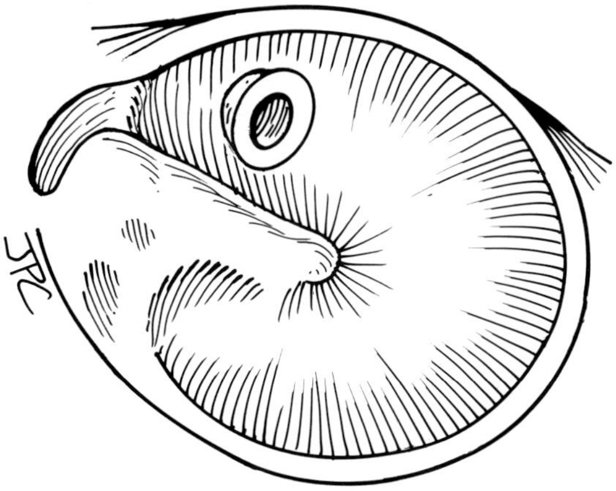

• FIGURE 3–6.

Tympanostomy tube in place.

tympanostomy tube placement can be helpful in selection of oral antimicrobial agents. We prefer to protect the ears when the child is bathing or swimming by using ear plugs. Patients are re-examined approximately 2 weeks after insertion of the tube, at which time another audiogram is obtained and compared with the preoperative test. If hearing is normal and the tympanostomy tubes are patent, based on our studies, the child can be re-examined in 6 months and then every 3 to 4 months until spontaneous extrusion occurs.

- Because episodes of acute otorrhea are common during the life of indwelling and patent tympanostomy tubes, early treatment of these infections with systemic antimicrobial therapy, ototopical agents, or both appears not only to decrease the duration and severity of the infection but also to prevent progression to the chronic stage.

PERMANENT TYMPANOSTOMY TUBE INSERTION

Indications

- For eustachian tube obstruction that has been determined to be "permanent," (i.e., otitis media/eustachian tube obstruction) and will most likely not improve with advancing age

- For conditions such as congenital or acquired eustachian tube stenosis, fracture through the tube following skull-base surgery, or benign neoplasms. These conditions are rare but can lead to chronic, potentially life-long eustachian tube obstruction; eustachian tube testing can aid in making the diagnosis (see *Pediatric Otolaryngology*)[5]

Anesthetic considerations

Anesthetic considerations are similar to those described for myringotomy and tympanostomy tube insertion.

Procedure (see also Myringotomy and Tympanostomy Tube sections)

- An incision is made with a myringotomy knife immediately anterior to the body of the malleus (Fig. 3–7).

- A Per-Lee tube is preferred (Fig. 3–8).[14] The tube should be shortened and a wide flange cut to fit posterior to the malleus; the wide flange is posterior behind the malleus, and a shorter anterior flange is cut to fit behind the anterior quadrant of the tympanic membrane.

- The tube is inserted using alligator forceps. Compression of flanges with alligator or cup forceps aids in insertion of the tube (Fig. 3–9).

- The tube is in place. Note the posterior flange behind the malleus (Fig. 3–10).

Postoperative care

Postoperative care is similar to that described for myringotomy and tympanostomy tube insertion.

• FIGURE 3-7.

An incision is made anterior to the body of the malleus.

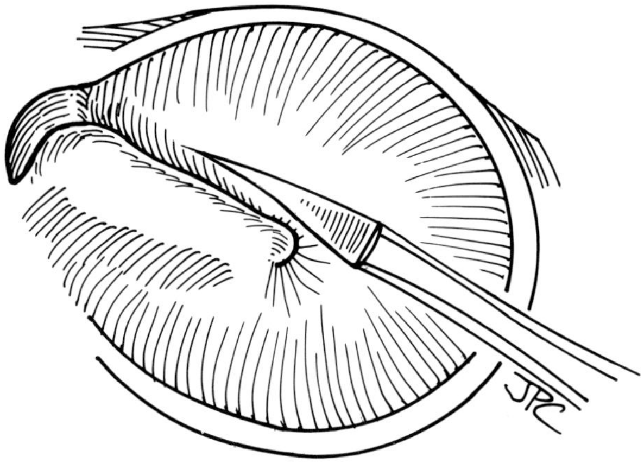

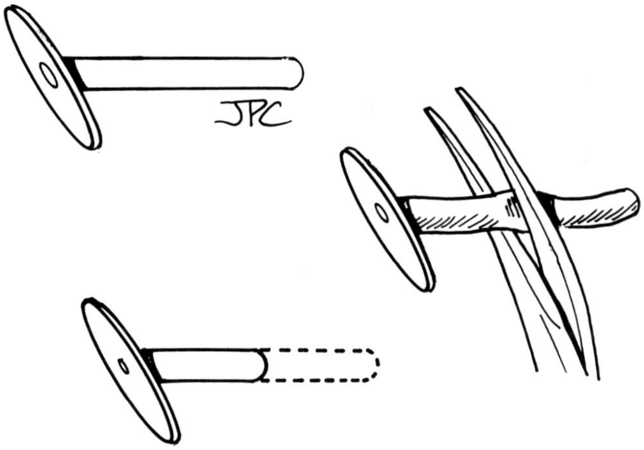

• FIGURE 3-8.

A Per-Lee tube (Xomed-Treace, Inc., Jacksonville, FL) is shortened.

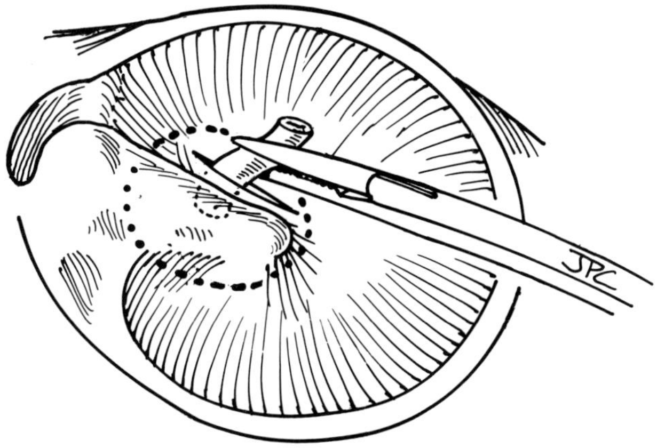

• FIGURE 3-9.

The tube is inserted using an alligator forceps.

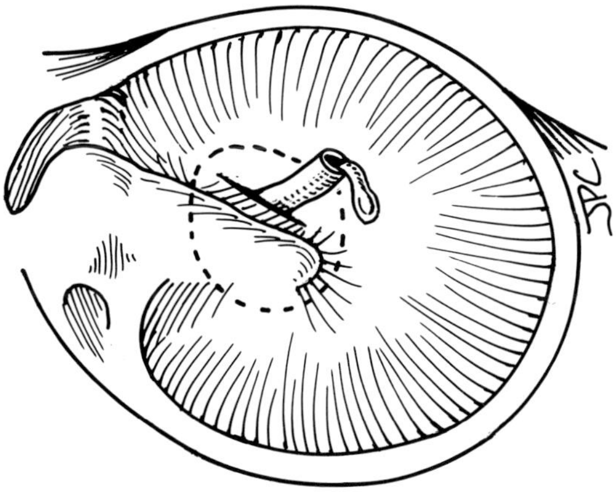

• FIGURE 3-10.

The tube in place.

REPAIR OF TYMPANIC MEMBRANE PERFORATION: REMOVAL OF TYMPANOSTOMY TUBES AND MYRINGOPLASTY

Tympanostomy tubes can be removed as an office procedure without the aid of either local or general anesthesia, especially when the tube is partially extruded or if there is chronic infection involving the tympanic membrane. In children, however, tympanostomy tubes are frequently removed under general anesthesia in the operating room, because the procedure is usually painful and because the rim of the perforation can be denuded of epithelium and the defect closed (i.e., myringoplasty) following the removal of the tube (more complete discussion of when to remove tympanostomy tubes is found in *Pediatric Otolaryngology*).[5] This method, although not tested in a clinical trial, appears to result in a higher rate of closure of the perforation than when the tube is removed with no attempt to close the defect. Because the decision-making process involved in removal of the tympanostomy tube is similar to the decision to close a relatively small perforation of the tympanic membrane, myringoplasty using a medial graft is included in this section. (Indications for myringoplasty are described more extensively in *Pediatric Otolaryngology*.[5])

TYMPANOSTOMY TUBE REMOVAL AND REPAIR OF THE DEFECT WITH STERI-STRIP PATCH MYRINGOPLASTY

Our studies of tympanostomy tubes indicate that the Armstrong-type tube usually lasts about 1 year, with the range being 6 to 18 months.[11–13] Tubes that remain in place longer than that period may require removal on an individualized basis and depend on several factors, such as the following:

- Age of the child
- Amount of time that the tube has remained in place
- Unilateral versus bilateral tubes
- Status of the contralateral ear when that tympanic membrane is intact
- Eustachian tube function
- Presence or absence of recurrent or chronic otorrhea (and frequency, severity, and duration of otorrhea)
- Patency of the tube
- Season of the year

The age of the child is one of the most important factors, because most studies of the epidemiology of otitis media show that the disease has a peak in infancy and declines rapidly after about 6 years of age. In addition, the structure and function of the eustachian tube and the child's immunity are usually more mature after 6 years of age. Therefore, removal of tubes in children who are 6 years of age and older is more desirable than in children who are younger. However, removal of the tube in selected children who are younger may be beneficial, such as when there is unilateral recurrent otorrhea through a tube—apparently owing to reflux of nasopharyngeal secretions into the middle ear—that is not controlled medically and when the contralateral tympanic membrane is intact (no tube is present) and that ear has been free of middle ear disease for 1 year or more (see *Pediatric Otolaryngology*).[5]

Indications

- Presence of a retained unilateral tympanostomy tube in children who are 6 years of age or older, when the contralateral tympanic membrane is intact and the middle ear has been free of disease for 1 year or more
- Selected similar children younger than 6 years of age, depending on the factors listed earlier
- Presence of retained bilateral tympanostomy tubes in children in whom eustachian tube function is now considered within normal limits owing to growth and development, or when a nonsurgical (e.g., allergy control or treatment) or surgical (e.g., adenoidectomy; repair of cleft palate) management may have improved eustachian tube function
- Presence of frequently recurrent otorrhea through a tympanostomy tube that is not prevented by antimicrobial prophylaxis; important factors in decision-making are frequency, severity, and duration of the episodes; age of the patient; and duration that the tube has been in place
- Following chronic otorrhea, especially when the criteria described in the first two points are met
- When the tympanostomy tube is imbedded in granulation tissue, which is unresponsive to medical treatment

Anesthetic considerations

- In children, general anesthesia is usually required. For selected children, especially teenagers, no anesthesia is needed.

Procedure

- The myringotomy tube is removed gently using an alligator forceps (Fig. 3–11).

- Epithelium from the rim of the perforation is removed using a right-angled pick or using a gently curved pick to split the layers of tympanic membrane and a cup forceps to remove the tissue (Fig. 3–12).

- A circular portion of Steri-Strip is cut and placed over the perforation. The operative site must be free of any bleeding prior to placement of the patch; application of epinephrine on Gelfoam for 5 minutes is adequate (Fig. 3–13).

- An antibiotic ointment (e.g., polymyxin B sulfate, zinc bacitracin, neomycin sulfate [Neosporin ointment]) is instilled into the external auditory canal using a syringe and a plastic needle tip (Fig. 3–14).

Postoperative care

- The patient is re-examined after 1 month. At that time, the Steri-Strip patch is usually off the tympanic membrane and the perforation is healed. If the patch is not displaced, an ototopical agent is instilled for several days and the child is re-examined. Confirmation of closure of the tympanic membrane can be achieved using pneumatic otoscopy or more precisely with the aid of the otomicroscope and a Bruening otoscope with a nonmagnifying lens. A microscopic defect, however, may still be present despite seemingly good tympanic mobility as observed during pneumatic otoscopy. Tympanometry is the most sensitive method to confirm that the tympanic membrane is intact.

- In the absence of a tympanostomy tube, we use the Steri-Strip myringoplasty technique when a small perforation is present secondary to a previously extruded tympanostomy tube, as a complication of otitis media, or following trauma. The surgical procedure is the same as that described earlier, and the indications are similar to those described below, when a myringoplasty is performed using a medial graft. When the Steri-Strip technique is used, however, the perforation should be small.

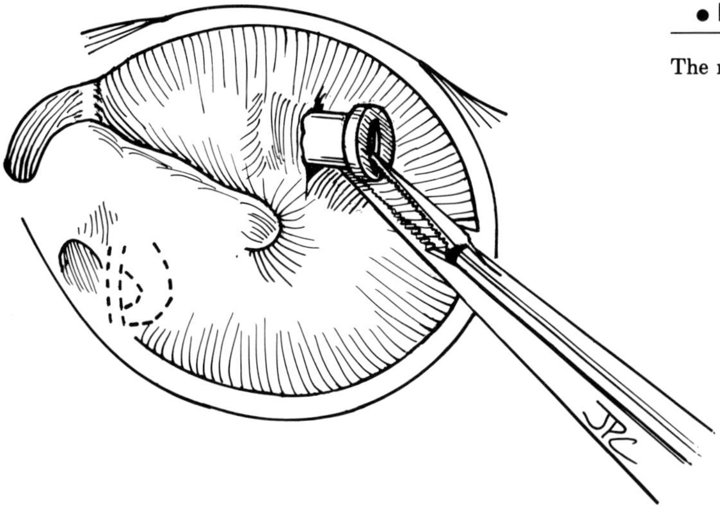

• FIGURE 3–11.

The myringotomy tube is removed gently using an alligator forceps.

• FIGURE 3-12.

Epithelium from the rim of the perforation is removed using a right-angled pick.

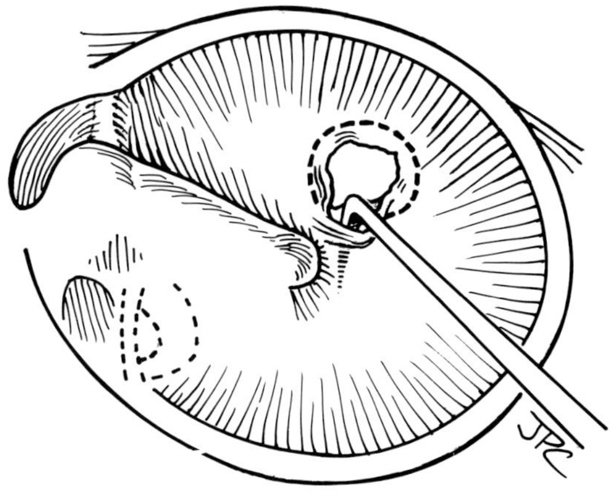

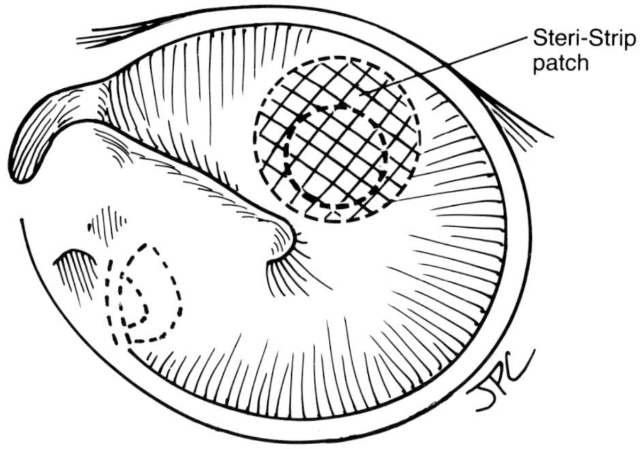

• FIGURE 3-13.

A circular portion of Steri-Strip (Medical-Surgical Division/3M, St. Paul, MN) is cut and placed over the perforation.

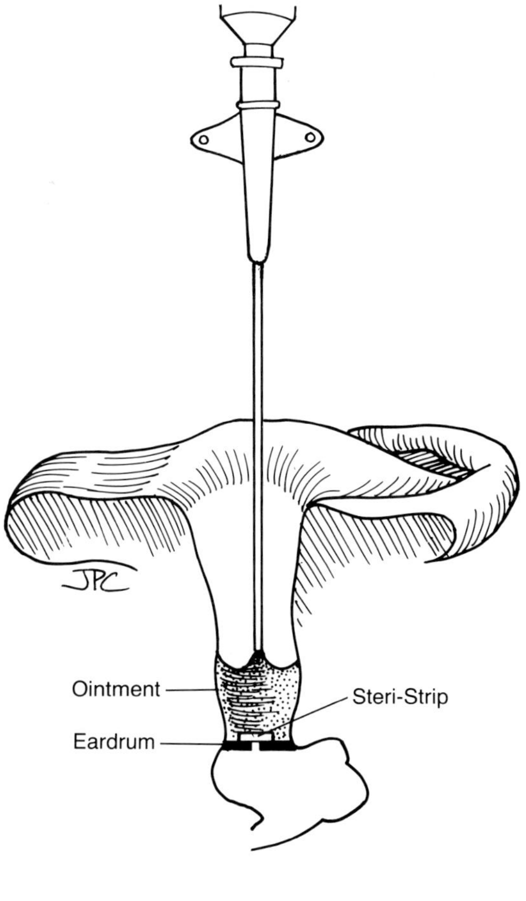

• FIGURE 3-14.

Instillation of an antibiotic ointment into the external auditory canal using a syringe and a plastic needle tip (Quik-Cath, Baxter Healthcare Corporation, Deerfield, IL).

MYRINGOPLASTY WITH MEDIAL TISSUE GRAFT

Myringoplasty is a procedure used to repair a tympanic membrane perforation, without the need to examine the middle ear. The procedure should be limited to patients with relatively small central perforations in whom the tympanic membrane is translucent and no middle ear disease is suspected and when hearing is within normal limits. When these conditions are not met, a tympanoplasty is indicated to facilitate the repair and to explore the middle ear (see *Pediatric Otolaryngology*).[5]

Indications

Indications for myringoplasty with medial tissue graft are similar to those described when removal of a tympanostomy tube is being considered, but there are a few notable differences:

- Site of the perforation: The perforation should not be in the anterosuperior quadrant of the pars tensa (unless the defect is very small); when it is in this site, the simpler Steri-Strip technique is usually successful. Placement of a medial graft through an anterosuperior perforation is difficult owing to the constricted space. Perforations in this quadrant are repaired more effectively using the endaural tympanoplastic technique described later under Anterosuperior Perforation: Endaural Approach, Medial Graft.

- Etiology: Chronic traumatic perforations can be repaired in infants and young children as well as in older children and adolescents, as long as recurrent or chronic middle ear infection does not coexist.

Anesthetic considerations

- In children, the procedure is performed under general anesthesia. Infiltration of a local anesthetic (1% Xylocaine with 1:100,000 epinephrine) is also preferred.

Preparation

- If a large speculum does not fit snugly into the external canal so that both of the surgeon's hands are free to perform the procedure, a speculum holder attached to the operating table should be used. The tissue graft that we use is either perichondrium removed from the tragus or fascia removed from the temporalis muscle. A small portion of the hair is shaved just above the pinna, if a temporalis graft is to be used.

Procedure

- Sites of injection of the local anesthetic agent: A needle is inserted at the bony cartilaginous junction at 3, 6, 9, and 12 o'clock (Fig. 3–15).

- An incision for a fascia graft is made superior to the pinna just above the hairline (Fig. 3–16*A*), and the graft is excised (Fig. 3–16*B*).

• FIGURE 3-15.

Sites of injection of the local anesthetic agent.

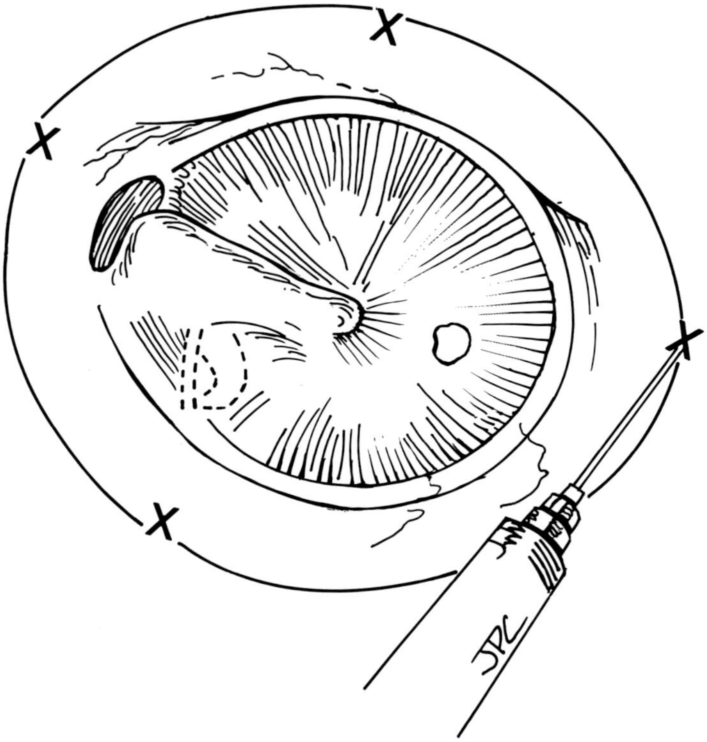

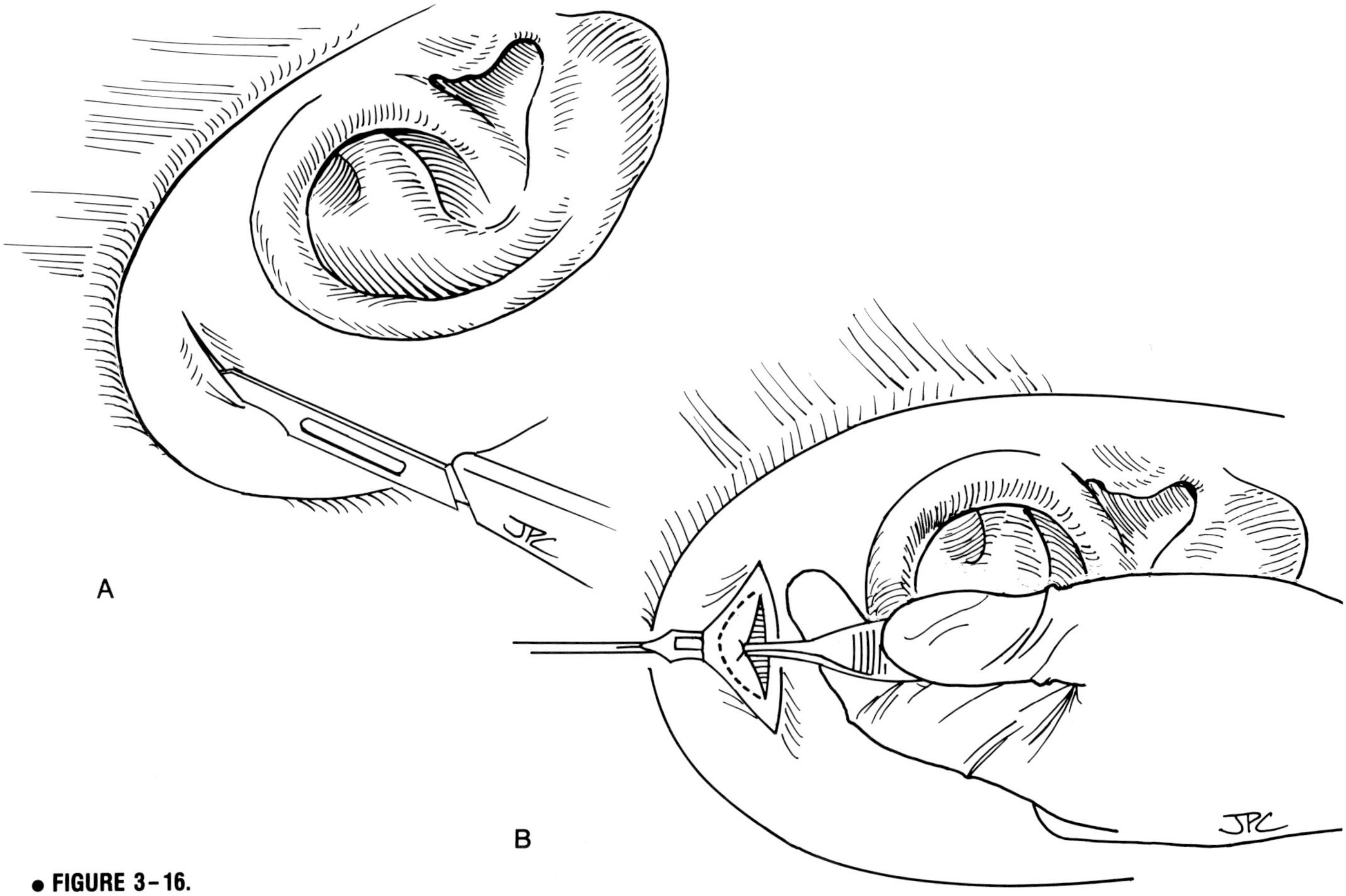

• FIGURE 3-16.

A, An incision for a fascia graft is made superior to the pinna just above the hairline. *B*, The fascia graft is excised.

• As an alternative to a fascia graft, a perichondrial graft can also be used. An incision for the perichondrial graft is made in the tragus, slightly toward the meatus (Fig. 3–17*A*), and the perichondrial graft excised (Fig. 3–17*B*).

• A small central perforation is ideal for this procedure (Fig. 3–18).

• The rim of the epithelium at the edge of the perforation is removed with a pick. A cup forceps will also facilitate this stage (Fig. 3–19).

• The middle ear is filled with Gelfoam (Fig. 3–20). A tissue graft is placed medial to the tympanic membrane (Fig. 3–21).

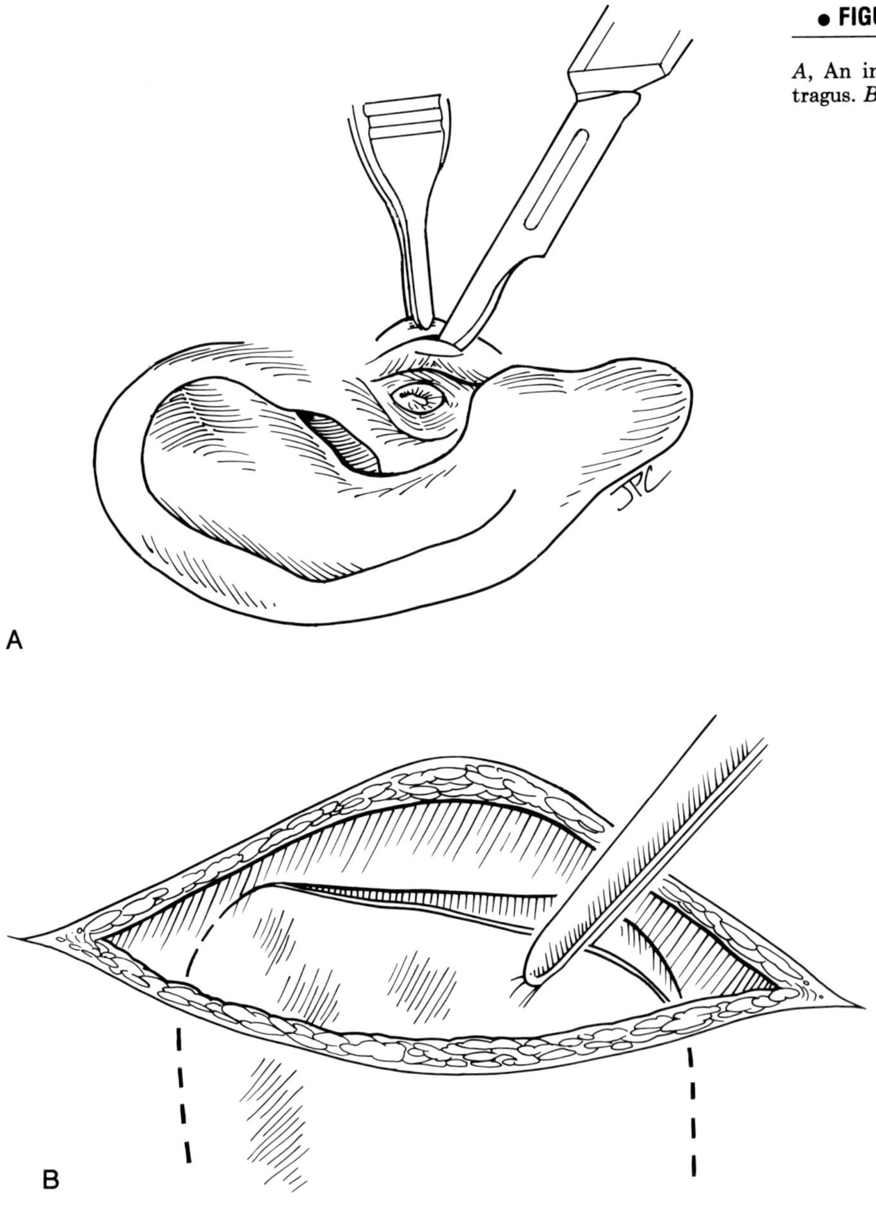

A

B

• FIGURE 3–17.

A, An incision for perichondrial graft is made in the tragus. *B*, The fascia graft is excised.

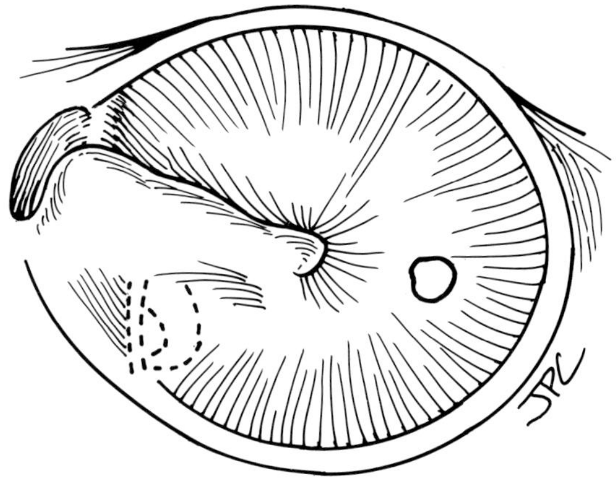

• FIGURE 3-18.

A small central perforation is present.

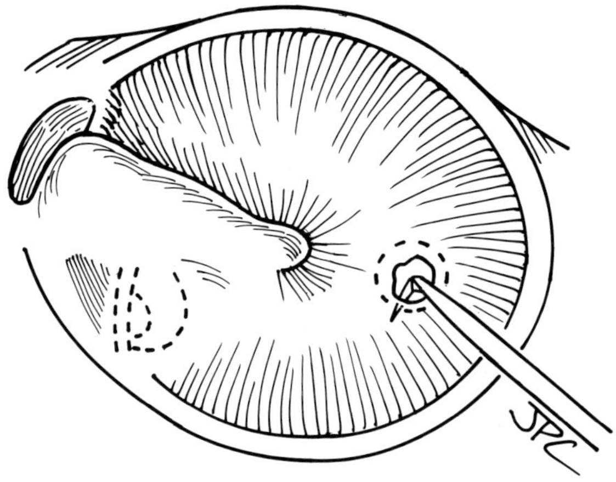

• FIGURE 3-19.

The rim of the epithelium at the edge of the perforation is removed with a pick.

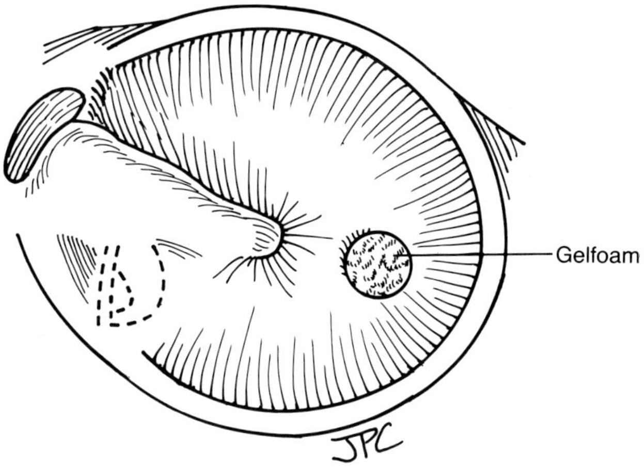

• FIGURE 3-20.

The middle ear is filled with absorbable gelatin sponge (Gelfoam) (The Upjohn Company, Kalamazoo, MI).

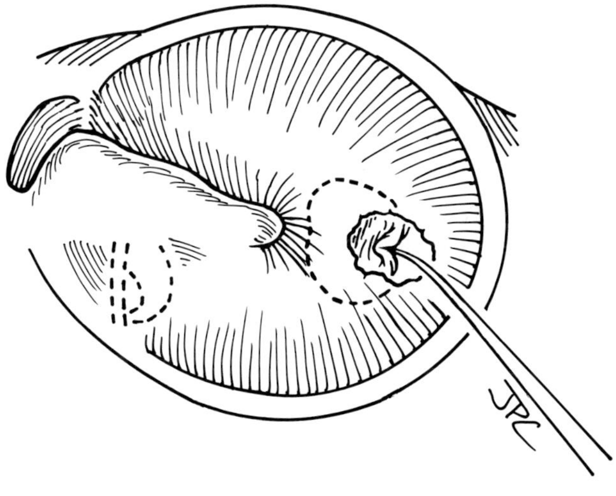

• FIGURE 3-21.

A tissue graft is placed medial to the tympanic membrane.

• A Steri-Strip is placed over the perforation and tissue graft (Fig. 3–22). If any bleeding occurs in the operative site, epinephrine applied to a piece of Gelfoam is used prior to placement of the Steri-Strip.

• An antibiotic ointment is instilled into the external auditory canal using a syringe and plastic needle tip (Fig. 3–23).

Postoperative care

• Postoperative care is similar to that described earlier under Tympanostomy Tube Removal and Repair of the Defect with Steri-Strip Patch Myringoplasty.

INCISIONS AND APPROACHES TO THE MIDDLE EAR AND MASTOID

There are three commonly used incisions and approaches to the middle ear: transcanal, endaural, and postauricular. The most commonly used approach to the mastoid is through a postauricular incision. Even though the endaural incision can be used to approach the mastoid, it does not provide as good exposure of the mastoid as the postauricular incision.

TRANSCANAL APPROACH

The transcanal approach is not used as commonly in children as it is in adults owing to the relatively small ear canal in infants and young children. When the external canal is too small, the endaural or postauricular approach is used. The tympanomeatal flap that is developed provides excellent exposure of the mesotympanum. The approach is one that was described by Rosen.[15]

Indications

• Tympanoplasty: Repair of tympanic membrane perforations when the canal is large enough for adequate exposure (an endaural or postauricular approach is indicated when the canal is too small) and when there is a need to examine the middle ear (see *Pediatric Otolaryngology*).[5]

• Cholesteatoma surgery: When a congenital or acquired cholesteatoma is localized to the tympanic membrane, mesotympanum, and hypotympanum. Also, cholesteatoma that is localized to the attic can be removed using this approach if the superior portion of the tympanomeatal incision is elongated into the superior and anterosuperior portions of the canal wall (see later).

• "Second look" tympanotomy: This procedure is usually performed approximately 6 months after surgery for cholesteatoma, in which the tympanic membrane is present and prevents adequate postoperative examination to determine if there is residual cholesteatoma. On occasion, a "third look" is indicated 6 months after a "second look" procedure if that operation uncovers a residual cholesteatoma; rarely, a "fourth look" is required.[19]

• FIGURE 3-22.

A Steri-Strip is placed over the perforation and tissue graft.

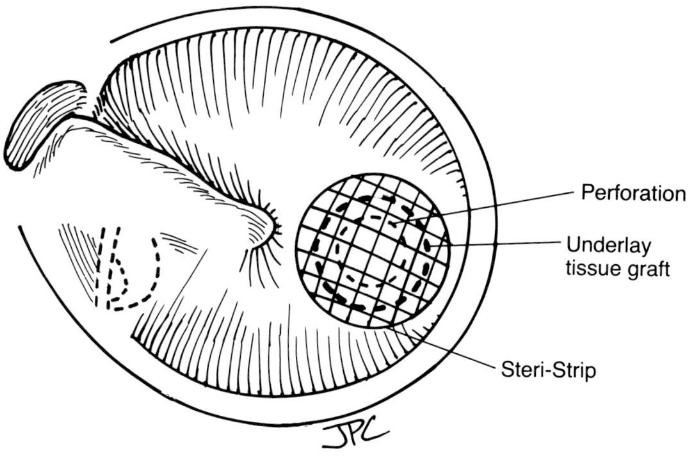

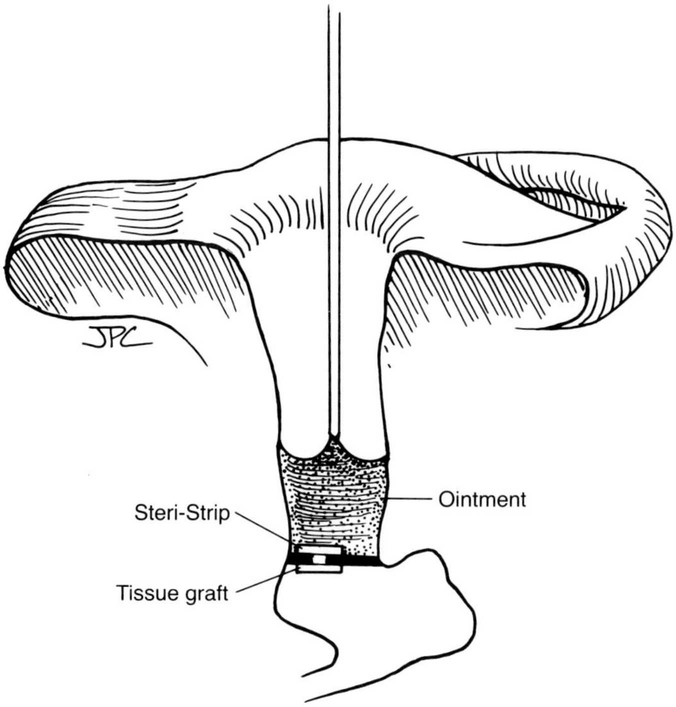

• FIGURE 3-23.

An antibiotic ointment is instilled into the external auditory canal using a syringe and plastic needle tip.

- Ossiculoplasty: Repair of congenital or acquired defects of the ossicular chain (see *Pediatric Otolaryngology*).[5]

- Otosclerosis surgery: When stapedectomy or stapedotomy is to be performed and the external canal is large enough to provide adequate visualization of the operative site (see *Pediatric Otolaryngology*).[5]

- Exploratory tympanotomy: When an examination of the middle ear is indicated to determine the cause of diseases and disorders of the middle ear that are not evident by other diagnostic methods, such as when there is a conductive or mixed hearing loss of undetermined origin or when a perilymphatic fistula is suspected (see *Pediatric Otolaryngology*).[5]

- Other procedures, such as labyrinthectomy, obliteration or closure of the eustachian tube (see later), and section of the tensor tympani or stapedius muscles, which are rarely indicated in children.

Anesthetic considerations and preparation

- The anesthesia and preparation for this procedure are identical to those described for myringoplasty with medial tissue graft (see earlier under Myringoplasty With Medial Tissue Graft).

Procedure

- This incision is used when the mesotympanum and hypotympanum are the surgical sites (Fig. 3–24*A*).

- An extended incision is made when greater exposure is desired, such as when disease involves the epitympanum (i.e., superior tympanomeatal flap) (Fig. 3–24*B*). The incision is made more lateral and anterior.

- The tympanomeatal flap is elevated to the annulus. Bleeding, if present, is controlled at this stage by application of cotton pledgets or by a Super Sorb Micro Eye Sponge (Storz Ophthalmics, Inc., St. Louis, MO) soaked in epinephrine prior to entering the middle ear (Fig. 3–25).

- The middle ear is entered by elevating the annulus just below the chorda tympani nerve (Fig. 3–26).

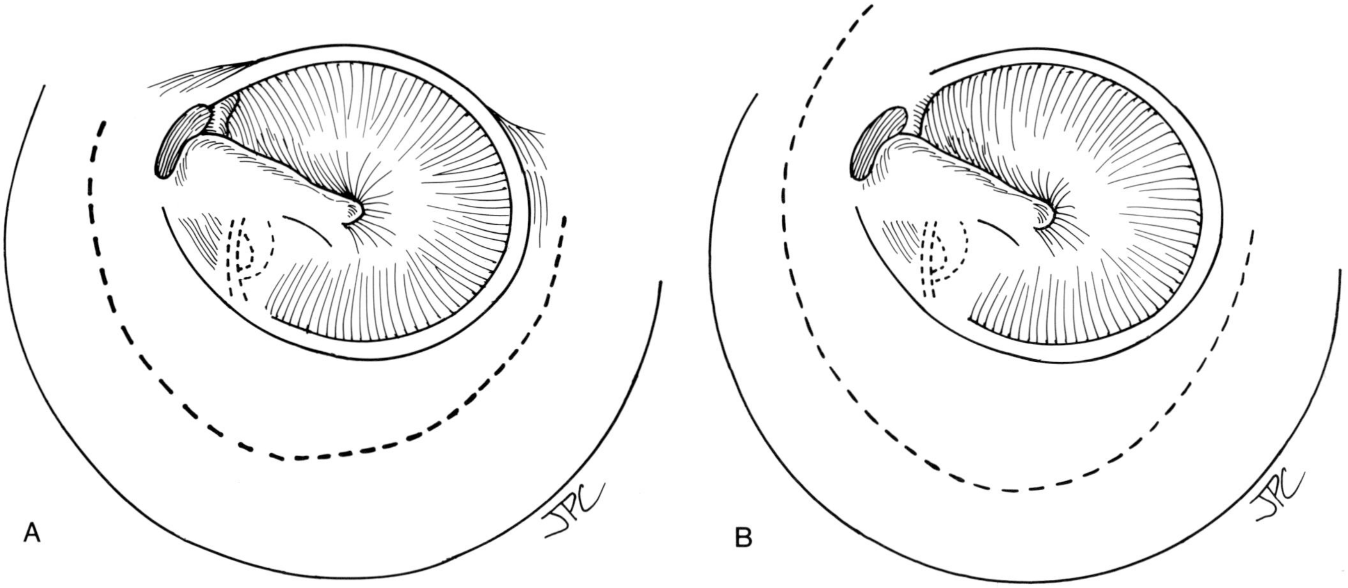

• FIGURE 3-24.

A, An incision is used only when the mesotympanum and hypotympanum are surgical sites. *B*, An extended incision is made when greater exposure is desired.

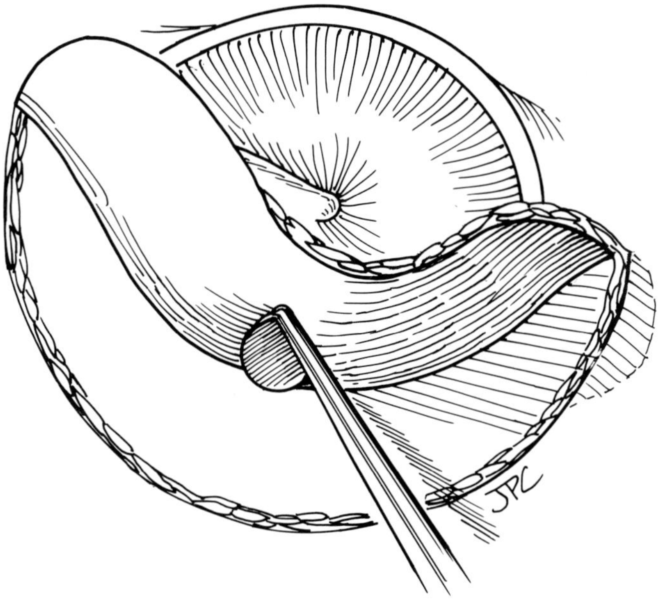

• FIGURE 3-25.

The tympanomeatal flap is elevated to the annulus with a moon elevator.

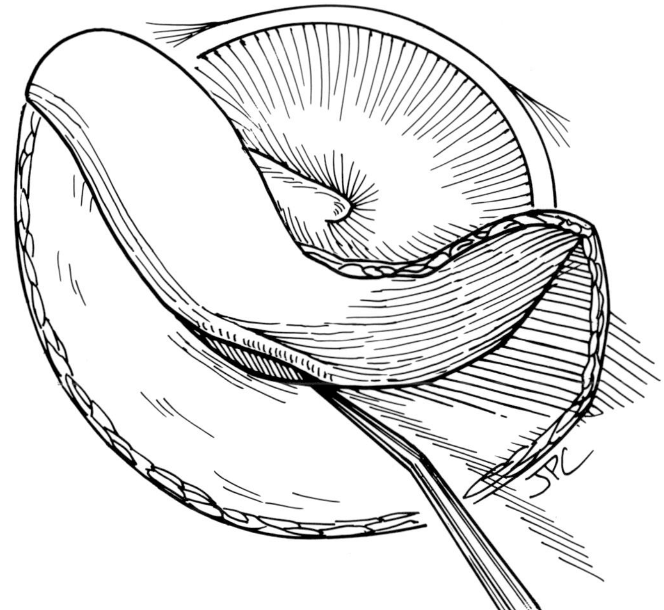

• FIGURE 3-26.

The middle ear is entered by elevating the annulus.

- The superior portion of the tympanomeatal flap is completed using a microscissors (Fig. 3–27).

- Curettage of the posterosuperior canal wall scutum to visualize the long process of the incus, stapes, and stapedius tendon may be necessary in many cases (Fig. 3–28).

- The tympanomeatal flap is completed when the posterior edge of the long process of the malleus, the long process of the incus, the stapes, the stapedius tendon, and the round window are visible, and the flap is reflected anteriorly without tension (Fig. 3–29).

Postoperative care

- Postoperative care depends on the final procedure performed. For example, if only a tympanoplasty was performed, the canal is filled with an antibiotic ointment, as described for myringoplasty (see earlier under Myringoplasty With Medial Tissue Graft). In such cases, the child can be re-examined 4 to 6 weeks later.

Endaural Approach

- The endaural approach is commonly used in children, because their ear canals are often too small to permit adequate exposure for the transcanal approach. Another advantage of the endaural approach is the accessibility of temporalis fascia (and muscle) in the operative field. The procedure described is a modification of the one described originally by Lempert.[16] In addition to differences in the canal incisions, the incision in the incisura of the pinna is shorter and only a small portion of the mastoid bone is exposed, because this approach is not usually used when a mastoidectomy is planned.

Indications

- Tympanoplasty: Repair of perforation in the anterosuperior quadrant of the pars tensa (see later).

- Attic retraction pocket: When the extent of the retraction pocket cannot be fully visualized using the otomicroscope, when there has been recurrent infection within it, when the pocket is progressively enlarging, or when placement of a tympanostomy tube fails to reverse an extensive pocket. Distinction among these types of retraction pockets and acquired cholesteatoma is frequently difficult (see later and also *Pediatric Otolaryngology*).[5]

- Congenital and acquired cholesteatoma: When the disease is localized to the anterior epitympanum and the mesotympanum (see later).

- Closure or obliteration of the eustachian tube: When adequate access is not possible employing the transcanal approach and an anterior tympanomeatal flap (see later).

Anesthetic considerations

General anesthesia is almost always required, and local infiltrative anesthesia is also used; injection sites are the same as those described for myringoplasty and transcanal tympanoplasty (see later), but additional injections are placed in the incisura of the pinna.

• FIGURE 3-27.

The superior portion of the tympanomeatal flap is completed using microscissors.

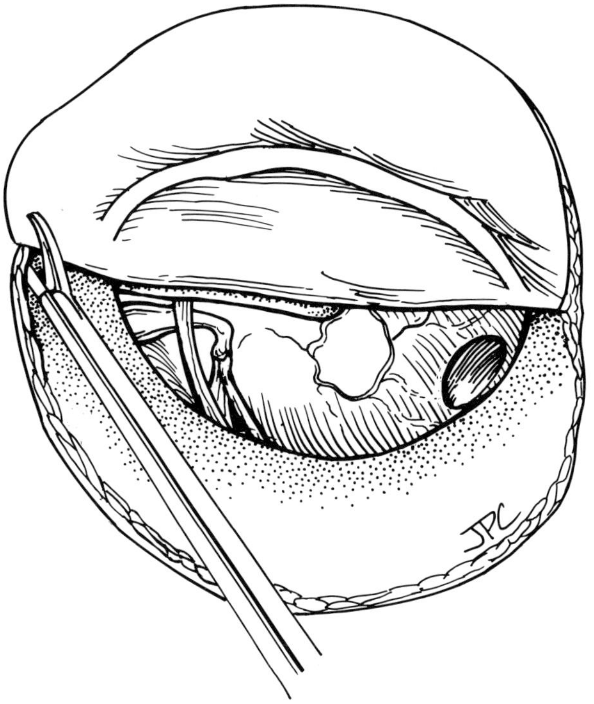

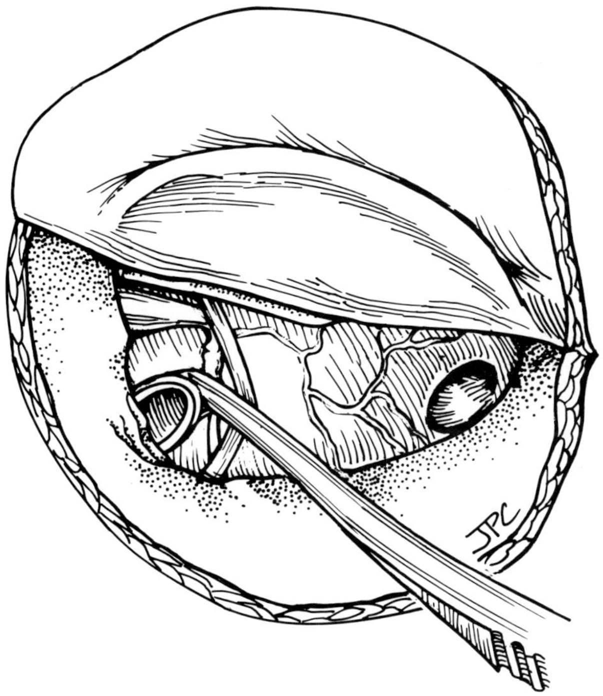

• FIGURE 3-28.

Curettage of the scutum.

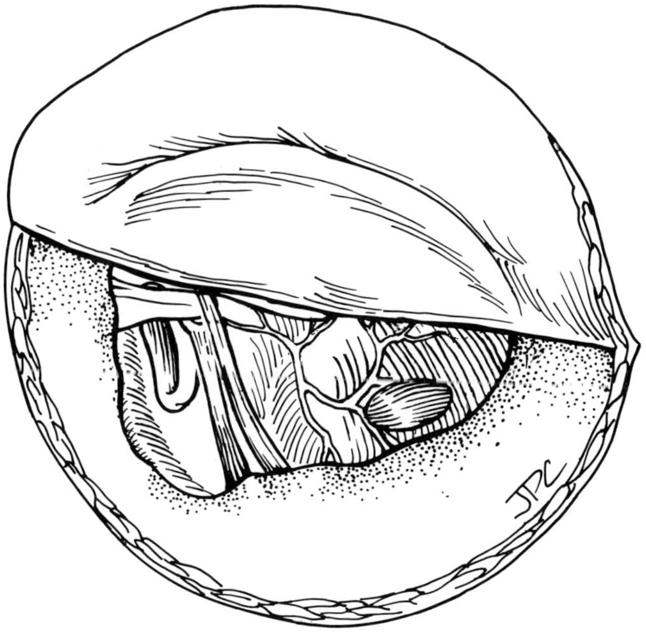

• FIGURE 3-29.

The tympanomeatal flap is completed.

Preparation

- Because the incision is carried into the incisura of the pinna, a small area of scalp hair may have to be shaved anterosuperior to the pinna.

Procedure

- A Lempert speculum exposes the bony cartilaginous junction (Fig. 3–30). Injection sites are just lateral to the junction but directed toward the bony canal and into the incisura of pinna.
- A posterior canal incision with a Rosen knife (a Bard-Parker blade is too large) is made slightly medial to the bony cartilaginous junction, so that the medial (i.e., tympanomeatal) flap is thin (Fig. 3–31).
- The incision is continued into the incisura of the pinna but superficial to the temporalis muscle, using a No. 15 Bard-Parker knife blade (Fig. 3–32).
- An anterior incision in the canal is connected to, and is a continuation of, the posterior canal incision (Fig. 3–33).

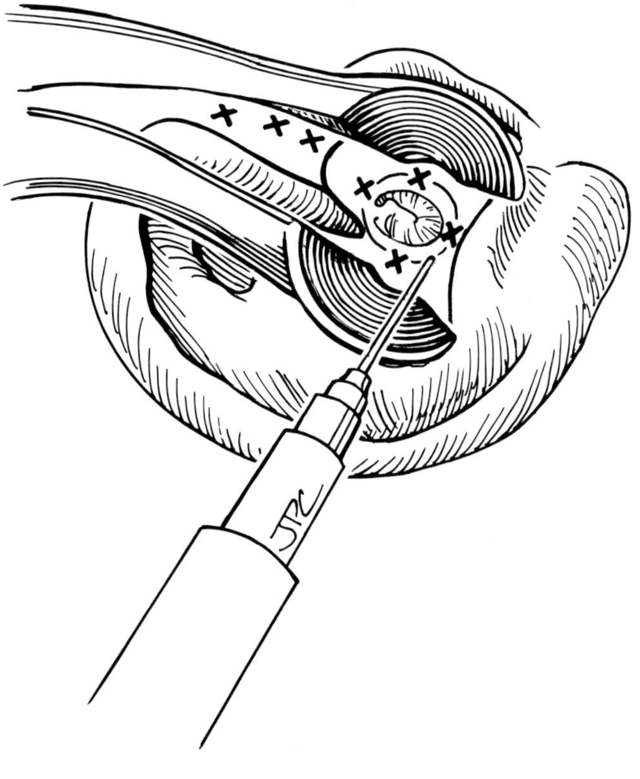

• FIGURE 3–30.

A Lempert speculum exposes the bony cartilaginous junction for injection of a local anesthetic agent.

• FIGURE 3-31.

A posterior canal incision is made with a Rosen knife.

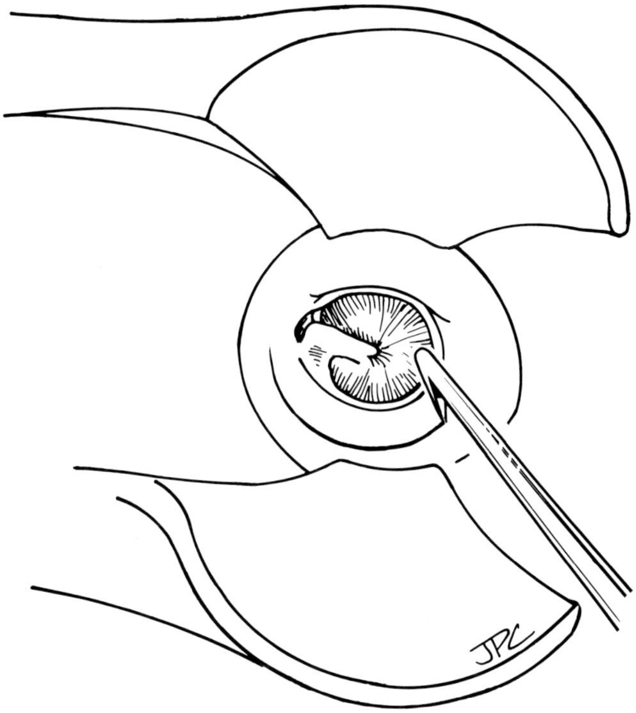

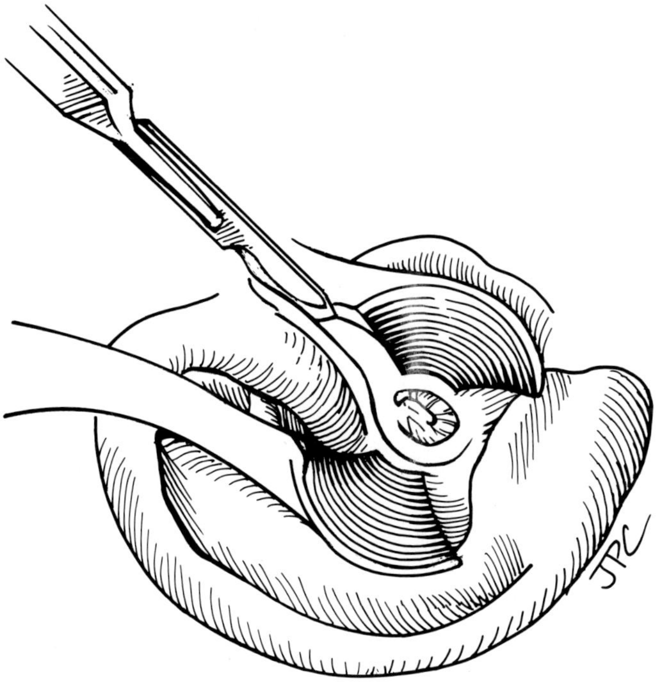

• FIGURE 3-32.

The incision is continued into the incisura of the pinna but superficial to the temporalis muscle.

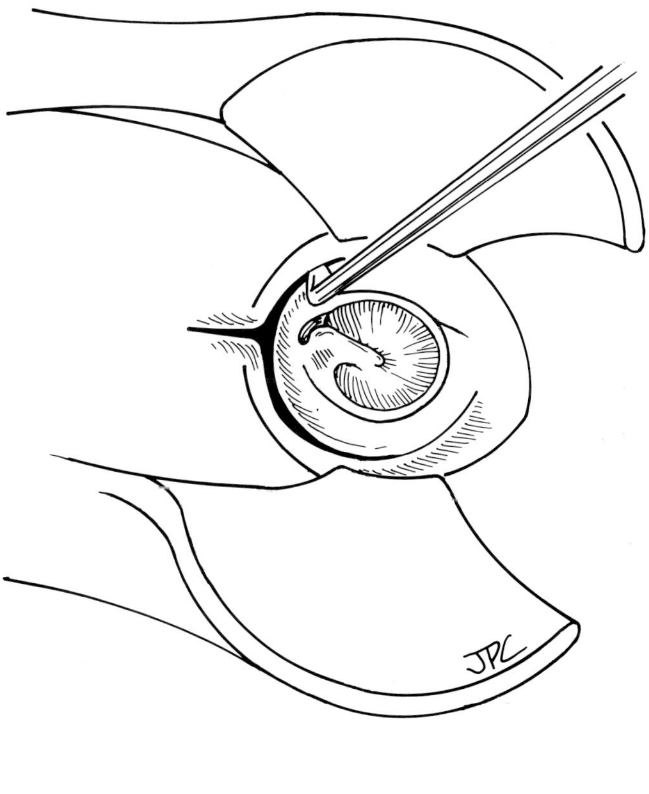

• FIGURE 3-33.

An anterior relaxing incision in the canal.

- The lateral posterior and anterior flaps are elevated with a periosteal elevator to permit insertion of the self-retaining retractor (Fig. 3–34).
- The tympanomeatal flap, tympanic membrane, and temporalis muscle are exposed (Fig. 3–35).
- The tympanomeatal flap is elevated (Fig. 3–36).
- When indicated, the flap is dissected off the malleus (Fig. 3–37).
- The flap is elevated exposing the middle ear (Fig. 3–38).

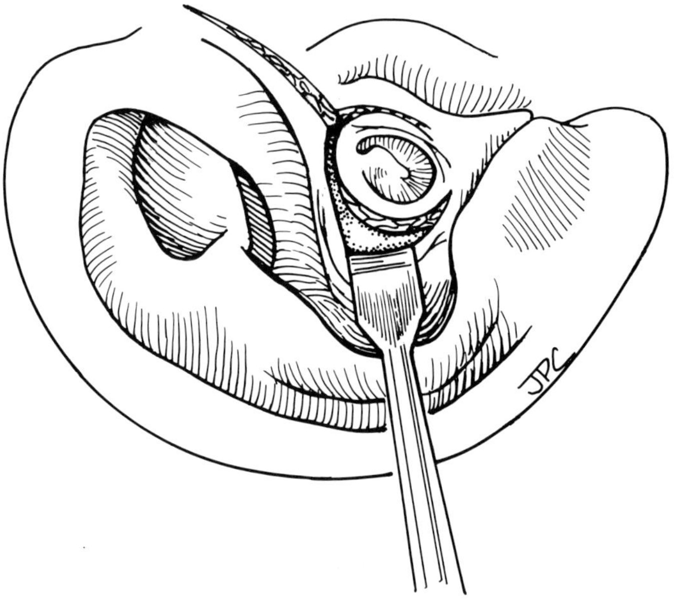

• FIGURE 3–34.

The lateral posterior and anterior flaps are elevated.

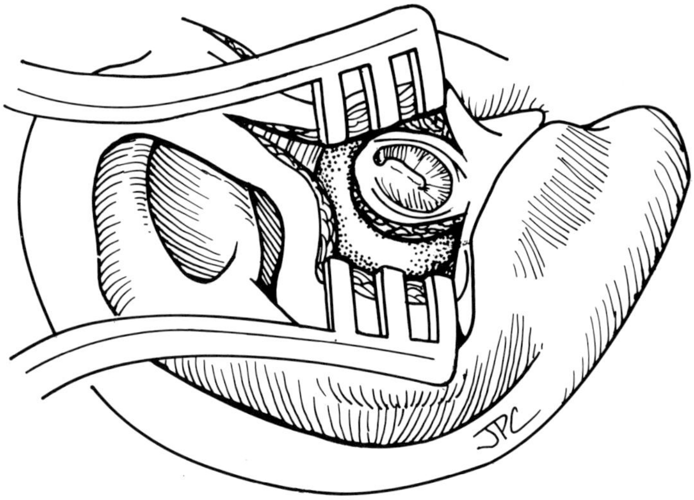

• FIGURE 3–35.

The tympanomeatal flap, tympanic membrane, and temporalis muscle are exposed with the aid of a self-retaining retractor.

• FIGURE 3-36.

The tympanomeatal flap is elevated.

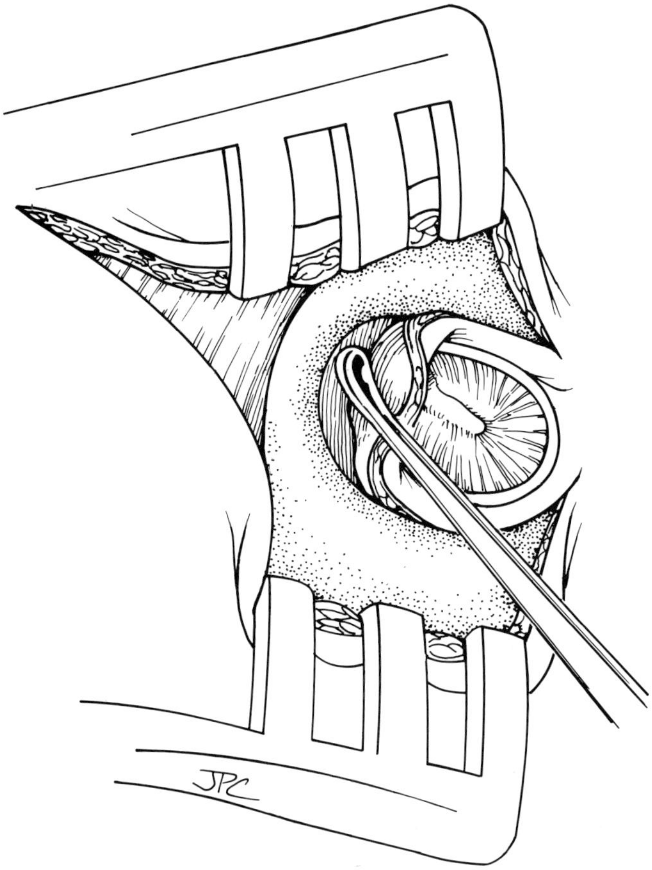

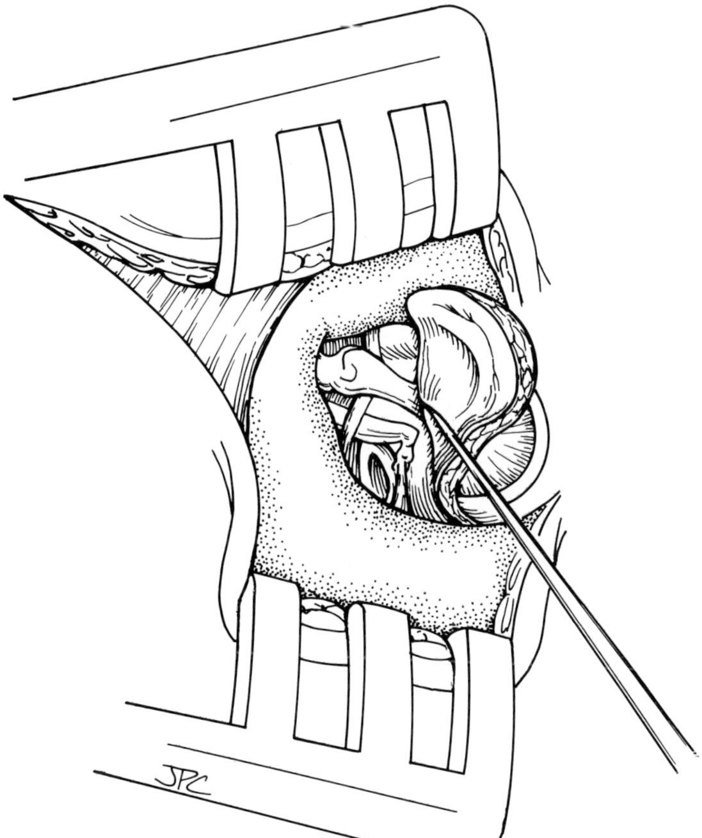

• FIGURE 3-37.

Dissection of the flap off the malleus using a curved pick.

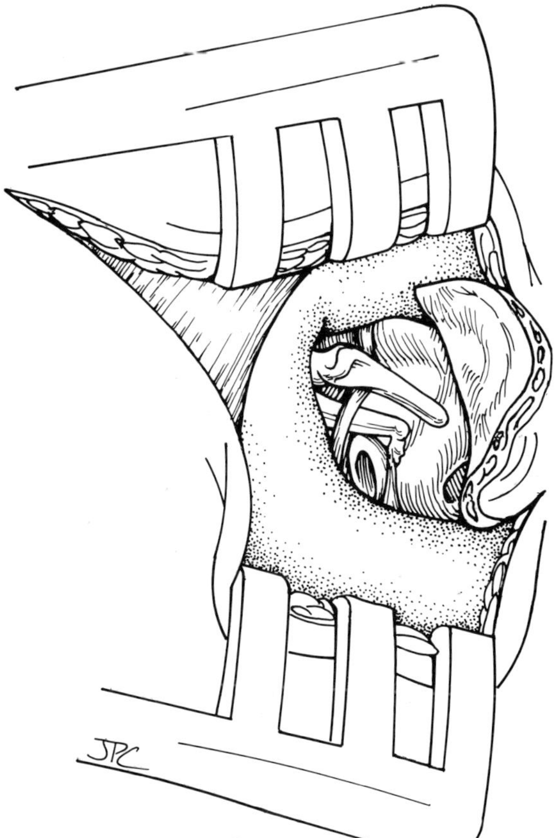

• FIGURE 3-38.

The middle ear is exposed.

Postoperative care

• Following a procedure that uses the endaural approach, the ear canal is packed with two strips (one medial and one lateral) of Adaptic gauze impregnated with an antibiotic ointment; two strips are used to prevent accidental removal of all the packing by the child during the postoperative period. A Glasscock pressure dressing is used for the first postoperative day. The Adaptic packing is removed after 1 week, and cotton is inserted into the meatus; cotton is changed whenever it becomes soiled or at least once a day and may be left out once there is no further drainage. Application of an antibiotic ointment into the edge of the wound in the incisura prevents the cotton from adhering to it. The child is re-examined in about 1 month.

POSTAURICULAR APPROACH

Indications

• The postauricular incisions and approach are indicated when there is disease that involves the mastoid, but it is also used to provide access to the middle ear when neither the transcanal approach nor the endaural approach is appropriate (see later). This approach is also used when tympanoplasty is required for a large perforation; both medial and lateral graft techniques can use this approach (see later).

Anesthetic considerations

• The anesthesia is the same as that described for the transcanal and endaural approaches, but additional injection sites are required in the postauricular area (Fig. 3–39).

Preparation

• A small area of the hair is shaved posterior and superior to the planned postauricular incision.

Procedure

• An incision is made a few millimeters posterior to the postauricular crease (Fig. 3–40). In children younger than 4 years of age, the incision is made away from the stylomastoid foramen and the facial nerve; injection sites are altered accordingly (Fig. 3–40*B*).

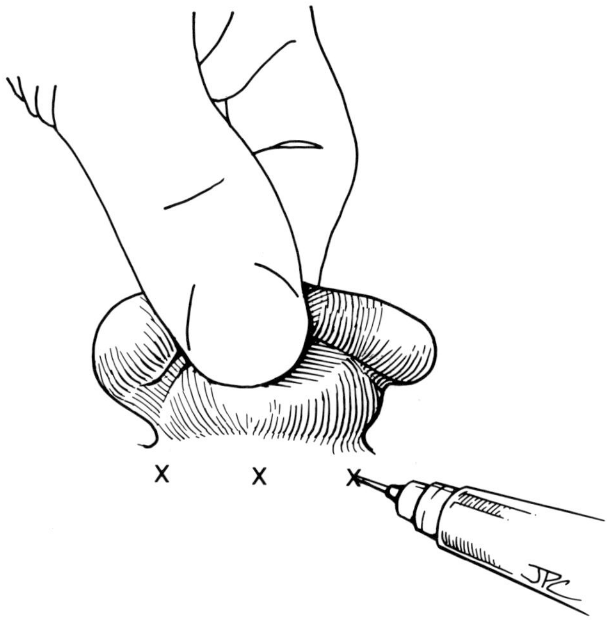

• FIGURE 3–39.

Injection sites in the postauricular area in addition to those in the canal.

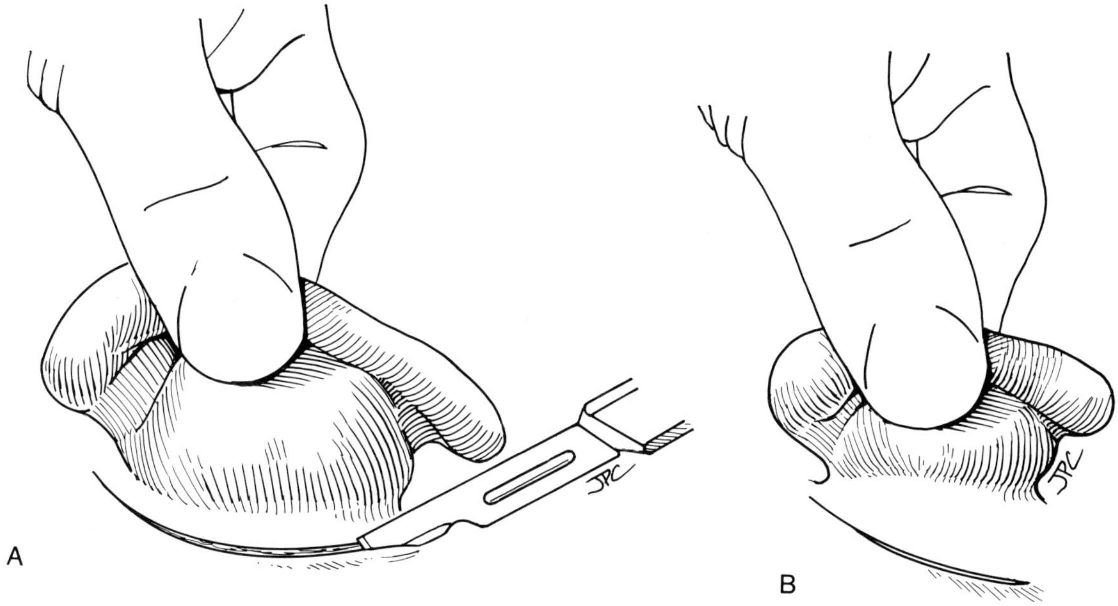

• FIGURE 3–40.

A, An incision is made just a few millimeters posterior to the postauricular crease. *B*, An incision used for children younger than 4 years of age.

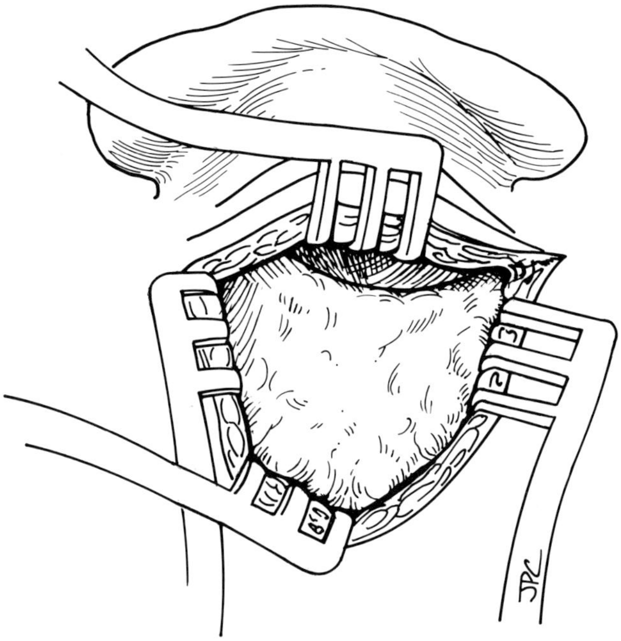

• FIGURE 3-41.

The postauricular soft tissue is exposed.

• FIGURE 3-42.

A transcanal incision is made to create a Koerner flap.

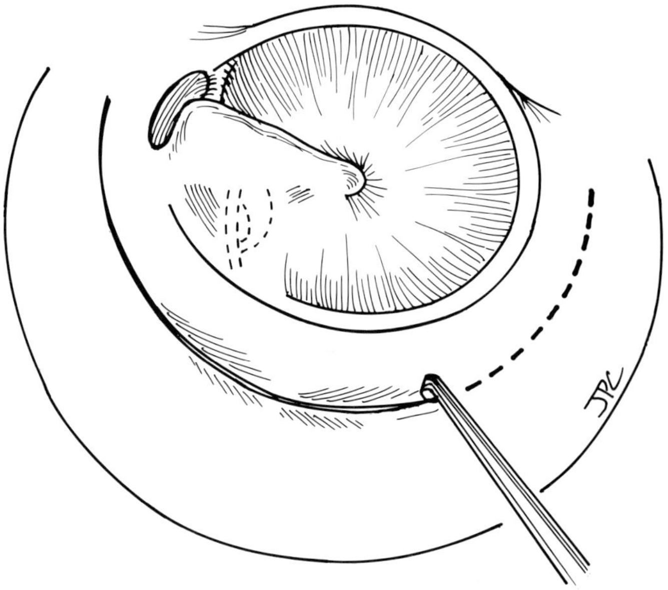

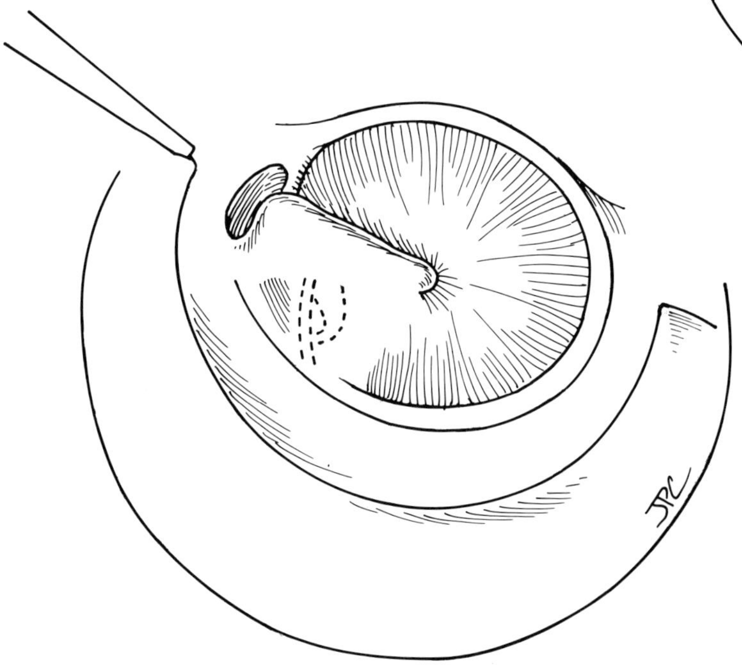

• FIGURE 3-43.

Canal incisions are extended laterally.

• FIGURE 3-44.

The Koerner flap is elevated a few millimeters laterally in the canal.

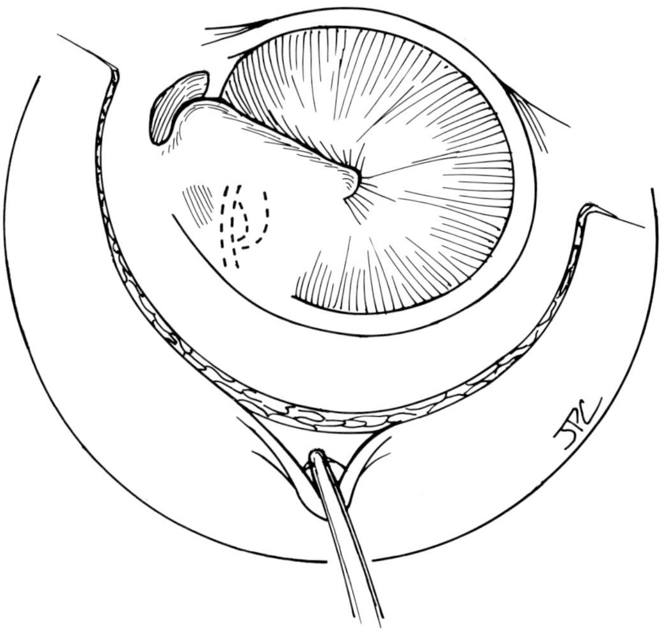

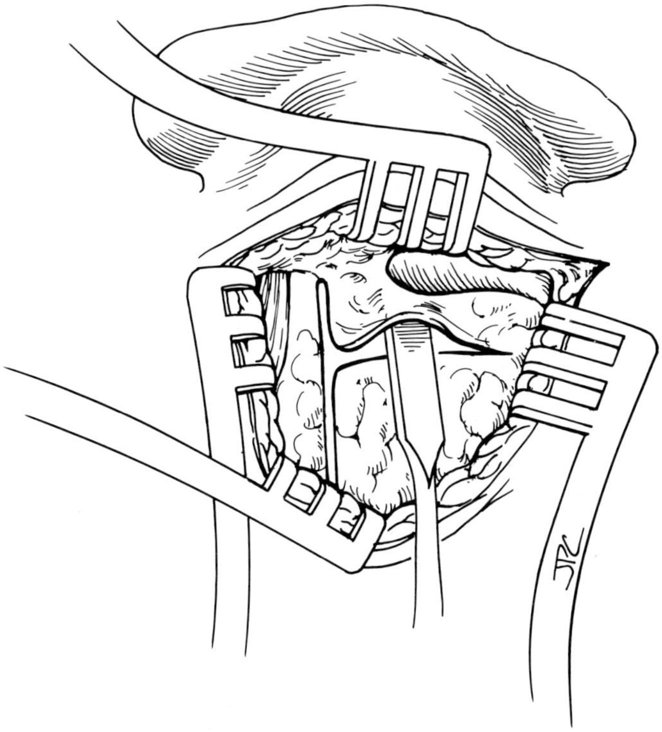

• FIGURE 3-45.

A "T" incision is made in postauricular soft tissue and is elevated.

• The postauricular soft tissue is exposed (Fig. 3-41).

• A transcanal incision is made from 6 o'clock to 12 o'clock to create a Koerner flap (the transcanal incision usually precedes the postauricular incision) (Fig. 3-42).

• Canal incisions are extended laterally (Fig. 3-43).

• A Koerner flap is elevated a few millimeters laterally in the canal to facilitate elevation from the postauricular approach (Fig. 3-44).

• A "T" incision is made in postauricular soft tissue and is elevated (Fig. 3-45).

- The Koerner flap is elevated through postauricular exposure (Fig. 3–46).
- The tympanic membrane, tympanomeatal flap, and mastoid are exposed (Fig. 3–47).
- A Penrose drain is used to retract the Koerner flap anteriorly, which is fastened to the surgical drape in front of the ear; the Penrose drain also protects the Koerner flap if a self-retaining retractor is used (Fig. 3–48).
- The tympanomeatal flap is elevated and reflected anteriorly to expose the mesotympanum, similar to that described for the transcanal approach (Fig. 3–49).

Postoperative care

- The postauricular wound is closed with an absorbable suture; a drain is optional. Two strips of Adaptic gauze impregnated with antibiotic ointment are used to pack the ear canal. A Glasscock pressure dressing is applied for 1 day. The packs are removed in 1 week, and the child is re-examined in about 1 month.

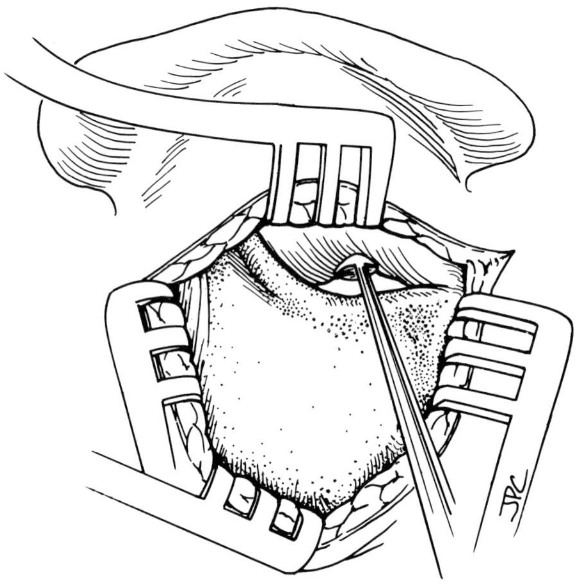

• FIGURE 3–46.

The Koerner flap is elevated.

• FIGURE 3-47.

The tympanic membrane, tympanomeatal flap, and mastoid are exposed.

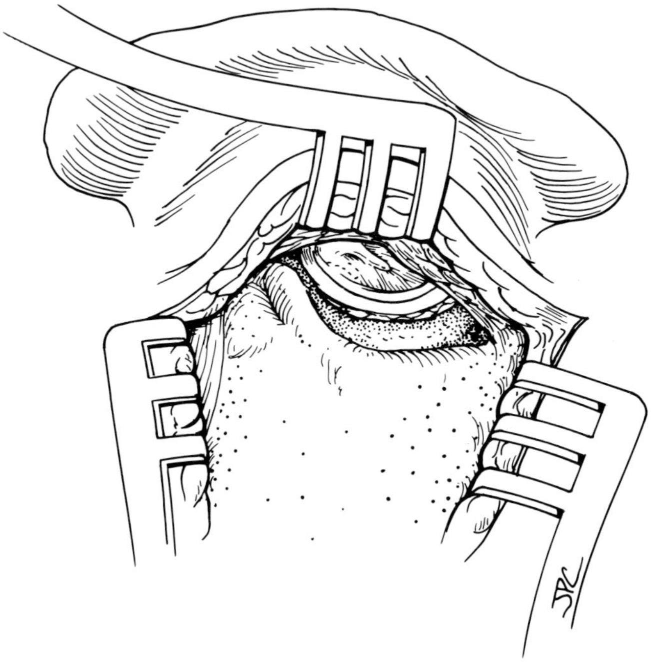

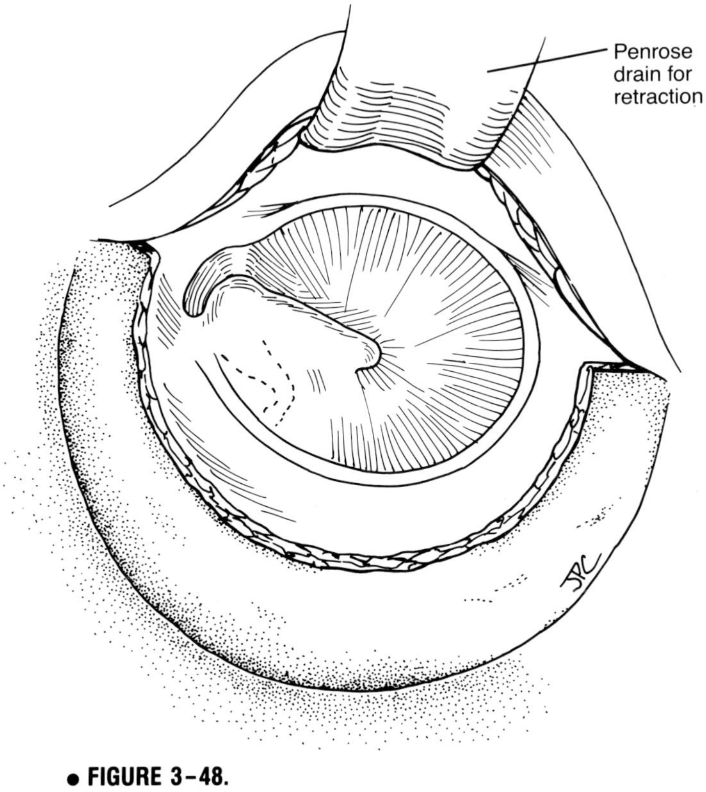

• FIGURE 3-48.

A Penrose drain is used to retract the Koerner flap anteriorly.

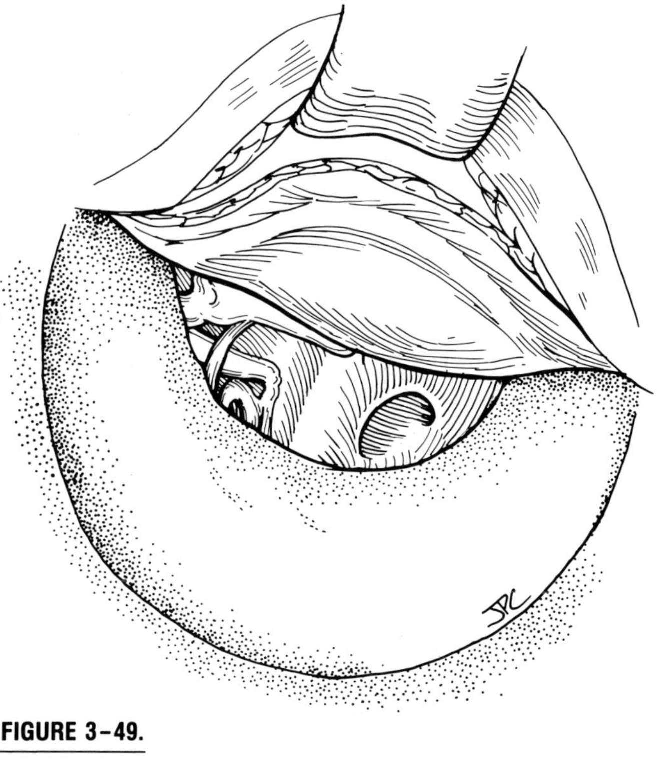

• FIGURE 3-49.

The tympanomeatal flap is elevated and reflected anteriorly to expose the mesotympanum.

TYMPANOPLASTY

Many techniques are advocated to repair perforations of the tympanic membrane. As described previously, relatively small central perforations can be repaired successfully using either a Steri-Strip or a medial tissue graft myringoplasty, as long as there is no desire to inspect the middle ear. A tympanoplasty should be performed, however, when there is a need to examine the middle ear, such as when there is conductive hearing loss that cannot be attributed to the size and position of the perforation or when an occult middle ear cholesteatoma is suspected. Additional indications would be when the perforation is large or is in a site that is difficult to repair using a myringoplasty procedure (e.g., when the perforation is in the anterosuperior quadrant). When the perforation is relatively small and exploration of the middle ear is desired, a transcanal approach can be used and a medial tissue graft can be employed in a manner similar to that described for a myringoplasty; the graft is more easily placed medial to the perforation from behind the tympanomeatal flap than through the perforation, as is done during a myringoplasty. When the perforation is in the anterosuperior quadrant and is relatively large, or when there is a defect (i.e., retraction pocket or "marginal" perforation) in the posterosuperior quadrant, one of the following procedures is used.

ANTEROSUPERIOR PERFORATION (AND RETRACTION POCKET): ENDAURAL APPROACH, MEDIAL GRAFT

Attempts to close perforations in this area using traditional transcanal myringoplasty or tympanoplasty procedures frequently fail, because they are difficult to perform in the constricted space. The endaural approach is the most successful method, because it provides excellent access to the area and the exposure provides an opportunity to visualize the mesotympanum as well as places a medial graft on three areas of attachment — the anterior and superior canal walls and the malleus. In addition, the fascia graft from the temporalis muscle can be harvested from the operative site. This technique is also used to repair a retraction pocket in the anterosuperior quadrant of the pars tensa, which is usually a sequela of a tympanostomy tube. Presumably, if a dimeric membrane is present and the child has a persistent eustachian tube dysfunction, a chronic retraction pocket can develop. The indications for surgical repair of a retraction pocket are as follows:

- Inability to fully visualize the extent with the otomicroscope
- Inability to expand the pocket using the Bruening otoscope, with the nonmagnifying lens and the otomicroscope (see *Pediatric Otolaryngology*)[5]
- Failure to expand the pocket during nitrous oxide anesthesia
- Following the insertion of a tympanostomy tube placed in another site
- Recurrent or chronic infection within the pocket
- Difficulty in determining whether a cholesteatoma is present (see *Pediatric Otolaryngology*)[5]

When a retraction pocket is repaired and eustachian tube dysfunction is expected to persist postoperatively, a tragal cartilage–perichondrial graft is placed medial to the fascia graft, and a tympanostomy tube is inserted into the anteroinferior quadrant of the drum (see later).

• FIGURE 3-50.

Perforation in the anterosuperior quadrant of the pars tensa.

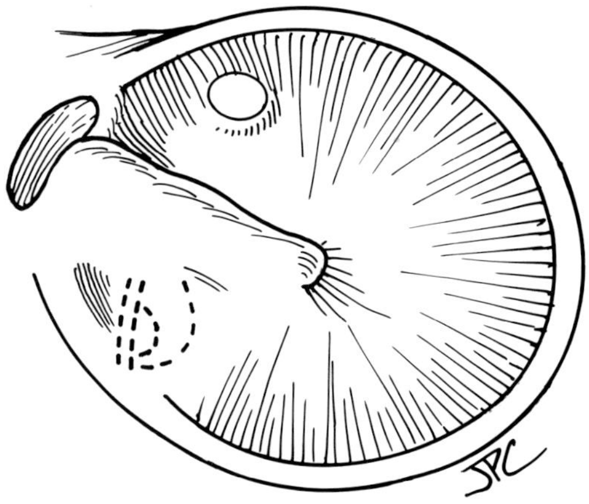

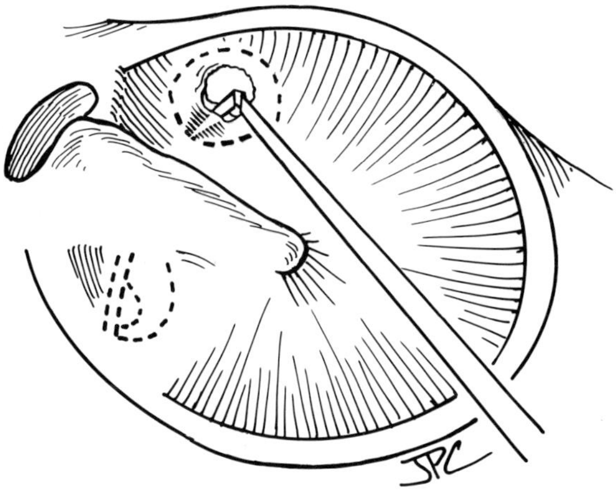

• FIGURE 3-51.

The epithelium at the rim of the perforation dissected with pick.

Indications

- Perforation in the anterosuperior quadrant of the pars tensa
- Retraction pocket in the anterosuperior quadrant of the pars tensa

Anesthetic considerations and preparation

- The anesthesia and the preparations for this procedure are described earlier under the Endaural Approach.

Procedure

- Perforation occurs in the anterosuperior quadrant of the pars tensa (Fig. 3–50).
- The epithelium at the rim of the perforation is removed with a pick, and a cup forceps is also used (Fig. 3–51).

- An endaural incision and approach are completed; the anterior relaxing incision is extended inferiorly on the anterior canal wall (see earlier under Endaural Approach) (Fig. 3–52).
- The fascia graft is harvested from the temporalis fascia (Fig. 3–53).
- The tympanomeatal flap is elevated from the superior posterior, and anterior canal walls (Fig. 3–54).
- The tympanic membrane is elevated and dissected off the malleus and reflected inferiorly to visualize the mesotympanum and the rest of the ossicular chain (Fig. 3–55).

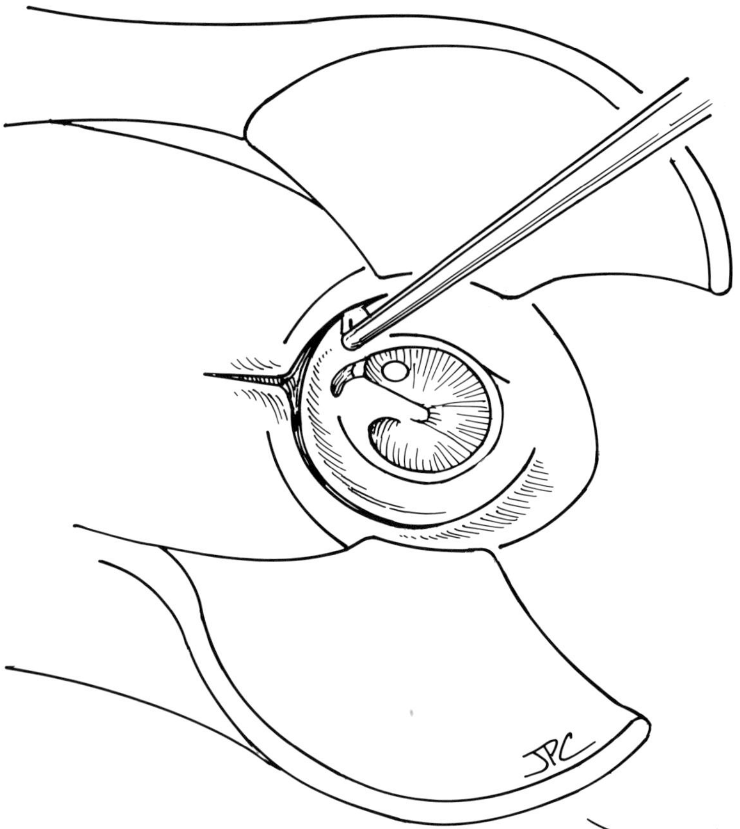

• FIGURE 3–52.

An endaural incision and approach are completed.

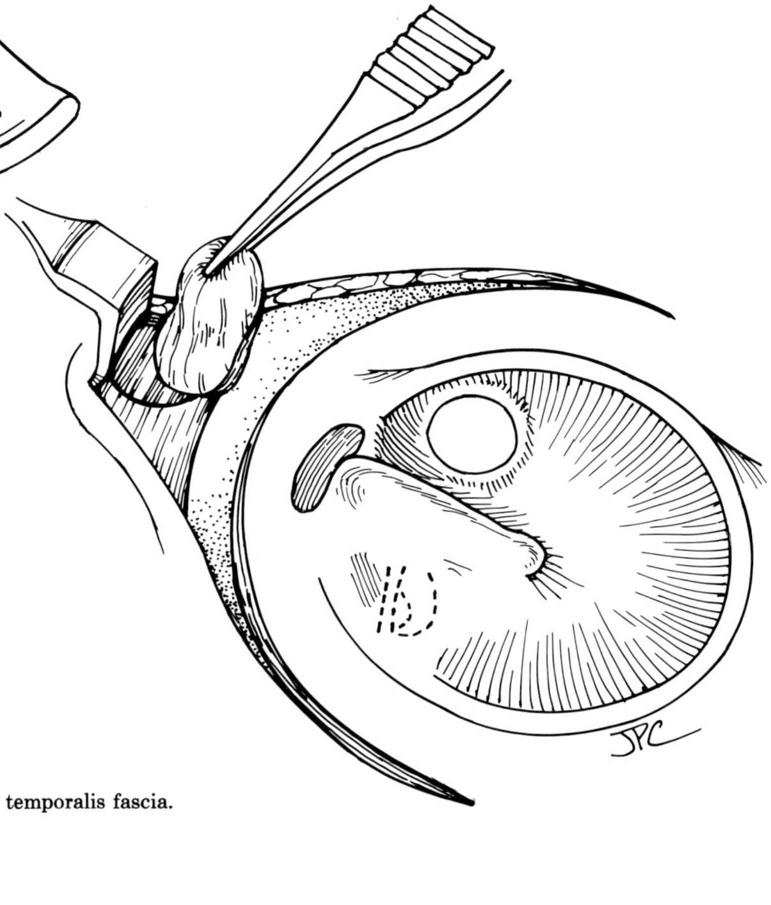

• FIGURE 3–53.

The fascia graft is harvested from the temporalis fascia.

• FIGURE 3-54.

The tympanomeatal flap is elevated from the canal walls.

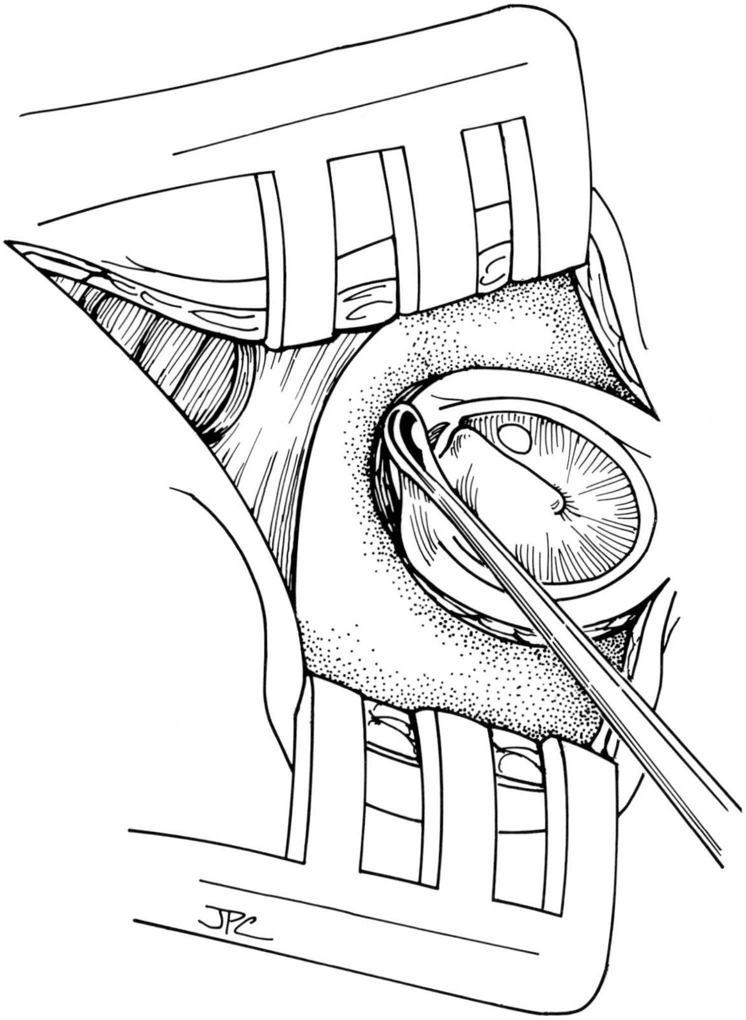

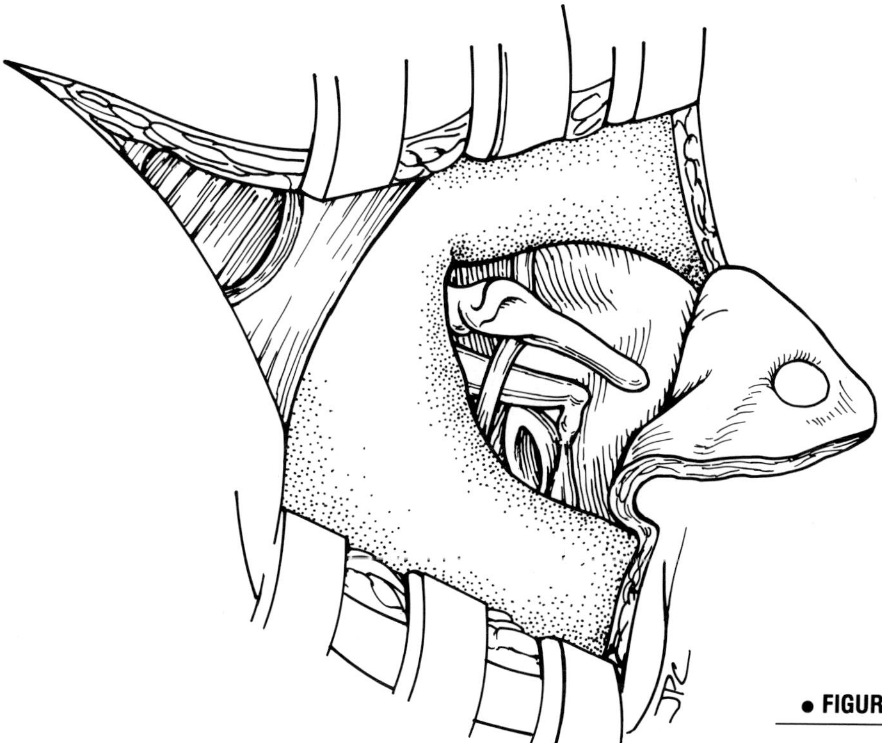

• FIGURE 3-55.

The tympanic membrane is elevated and may be reflected inferiorly to visualize the mesotympanum.

- A fascia graft is placed over the superior and anterosuperior canal walls and the malleus; Gelfoam fills the middle ear (Fig. 3–56).
- The tympanomeatal flap is replaced (Fig. 3–57).
- Adaptic packing is inserted into the external canal; a layer of Gelfoam is placed over the tympanic membrane (Fig. 3–58).
- The endaural incision is closed with an absorbable suture (Fig. 3–59).

Postoperative care

- The postoperative care is described earlier under Endaural Approach.

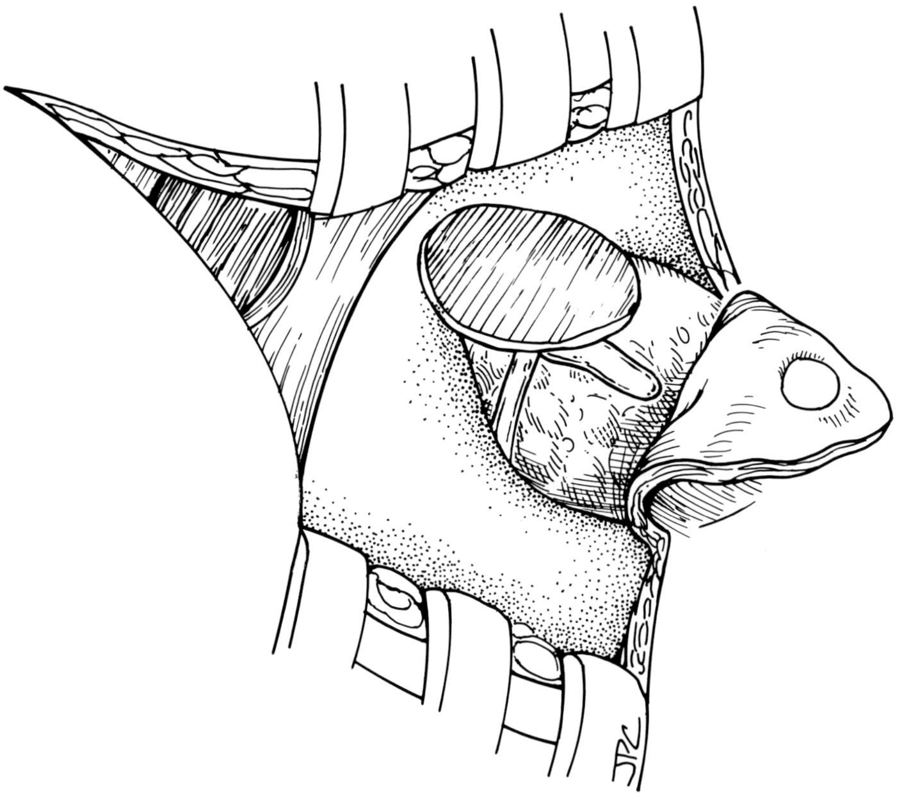

• FIGURE 3–56.

A fascia graft is placed over the superior and anterosuperior canal walls and the malleus.

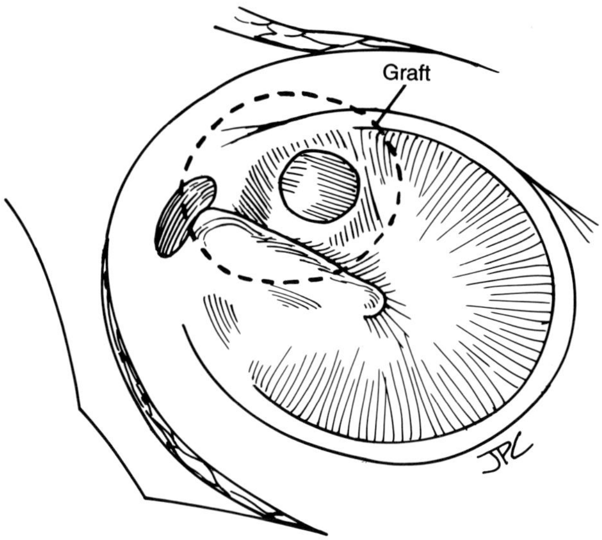

• FIGURE 3-57.

The tympanomeatal flap is replaced.

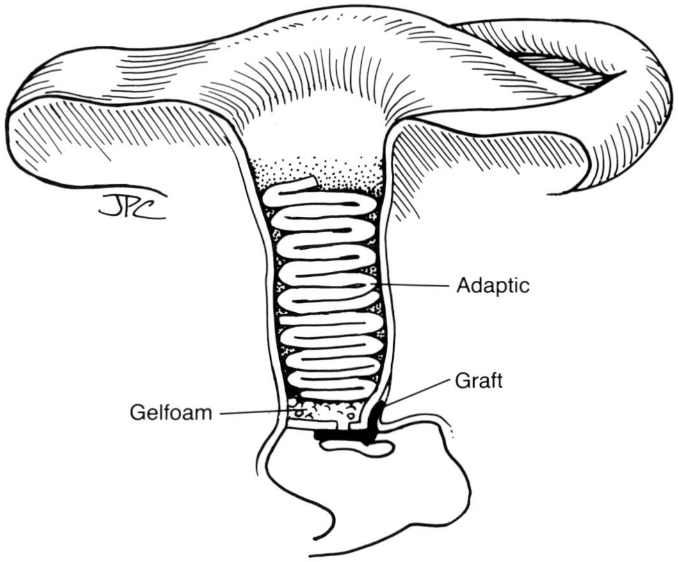

• FIGURE 3-58.

A layer of Gelfoam is placed over the tympanic membrane, and adaptic packing (Johnson & Johnson Medical, Inc., Arlington, TX) is inserted into the external canal.

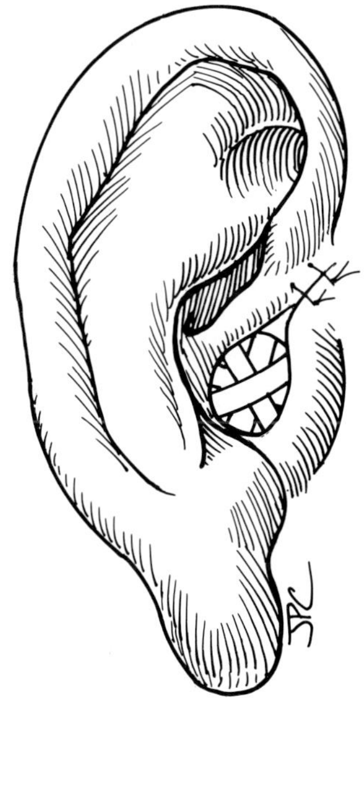

• FIGURE 3-59.

The endaural incision is closed.

LARGE CENTRAL PERFORATION: POSTAURICULAR APPROACH, LATERAL GRAFT

This method to close relatively large central perforations in children has been found to be more successful than medial graft techniques.[3] The reasons why the lateral graft technique has a better long-term success rate than the medial graft technique are probably related to the wider attachment of the lateral graft to the canal walls and the fact that persistent or recurrent negative middle ear pressure, which is usually present in children who have middle ear disease, is probably deleterious to a medial graft during the immediate postoperative period, whereas negative middle ear pressure is an advantage when a lateral graft is used. An additional application is when there is generalized atelectasis of the pars tensa.

This procedure uses the postauricular incision and approach, but the Koerner flap is longer than that described earlier. The posterior canal incision is made only a few millimeters from the annulus, because the skin adjacent to the annulus and the outer epithelial layer of the tympanic membrane are discarded; as little skin as possible is removed from the external canal, to facilitate rapid postoperative healing. The procedure is designed to create two laterally based pedicle flaps, one posterior (i.e., the "long" Koerner flap) and one anterior. The entire external canal is exposed, which facilitates the procedure. Also, if needed, a canaloplasty can be performed. Postoperative "blunting" in the anterior sulcus and lateralization of the graft are rarely observed, but an iatrogenic implantation cholesteatoma, between the graft and the tympanic membrane or in the canal wall, is not an uncommon postoperative sequela; the occurrence is related frequently to the inexperience of the surgeon.

Indications

- Large central perforations of the pars tensa
- Extensive atelectasis of the pars tensa, in which most of the tympanic membrane is replaced with tissue graft

Anesthetic considerations and preparation

- The anesthesia and the preparations for this procedure are described earlier under Postauricular Approach.

Procedure

- This procedure is ideal for a large central perforation (Fig. 3–60).
- An incision for a "long" Koerner flap is made closer to the posterior annulus (approximately 2 mm) than the usual incision (Fig. 3–61).
- The postauricular incision and approach are completed (see earlier), and a fascia graft is taken from the temporalis muscle (Fig. 3–62).

• FIGURE 3-60.

This is the typical size of a central perforation to be repaired.

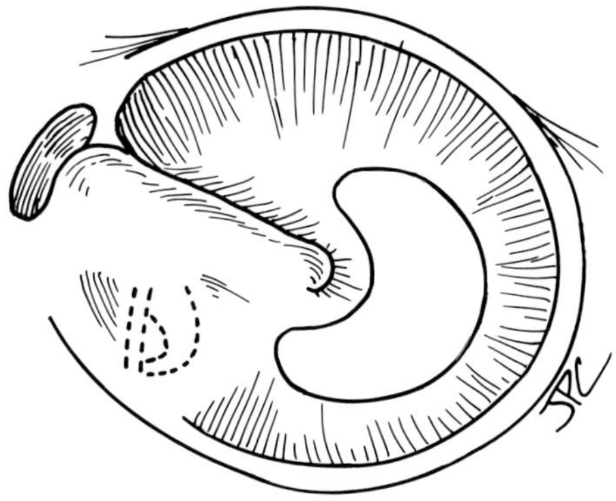

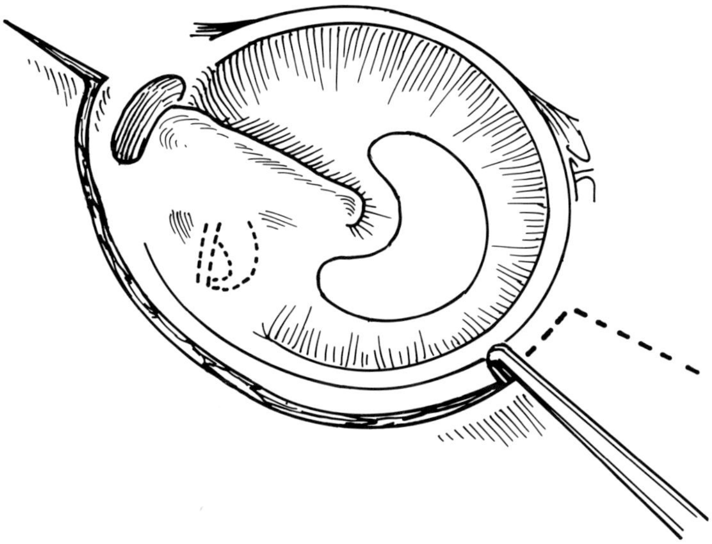

• FIGURE 3-61.

An incision for a "long" Koerner flap is made closer to the posterior annulus.

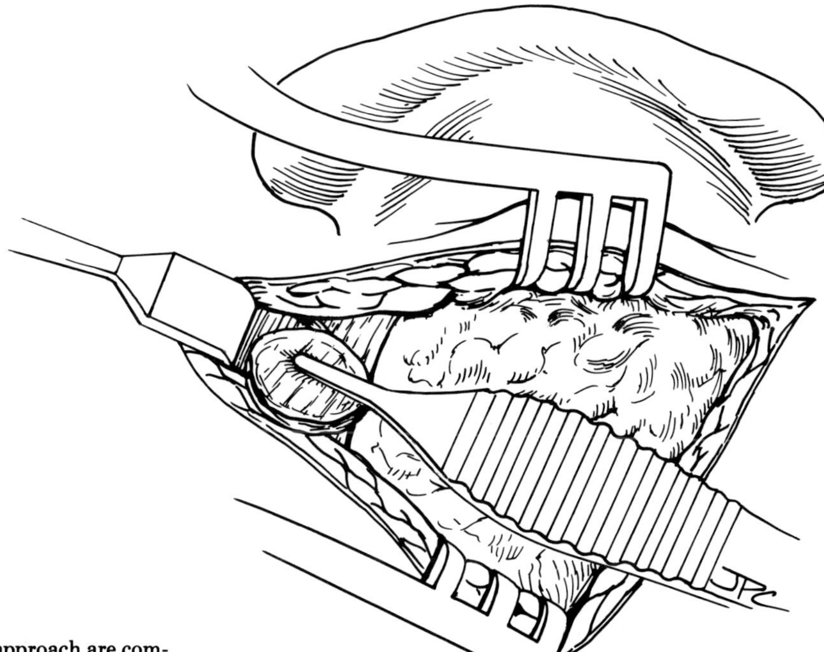

• FIGURE 3-62.

The postauricular incision and approach are completed, and a fascia graft excised.

- A "T" incision is made in the postauricular soft tissue (Fig. 3–63).
- A Penrose drain is placed for retraction of the Koerner flap (Fig. 3–64).
- An anterior incision for the anterior flap is made approximately 2 mm lateral to the anterior annulus and is connected to the Koerner flap incision (Fig. 3–65).
- The anterior flap is elevated, rolled, and tucked laterally out of the medial portion of the canal (Fig. 3–66)

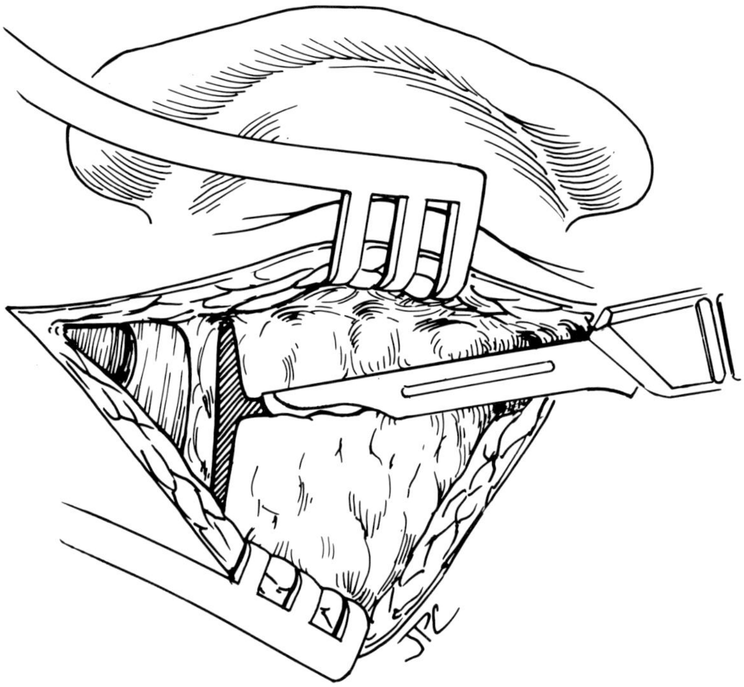

• FIGURE 3–63.

A "T" incision in the postauricular soft tissue.

• FIGURE 3-64.

A Penrose drain is placed for retraction of the "long" Koerner flap.

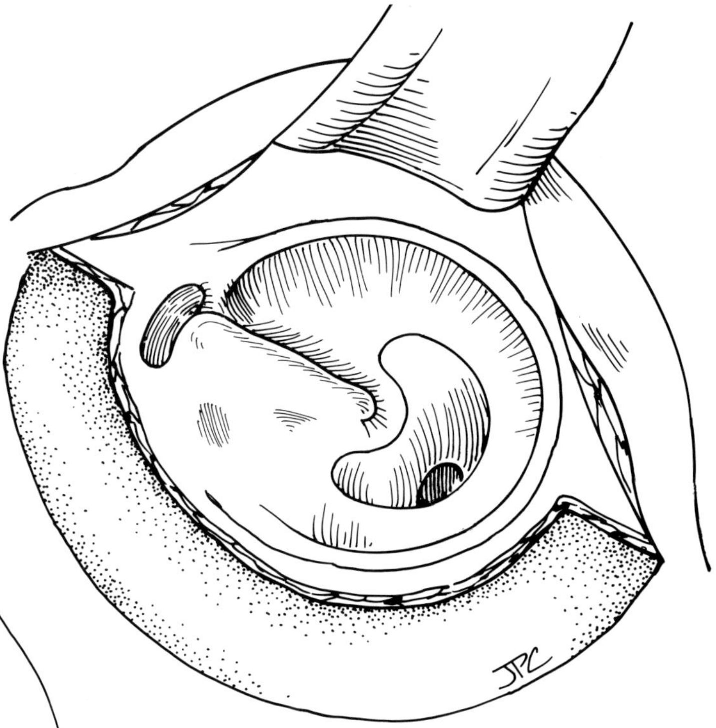

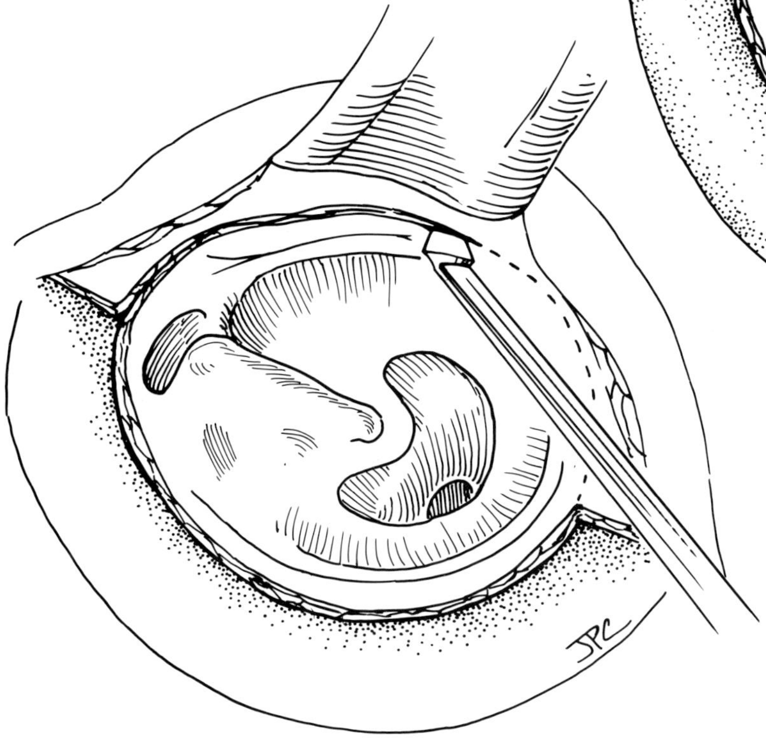

• FIGURE 3-65.

An anterior incision is made approximately 2 mm lateral to the anterior annulus.

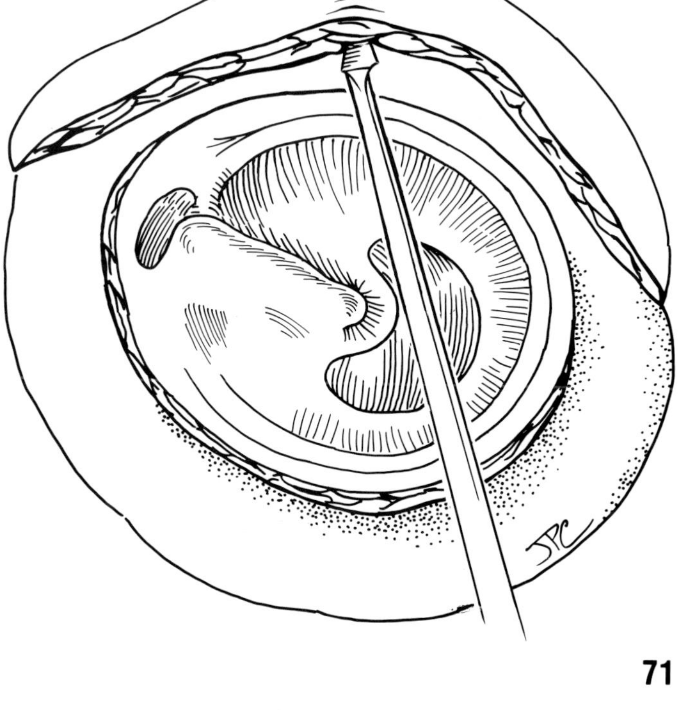

• FIGURE 3-66.

The anterior flap is elevated.

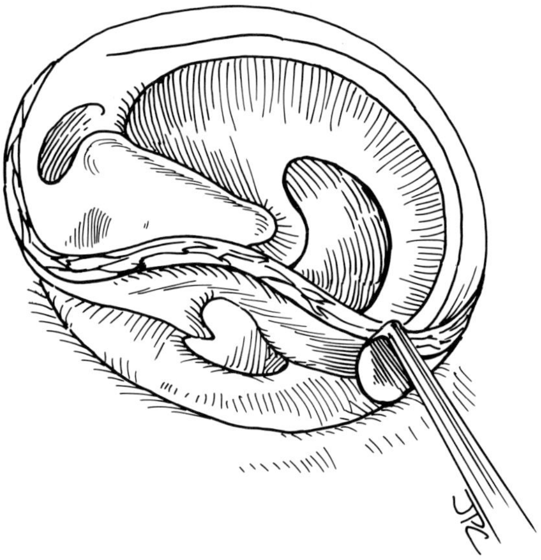

• FIGURE 3-67.

A medial strip of canal skin and the entire outer epithelial layer of the tympanic membrane are removed.

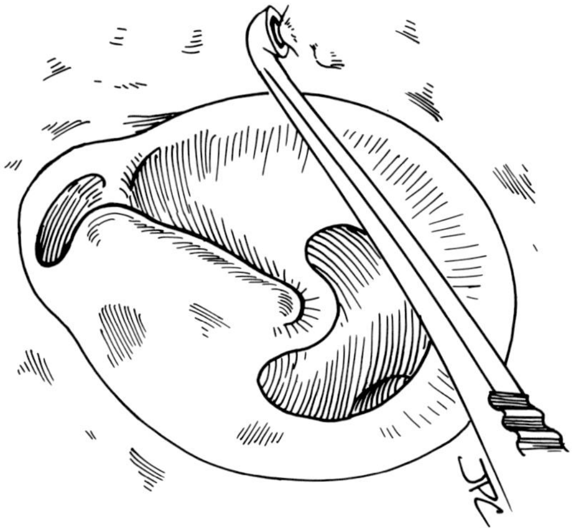

• FIGURE 3-68.

The canal wall is curetted to remove any remnants of canal skin.

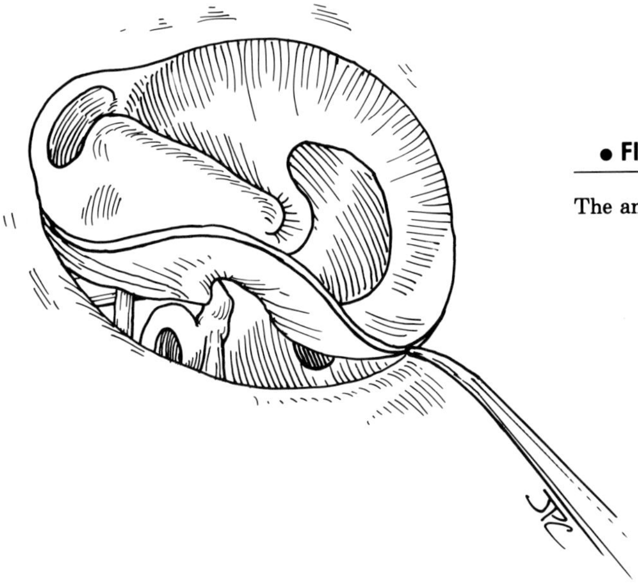

• FIGURE 3-69.

The annulus is elevated to examine the mesotympanum and the ossicles.

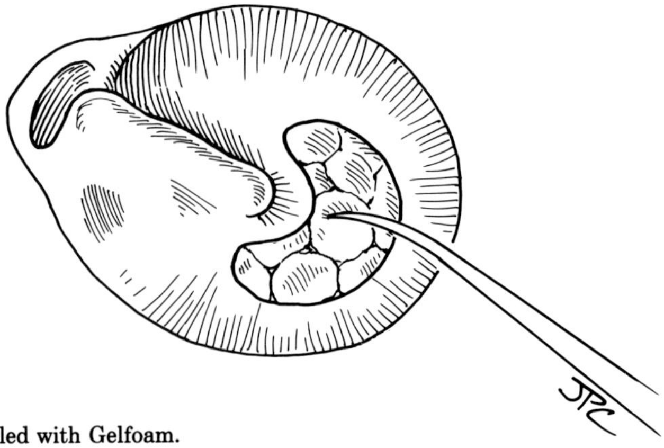

• FIGURE 3-70.

The middle ear is filled with Gelfoam.

• FIGURE 3-71.

A fascia graft is placed over the medial canal wall; four pieces of Surgicel (Johnson & Johnson Medical, Inc., Arlington, TX) are placed over the edge of the graft and onto the canal wall.

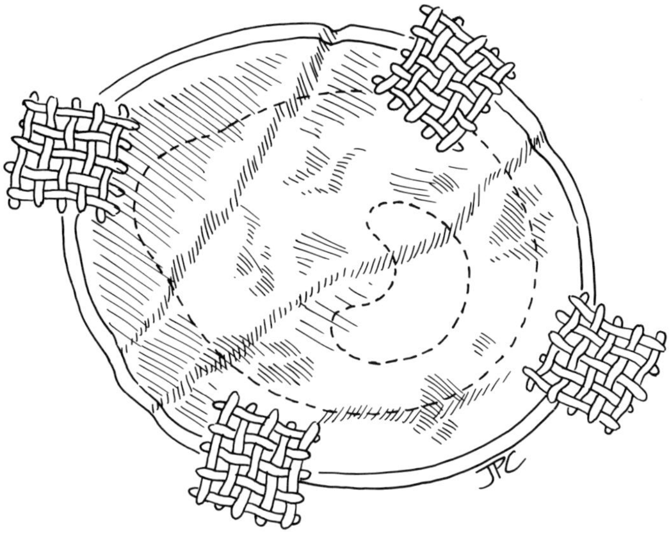

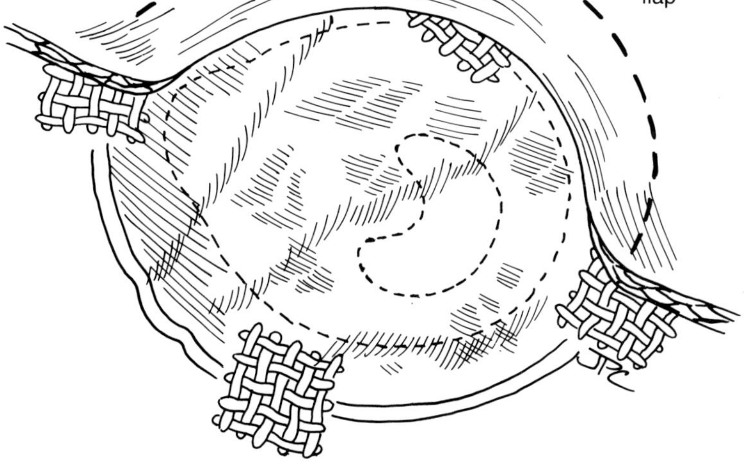

• FIGURE 3-72.

The anterior pedicle flap is replaced and overlaps the lateral edge of the graft.

• A medial strip of canal skin is adjacent to the annulus, and the entire outer epithelial layer of the tympanic membrane is elevated using a moon elevator and discarded (Fig. 3-67).

• The canal wall is curetted to remove any remnants of canal skin; a microdrill is another option; when indicated, a canalplasty can be performed at this stage (Fig. 3-68).

• The annulus is elevated to examine the mesotympanum and the ossicles (Fig. 3-69).

• The middle ear is filled with Gelfoam (Fig. 3-70).

• A fascia graft is placed over the tympanic membrane remnant, overlapping onto the medial canal wall; four pieces of Surgicel are placed over the edge of the graft and onto the canal wall to "fix" the graft (Fig. 3-71).

• The anterior pedicle flap is replaced and overlaps the lateral edge of the anterior portion of the fascia graft (Fig. 3-72).

- The Penrose drain is removed, and the Koerner flap, which overlaps the lateral edge of the posterior portion of the fascia graft, is replaced (Fig. 3–73).

- A layer of Gelfoam is placed over the tympanic membrane remnant and graft, and two strips of Adaptic gauze impregnated with antibiotic ointment are inserted into the external canal (Fig. 3–74).

Postoperative care

- The postauricular wound is closed with an absorbable suture, and a Glasscock pressure dressing is applied. The postoperative care is described earlier under Postauricular Approach.

POSTEROSUPERIOR QUADRANT DEFECTS OF PARS TENSA: POSTAURICULAR APPROACH, MEDIAL FASCIA AND CARTILAGE-PERICHONDRIAL GRAFTS

Retraction pockets frequently occur in the posterosuperior quadrant of the pars tensa. These defects can progress into a cholesteatoma, and the two are often indistinguishable. Retraction pockets in this area are most likely the result of two major factors—anatomy of the tympanic membrane and middle ear, and eustachian tube dysfunction. The posterosuperior quadrant is the most compliant part of the pars tensa,[17] probably owing to the long distance between the attachment of the tympanic membrane to the malleus and the posterior annulus. Thus, persistent high negative pressure could cause retraction in this area and, because the long processes of the incus and the stapes are immediately medial, the tympanic membrane can become adherent to these structures.

The most effective approach to this area is postauricular. Elevation of the Koerner and tympanomeatal flaps provides adequate exposure to visualize a small retraction pocket, but if there is an extension into the facial recess and sinus tympani, as is commonly encountered, a 3-mm 70-degree Hopkins rod lens telescope is placed in the hypotympanum to visualize these areas; a less effective alternative is the use of the Buckingham mirror. A medial fascia graft is placed to close the defect. To prevent a recurrence of the retraction pocket, a tragal cartilage–perichondrial graft (conchal cartilage–perichondrial graft can also be used, because it is in the surgical field) is placed medial to the tympanic membrane. A tympanostomy tube is also usually inserted. Eustachian tube dysfunction has been found to be present in children who have retraction pockets (see *Pediatric Otolaryngology*).[5]

Indications

- Indications for surgically correcting a retraction pocket are listed earlier under Anterosuperior Perforation (and Retraction Pocket): Endaural Approach, Medial Graft.

Anesthetic considerations and preparation

- The anesthesia and the preparations for this procedure are described earlier under Postauricular Approach. If relatively extensive disease is anticipated, a facial nerve monitor is used during the procedure.

• FIGURE 3-73.

The Penrose drain is removed, and the Koerner flap is replaced.

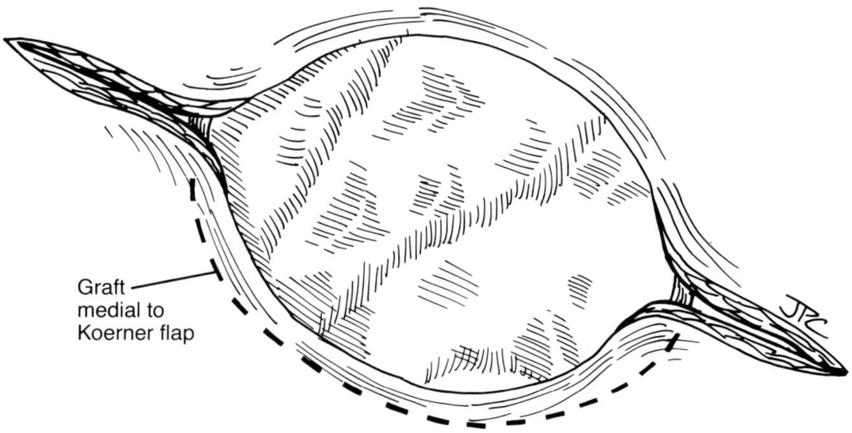

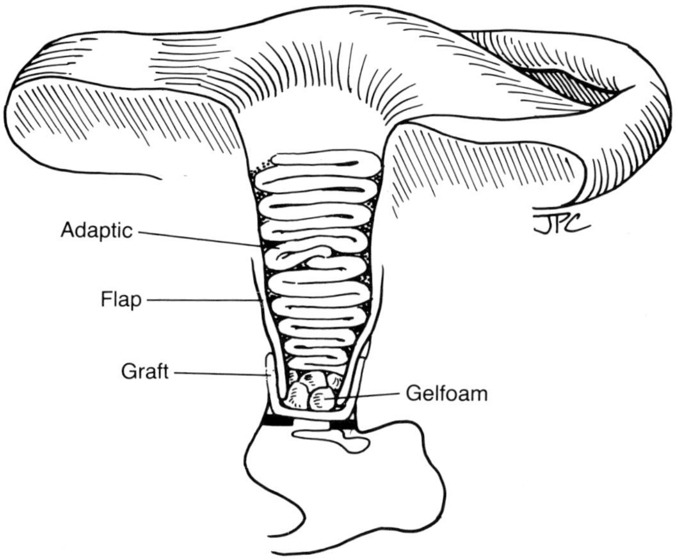

• FIGURE 3-74.

A layer of Gelfoam is placed over the tympanic membrane remnant and the graft, and two strips of Adaptic are inserted into the external canal.

Procedure

- A retraction pocket defect is identified in the posterosuperior quadrant of the pars tensa, with a probable extension into the facial recess and the sinus tympani (Fig. 3–75).
- Incisions for the Koerner flap are made (Fig. 3–76).
- The postauricular approach is completed, and the Koerner flap is retracted anteriorly (Fig. 3–77).
- The tympanomeatal flap and retraction pocket are elevated (Fig. 3–78).

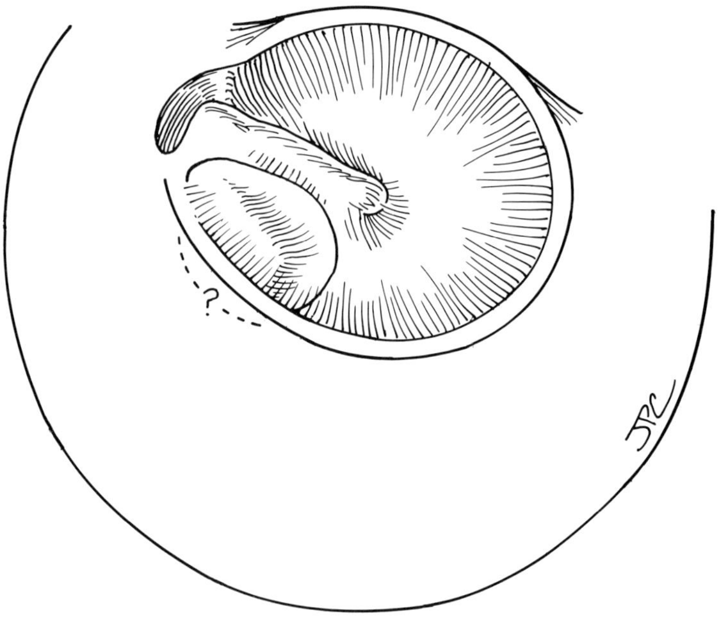

• FIGURE 3–75.

Retraction pocket defect in the posterosuperior quadrant of the pars tensa; posterior extension is unknown.

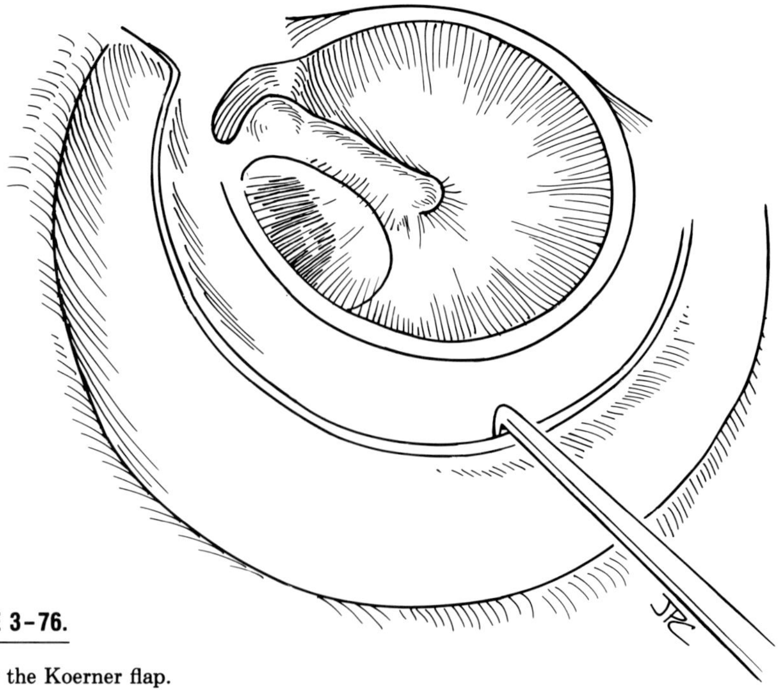

• FIGURE 3–76.

Incisions for the Koerner flap.

• FIGURE 3-77.

The postauricular approach is completed, and the Koerner flap is retracted anteriorly.

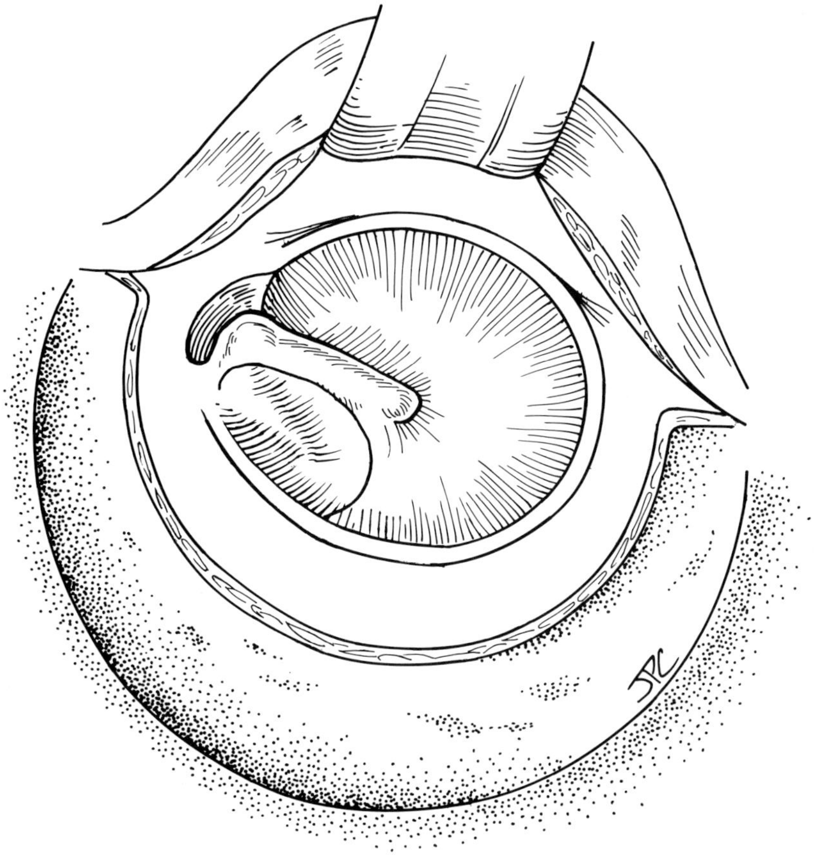

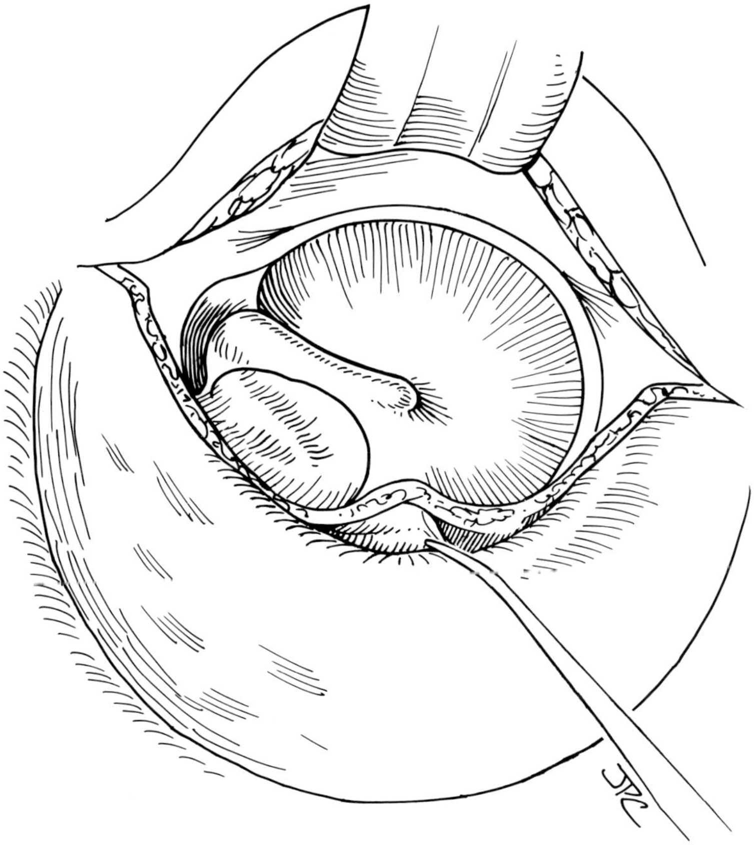

• FIGURE 3-78.

The tympanomeatal flap is elevated.

• A portion of the posterosuperior canal wall is removed with a curette to visualize the ossicles and the surrounding area. The tympanic membrane and the retraction pocket are dissected from attachments medial and posterior to the annulus (Fig. 3–79).

• A telescope is placed in the hypotympanum to visualize the facial recess and the sinus tympani for residual epithelium (Fig. 3–80).

• A Buckingham mirror is used as an alternative to the telescope (Fig. 3–81).

• An incision is made in the tragus to harvest a piece of cartilage; a conchal cartilage–perichondrial graft is an alternative donor site (Fig. 3–82).

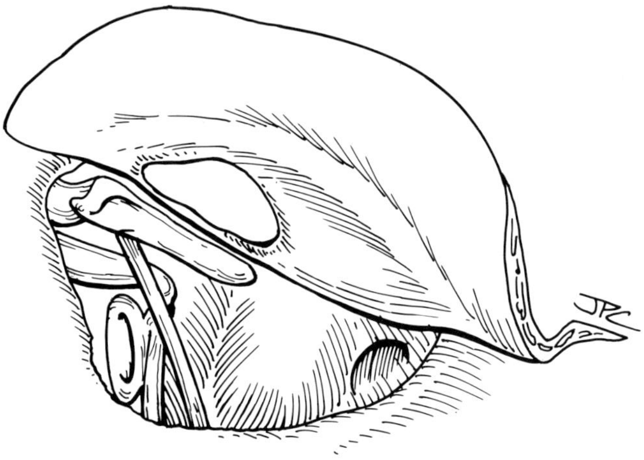

• FIGURE 3–79.

A portion of the posterosuperior canal wall is removed with a curette.

• FIGURE 3-80.

A telescope is placed in the hypotympanum to visualize the facial recess and the sinus tympani.

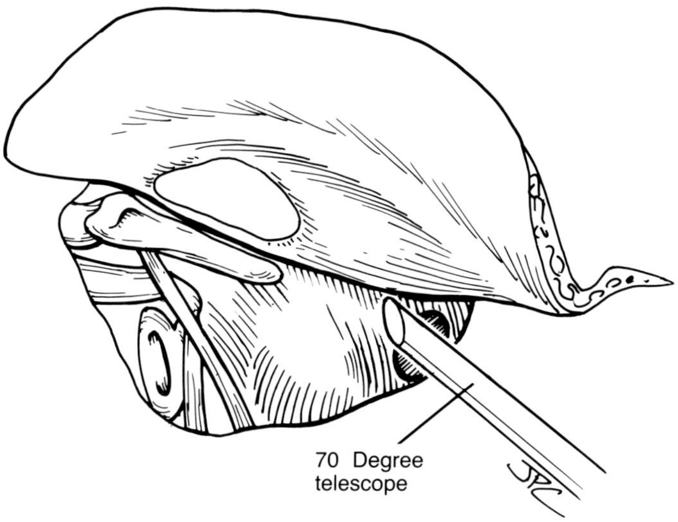

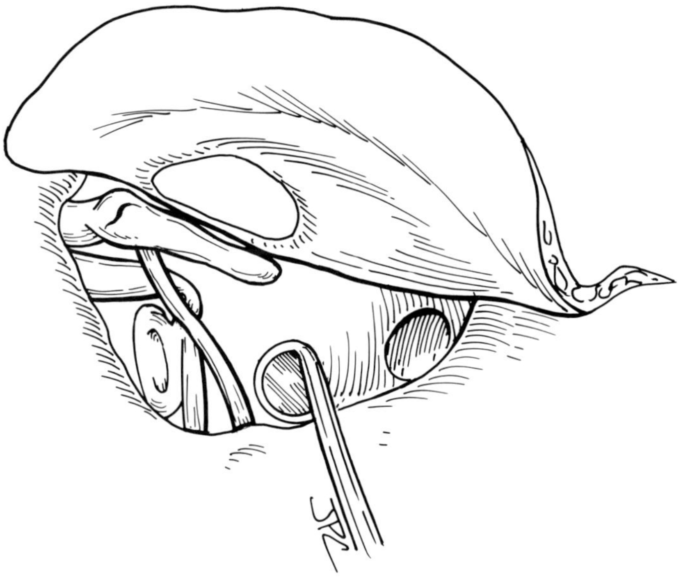

• FIGURE 3-81.

A Buckingham mirror is used as an alternative to the telescope.

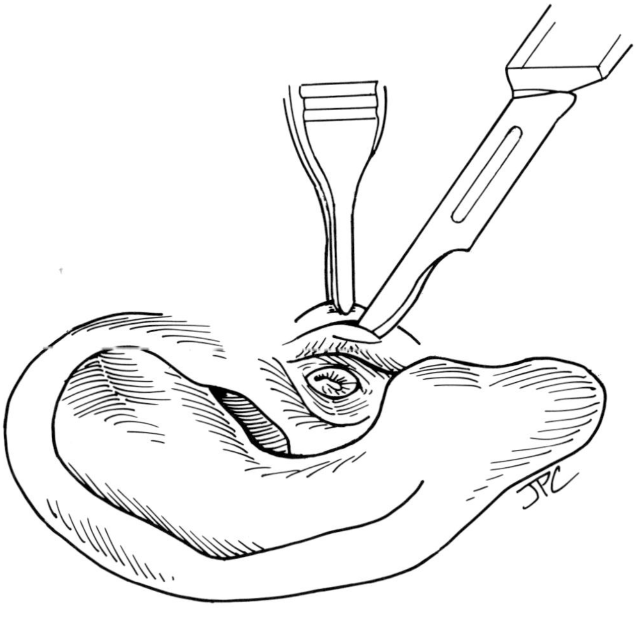

• FIGURE 3-82.

An incision is made in the tragus to harvest a cartilage-perichondrial graft.

- The tragal cartilage–perichondrial graft is excised, maintaining the lateral edge of the tragus to prevent a postoperative cosmetic deformity (Fig. 3–83).
- The tragal cartilage is placed over the long process of the malleus and overlapping the posterior canal wall. A fascia graft is also used to repair the defect and is lateral to the cartilage graft, but medial to the tympanic membrane (Fig. 3–84).
- A tympanostomy tube is inserted into the tympanic membrane (Fig. 3–85).

Postoperative care

- A layer of Gelfoam is placed over the tympanic membrane and graft. Two strips of Adaptic gauze impregnated with antibiotic ointment are inserted into the external canal.
- The postoperative care is the same as that described earlier under Postauricular Approach.

MASTOIDECTOMY

Many procedures include a mastoidectomy, but the most common indication to perform a mastoidectomy in infants and children is for acute and chronic mastoiditis, when cholesteatoma is present, or when both diseases coexist. There are three traditional procedures: complete simple mastoidectomy, modified radical mastoidectomy, and radical mastoidectomy. A tympanomastoidectomy (tympanoplasty with mastoidectomy) combines a simple mastoidectomy or modified radical mastoidectomy with a middle ear surgical procedure that frequently includes a tympanoplasty. The following is a description of the basic steps in performing these procedures, which are covered in greater detail in current standard atlases. The approach for all three is postauricular. The section on Cholesteatoma shows how these procedures are used in surgery for cholesteatoma (see later), and Chapter 8 shows the method to perform a posterior tympanotomy (see *Pediatric Otolaryngology*).[5]

SIMPLE (CORTICAL; COMPLETE) MASTOIDECTOMY

This procedure is indicated when acute mastoiditis, or more correctly termed acute mastoid osteitis (also called acute "coalescent" mastoiditis or acute surgical mastoiditis), is present (see *Pediatric Otolaryngology*).[5] The procedure can also be part of the canal wall-up tympanomastoidectomy (see later under Acquired Cholesteatoma).

Indications

- Acute mastoiditis: When osteitis or a subperiosteal abscess (and other extensions into temporal bone and deep neck) is present (see *Pediatric Otolaryngology*)[5]
- Chronic suppurative otitis media and mastoiditis: When nonsurgical management fails (see *Pediatric Otolaryngology*)[5]

• FIGURE 3-83.

The tragal cartilage–perichondrial graft is excised.

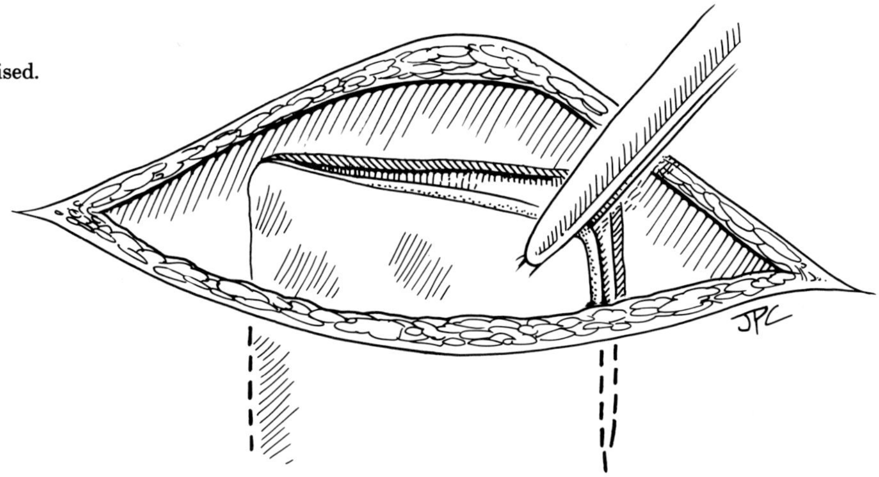

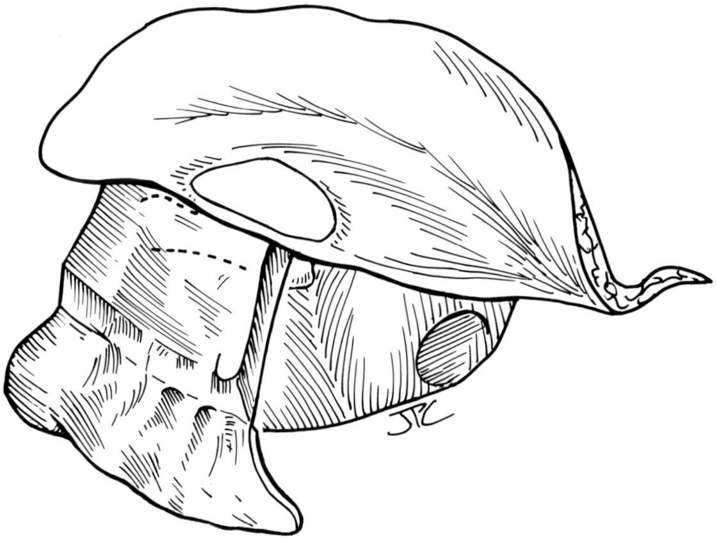

• FIGURE 3-84.

The tragal cartilage is placed over the long process and onto the posterior canal wall.

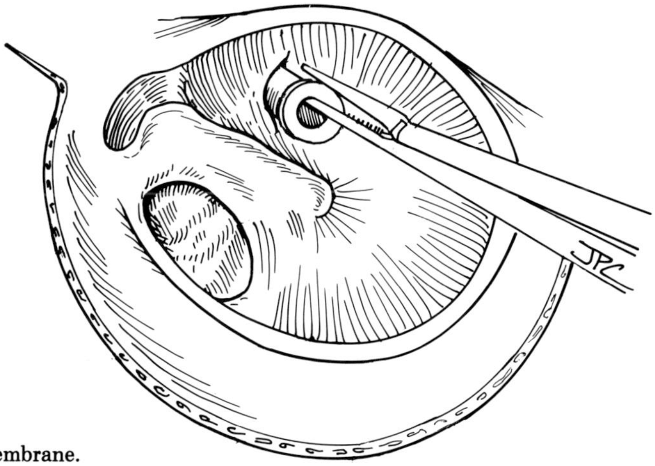

• FIGURE 3-85.

A tympanostomy tube is inserted into the tympanic membrane.

- Cholesteatoma (with or without chronic suppurative otitis media and mastoiditis): When the cholesteatoma extends into the mastoid air cells (see later)
- Cochlear implant: With posterior tympanotomy (see *Pediatric Otolaryngology*)[5]
- Others, such as facial nerve decompression, translabyrinthine labyrinthectomy, neoplasm, and mastoid trauma, which are relatively uncommon in infants and children

Anesthetic considerations

- The anesthesia and the preparation for this procedure are described earlier under Postauricular Approach. A facial nerve monitor is used during the procedure.

Procedure

- A postauricular approach and a drill are used to uncover the mastoid antrum (Fig. 3–86).
- The mastoid antrum is identified (Fig. 3–87).
- A curette removes the thinned bone over the incus (Fig. 3–88); drilling at this stage could injure the incus and result in conductive, sensorineural (due to acoustic trauma), or mixed hearing loss.
- Dissection is complete when the epitympanum, zygomatic cells, and heads of the incus and malleus are identified (Fig. 3–89).

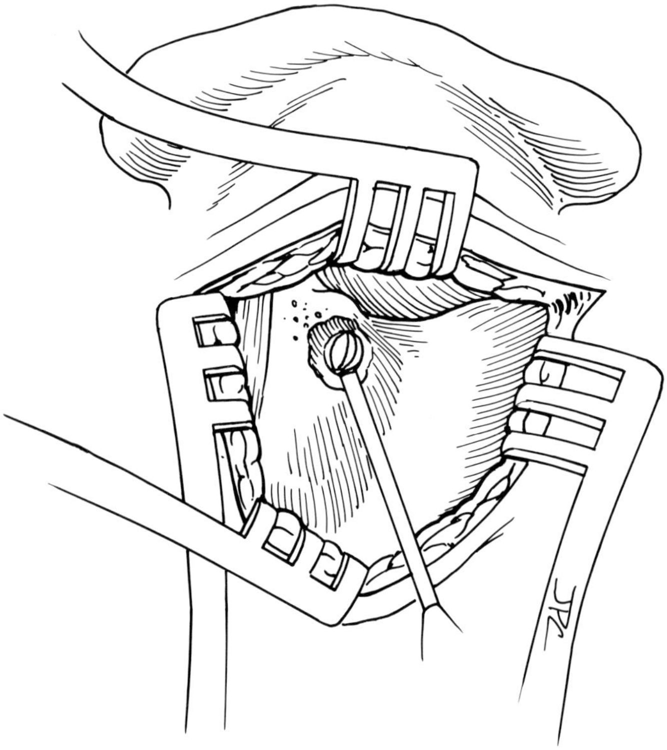

• FIGURE 3–86.

A postauricular approach and drill are used to uncover the mastoid antrum.

• FIGURE 3-87.

The mastoid antrum is identified.

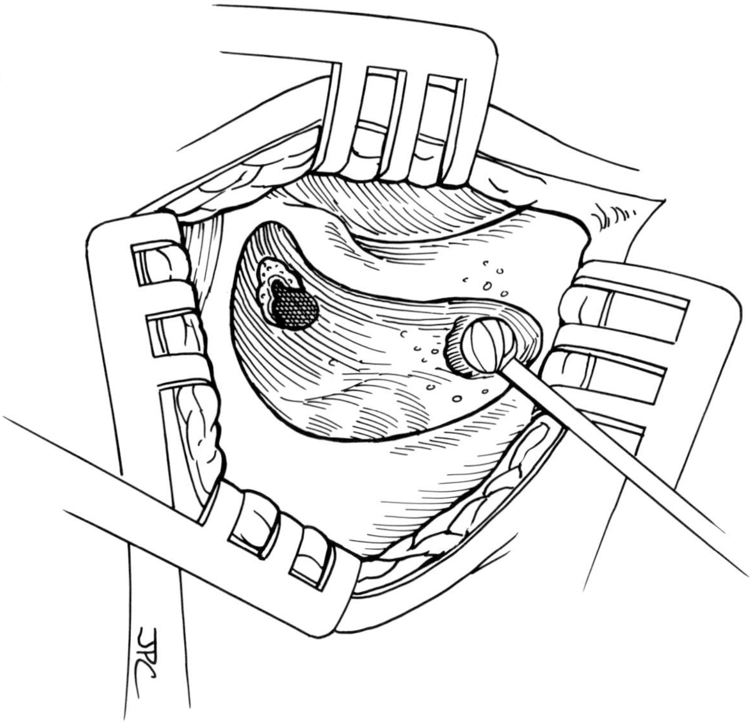

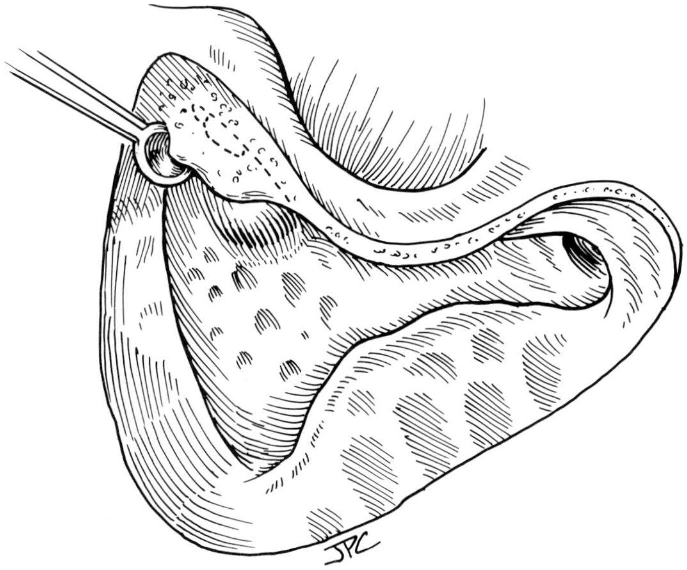

• FIGURE 3-88.

A curette removes the thinned bone over the incus.

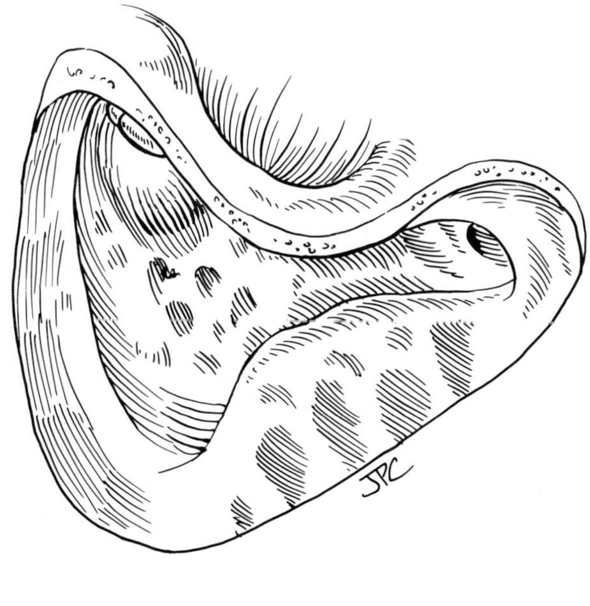

• FIGURE 3-89.

Dissection is complete when the epitympanum, zygomatic cells, and heads of the incus and malleus are identified.

- Tympanostomy tube and wide-field myringotomy are used when acute mastoiditis is an indication for surgery (Fig. 3–90).

- The postauricular wound is closed with an absorbable suture. A plastic drain, with holes cut into the portion that is in the mastoid cavity, is placed in the mastoid cavity (Fig. 3–91).

Postoperative care

- When the procedure is performed for acute mastoiditis, no packing is inserted into the external canal. The child is maintained on intravenous antimicrobial therapy, which can be adjusted after the results of the culture and susceptibility studies are available; specimens for culture and susceptibility are taken intraoperatively from the mastoid mucosa and bone, as well as from the middle ear and mastoid purulent material. The drain is removed when there is no further drainage from the wound. The child can be discharged on an oral antimicrobial agent when the patient is afebrile and when there is no further discharge from the middle ear or mastoid wound.

MODIFIED RADICAL MASTOIDECTOMY

A modified radical mastoidectomy is most commonly performed to eradicate disease from the mastoid that is due to congenital or acquired cholesteatoma, chronic suppurative otitis media and mastoiditis, or both. The mastoid cavity, the epitympanum, and the external canal are exteriorized into a common cavity. The tympanic membrane or graft is present. In a study of 232 children in Pittsburgh who were operated on for cholesteatoma, there were 244 surgical procedures, of which 24% were modified radical mastoidectomies.[4] A Bondy modified radical mastoidectomy is performed in selected cases (e.g., small, constricted mastoid) in which cholesteatoma is localized to the epitympanum and the mastoid air cells but is not present in the middle ear. When chronic suppurative otitis media and mastoiditis fail to improve after intensive medical management, a complete "simple" mastoidectomy is usually the next step in management. If, during surgery, there appears to be a persistent obstruction between the middle ear and the mastoid cavity following the simple mastoidectomy (i.e., irrigation fluid fails to flow freely between the two areas), then the canal wall may have to be removed and the operation converted into a modified radical mastoidectomy. An alternative would be to try a posterior tympanotomy approach to the facial recess, but this technique is not as effective in controlling and preventing the infection as removing the canal wall. An alternative to removing the posterior canal wall would be to remove the incus (see *Pediatric Otolaryngology*).[5]

Indications

- Cholesteatoma: When disease extends to the mastoid air cells and cannot be effectively managed employing an intact canal wall-up procedure (see page 98)

- Chronic suppurative otitis media and mastoiditis: When nonsurgical methods fail and a complete "simple" mastoidectomy will most likely be, or has been, unsuccessful in providing adequate aeration between the middle ear and the mastoid cavity

• FIGURE 3–90.

Tympanostomy tube and wide-field myringotomy.

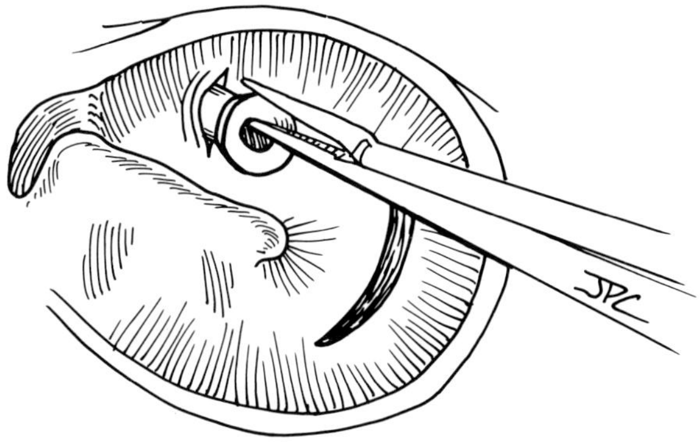

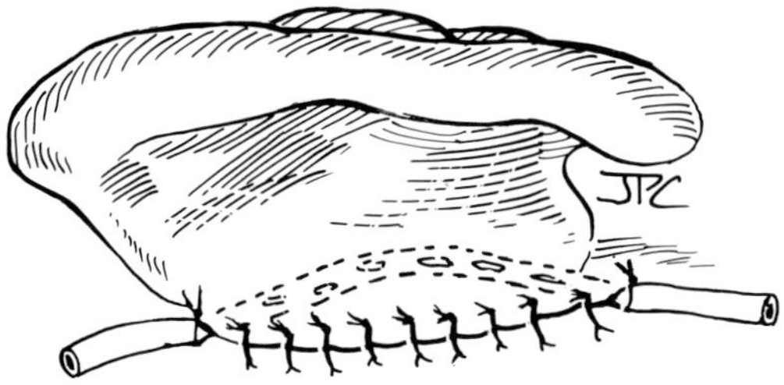

• FIGURE 3–91.

The postauricular wound is closed with an absorbable suture and drain inserted.

Anesthetic considerations and preparation

- The anesthesia and the preparation for this procedure have been described earlier, but when chronic suppurative disease (with or without cholesteatoma) is present, perioperative antimicrobial therapy is usually administered; an agent effective against *Pseudomonas aeruginosa* is recommended. A facial nerve monitor is used during the procedure.

Procedure

- A complete "simple" mastoidectomy is usually performed first (Fig. 3–92).
- The posterior canal wall is taken down to the facial ridge (Fig. 3–93).
- The tympanic membrane is replaced; the epitympanum and the mastoid cavity are exteriorized (Fig. 3–94).

Postoperative care

- In children, the mastoid cavity is usually not grafted or obliterated, because residual disease may be obscured, and the cavity frequently becomes smaller with advancing age. A layer of Gelfoam is placed on the tympanic membrane/graft, and two strips of Adaptic are lightly packed into the canal and mastoid cavity.
- The postoperative care is similar to that described for a lateral graft tympanoplasty (see earlier under Large Central Perforation; Postauricular Approach, Lateral Graft). When the indication is chronic suppurative mastoiditis, perioperative intravenous antimicrobial therapy is usually administered.
- Cavity care is more difficult in the child, and the procedure may have to be performed in the operating room with the patient under general anesthesia, especially when residual cholesteatoma is present.

RADICAL MASTOIDECTOMY

- Radical mastoidectomy creates a common cavity that consists of the middle ear, epitympanum, mastoid cavity, and external canal. The operation is not performed as frequently today as it was in the preantibiotic era; however, it is performed when extensive cholesteatoma that cannot be controlled with a less radical procedure is present. In children, an extensive rapidly growing cholesteatoma is not uncommon, and radical mastoidectomy is still performed in selected cases. In our series of 244 surgical procedures for cholesteatoma, 26% were radical mastoidectomies.[4] In the past, this procedure had also been advocated when a suppurative intracranial complication developed in a patient who had acute or chronic otitis media and mastoiditis, but today a lesser procedure may be effective in individualized patients, such as when cholesteatoma is absent. With the advent of the telescope to aid in removal of the cholesteatoma, it is hoped that radical mastoidectomy will be less commonly needed in the future.
- Closure of the eustachian tube at the bony (protympanic) portion can prevent troublesome postoperative recurrent or chronic otorrhea caused by reflux of nasopharyngeal secretions (see later under Obliteration of the Eustachian Tube). I do not routinely perform this part of the procedure, because all patients do not have postoperative drainage and, more important, future reconstruction of an aerated middle ear space is not possible, unless a tube is inserted or a perforation is present in the reconstructed tympanic membrane.

• FIGURE 3-92.

A complete "simple" mastoidectomy is usually performed first.

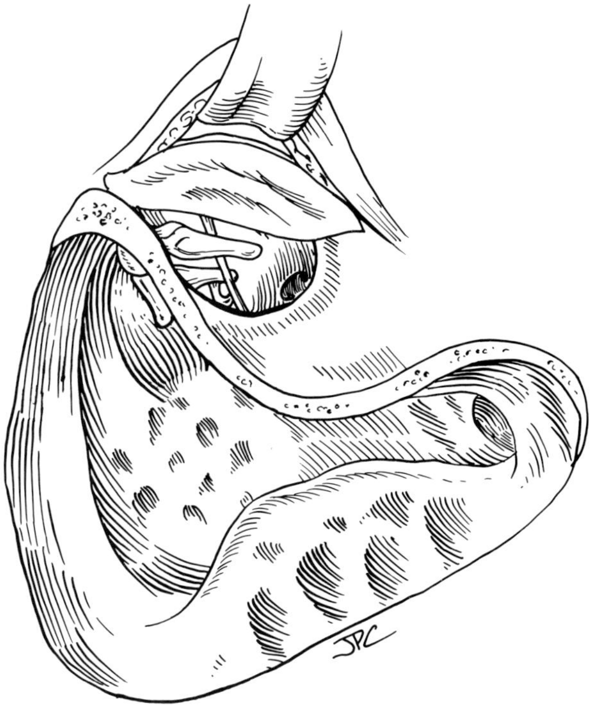

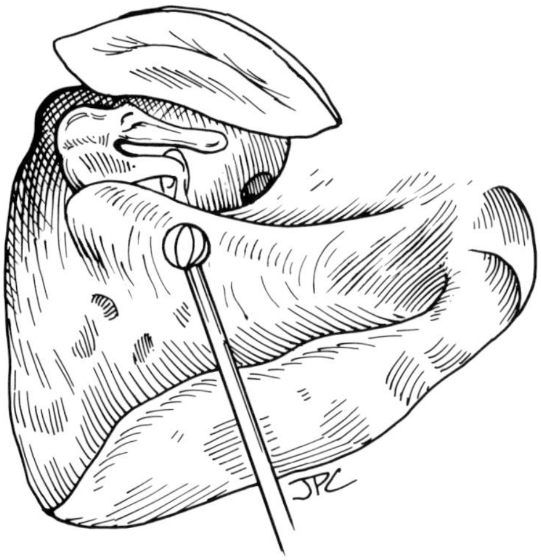

• FIGURE 3-93.

The posterior canal wall is taken down to the facial ridge.

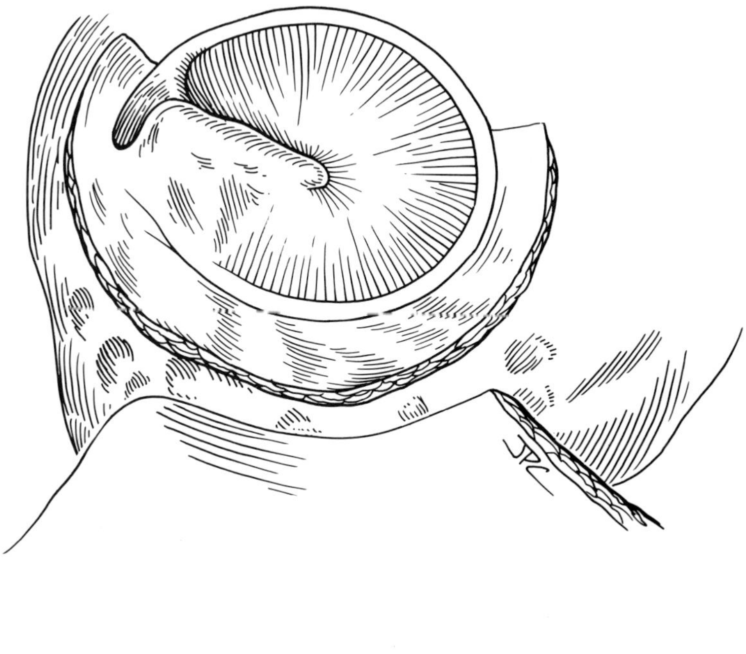

• FIGURE 3-94.

The tympanic membrane is replaced.

Indications

- Extensive congenital or acquired cholesteatoma: When a less radical procedure is not possible
- Suppurative intracranial complications of cholesteatoma, or for selected children who have acute and chronic suppurative otitis media and mastoiditis: When a less radical procedure is not likely to control the disease process

Anesthetic considerations and preparation

- When suppurative disease is present within the middle ear cleft, intravenous antimicrobial therapy is often administered perioperatively and should be given when there is a suppurative complication of ear disease.
- The anesthesia and the preparation for this procedure are the same as described earlier—except when an intracranial procedure is to be performed in addition to the mastoidectomy; then, the patient should also be prepared for that procedure. A facial nerve monitor is used during the procedure.

Procedure

- The posterior auditory canal is taken down and a facial ridge is created as in a modified radical mastoidectomy (Fig. 3–95).
- The tympanic membrane, malleus, and incus are removed; a meatoplasty is usually performed (Fig. 3–96).

Postoperative care

- The postoperative care is similar to that described following a modified radical mastoidectomy.

• FIGURE 3-95.

The posterior auditory canal is taken down, and a facial ridge is created.

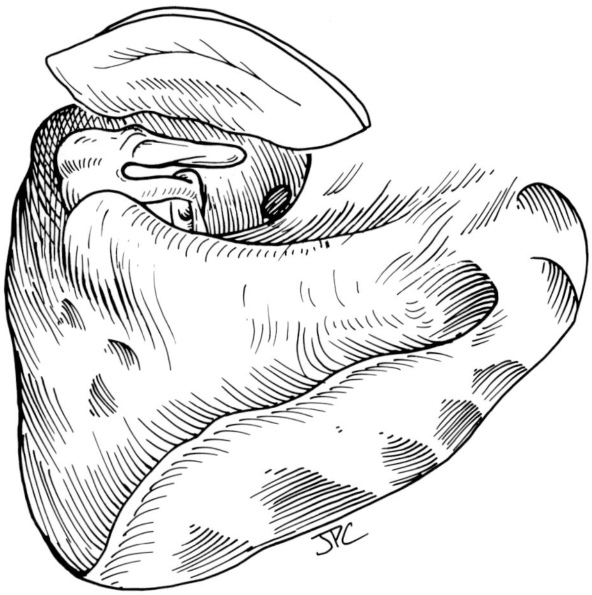

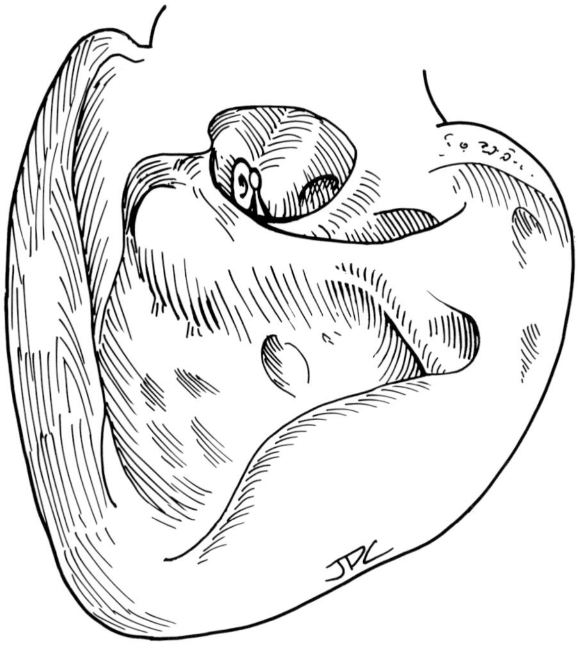

• FIGURE 3-96.

The tympanic membrane, malleus, and incus are removed.

ACQUIRED CHOLESTEATOMA

The most frequent anatomic site in which we encounter an acquired cholesteatoma in children is in the posterosuperior quadrant of the pars tensa, and the second most common site is in the pars flaccida area. Frequently, the distinction between congenital and acquired cholesteatoma is not possible because of the extent of the disease; however, when a cholesteatoma is within the middle ear (and mastoid air cells), the tympanic membrane is intact, and there is no defect (e.g., perforation or retraction pocket) in the eardrum, one can assume that the cholesteatoma is congenital. On the other hand, when there is a defect in an area of the tympanic membrane that is susceptible to a retraction pocket, one can assume that the cholesteatoma is acquired. When most of the tympanic membrane is absent, the cholesteatoma is of uncertain origin.

As stated earlier, we individualize each child's final procedure depending on several factors. One surgical procedure is not advocated for all cholesteatomas. The following factors are important in the preoperative planning and the intraoperative decision-making process:

- Anatomic site
- Extent of disease
- Condition of ossicular chain and tympanic membrane
- Presence or absence of chronic suppurative otitis media and mastoiditis
- Presence or absence of suppurative or nonsuppurative complications
- Anatomy of the temporal bone and the middle ear cleft
- Status of eustachian tube function
- Age and general health of the child
- Findings on computed tomography (CT) scans
- Availability of postoperative follow-up care

The long-standing goals of surgery for cholesteatoma are eradication of the disease, reconstruction of the tympanic membrane, maintenance of the anatomy of the middle ear cleft, and preservation (restoration) of hearing. We hope to preserve the external auditory canal and to prevent the potential morbidity of an exposed mastoid cavity. Unfortunately, this is not always possible when cholesteatoma is present in children, because it is frequently more invasive, grows more rapidly, and is associated with a higher residual or recurrence rate than when cholesteatoma is present in adults. Other factors that may be related to this difference are the higher rate of recurrent and chronic otitis media and poor eustachian tube function in the pediatric population. Of the 199 procedures performed for acquired cholesteatoma (or cholesteatoma of uncertain etiology) at Children's Hospital, 28% were only a middle ear procedure, 20% were canal wall-up mastoidectomy, 25% were modified mastoidectomy, and 28% were radical mastoidectomy.[4]

The following are two examples of the most common types of acquired cholesteatoma that we encounter in children. Each example includes the common sites of extension of the cholesteatoma and the final procedure selected, depending on the extent of the disease. There is a logical progression of the operation, and the reader can follow the decision-making process. Preoperative evaluation of the CT scan can be helpful in planning the procedure and discussing the informed consent with the parents. The CT scan does not have high enough sensitivity to accurately identify the extent of the cholesteatoma in many patients, but it is a valuable diagnostic aid.

These procedures are not reserved only for presumed acquired cholesteatoma: They can also be used when cholesteatomas are congenital or of uncertain etiology. In addition, there are several other procedures designed to eradicate cholesteatoma that are not described in this section but are adequately described in other atlases.

POSTEROSUPERIOR QUADRANT ACQUIRED CHOLESTEATOMA ("MARGINAL PERFORATION")

Cholesteatoma that occurs in the posterosuperior quadrant of the pars tensa of the tympanic membrane has been called a "marginal perforation," but this is in almost all cases a misnomer or misconception, because there is no perforation, at least when encountered in children. It is most likely to be the result of recurrent or persistent middle ear negative pressure, due to eustachian tube functional obstruction, and immediately preceded by a retraction pocket (see *Pediatric Otolaryngology*).[5]

The following surgical description consists of examples of a possible extension of this type of cholesteatoma into the following areas:

- Confined to the posterior mesotympanum, facial recess, and sinus tympani
- Extending into the superior portion of the facial recess and epitympanum
- Extending into the aditus ad antrum and mastoid air cells
- Extending into the remaining portion of the middle ear in addition to other areas

Indications

- Cholesteatoma in the posterosuperior quadrant, with and without extension into the epitympanum, mastoid air cells, and middle ear (Fig. 3–97)

Anesthetic considerations and preparation

- The anesthesia and the preparation for this procedure are the same as for a postauricular approach (see earlier); a facial nerve monitor is used during the procedure.

Procedure

- Incisions for a Koerner flap and postauricular approach are completed (see earlier under Postauricular Approach) (Fig. 3–98).

NO. 1: CHOLESTEATOMA IN THE POSTERIOR MESOTYMPANUM, FACIAL RECESS, AND SINUS TYMPANI

- The tympanomeatal flap is elevated to reveal a cholesteatoma confined to the posterior mesotympanum, facial recess, and sinus tympani (Fig. 3–99).

- The posterosuperior portion of the canal wall scutum is removed with a curette to further visualize the cholesteatoma and the long process of the incus (eroded) and stapes (Fig. 3–100). The cholesteatoma in the facial recess is removed, and the sinus tympani is enhanced with the aid of a telescope (see Fig. 3–80).

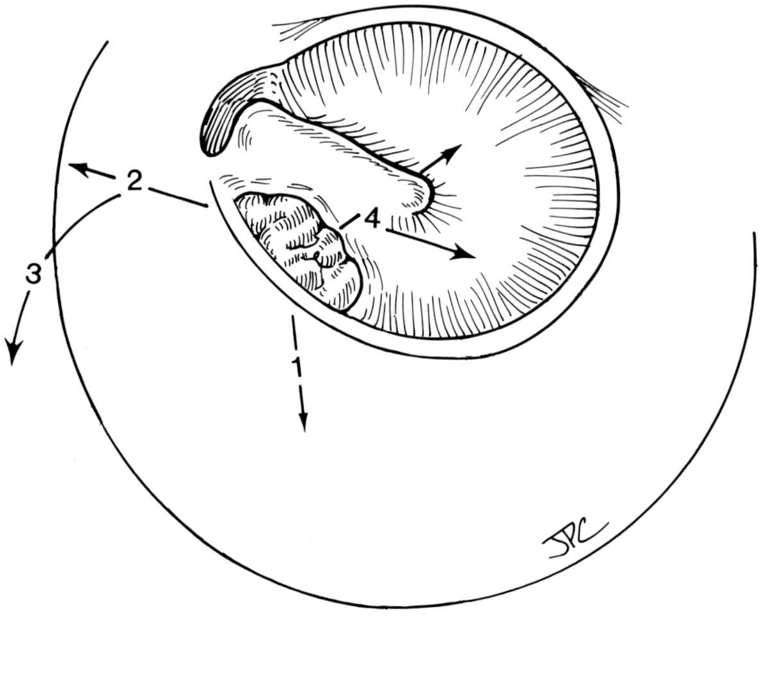

• FIGURE 3-97.

Posterosuperior quadrant cholesteatoma of uncertain extension into one or more of four possible areas.

• FIGURE 3-98.

Incisions for a Koerner flap are made approximately one third of distance from annulus to meatus.

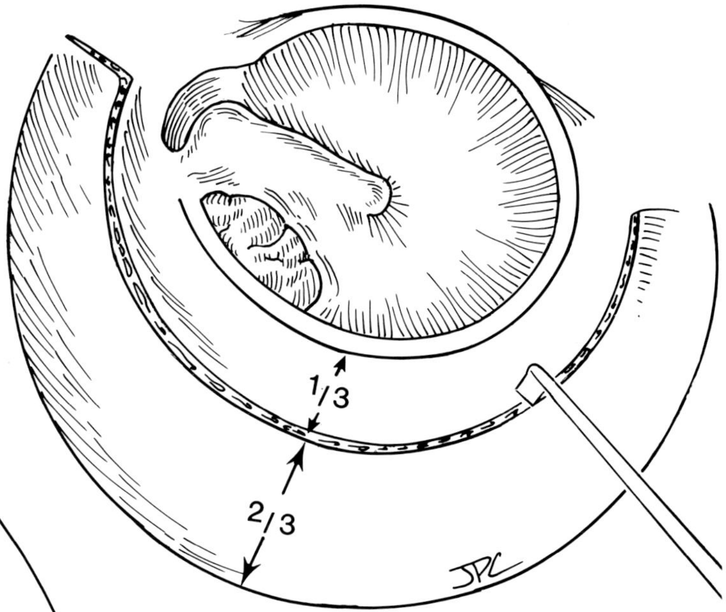

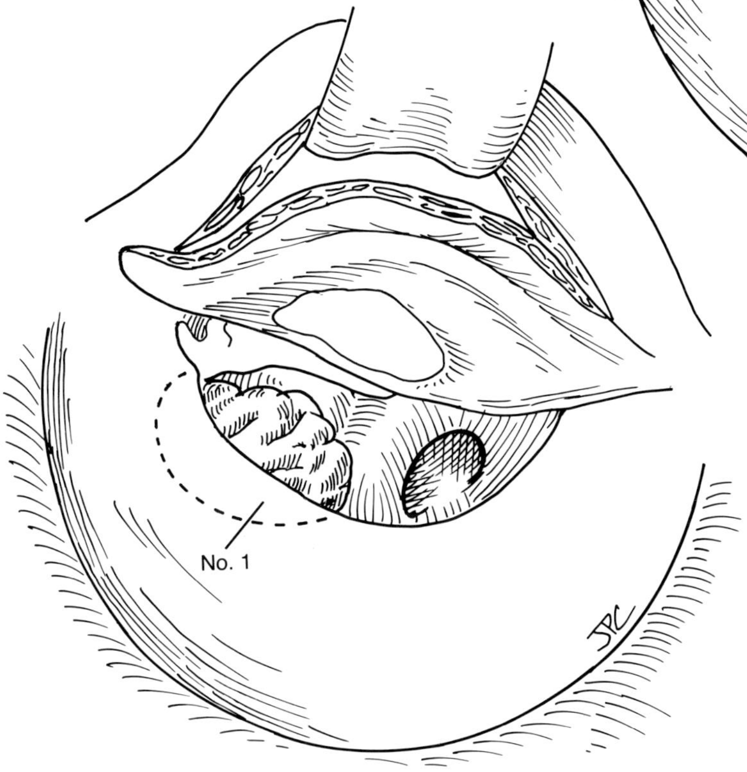

• FIGURE 3-99.

The tympanomeatal flap is elevated to reveal a cholesteatoma confined to the posterior mesotympanum, facial recess, and sinus tympani.

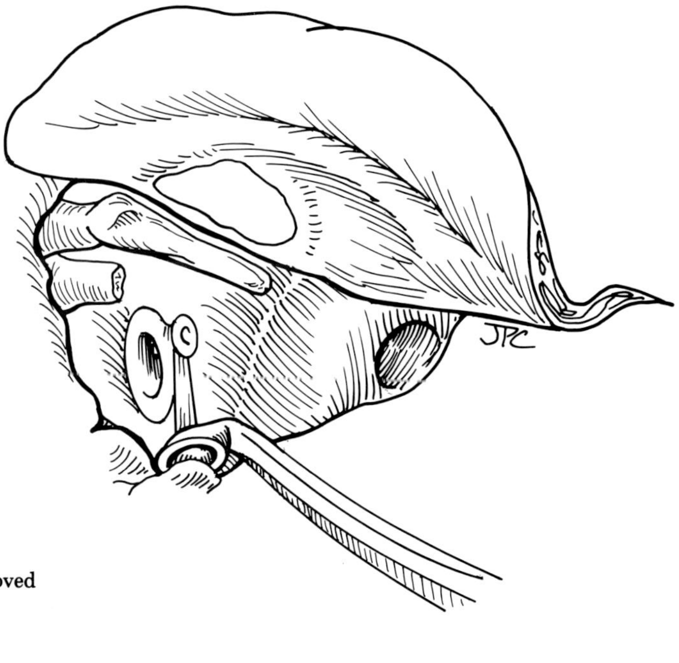

• FIGURE 3-100.

The posterosuperior portion of the canal wall scutum is removed with a curette.

- The incus is removed and sculpted (Fig. 3–101).
- The incus is inserted between the malleus and the stapes (Fig. 3–102).
- Gelfoam is placed in the middle ear; a cartilage-perichondrial graft (harvested from the tragus or concha; see Figs. 3–82 and 3–83) is placed over the defect (Fig. 3–103).
- A tympanostomy tube is inserted into the anterior portion of the tympanic membrane (Fig. 3–104).

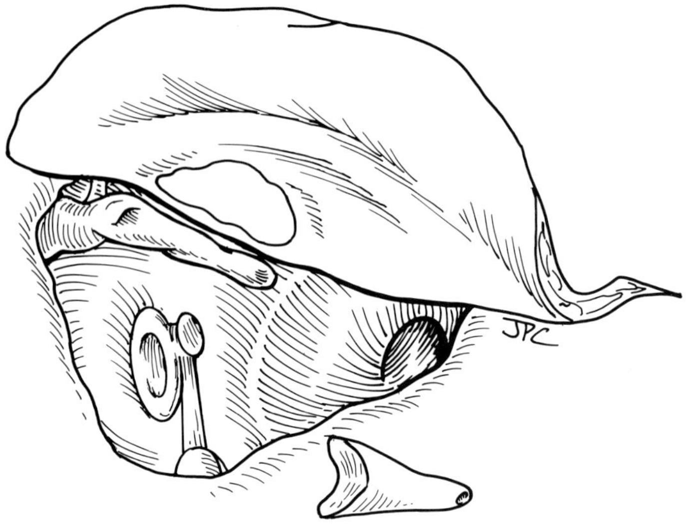

• FIGURE 3–101.

The incus is removed and sculpted.

• FIGURE 3-102.

The incus is inserted between the malleus and the stapes.

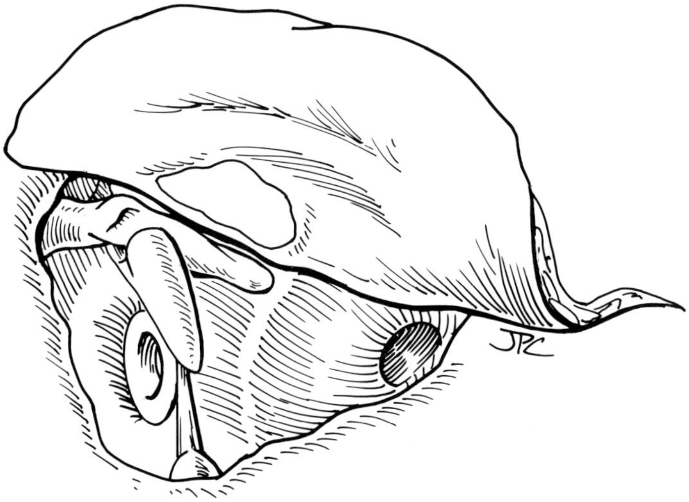

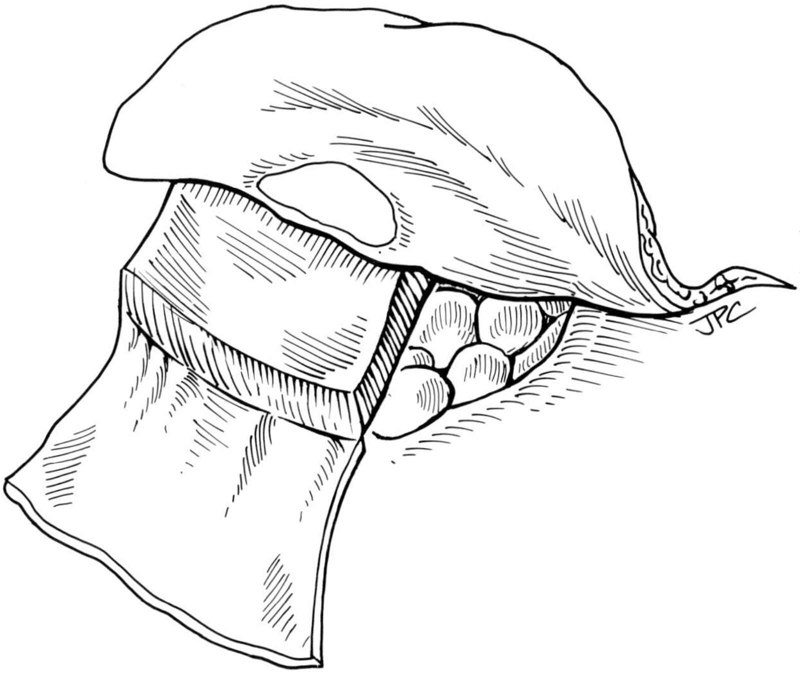

• FIGURE 3-103.

A cartilage-perichondrial graft is placed over the defect.

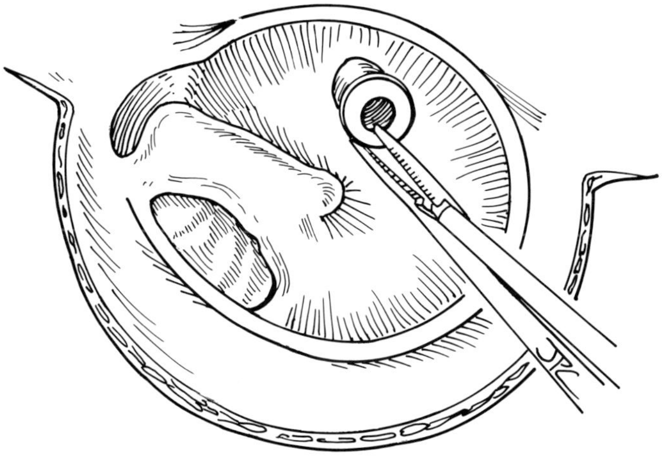

• FIGURE 3-104.

A tympanostomy tube is inserted into the anterior portion of the tympanic membrane.

NO. 2: CHOLESTEATOMA EXTENDING INTO THE EPITYMPANUM

- The tympanomeatal flap is elevated to reveal that the cholesteatoma extends into the epitympanum (Fig. 3–105).

- Atticotomy is performed with a microdrill. The incus and the head of the stapes are removed (Fig. 3–106).

- Incus interposition is one option, but removal of the entire malleus and a myringostapediapexy is an alternative. A cartilage-perichondrial graft and a fascia graft are placed medial to the tympanic membrane remnant (Fig. 3–107).

NO. 3: CHOLESTEATOMA EXTENDING INTO MASTOID AIR CELLS

- Atticotomy reveals that cholesteatoma extends superiorly and posteriorly into the attic and the area of the aditus ad antrum (Fig. 3–108).

- The mastoid cortex is entered and, if a cholesteatoma can be removed without taking the canal wall down, a complete "simple" mastoidectomy is performed (see earlier under Simple Mastoidectomy). The defect is repaired as described in Figure 3–107 (Fig. 3–109).

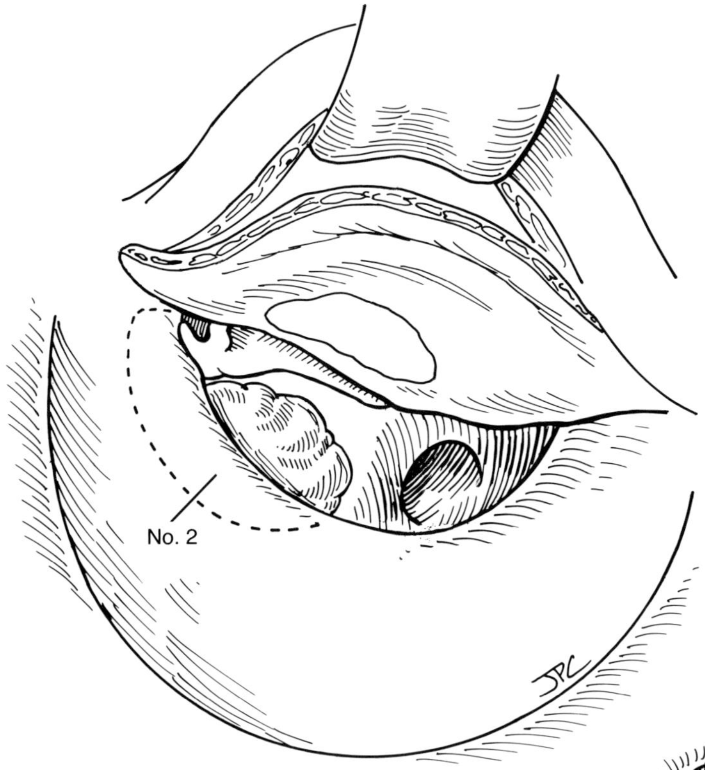

• FIGURE 3–105.

The cholesteatoma extends into the epitympanum.

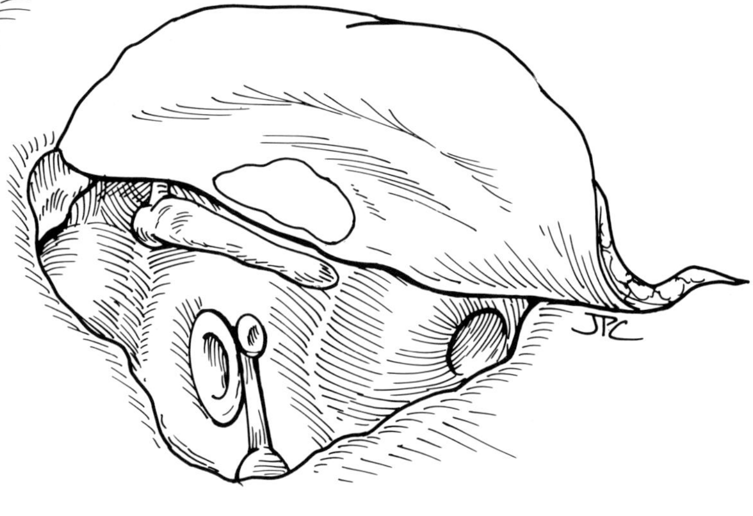

• FIGURE 3–106.

Atticotomy is performed.

• FIGURE 3-107.

A cartilage-perichondrial graft and a fascia graft are placed medial to the tympanic membrane remnant.

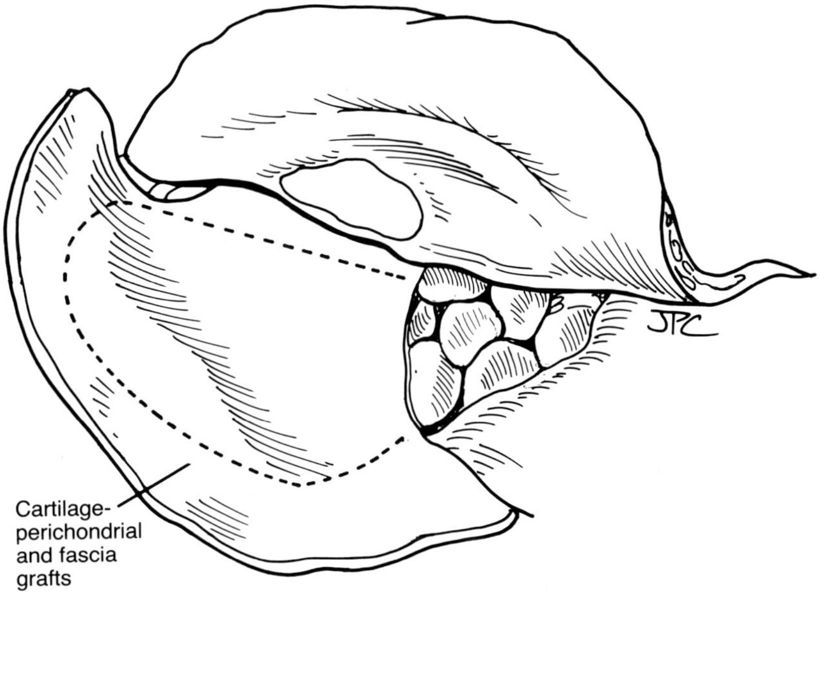

• FIGURE 3-108.

The cholesteatoma extends posterosuperiorly.

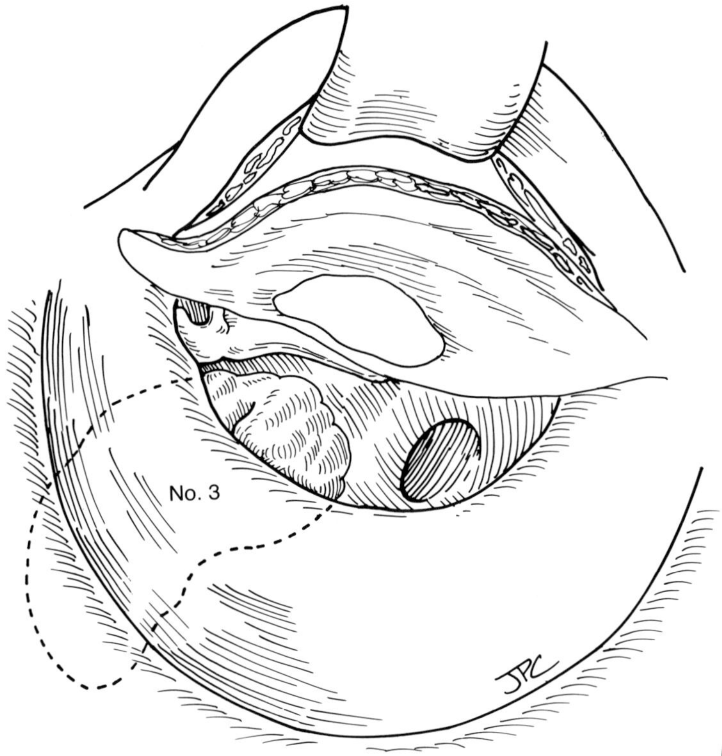

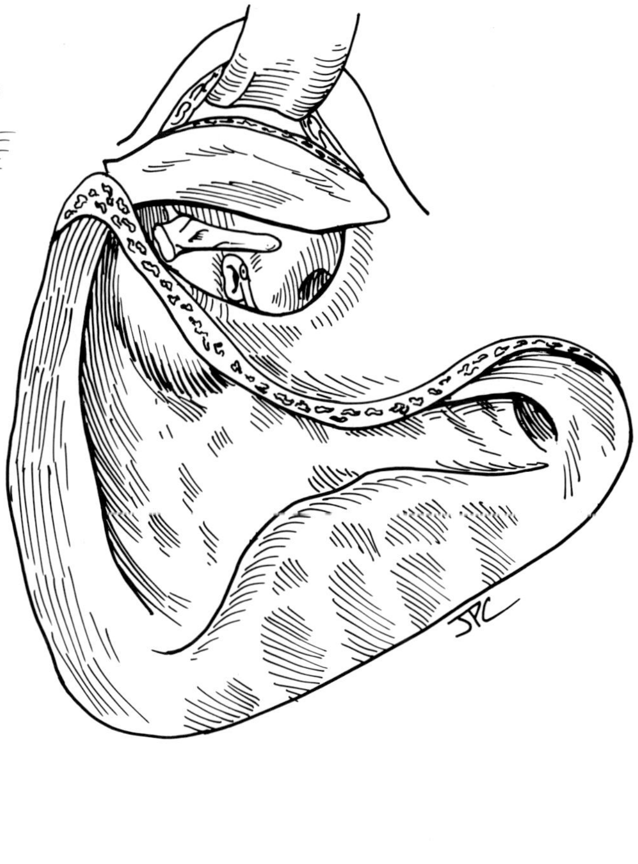

• FIGURE 3-109.

"Simple" mastoidectomy is completed.

NO. 4: EXTENSIVE CHOLESTEATOMA

- Mastoidectomy and middle ear examination reveal extensive cholesteatoma that cannot be adequately removed without removal of the posterior and superior canal walls (Fig. 3–110). A modified radical can be successful in selected cases with this extent of disease. However, the use of the telescope may enhance removal of the cholesteatoma and obviate a canal wall-down procedure.

- A radical mastoidectomy is performed when cholesteatoma is so extensive that a canal wall-up procedure or even a modified radical will not safely control the disease (Fig. 3–111).

Postoperative care

The early postoperative care is as described earlier; however, the patient is re-examined periodically for up to 5 years if a cholesteatoma has been removed. There are two major concerns: residual cholesteatoma that persists following the initial surgical procedure, and occurrence of a new cholesteatoma (i.e., recurrent cholesteatoma), which can be the result of persistent eustachian tube dysfunction and a new retraction pocket in an anatomic site similar to the original one or in another area of the tympanic membrane. In addition, implantation (iatrogenic cholesteatoma) can develop following this type of middle ear and mastoid surgery. In children who have had cholesteatoma surgery that results in a procedure that prevents adequate postoperative examination to determine if a residual cholesteatoma persists (e.g., a canal wall-up tympanomastoidectomy), a "second look" exploratory tympanotomy is performed about 6 months after the initial mastoid procedure; 6 months appears to be the most appropriate time interval in children. In our study that involved 232 children who had 244 surgical procedures, residual or recurrent cholesteatoma developed in 38%, and 23% of those cholesteatomas were detected at the time of the "second look" procedure. Development of residual or recurrent disease was statistically associated with the presence of erosion of the ossicles at the time of the original surgery. At the time of the "second look" exploratory tympanotomy, I also use the 3-mm, 70-degree Hopkins rod lens telescope to inspect the middle ear for residual or recurrent disease.

• FIGURE 3-110.

Mastoidectomy and middle ear examination reveal extensive cholesteatoma in the mastoid and entire middle ear.

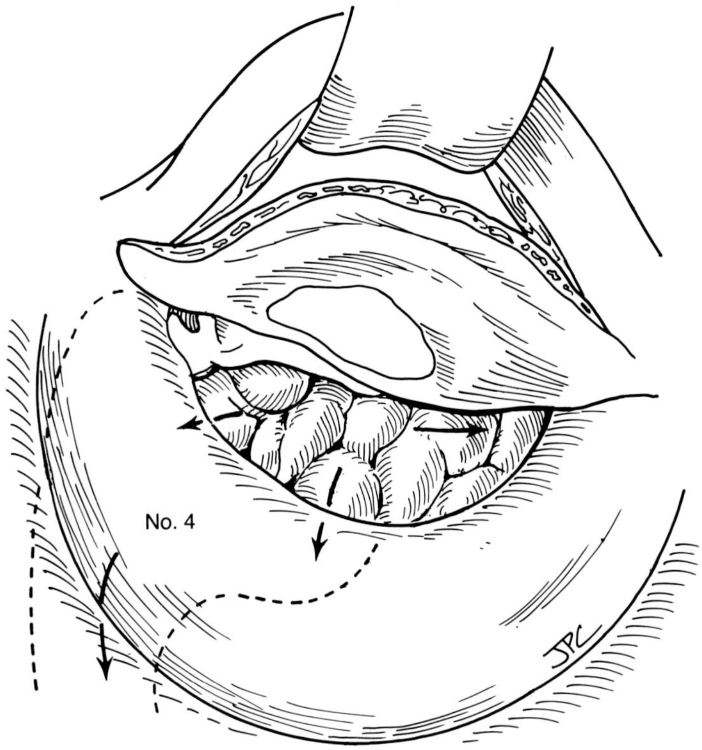

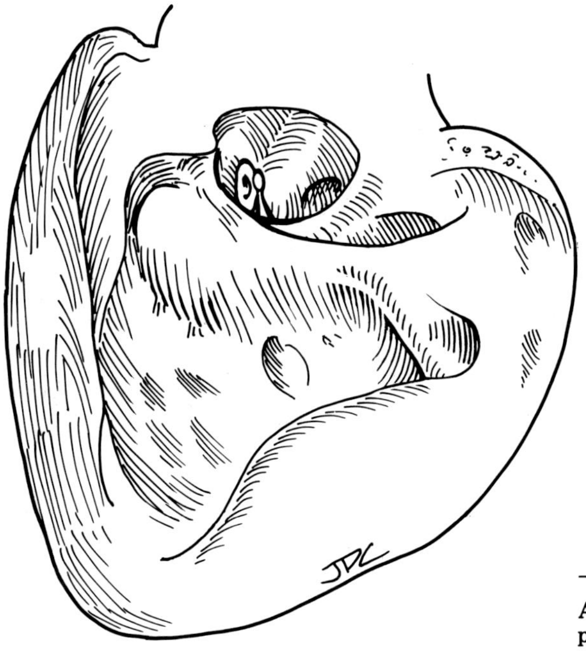

• FIGURE 3-111.

A radical mastoidectomy is performed when disease is too extensive to perform a less radical procedure.

PARS FLACCIDA CHOLESTEATOMA ("ATTIC CHOLESTEATOMA")

A cholesteatoma that is visualized otoscopically as occurring in the pars flaccida area has been inappropriately termed an "attic perforation," when in reality there is no perforation but a cholesteatoma (or retraction pocket). The etiology and pathogenesis are most likely similar to cholesteatoma that develops in the posterosuperior quadrant of the pars tensa and, as described earlier, a retraction pocket precedes the cholesteatoma.

The following is an example of a cholesteatoma in the pars flaccida that has three possible extensions:

- Confined to anterior epitympanum
- Extending into the aditus ad antrum and mastoid
- Extensive cholesteatoma

The preoperative evaluation of the CT scan can be helpful in deciding to use an endaural or postauricular approach. When the cholesteatoma is considered to be confined to the epitympanum, the endaural approach is used, whereas if the cholesteatoma has most likely extended into the mastoid, a postauricular approach is employed. An alternative is to plan to use the endaural approach. If the cholesteatoma does indeed extend into the mastoid, then a classical Bondy modified radical mastoidectomy is performed in selected cases; however, this approach is not effective when there is extensive disease in the mastoid. The postauricular approach is more feasible.

Indications

- Cholesteatoma in the pars flaccida, with and without extension into mastoid air cells and middle ear (Fig. 3–112)

Anesthetic considerations and preparation

- The anesthesia and the preparation are dependent on the surgical approach, which will be endaural when the cholesteatoma is relatively small and confined to the epitympanic space or when a Bondy modified radical mastoidectomy is performed (see earlier). If the cholesteatoma is thought to be extensive, as evaluated preoperatively on the CT scan, the postauricular approach is used (see earlier).

Procedure

NO. 1: CHOLESTEATOMA CONFINED TO THE ANTERIOR EPITYMPANUM

- Endaural incisions and the approach (see earlier under Endaural Approach) are completed to visualize cholesteatoma (Fig. 3–113).

• FIGURE 3-112.

Cholesteatoma in the pars flaccida with three possible extensions.

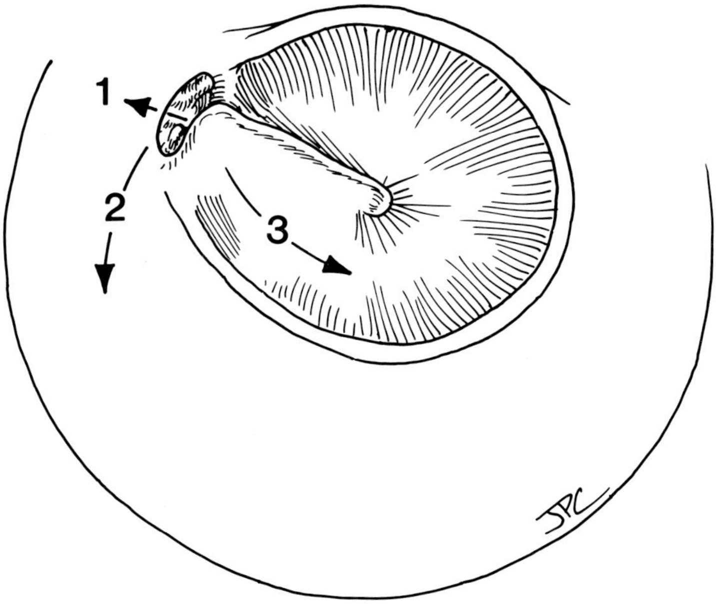

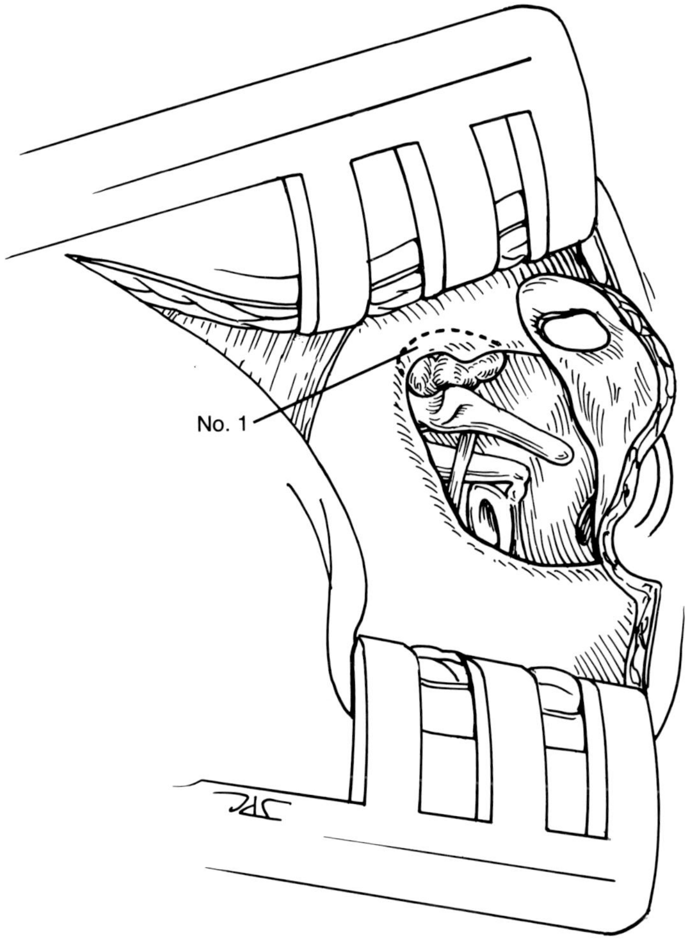

• FIGURE 3-113.

Endaural incisions and the approach are completed.

- An anterior atticotomy is completed with a microdrill (Fig. 3–114).

- Cholesteatoma is removed, and the defect is repaired using tragal cartilage–perichondrial and fascia grafts medial to the tympanic membrane (see earlier under Anterosuperior Perforation [and Retraction Pocket: Endaural Approach, Medial Graft]) (Fig. 3–115).

- A tympanostomy tube is inserted into the anteroinferior quadrant of the tympanic membrane (Fig. 3–116).

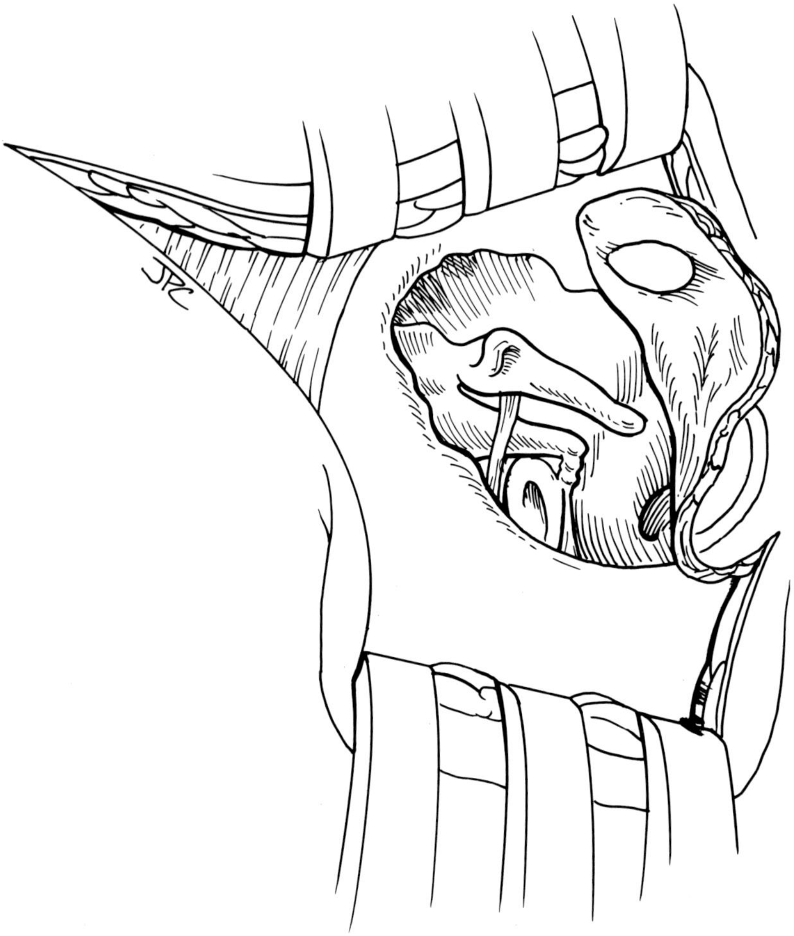

• FIGURE 3–114.

An anterior atticotomy is completed.

• FIGURE 3-115.

Defect is repaired using tragal cartilage–perichondrial and fascia grafts.

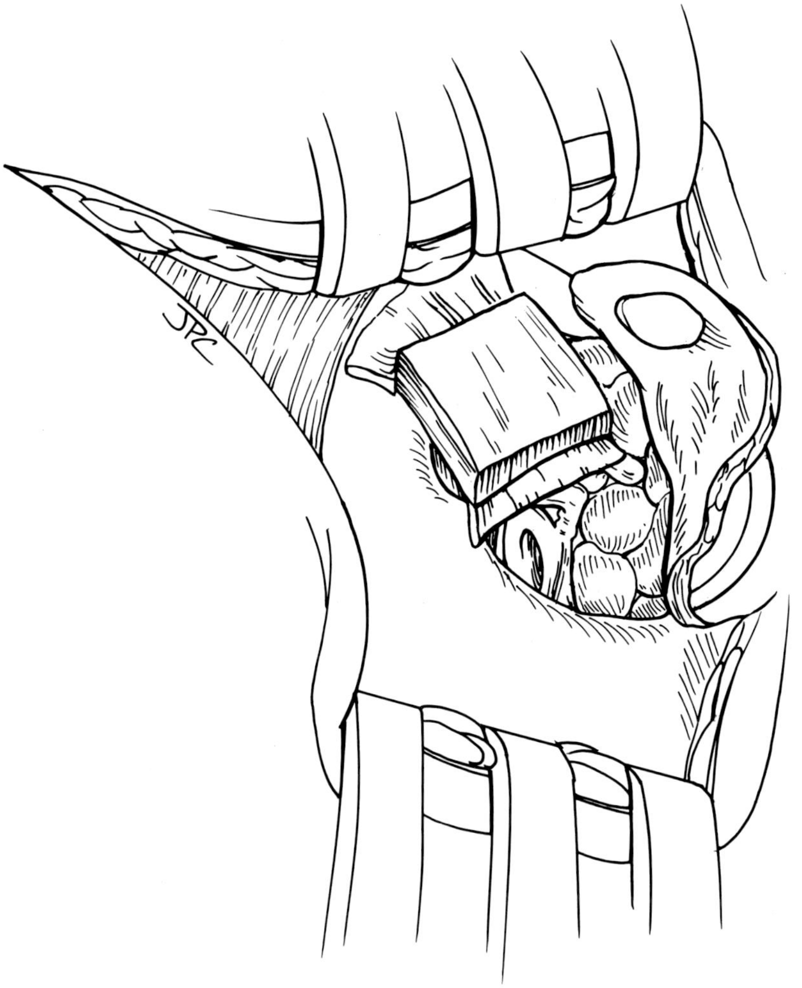

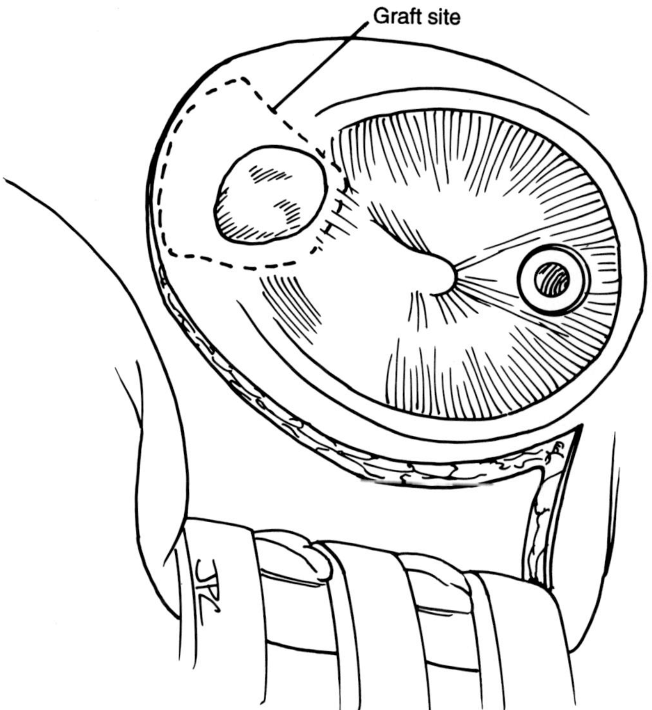

• FIGURE 3-116.

A tympanostomy tube is inserted into the tympanic membrane.

NO. 2: CHOLESTEATOMA EXTENDING MASTOID AIR CELLS

- An endaural approach and an atticotomy reveal that cholesteatoma extends posteriorly into the aditus ad antrum and possibly into the mastoid air cells (Fig. 3–117).

- If cholesteatoma is lateral to the ossicles and is not in the middle ear but is in the mastoid, a modified radical approach mastoidectomy is one option (Fig. 3–118); if possible, a canal wall-up procedure is another option (Fig. 3–118). A postauricular approach would be a more feasible approach.

NO. 3: EXTENSIVE CHOLESTEATOMA

- Extensive cholesteatoma is anticipated from the CT scan. A postauricular approach is indicated, and the final procedure is dependent on the extent (Fig. 3–119).

Postoperative care

- The postoperative care is similar to that described earlier under Endaural, and Postauricular Approach.

EUSTACHIAN TUBE DYSFUNCTION

Unfortunately, there are no surgical procedures to correct the most common type of eustachian tube dysfunction—functional obstruction. Functional obstruction and its attendant middle ear disease, however, are most common in infants and young children, but the condition improves with advancing age. For adolescents and adults whose functional obstruction persists, a definitive operative procedure to improve function is a goal of future research. Presently, we have only a bypass procedure, myringotomy with tympanostomy tube insertion; however, there are certain indications to obstruct the eustachian tube, and for these patients we do have effective surgical procedures.

• FIGURE 3-117.

An endaural approach and an atticotomy reveal that cholesteatoma extends posterior toward the mastoid air cells.

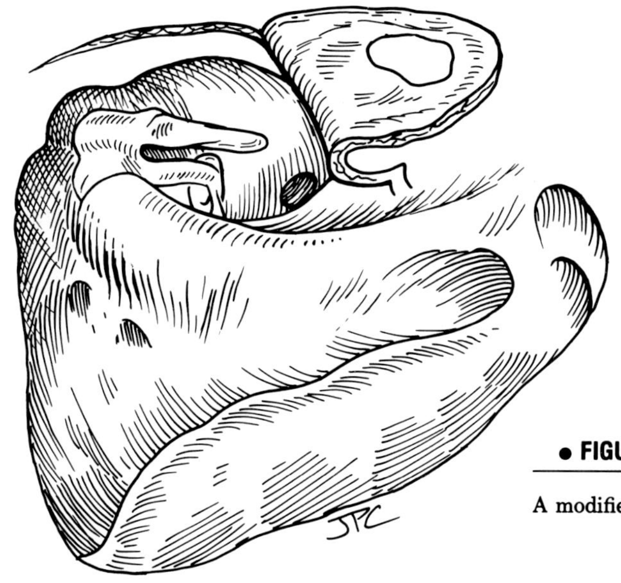

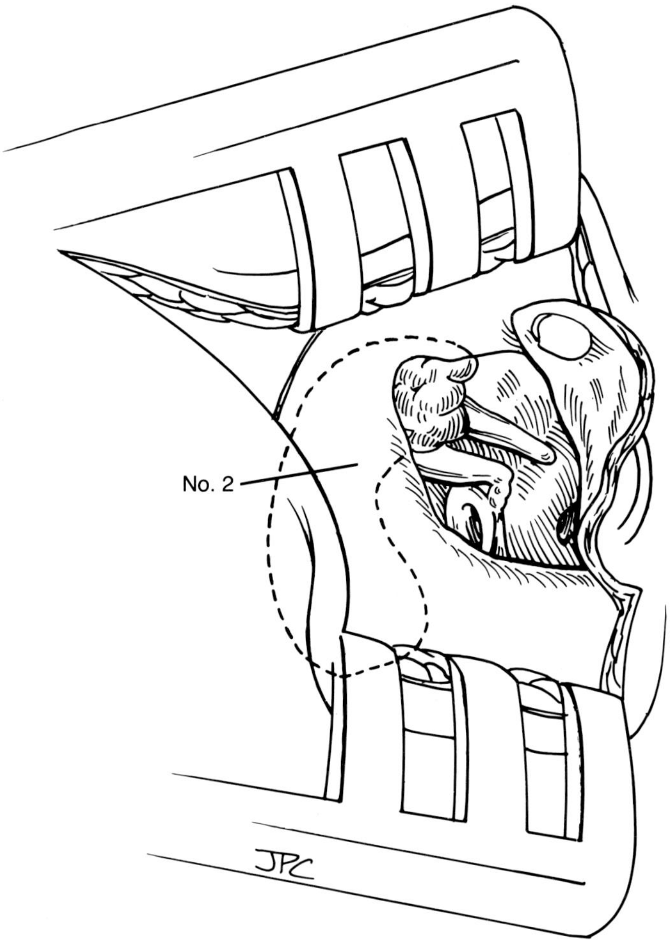

• FIGURE 3-118.

A modified radical mastoidectomy is one option.

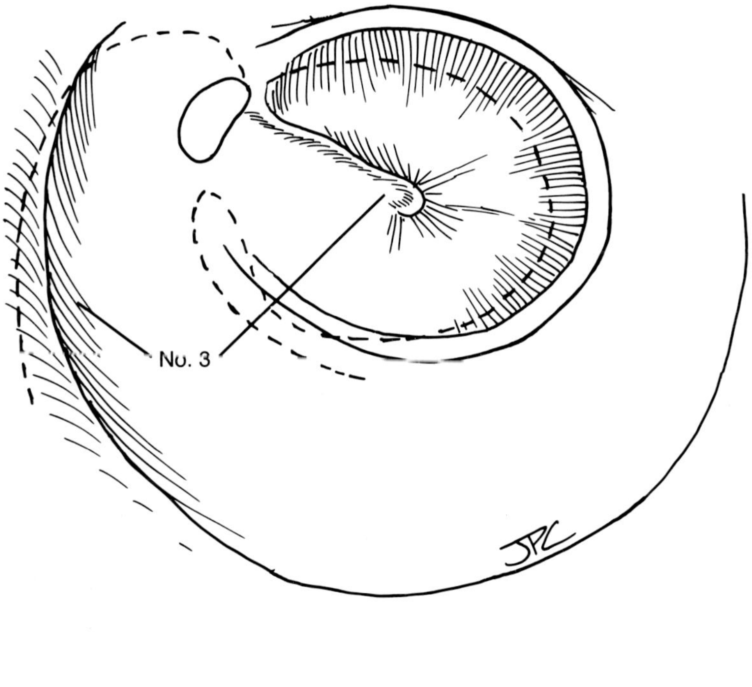

• FIGURE 3-119.

Extensive cholesteatoma is anticipated from the computed tomography scan.

OBLITERATION OF THE EUSTACHIAN TUBE

Otorrhea is a common problem following mastoidectomy and is seen most frequently when there is a large perforation of the tympanic membrane or when the eardrum has been removed completely as part of a radical mastoidectomy. The discharge can usually be controlled medically or by repairing the tympanic membrane and by providing a closed middle ear space. In the absence of contamination from water entering the external canal, the ear discharge is caused by unwanted nasopharyngeal secretions refluxing through the eustachian tube and into the middle ear, resulting from the lack of the middle ear air cushion. Occasionally, a patient (usually one who has had a radical mastoidectomy) has significant morbidity from otorrhea and medical management fails to prevent the recurrent or chronic aural discharge. In this patient, reconstruction of the middle ear is an unlikely possibility. Obliteration of the eustachian tube is a reasonable alternative, as long as the patient and the parents are fully informed concerning the benefits (i.e., prevention of otorrhea) and costs (e.g., inability to reconstruct a functioning gas-filled middle ear with an intact eardrum). The most likely candidates are those who have no serviceable hearing in the affected ear, and for them, obliteration of the entire middle ear cleft should also be considered (see *Pediatric Otolaryngology*).[5]

Indications

- Presence of postoperative recurrent or chronic otorrhea following mastoidectomy, and reconstruction of the middle ear and tympanic membrane is not feasible or indicated.

Anesthetic considerations and preparation

The anesthesia and the preparation for this procedure are the same as those described earlier under Radical Mastoidectomy.

Procedure

- The middle ear and the mastoid are approached through postauricular incision when mastoidectomy is to be revised. Bone paté is harvested from an uninvolved area of the cortex with a drill and is collected in a Lukens (bronchoscopic) trap (Fig. 3–120).

- A small piece of temporalis muscle, bone paté, and a temporalis fascia graft are used to obliterate the protympanic (i.e., bony or middle-ear portion) of the eustachian tube (Fig. 3–121). Careful removal of mucosa of the eustachian tube precedes obliteration.

Postoperative care

- A layer of Gelfoam is placed over the fascia graft and in the middle ear, and a small strip of Adaptic impregnated with an antibiotic ointment is placed in the ear canal; the Adaptic strip is removed in 1 week.

• FIGURE 3-120.

Bone paté is harvested and aspirated into a trap.

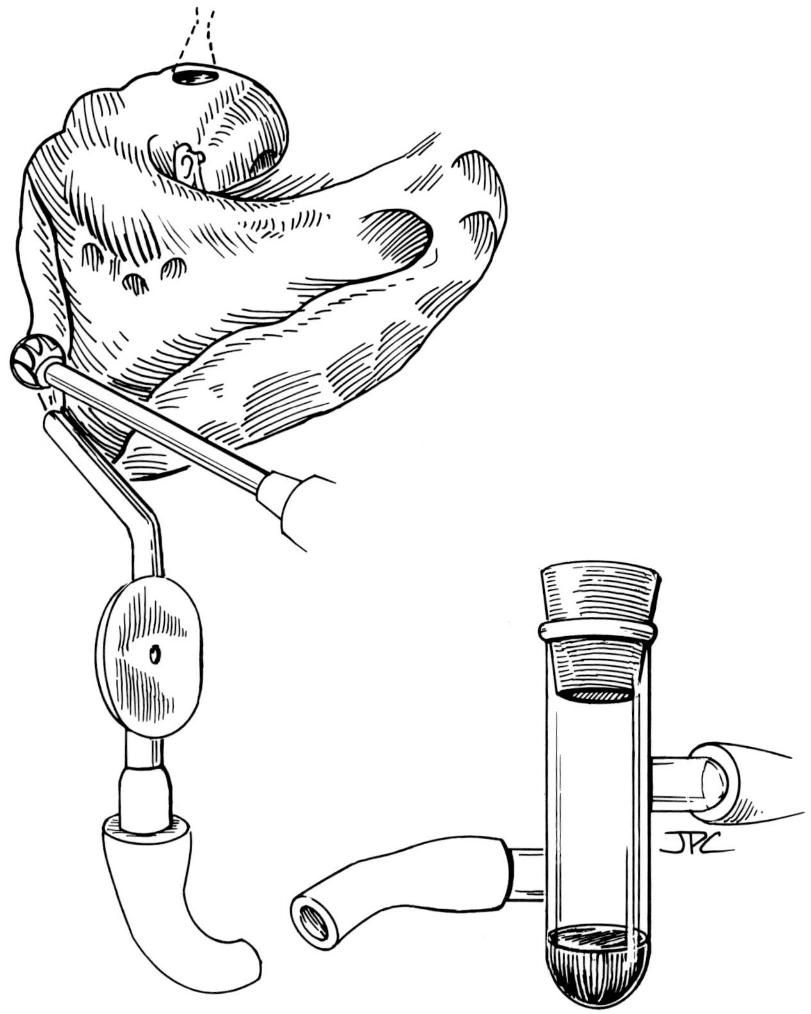

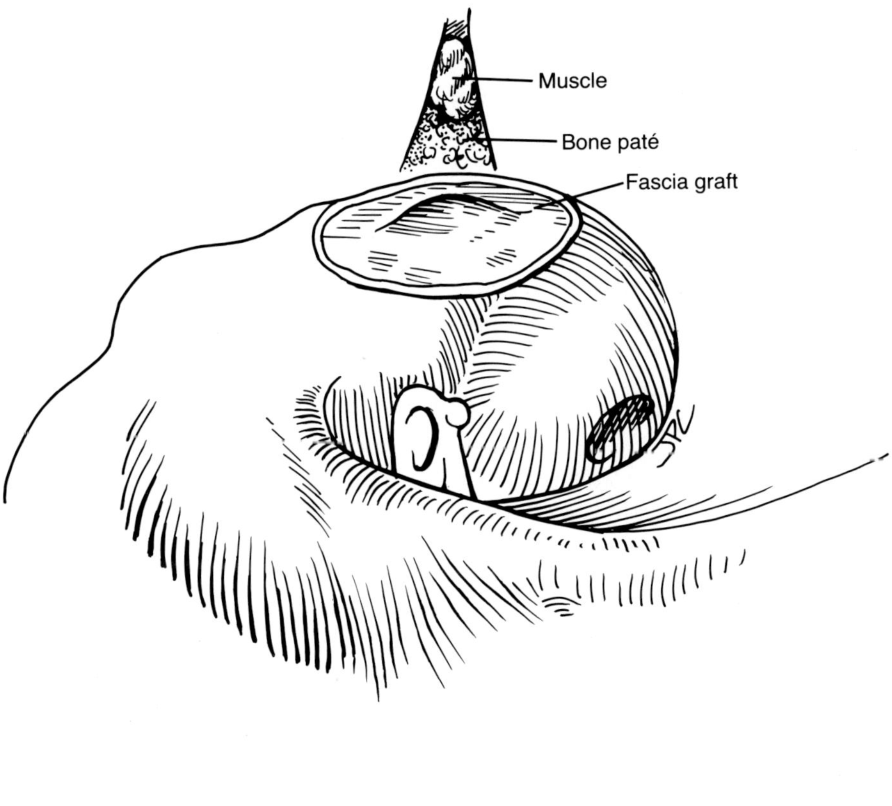

• FIGURE 3-121.

A small piece of temporalis muscle, bone paté, and temporalis fascia are used to obliterate the protympanic of the eustachian tube.

PATULOUS EUSTACHIAN TUBE: CATHETER OBSTRUCTION

A continuously open eustachian tube is termed patulous, and some patients (most frequently adults) complain of autophony and of hearing their own breathing (see *Pediatric Otolaryngology*).[5] Rapid loss of weight is often the predisposing factor in some, but by no means all, patients. In 1981, we reported on a surgical procedure to obstruct the tube in selected patients who had been unsuccessfully treated medically and who were relieved of their symptoms by the procedure.[18] More recently, we reported on nine patients who had had the procedure and whose follow-up ranged from 4 months to 15 years. Six of the nine patients had no further or infrequent symptoms, and three reported no relief.[19]

The procedure has undergone some modifications during the last 10 years and now has a better chance of success than the technique originally described. When the external auditory canal is relatively small, an endaural approach is employed, but if the anterior canal wall and tympanic membrane are completely seen, the transcanal approach is used and an anterior tympanomeatal flap is elevated to visualize the middle ear orifice of the eustachian tube. We now use a pressure manometer intraoperatively. Prior to replacing the tympanomeatal flap, the manometer (or tympanometer) is used to assess the opening pressure of the now-occluded eustachian tube. A sterile olive tip probe is introduced into the external auditory canal, and the pressure is raised to 400 to 600 mm of H_2O. Maintenance of pressure in this range represents adequate occlusion of the tubal lumen. If there is a low opening pressure, there is usually an open space somewhere around the tube, and a small amount of bone paté (or bone wax) is used to fill the gap.

Indications

- Patulous eustachian tube: When the symptoms are debilitating and unrelieved by nonsurgical measures.

Anesthetic considerations and preparation

- When the transcanal approach is used, the anesthesia and the preparation are as described earlier under Transcanal Approach.

- If the endaural approach is used, the anesthesia and the preparation are as described under Endaural Approach.

Procedure

- An incision is made for an anterior tympanomeatal flap; if the anterior canal wall obscures adequate visualization of operative site, a microdrill is used for an anterior canaloplasty, or the endaural approach is used (Fig. 3–122).

- The anterior tympanomeatal flap is elevated, and the orifice of the eustachian tube is identified (Fig. 3–123).

- A small-bore polyethylene tube (e.g., No. 90) is introduced into the orifice of the eustachian tube to determine the site, direction, and approximate length of the Medicut angiocatheter to be inserted (Fig. 3–124).

• FIGURE 3-122.

An incision is made for an anterior tympanomeatal flap.

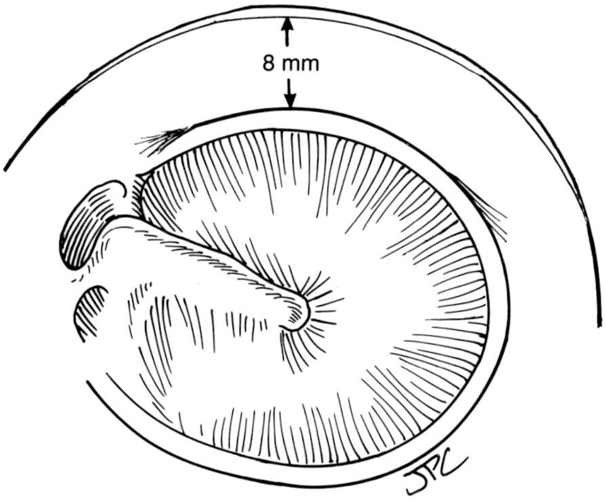

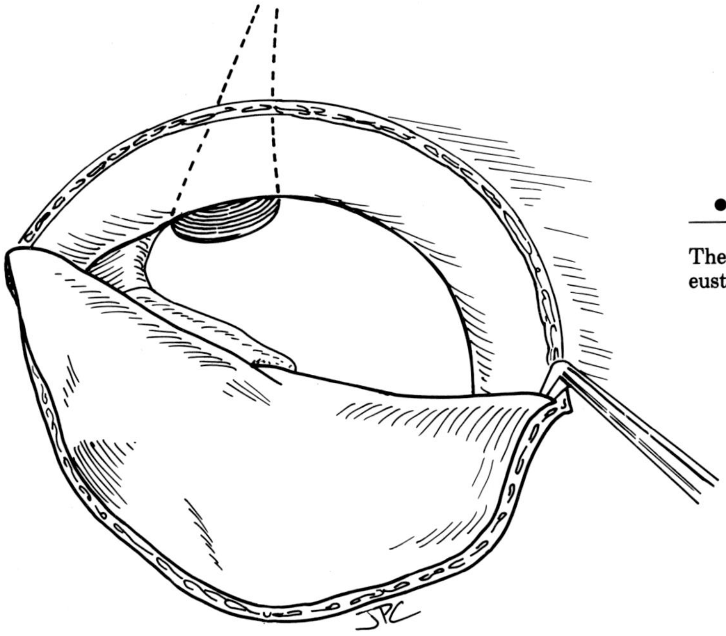

• FIGURE 3-123.

The anterior tympanomeatal flap is elevated, and the orifice of the eustachian tube is identified.

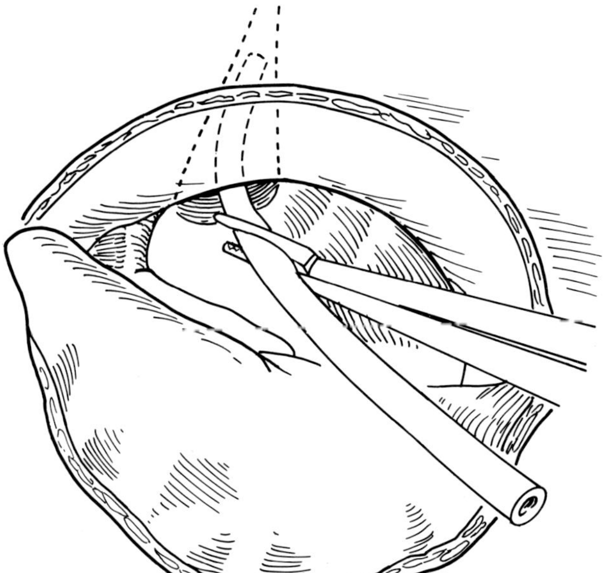

• FIGURE 3-124.

A small-bore polyethylene tube is introduced into the orifice of the eustachian tube.

- A small length of Medicut catheter is cut; a portion of the flared tip of the catheter is maintained (Fig. 3–125).
- Bone wax is inserted into the lumen of the catheter (Fig. 3–126).
- The narrow end of a Medicut catheter is inserted into the orifice of the eustachian tube until it is tightly in place and the flared end is in the middle ear but not touching the malleus (Fig. 3–127). A pressure manometer tests whether the eustachian tube is obstructed at this stage.
- A tympanostomy tube is inserted into the anteroinferior portion of the tympanic membrane (Fig. 3–128).

Postoperative care

- The immediate postoperative care is as described for either a transcanal or an endaural approach (see earlier under Transcanal Approach or Endaural Approach). The tympanostomy tube should be left in place until it spontaneously extrudes. Some patients will not require replacement of the tympanostomy tube, if their middle ear remains aerated and they are without middle ear symptoms; apparently, there is sufficient gas passing from the nasopharynx around the catheter and into the middle ear, but their eustachian tube is no longer patulous. If there is any postoperative problem with the catheter (e.g., otorrhea), it can be removed, but this should be carried out by elevating the anterior tympanomeatal flap as an operative procedure.

• FIGURE 3-125.

A small length of Medicut angiocatheter (Argyle Medicut, Sherwood Medical Industries, St. Louis, MO) is cut.

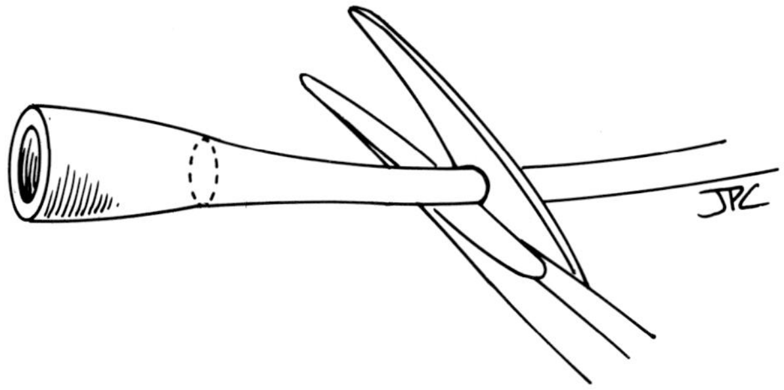

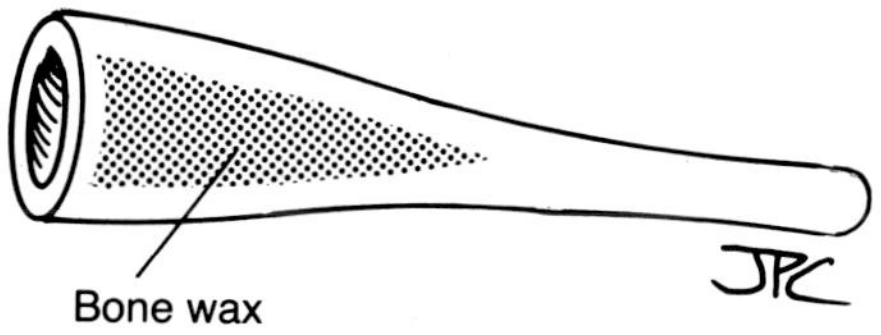

• FIGURE 3-126.

Bone wax is inserted into the lumen of the catheter.

• FIGURE 3-127.

A Medicut catheter is inserted into the orifice of the eustachian tube.

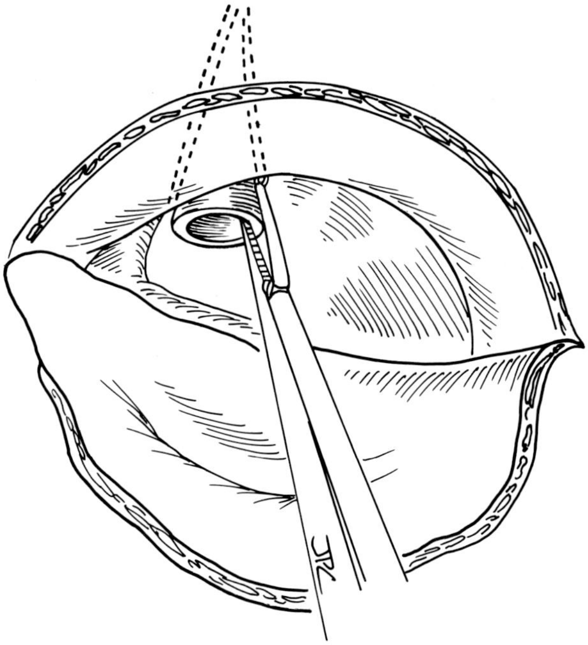

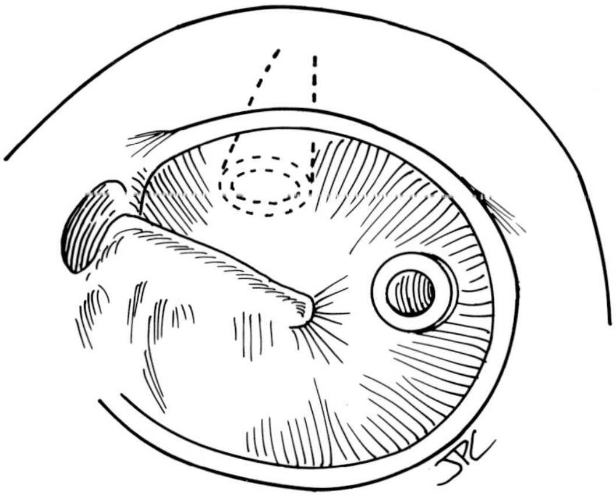

• FIGURE 3-128.

A tympanostomy tube is inserted into the tympanic membrane.

CONGENITAL DISORDERS

CONGENITAL PERILYMPHATIC FISTULA

Congenital perilymphatic fistula is a condition in which an abnormal communication between the inner and middle ears has been present since birth, which results in leakage of perilymphatic fluid (or cerebrospinal fluid) from the inner ear into the middle ear (see *Pediatric Otolaryngology*).[5] We described this condition in children originally in 1978 and subsequently in 1983.[20, 21] More recently, we reported on 94 children who had an exploratory tympanotomy for possible fistula at our hospital between 1980 and 1989.[22] Of these 94 children, 60 (63.8%) had a fistula identified at the time of surgery, and 86.3% of these patients had a congenital malformation of the middle ear (visualized at surgery), the inner ear (identified on CT scan), or both. The most common abnormality found was a congenital malformation of the stapes superstructure. We have also reported that an intraoperative test, β_2-transferrin, aids in the confirmation of some, but not all, of the leaks observed.[23] Further research is needed to determine if this test has a high enough sensitivity and specificity to warrant its routine use. In addition, the test results are available only in the postoperative period; an accurate intraoperative test is needed. Postoperatively, patients usually have no further hearing loss, and, if vertigo is present preoperatively, they are frequently asymptomatic postoperatively if a fistula is found at surgery.[21, 24]

Indications

- Congenital perilymphatic fistula: Suspected preoperatively from the history, physical findings, serial audiometry, and CT scans.

Anesthetic considerations and preparation

- The usual approach is transcanal, and the anesthesia and the preparation are as described earlier under Transcanal Approach. In infants and young children, the external canal may be too narrow for a transcanal approach, in which case we use the endaural approach (see earlier under Endaural Approach). A small area of hair is shaved above the pinna where the temporalis muscle graft is to be obtained.

Procedure

- The tympanomeatal flap is elevated for an exploratory tympanotomy (Fig. 3–129).
- Three types of malformations of stapes are frequently encountered: a posteriorly positioned anterior crus, no anterior crus, or a monopod stapes (Fig. 3–130).
- Because the anatomy of the stapes superstructure is difficult to visualize, a 90-degree pick is used to palpate the crura and obturator foramen to determine if an abnormality is present (Fig. 3–131). A leak is frequently seen in the anterior footplate area.

• FIGURE 3-129.

The tympanomeatal flap is elevated for an exploratory tympanotomy.

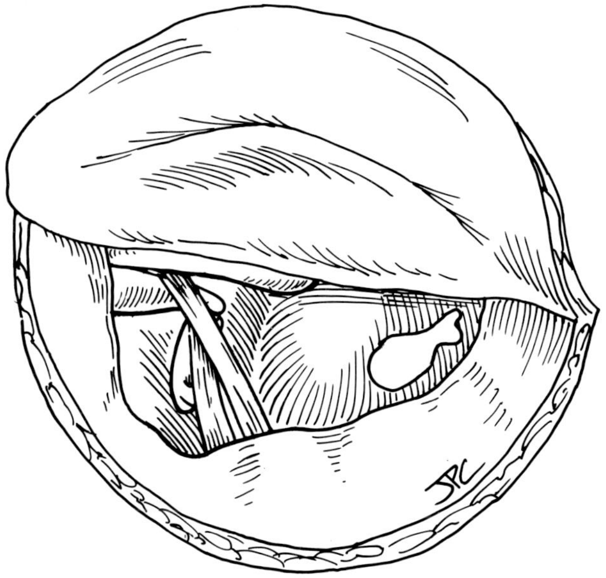

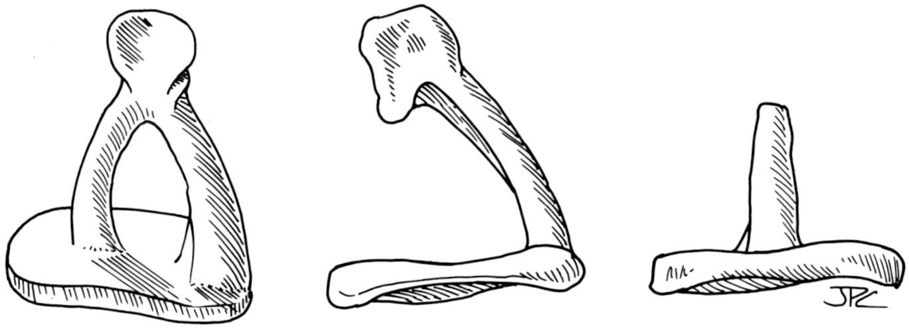

• FIGURE 3-130.

Three types of malformations of stapes are frequently encountered.

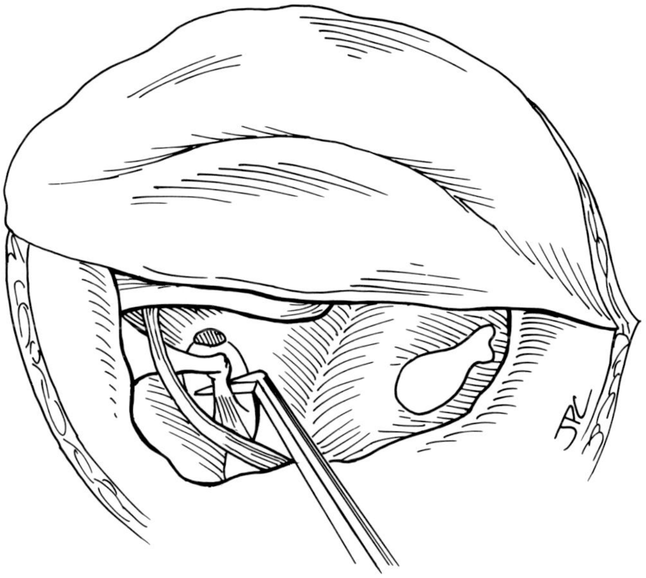

• FIGURE 3-131.

A 90-degree pick is used to palpate the crura and obturator foramen.

- A small pledget of Gelfoam is placed over the stapes footplate, and another pledget is placed over the round window; both remain in place for a few minutes and then are sent to the immunopathology laboratory for β_2-transferrin test (Fig. 3–132).

- An incision is made slightly above the hairline to remove a small piece of temporalis muscle for a graft (Fig. 3–133). The donor site is closed with absorbable suture.

- Mucosa around the stapes footplate and the round window niche is denuded for the graft site (Fig. 3–134).

- Small pieces of muscle are laid over the stapes footplate and in and around the round window niche. A layer of Gelfoam is placed over the muscle grafts, and the tympanomeatal flap is replaced (Fig. 3–135).

Postoperative care

- If a perilymphatic fistula is identified at surgery, the child is kept at bedrest overnight, and the patient and parents are counseled about the type of physical activity permitted in the future to prevent a recurrence of the fistula. In general, we recommend avoiding activities that grossly elevate cerebrospinal fluid pressure (e.g., weight-lifting, pushups, situps) and activities that rapidly alter middle ear pressure, such as diving in water (especially scuba) and flying in unpressurized cabins of airplanes.

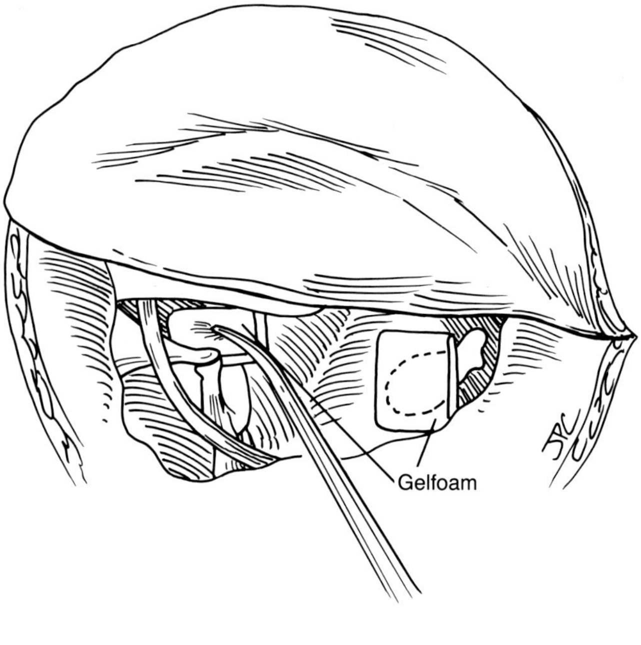

• FIGURE 3–132.

Small pledgets of Gelfoam are placed over the stapes footplate and the round window.

• FIGURE 3-133.

An incision is made slightly above the hairline to remove a small piece of temporalis muscle for a graft.

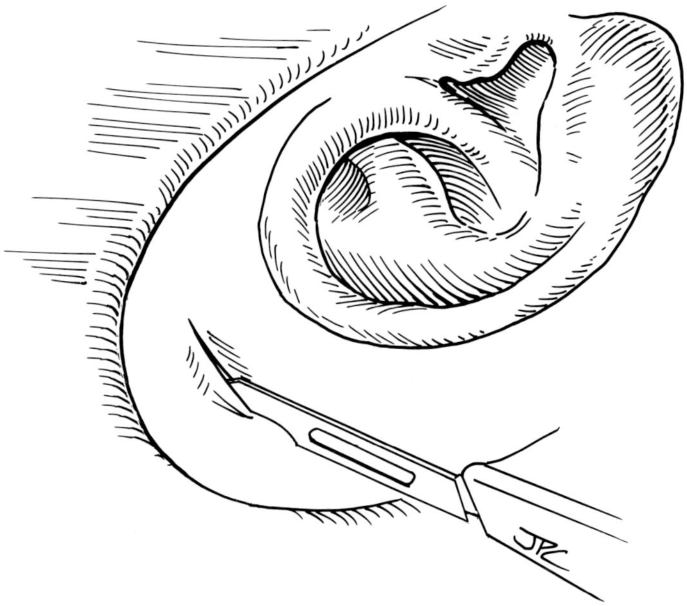

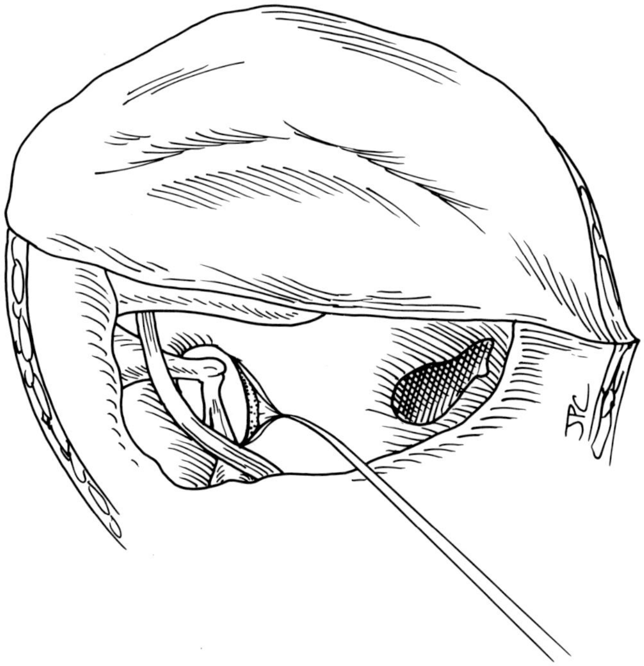

• FIGURE 3-134.

The mucosa around the stapes footplate and the round window niche is denuded for the graft site.

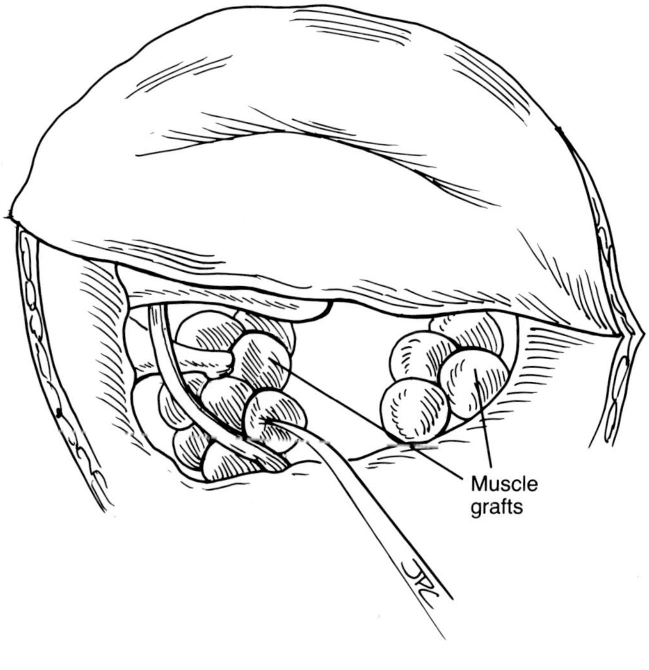

• FIGURE 3-135.

Small pieces of muscle are laid over the stapes footplate and in and around the round window niche.

CONGENITAL CHOLESTEATOMA

In general, the surgical procedures that are performed to remove an acquired cholesteatoma are employed when a congenital cholesteatoma is diagnosed; often, the cause of the cholesteatoma is uncertain when the disease is far advanced. However, because the tympanic membrane is intact when a congenital cholesteatoma is diagnosed early, there are two anatomic sites and procedures that are used that are not described in the section on Acquired Cholesteatoma (see earlier): (1) intratympanic membrane cholesteatoma; and (2) cholesteatoma posterior to the anterosuperior quadrant of an intact tympanic membrane. Both of these anatomic sites are relatively frequently encountered in infants and children. In our study of 45 surgical procedures for congenital cholesteatoma (intratympanic membrane cholesteatoma was excluded from the analysis), 56% were only middle ear procedures (with and without atticotomy), 13% were canal wall-up tympanomastoidectomies, 9% were modified radical mastoidectomies, and 20% were radical mastoidectomies to eradicate the disease.[4]

Indications

- Intratympanic membrane congenital cholesteatoma
- Congenital cholesteatoma medial to the anterosuperior quadrant of the pars tensa of the intact tympanic membrane

Anesthetic considerations and preparation

- The anesthesia and the preparation depend on the site and the approach. For an intratympanic membrane cholesteatoma, the anesthesia and preparation are similar to those described earlier under Tympanostomy Tube Insertion. For a congenital cholesteatoma that is within the middle ear and epitympanum, the anesthesia and preparations are the same as described earlier under Endaural Approach or Transcanal Approach.

Procedure

CONGENITAL CHOLESTEATOMA: INTRATYMPANIC MEMBRANE

- Congenital cholesteatoma within the intact tympanic membrane (Fig. 3–136).
- Cholesteatoma is removed with a pick; a cup forceps is also used (Fig. 3–137).
- A Steri-Strip patch is placed over the defect if a perforation is present and it is small. If the perforation is large, a tissue graft myringoplasty is performed (see earlier under Tympanostomy Tube Removal and Repair of the Defect with Steri-Strip Patch Myringoplasty) (Fig. 3–138).

CONGENITAL CHOLESTEATOMA: ANTEROSUPERIOR MESOTYMPANUM AND EPITYMPANUM MEDIAL TO THE INTACT TYMPANIC MEMBRANE

- A congenital cholesteatoma is visualized in the medial to anterosuperior quadrant of the intact tympanic membrane (Fig. 3–139).

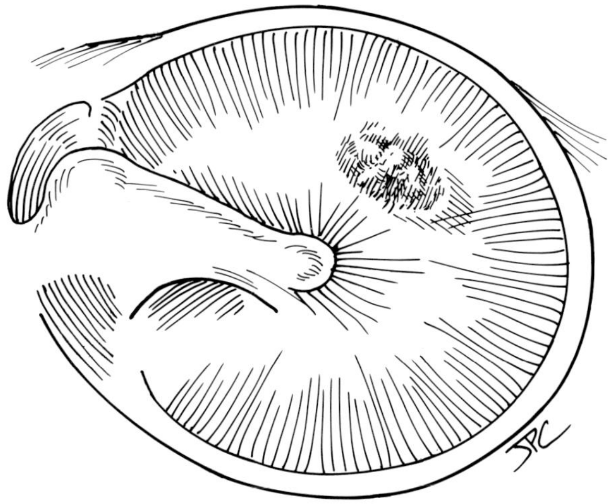

• FIGURE 3-136.

Congenital cholesteatoma within the intact tympanic membrane.

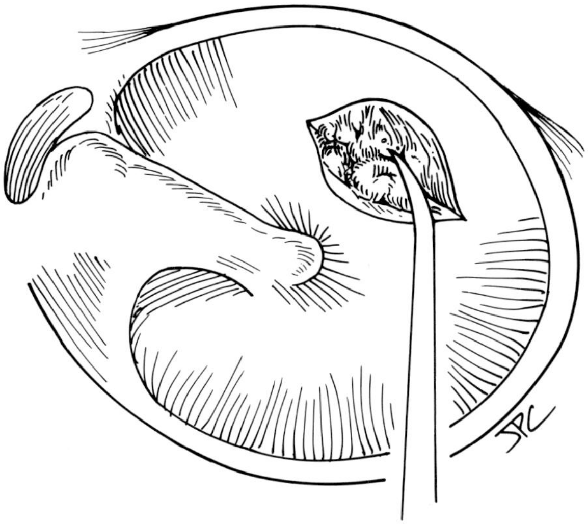

• FIGURE 3-137.

Cholesteatoma is removed with a curved pick.

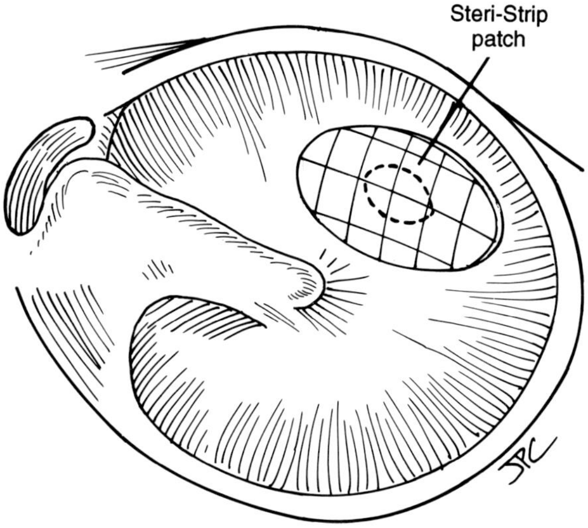

• FIGURE 3-138.

A Steri-Strip patch is placed over the defect.

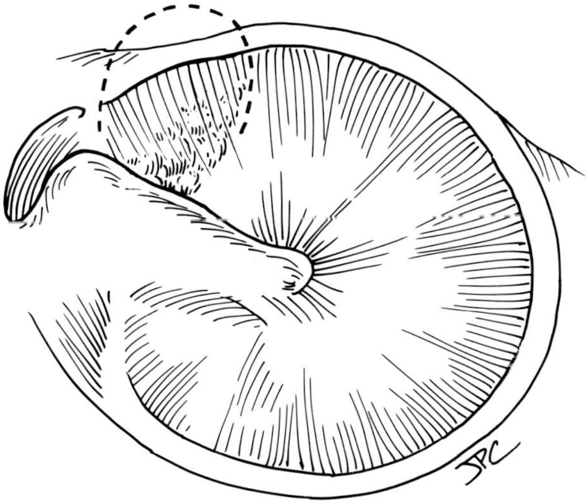

• FIGURE 3-139.

A congenital cholesteatoma is visualized in the medial to anterosuperior quadrant of the intact tympanic membrane.

- Endaural incisions (see earlier under Endaural Approach) and approach are used if the cholesteatoma is localized to the anterior mesotympanum and the anterior epitympanum (as noted on the CT scan) (Fig. 3–140*A*). A transcanal approach is used (see earlier under Transcanal Approach), if feasible; a modified tympanomeatal flap is extended onto the anterior canal wall for exposure (Fig. 3–140*B*).
- An anterior atticotomy is done with a microdrill, and the cholesteatoma is removed (for more extensive disease see earlier under Acquired Cholesteatoma) (Fig. 3–141).
- The tympanomeatal flap is replaced (Fig. 3–142).

Postoperative care

- The postoperative care is dependent on the approach used (see earlier under Endaural Approach and Transcanal Approach). A "second look" exploratory tympanotomy is usually performed 6 months after the procedure to remove a middle ear and epitympanic cholesteatoma, to determine if residual cholesteatoma is present; the site and extent of the cholesteatoma, the status of the hearing, and the degree of translucency of the tympanic membrane are key factors in recommending a "second look" operation (see earlier under Acquired Cholesteatoma).

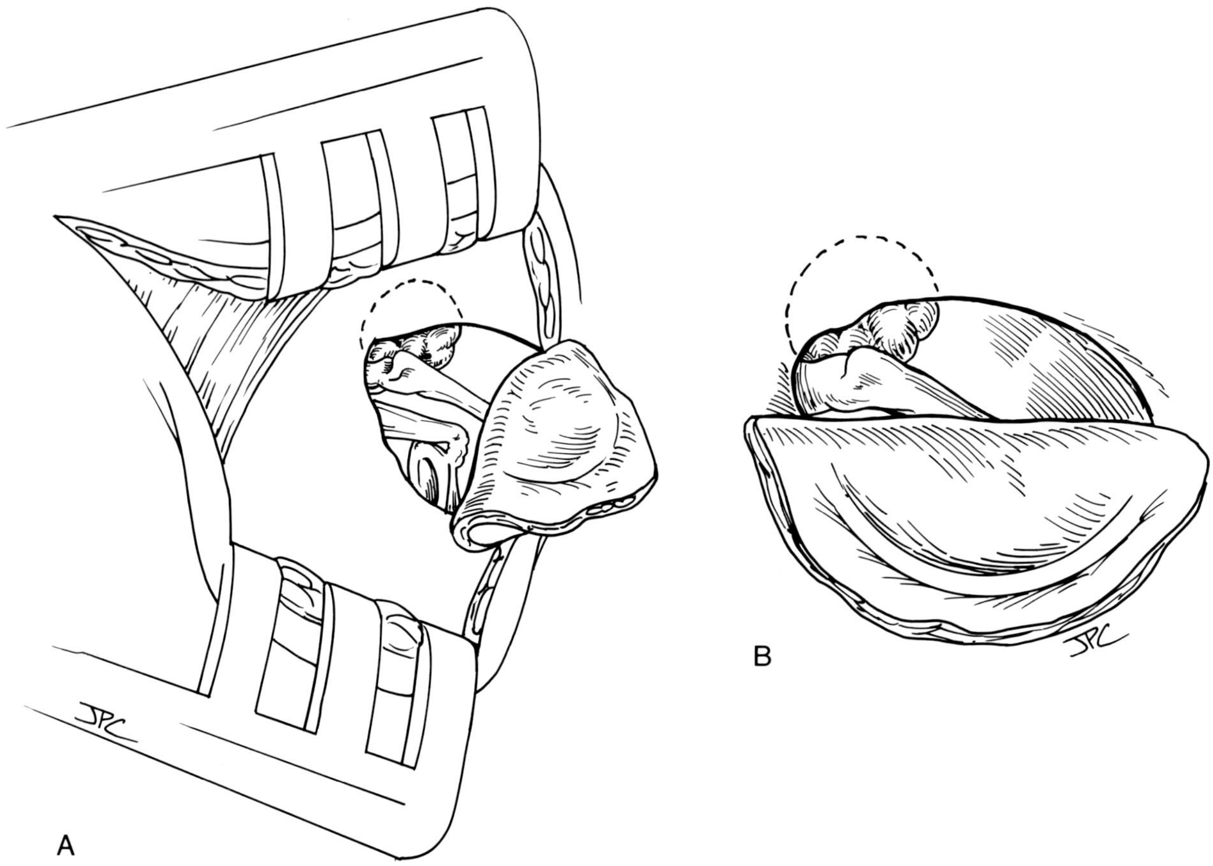

• FIGURE 3–140.

A, Endaural incisions and the approach when localized to the anterior mesotympanum and the anterior epitympanum. *B*, Transcanal approach is used, if feasible.

• FIGURE 3-141.

An anterior atticotomy is done with a microdrill, and cholesteatomas are removed.

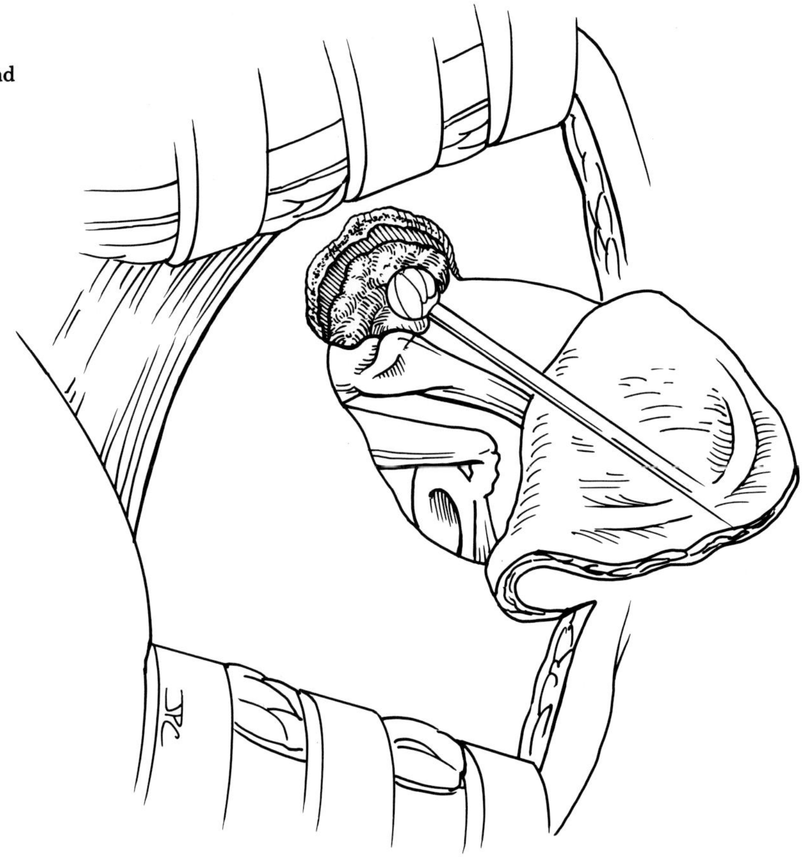

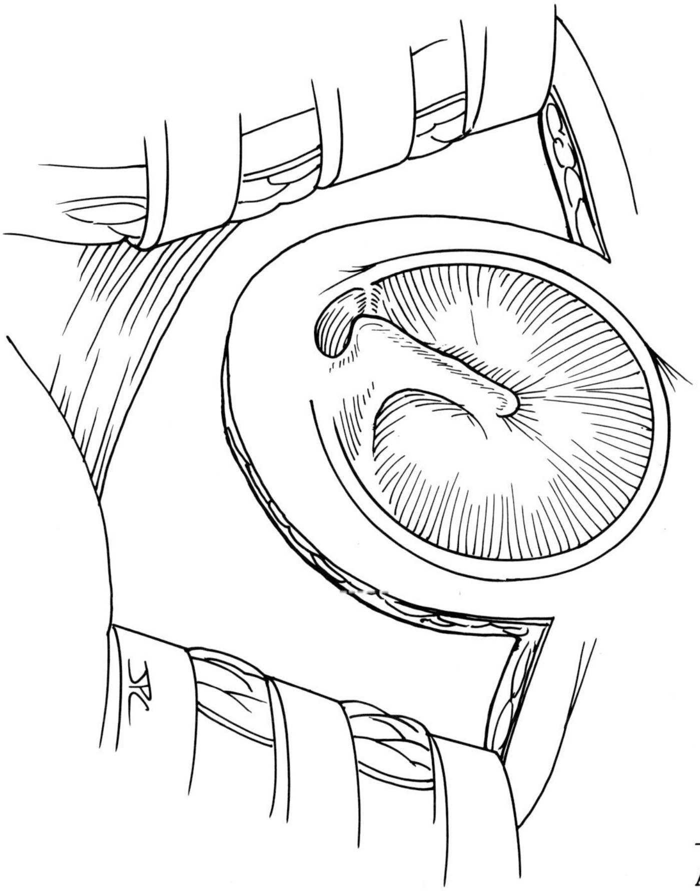

• FIGURE 3-142.

A tympanomeatal flap is replaced.

LOP EAR OTOPLASTY

A lop ear is the abnormal protrusion of the auricle, which is most commonly due to a poorly developed or an absent fold of the antihelix. The angle between the scapha and concha is produced by the antihelix. The goal of otoplasty for lop ear is to construct a normally appearing antihelix in which the superior crus of the antihelix is rounded and smooth, not sharp. Prior to undertaking surgery to correct lop ear, the surgeon should be fully familiar with the anatomy of both the anterior and posterior aspects of the cartilage of the auricle. The procedure that I use is a modification of the one originally described by Becker.[1]

Anatomy of Anterior and Posterior Auricular Cartilage

The anatomy of the auricular cartilage is shown (Figs. 3–143 and 3–144). The parts of the cartilage of the auricle that are prominent on the anterior surface will be depressions on the posterior surface, and vice versa. For example, the fossa triangularis on the anterior surface is the eminentia triangularis on the posterior surface of the auricle.

Indications

- Otoplasty is indicated when both the child and the parents agree that a lop ear deformity is causing psychologic disturbance to the child.
- The procedure is best performed when the auricle has reached maturation and the child is old enough to understand the problem, desires the operation, and can cooperate with the postoperative care, which is usually at 5 years of age and older.
- Caution should be exercised when recommending otoplasty if the child is known to form keloids or has a severe and extensive deformity of the auricle that involves more than just the antihelix.
- When the child has a unilateral moderate-to-severe deformity that is to be corrected and the contralateral ear appears normal, naturally only the deformed ear should be operated on. However, when the contralateral ear has even a mild deformity, a bilateral otoplasty should be performed to ensure postoperative symmetry of the ears.

• FIGURE 3-143.

The anatomy of the anterior surface of auricular cartilage.

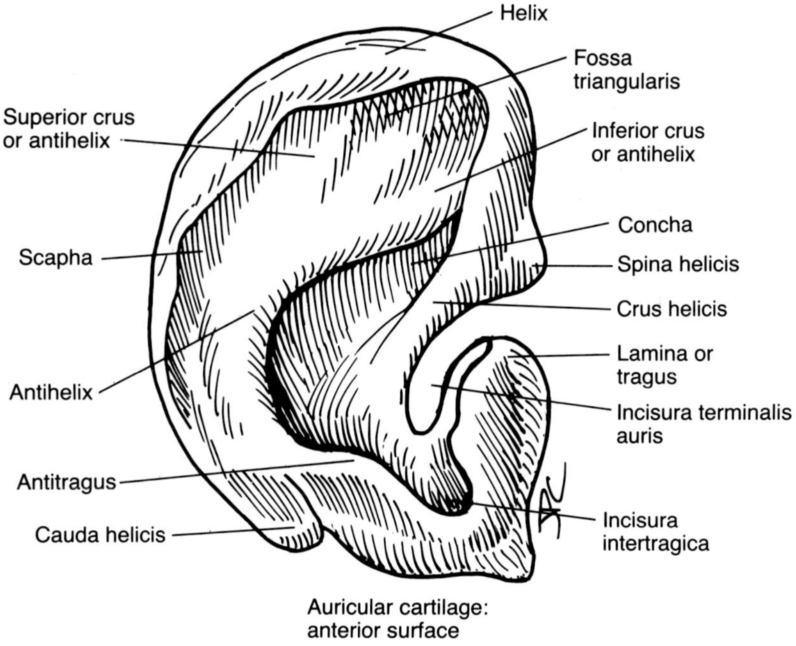

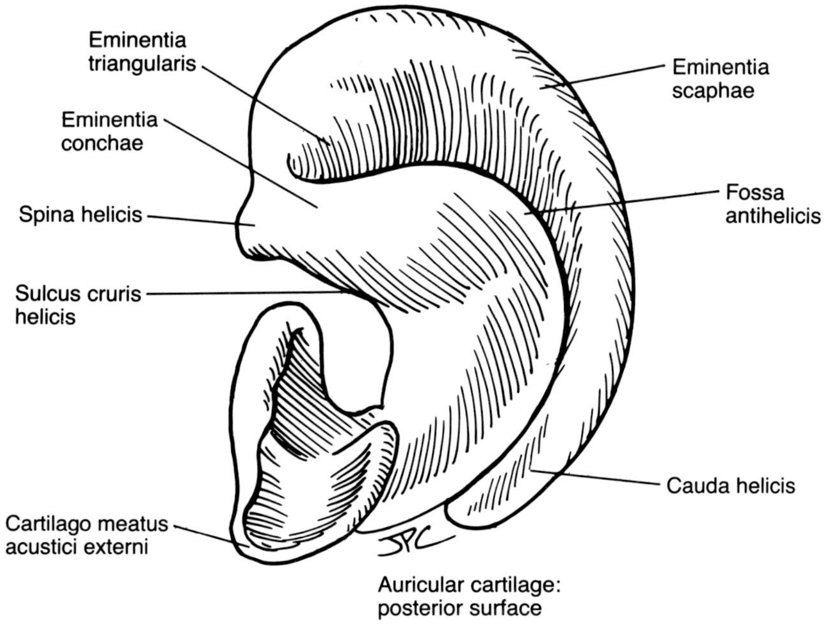

• FIGURE 3-144.

The anatomy of the posterior surface of auricular cartilage.

Anesthetic considerations

- The procedure in children is performed under general endotracheal anesthesia; however, in some adolescents, the operation can be carried out with only local infiltrative anesthesia and with the aid of intravenous analgesia.

- Infiltration of the postauricular skin using 1% lidocaine (Xylocaine) containing 1:100,000 epinephrine for hemostasis.

Preparation

- Prior to performing the procedure, photographs should be obtained that show the full head and ears of the patient. Frontal, posterior, and both right and left sides should be included. These preoperative photographs can then be compared with postoperative ones usually obtained 6 months after the operation.

- Following the usual preoperative sterilization of the auricle, the ear is draped. When both ears are to be operated on, both ears can be prepared and draped. However, care should be taken not to fold the first auricle forward toward the face when the contralateral ear is being operated on. Also, when both ears are to be corrected, the surgeon should try not to repeatedly turn the patient's head from side to side, because the larynx may become traumatized by these movements owing to the endotracheal tube's injuring the subglottic space.

- Cotton pledgets can be placed into the external auditory canal to prevent blood from entering and forming a clot, which, when present in the postoperative period, can be troublesome to both the surgeon and the patient.

Procedure

- By folding the pinna back into the desired position, the amount of redundant postauricular skin to be excised is estimated (Fig. 3–145).

- An elliptical portion of skin to be excised is outlined with methylene blue and injected with lidocaine and epinephrine (Fig. 3–146).

- The excess skin is excised from the postauricular incisions and discarded (Fig. 3–147).

• FIGURE 3-145.

The pinna folded back into desired position to estimate amount of redundant postauricular skin to be excised.

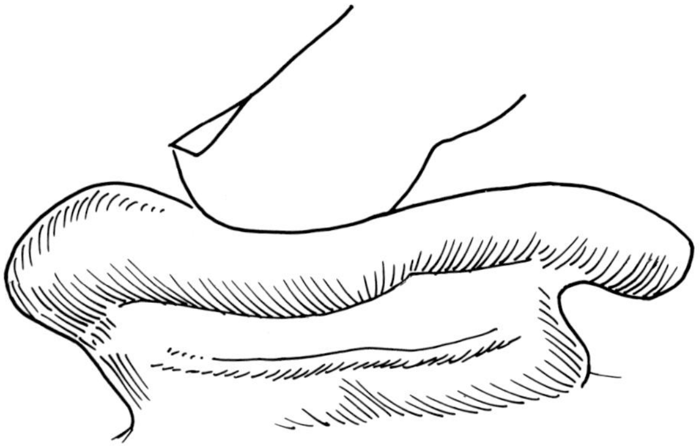

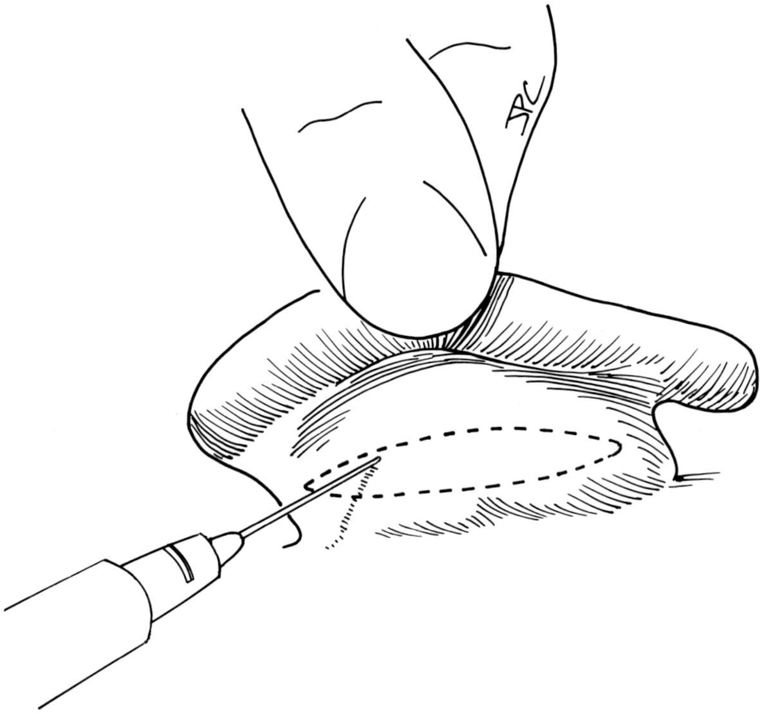

• FIGURE 3-146.

An elliptical portion of skin to be excised is outlined with methylene blue and injected with local anesthetic agent.

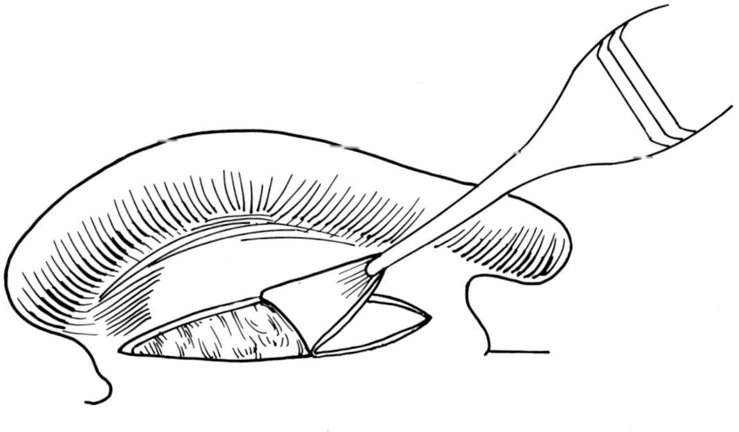

• FIGURE 3-147.

Postauricular skin is excised and discarded.

• Undermining of postauricular skin and the perichondrium to the eminentia scaphae is done, exposing the cauda helicus and fissura antiragohelicina (Fig. 3–148).

• Cartilage incisions are made along the outer edge of the eminentia scaphae (hidden anteriorly in the scapha under the helix), which is the outer border of new antihelix, and the eminentia conchae (hidden anteriorly under new antihelix), which is the inner border of the new antihelix (Fig. 3–149). This inner incision is carried through the middle of the cauda helicus. Incisions go through cartilage but not through skin on the anterior surface of the auricle (i.e., "button-hole"). Keith needles placed through the anterior surface of the auricle are used to identify where most appropriate outer and inner incisions (marked with methylene blue at the needle puncture sites on the posterior auricular surface) are to be made on the posterior surface of the auricle.

• A new antihelix is undermined partially on the outer and inner surfaces, leaving a new antihelix attached in the middle (Fig. 3–150).

• The outer and inner edges of the new antihelix are rolled to almost approximate each other and are sutured in place using a 4-0 white Mersolene suture (Fig. 3–151).

• About three to five sutures are used and inverted to bury the knot in the depths of the new antihelix (Fig. 3–152).

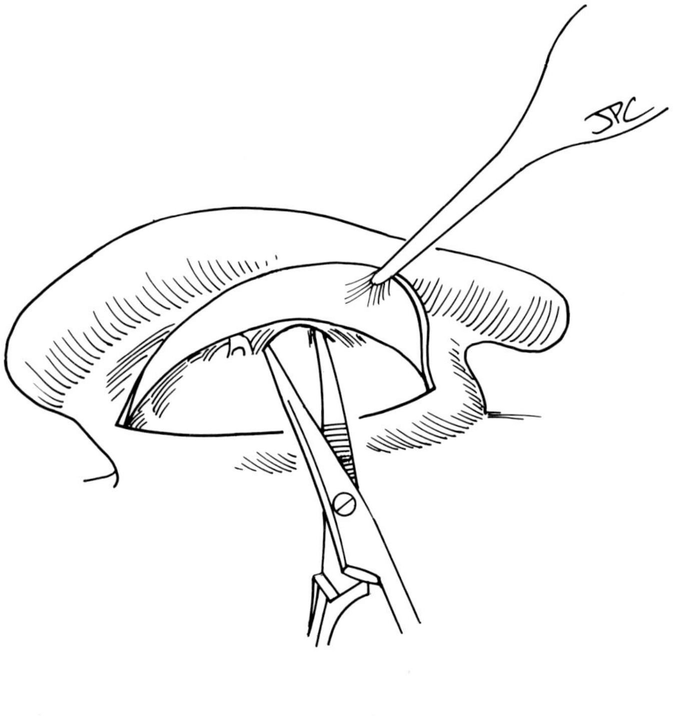

• FIGURE 3–148.

Undermining of the postauricular skin and the perichondrium.

• FIGURE 3-149.

Incisions are made along the outer edge of the eminentia scaphae and the eminentia conchae.

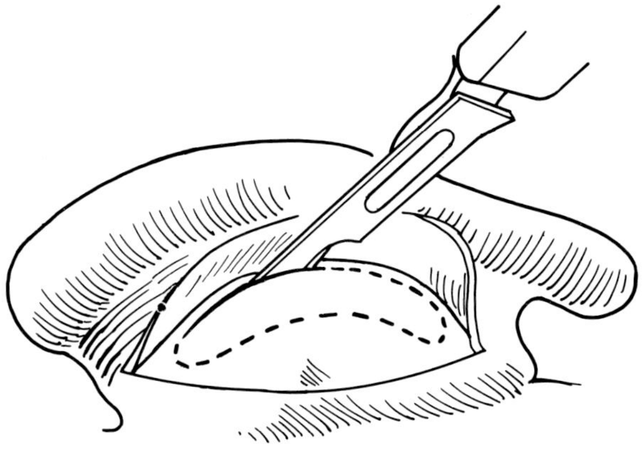

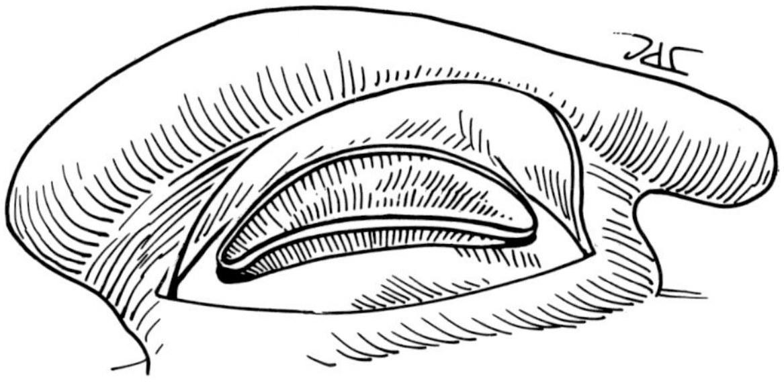

• FIGURE 3-150.

A new antihelix is undermined partially on the outer and inner surfaces.

• FIGURE 3-151.

The outer and inner edges of the new antihelix are rolled to almost approximate each other and sutured.

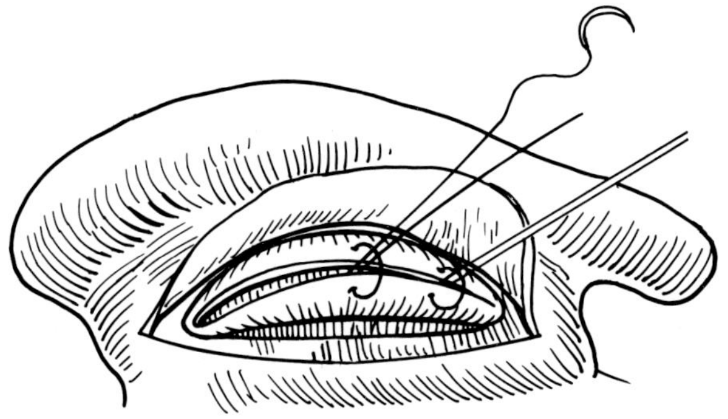

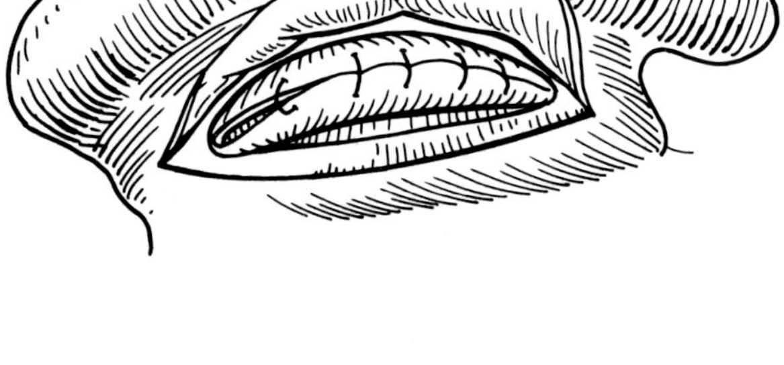

• FIGURE 3-152.

Sutures are used and inverted to bury the knot in the depths of the new antihelix.

- Two small bolsters made of Adaptic are placed on the anterior surface of the auricle on each side of the new antihelix and sutured in place with 4-0 silk mattress sutures (Fig. 3–153).

- The postauricular wound is closed with an interrupted absorbable suture; a drain is used only if bleeding has been a problem (Fig. 3–154).

Postoperative care

- Cotton impregnated with glycerine is inserted into the external meatus of the canal, concha, and scapha. A fluff dressing is placed over the anterior surface of the pinna, and a piece of Adaptic and one or two 4 × 4″ gauze pads are placed between the posterior surface of the auricle and the temporal bone.

- Bilateral mastoid pressure dressings are applied and changed the following day to determine if a hematoma has developed; if one has, it must be evacuated, or the auricle will have a permanent thickened appearance. The mastoid dressing is replaced and changed again 4 days following the surgery, at which time the bolsters are removed. The mastoid dressing remains for a total of 2 weeks, after which the child wears a stockinette over the ears for an additional 3 months when sleeping.

ACKNOWLEDGMENTS

I am indebted to Cuneyt Alper, M.D., for his assistance in the preparation of this chapter, and to my colleague and friend Herman Felder, M.D., for his innovative ideas in the development of the lateral graft tympanoplasty technique that is described in this chapter.

• FIGURE 3-153.

Two small bolsters made of Adaptic are placed on the anterior surface of the auricle on each side of the new antihelix.

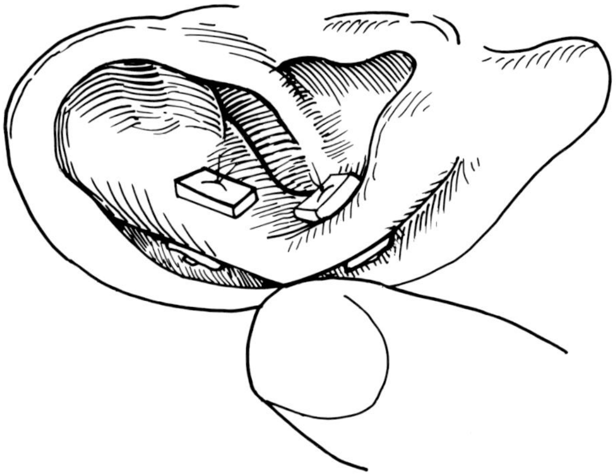

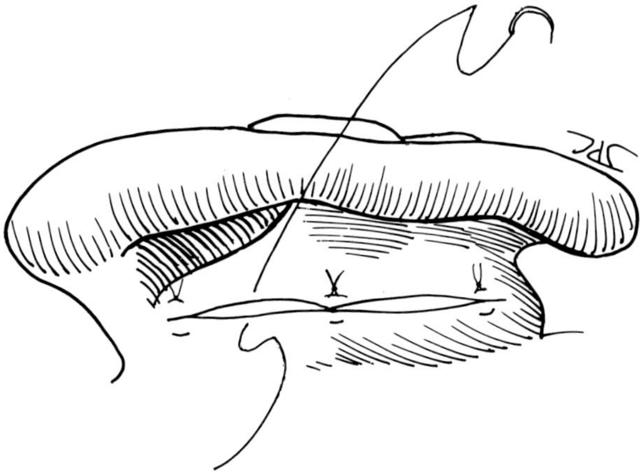

• FIGURE 3-154.

The postauricular wound is closed.

REFERENCES

1. Becker OJ: Surgical correction of the abnormally protruding ear. Arch Otolaryngol 50:541–560, 1949.
2. Bluestone CD, Cantekin EI, and Douglas GS: Eustachian tube function related to tympanoplasty in children. Laryngoscope 89:450–458, 1979.
3. Manning SC, Cantekin EI, Kenna MA et al: Prognostic value of eustachian tube function in pediatric tympanoplasty. Laryngoscope 97:1012–1016, 1987.
4. Rosenfeld RM, Moura RL, and Bluestone CD: Predictors of residual-recurrent cholesteatoma in children. Arch Otolaryngol Head Neck Surg 118:384–391, 1992.
5. Bluestone CD and Stool SE (eds): Pediatric Otolaryngology, 2nd ed., Vols 1 and 2. Philadelphia, WB Saunders, 1990; Bluestone CD, Stool SE, and Kenna MA (eds): Pediatric Otolaryngology, 3rd ed., vol 1: Philadelphia, WB Saunders, 1995 (in press).
6. Glasscock ME and Shambaugh GE: Surgery of the Ear, 4th ed. Philadelphia, WB Saunders, 1990.
7. Goycoolea MV, Paparella MM, and Nissen RL (eds): Atlas of Otologic Surgery. Philadelphia, WB Saunders, 1989.
8. Nadol JB and Schuknecht HF: Surgery of the Ear and the Temporal Bone. New York, Raven Press, 1993.
9. Arriaga MA, Bluestone CD, and Stool SE: The role of tympanocentesis in the management of infants with sepsis. Laryngoscope 99:1048–1051, 1989.
10. Kaleida PH, Casselbrant ML, Rockette HE et al: Amoxicillin or myringotomy or both for acute otitis media: Results of a randomized clinical trial. Pediatrics 87:466–474, 1991.
11. Casselbrant ML, Kaleida PH, Rockette HE, et al: Efficacy of antimicrobial prophylaxis and tympanostomy tube insertion for prevention of recurrent acute otitis media: Results of a randomized clinical trial. Pediatr Infect Dis J 11:278–286, 1992.
12. Mandel EM, Rockette HE, Bluestone CD et al: Myringotomy with and without tympanostomy tubes for chronic otitis media with effusion. Arch Otolaryngol Head Neck Surg 115:1217–1224, 1989.
13. Mandel EM, Rockette HE, Bluestone CD et al: Efficacy of myringotomy with and without tympanostomy tubes for chronic otitis media with effusion. Pediatr Infect Dis J 11:270–277, 1992.
14. Per-Lee JH: Long-term middle ear ventilation. Laryngoscope 91:1063–1073, 1981.
15. Rosen S: Mobilization of the stapes to restore hearing in otosclerosis. NY J Med 53:2650–2653, 1953.
16. Lempert J: Endaural, antauricular surgical approach to the temporal bone: Principles involved in this new approach. Summary report of 1,780 cases. Arch Otolaryngol Head Neck Surg 27:555–587, 1937.
17. Khanna SM and Tonndorf J: Tympanic membrane vibration in cats studied by time-averaged holography. J Acoust Soc Am 51:1904, 1972.
18. Bluestone CD and Cantekin EI: Management of the patulous eustachian tube. Laryngoscope 91:149–152, 1981.
19. Magit AE and Bluestone CD: Catheter occlusion of the patulous eustachian tube (Abstract). Proceedings of the American Otolaryngological, Rhinological, and Laryngological Society, Western Section Meeting, 1992.
20. Grundfast KM and Bluestone CD: Sudden or fluctuating hearing loss or vertigo in children due to perilymph fistula. Ann Otol Rhinol Laryngol 87:761–771, 1978.
21. Supance JS and Bluestone CD: Perilymph fistula in infants and children. Otolaryngol Head Neck Surg 91:663–671, 1983.
22. Weber PC, Perez BA, and Bluestone CD: Congenital perilymphatic fistula and associated middle ear abnormalities. Laryngoscope 103:160–164, 1993.
23. Weber PC, Kelly RH, Bluestone CD, and Bassiouny M: Beta-2 transferrin confirms perilymph fistula in children. Otolaryngol Head Neck Surg (In press).
24. Weber PC, Bluestone CD, and Perez B: Outcome of hearing and vertigo following surgery for congenital perilymphatic fistula in children. Abstract, presented at annual meeting of the American Society of Pediatric Otolaryngology, Los Angeles, CA, April 21, 1993.

chapter

4

The Facial Nerve

RAYMOND L. HILSINGER, JR., M.D.

Surgical procedures of or around the facial nerve epitomize much of what is challenging and intriguing about the specialty of otolaryngology–head and neck surgery. To be successful, the head and neck surgeon must have a precise knowledge of anatomy; the ability to handle traumatic, neoplastic, infectious, idiopathic, and congenital diseases; the skills to manage emergent, urgent, and routine situations; and the technical expertise to do both macroscopic and microscopic surgery in an open operative field as well as in a confined space.

For surgical purposes, the facial nerve can be divided into intracranial, intratemporal, and extratemporal segments. The intratemporal segment can be further divided into meatal (internal auditory canal), labyrinthine (petrous), tympanic (horizontal), and mastoid (vertical) subsegments (Fig. 4–1).[1]

The intracranial segment of the motor branch of the facial nerve emerges from the inferior border of the pons between the olive and the inferior cerebellar peduncle, medial to the vestibulocochlear nerve and the nervus intermedius (intermediate nerve).[1-3] The nerve then courses laterally in the cerebellopontine angle.

The intratemporal segment begins as the nerve enters the internal auditory meatus at the medial end of the internal auditory canal. The facial nerve occupies the anterior, superior area of the canal and courses laterally in a horizontal plane just superior to the cochlear nerve and anterior to the nervus intermedius. In its most lateral aspect, it is separated from the cochlear nerve by the falciform crest and from the superior vestibular nerve by the vertical crest, just before it passes through the orifice of the facial (fallopian) canal.[1-3]

The labyrinthine subsegment begins medially at the orifice of the facial canal and continues laterally but angles slightly anteriorly and inferiorly for 3 to 5 mm to the first turn (genu) just posterior to the geniculate fossa and geniculate ganglion.[1-3]

The facial nerve bends 75 degrees to course posteriorly and slightly laterally and inferiorly at about a 10-degree angle from horizontal for about 1 cm in its tympanic subsegment. From anterior to posterior, the tympanic subsegment is positioned just superior and posterior to the cochleariform process, superior to the oval window, and inferior and slightly medial to the lateral semicircular canal.[1-3]

The second turn (genu) begins at the posterior end of the tympanic subsegment (just posterior to the oval window) and bends from 95 to 125 degrees just inferior to the lateral semicircular canal, to begin the mastoid subsegment of the intratemporal segment of the facial nerve. In neonates and small children, the second turn of the nerve is more acute and courses in a more lateral fashion because of the incompletely developed mastoid bone. The mastoid subsegment runs inferiorly at an angle from 5 degrees to between 30 and 35 degrees from vertical and usually slightly laterally until it exits the stylomastoid foramen. The length of the mastoid subsegment varies depending on the development of the mastoid process and on the location of the stylomastoid foramen, from which the intratemporal facial nerve exits the temporal bone. In the newborn, the stylomastoid foramen may be at the level of the mastoid antrum, but as the squamous portion of the mastoid process grows, the foramen moves inferiorly, always posterior to the styloid process.[1-3]

After the facial nerve exits the stylomastoid foramen, the extratemporal segment of the nerve begins. The nerve courses anteriorly and slightly laterally to enter the parotid gland and then passes lateral to the mandible and masseter muscle within the gland, separating the gland into superficial and deep portions.

In small children, the nerve enters the parotid gland in a more anterior location because the parotid gland is smaller and located more anteriorly.[4]

At about the posterior border of the mandible, the facial nerve divides into temporofacial and cervicofacial branches. The temporofacial branch further divides into temporal (frontal), zygomatic, and buccal branches; the cervicofacial branch further divides into buccal, mandibular, and cervical branches. Many

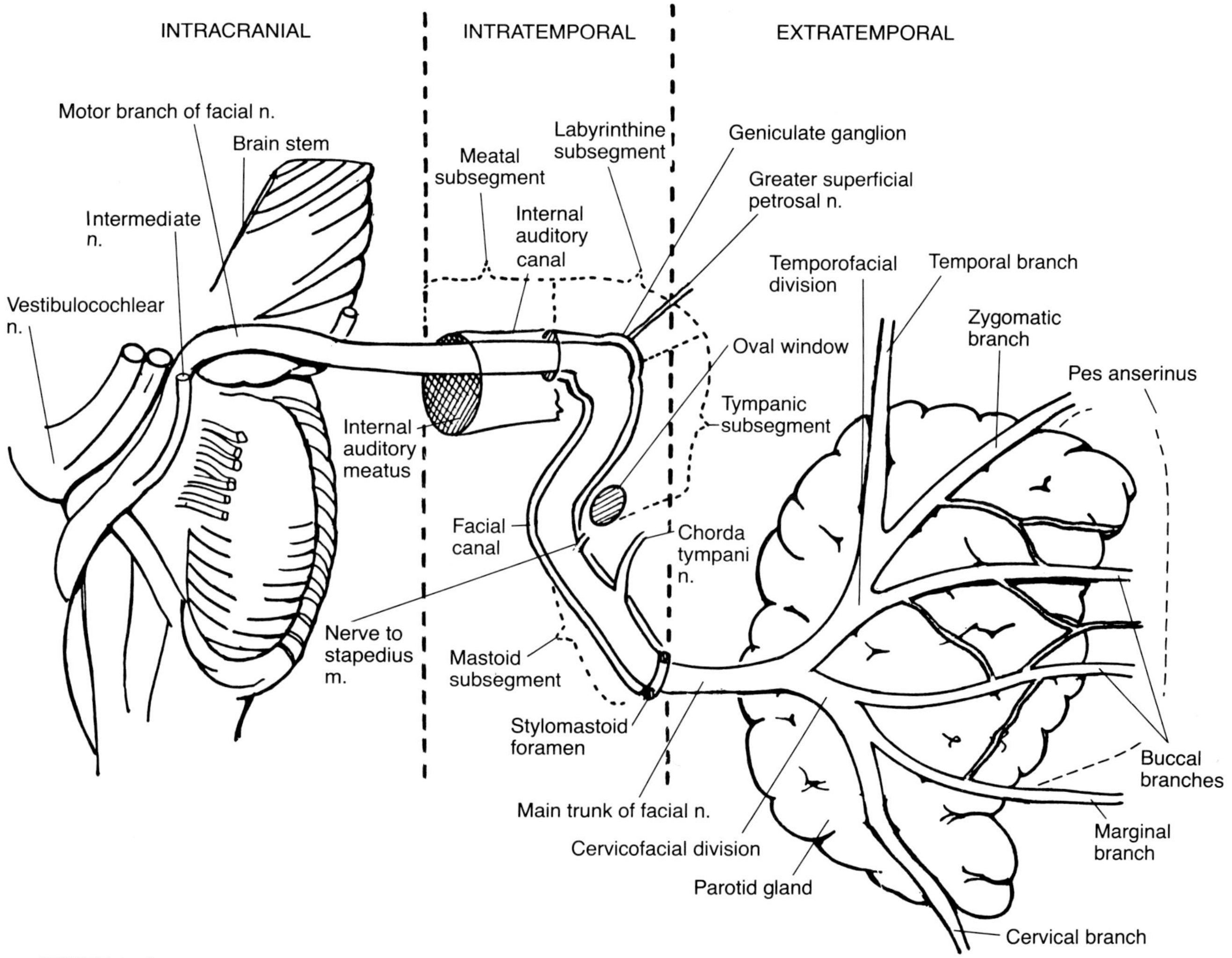

• FIGURE 4-1.

Schematic anatomy of the right facial nerve.

anatomic variations as well as multiple cross-anastomoses can be found (particularly between the buccal branches), and this interconnecting plexus of branches is called the pes anserinus.

Surgically, an intracranial, intratemporal, extratemporal, or combined approach can be used to expose the facial nerve. This chapter describes surgical approaches to the facial nerve from the geniculate ganglion peripherally.

INTRATEMPORAL BONE FACIAL NERVE PROCEDURES

EXPLORATION OR EXPLORATION WITH DECOMPRESSION

Intratemporal procedures are done to explore and visualize the course of the facial nerve or to decompress the nerve by removing the lateral bony facial canal wall. In cases of acute or chronic infection, a drainage procedure (mastoidectomy with enlargement of the aditus ad antrum, with or without a wide myringotomy and large tympanostomy tube) may suffice. A modified or radical mastoidectomy may be required when the surgeon needs to remove bony fragments, cholesteatoma, or extrinsic neoplasms compressing the nerve. When exploration reveals a missing nerve segment or when a facial nerve neuroma is excised, an interposition graft is often required.

Indications

- Peripheral facial nerve paralysis caused by
  - Blunt or penetrating head trauma (usually resulting in temporal bone fracture and immediate paralysis) with computed tomography (CT) scan or magnetic resonance imaging (MRI) evidence of disruption of the facial canal and compression or disruption of the facial nerve
  - Iatrogenic injury
    - Detected at the time of injury during middle ear or mastoid surgery
    - Noted after middle ear or mastoid surgery during which the facial nerve may not have been visualized
  - Prolonged labor or difficult vaginal delivery (or both), with or without the use of forceps and associated with
    - Hemotympanum or other evidence of temporal bone fracture
    - Complete immediate facial nerve paralysis or progression to complete loss of facial function
  - Acute otitis media that does not resolve in 4 to 6 weeks after wide myringotomy, simple mastoidectomy with enlargement of the aditus ad antrum, and use of antibiotics
  - Chronic suppurative otitis media with tympanic membrane perforation that does not resolve after mastoidectomy with enlargement of the aditus ad antrum and use of topical and parenteral antibiotics
  - Chronic suppurative otitis media with cholesteatoma
  - Congenital cholesteatoma or neoplasm in the temporal bone
  - Facial nerve neuroma

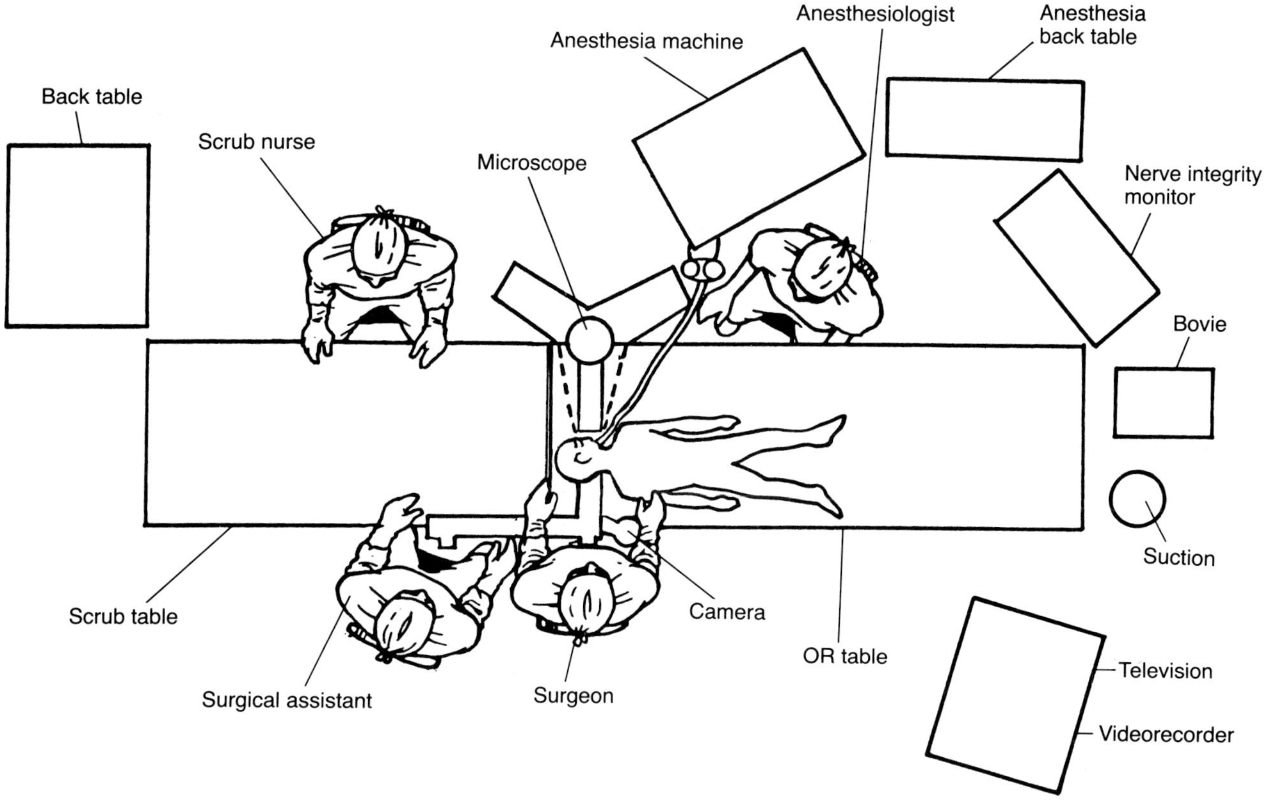

• FIGURE 4-2.

Operating room arrangement for a right ear intratemporal bone facial nerve procedure.

Anesthetic considerations

General endotracheal anesthesia should be used without anesthetic agents that interfere with nerve testing and monitoring. Careful control of fluid intake, using a volume control chamber, infusion pump, or similar device, is necessary. A warming blanket or warming lights (or both) and a fluid warmer are necessary for newborns and may be necessary for young infants. Appropriately sized breathing circuits, blood pressure cuffs, masks, laryngoscopes, and endotracheal tubes are necessary.

The anesthesiologist is positioned on the opposite side of the table from the surgeon, inferior to the patient's shoulder. The endotracheal tube is taped in position on the side of the mouth closest to the anesthesiologist (Fig. 4-2). An angled side bar is attached to the operating table on the side of the anesthesiologist to ensure easy access to the endotracheal tube and airway.

Preparation

The operating table can be reversed to more easily accommodate both the microscope base and the surgeon's legs. The patient is placed in the supine position as close as possible to the surgeon. The head is placed in a foam sponge head holder with the top of the head flush with the end of the operating table and the chin flexed on the neck to bring the ear into a vertical position. Alternatively, a Juers head holder can be attached to the end of the table. The head can be taped to the head holder or the table for further immobilization. In that case, the circulating nurse will rotate the table toward the surgeon for posterior visualization and away from the surgeon for anterior visualization.

Nerve integrity monitor electrodes are placed in the orbicularis oculi and orbicularis oris muscles, are connected to the unit, are tested for function, and are activated before surgery.

The ear canal and tympanic membrane are examined under the microscope. The canal skin and proposed postauricular incision are injected with a 1:100,000 epinephrine solution (0.1 ml of 1:1000 epinephrine in 10 ml of sterile saline) for increased vasoconstriction and subsequent improved visualization.

If a fascia graft is believed to be necessary, a sufficient amount of hair is shaved superior or posterior to the auricle (or both) for access to the temporalis fascia.

The entire auricle, ear canal, side of the face, and neck are sterilized with a surgical preparation.

A 3M 1030 Steri-Drape (3M, St. Paul, MN) is placed with the fenestration over the ear and the long end draped over the angled side bar. A thyroid sheet is then placed over the patient.

The side arm for viewing is positioned on the side of the microscope closest to the scrub table for ease of assistant viewing and retraction. The video camera attachment is positioned on the opposite side, toward the patient's feet.

The microscope is draped with a sterile cover and is positioned at the level of the patient's head with the long foot of the base pointed toward the surgeon for stability. The video camera attachments are connected to the videorecorder and viewing screen.

The scrub table extends from the top of the operating table and at an equal height. The scrub nurse sits facing the surgeon, at the opposite side of the table.

Procedure

The ear canal and tympanic membrane are examined for anatomic deformity. Wax and debris are removed.

The ear canal is irrigated with sterile saline if the tympanic membrane is intact. If the facial nerve is suspected to be in an abnormal position and the paralysis has been present less than 72 hours, a nerve stimulator can be used to map the approximate position of the main trunk and branches of that nerve. The course of the facial nerve can then be marked with a indelible surgical marker.

The mastoid tip is palpated, and an incision is made 1 to 2 cm posterior to the retroauricular fold, from the superior attachment of the auricle to the mastoid tip. If a great auricular nerve graft is needed, the incision can then be continued in a gradual curve onto the neck about 2 cm inferior to the margin of the mandible (Fig. 4–3).

In infants in whom a mastoid tip has not yet developed or in anyone in whom the course of the facial nerve is considered anomalous, an incision is made 1.5 to 2 cm posterior to and not inferior to the auricular attachment (Fig. 4–4). The skin is elevated by sharp and blunt dissection until the nerve is identified or the lateral extent of the external bony canal wall is reached.[4]

The postauricular skin and fibrofascial tissues are elevated anteriorly so that the suprameatal spine (the spine of Henle) at the superoposterior aspect of the lateral bony canal wall can be identified (Fig. 4–5). Further elevation can be done anterosuperior to the canal to expose the zygomatic root and inferiorly to expose the mastoid tip. If the facial nerve has been located in an anomalous lateral position, preservation of the nerve should be the primary consideration during elevation and dissection.

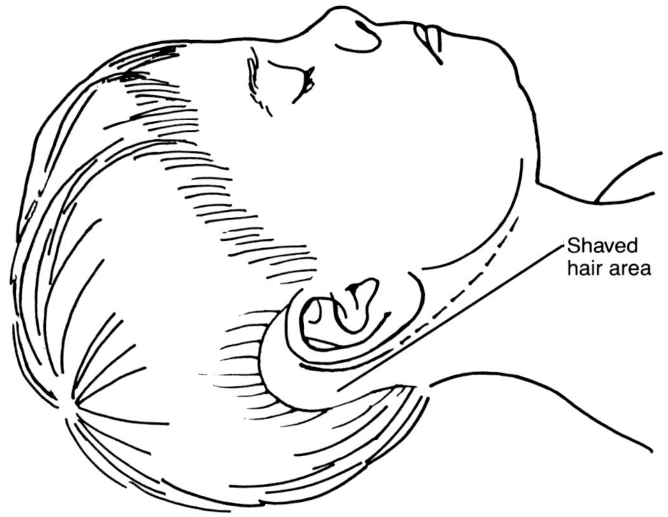

• FIGURE 4-3.

A postauricular incision, 1 to 2 cm posterior to the retroauricular sulcus, may be continued on to the upper neck 2 cm inferior to the mandible if a great auricular nerve graft is needed.

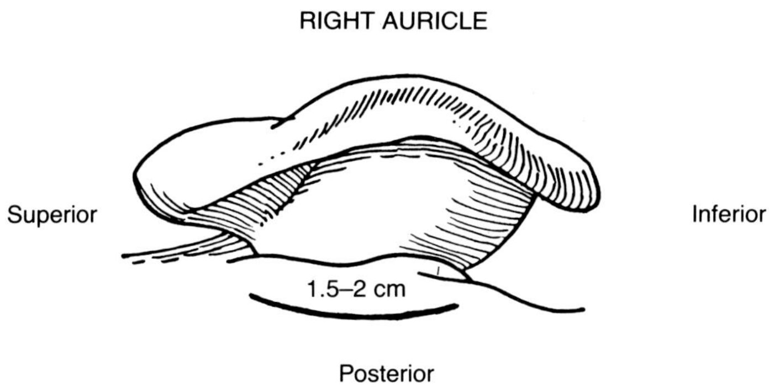

• FIGURE 4-4.

A postauricular incision in neonates and young infants is made 1.5 to 2 cm posterior to the retroauricular sulcus and not inferior to the auricular attachment.

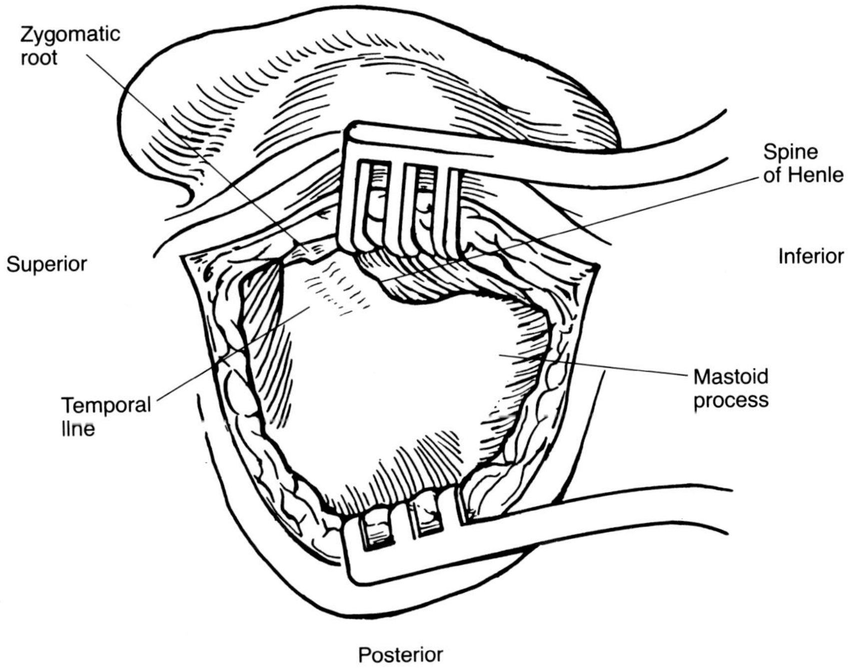

• FIGURE 4-5.

Postauricular elevation to expose the spine of Henle, zygomatic root, temporal line, and mastoid process.

An otosurgical drill with large burs is used in a horizontal direction just inferior to the temporal line to locate the mastoid air cells. The drill is then used in a vertical direction from the temporal line to the mastoid tip to enlarge the opening. The tegmen is located superior and posterior to the external canal at the temporal line (Fig. 4–6).

Constant suction irrigation is used during any mastoid and middle ear surgical drilling to improve visualization and drill performance and to prevent thermal injury to the facial nerve and inner ear.

The dissection is continued medially along the tegmen to identify Körner's septum and, more medially, the aditus ad antrum, the lateral (horizontal) semicircular canal, and the short process of the incus.

The mastoid cavity is enlarged by drilling the sinodural angle posteriorly and superiorly, the mastoid tip and digastric ridge inferiorly, and the zygomatic root anteriorly and by delineating the sigmoid (lateral) sinus posteriorly (Fig. 4–7).

The posterior bony external canal wall is thinned to expose more of the posterior and superior surfaces of the incus and the facial recess.

The posterior canal wall skin can be elevated to aid in visualization for thinning the posterior canal wall.

An exploratory tympanotomy incision can be made before or after mastoidectomy if the middle ear must be entered to localize the facial nerve or to visualize or manipulate the ossicular chain.

If the facial nerve has not been identified after enlarging of the mastoid cavity and thinning of the posterior canal, it can be identified at either its superior or inferior aspect in the mastoid cavity.

Superiorly, the facial nerve can be identified just inferior to the fossa incudis and anterior and, usually, medial to the lateral semicircular canal. Identification or further delineation can be obtained by making a triangular opening in the facial recess by using smaller burs and by drilling parallel to the expected course of the nerve (Fig. 4–8).

• FIGURE 4-6.

A T-shaped opening is made to begin the mastoidectomy.

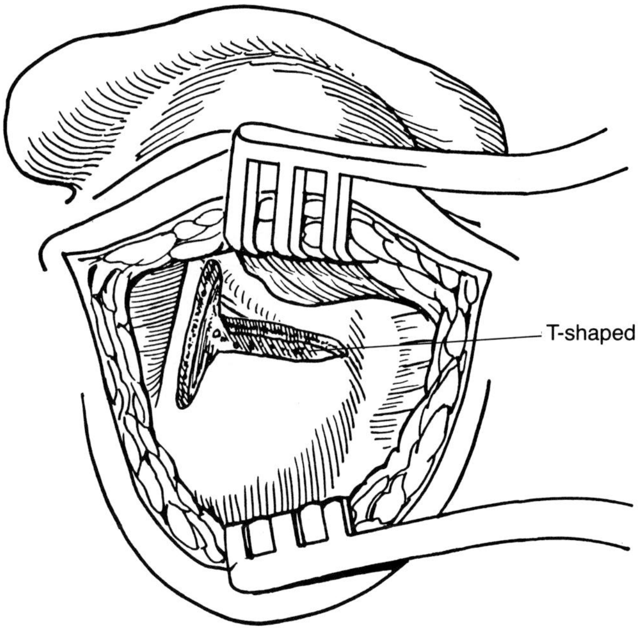

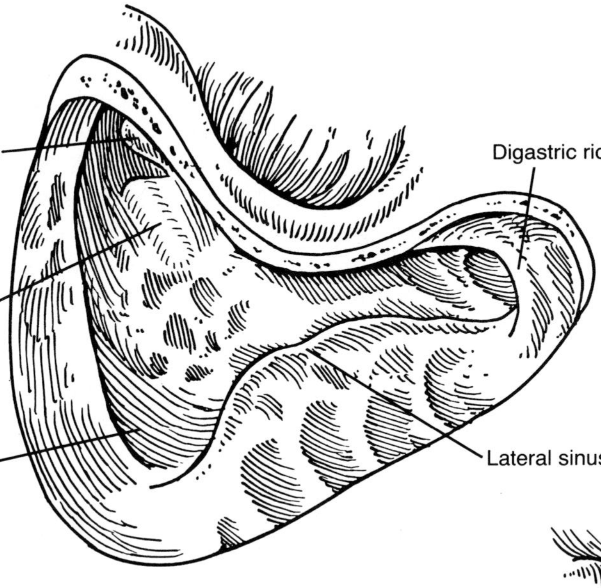

• FIGURE 4-7.

Exposure of the lateral semicircular canal, short process of incus, sinodural angle, lateral sinus, and digastric ridge.

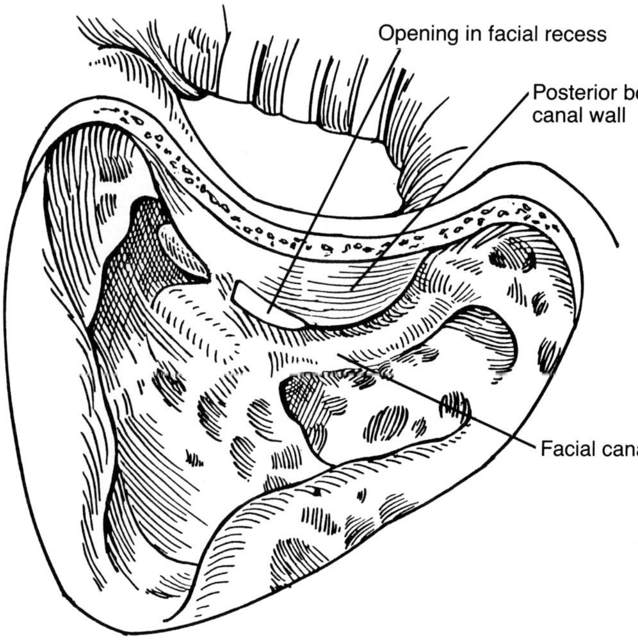

• FIGURE 4-8.

A facial recess approach to locate the facial nerve.

A small bridge of bone is left intact inferior to the fossa incudis to protect the short process of the incus at the base of the facial recess triangle. The lateral side of the triangle is the annulus; the medial side is the facial nerve.

The chorda tympani nerve originates at the apex of the triangle and continues as part of the lateral side. If located, it can be followed inferiorly and posteriorly to the mastoid subsegment of the facial nerve (Fig. 4–9).

Enlarging the facial recess and the epitympanum and working through the tympanotomy incision facilitates exposure of the tympanic subsegment of the facial nerve. This approach can help to determine the continuity of the ossicular chain, the extent of cholesteatoma or neoplasm, or the extent of temporal bone fracture or trauma.

Some cases may necessitate disarticulating the incudostapedial and incudomalleolar joints and either rotating the incus medially or laterally for improved visualization or removing the incus to maximize visualization. To expose the tympanic subsegment of the facial nerve, small burs are used to work through the facial recess or, occasionally, through the external canal. At the end of the procedure, the incus is either returned to its anatomic position or interposed between the malleus and stapes and stabilized with small pieces of absorbable gelatin sponge.[5]

Inferiorly, the nerve can be located at the stylomastoid foramen by following the digastric ridge anteriorly and superiorly, staying on the lateral margin to minimize trauma to the nerve.

In traumatic paralysis, if no fracture or trauma site is seen, the mastoidectomy procedure can be terminated.

When a trauma site is identified, the facial nerve is explored both proximally and distally. The largest possible diamond burs are used. A thin bony covering is left to protect the nontraumatized nerve in the facial canal. Bony fragments are lifted carefully off the damaged nerve area, a few millimeters proximal and distal to the site of injury, with angled picks and elevators (Fig. 4–10). To minimize additional nerve trauma and to maintain as much normal blood supply as possible, the area of nerve exposure is limited to the trauma site. The nerve sheath is not incised; it serves as a protective layer for the nerve and facilitates axonal regeneration.

For avulsed nerve segments or for excision of facial nerve neuroma, interposition grafting is necessary, as is described in the section on facial nerve approximation, rerouting, and grafting.

The cavity is irrigated with saline solution after the completion of drilling and before any grafting procedure. If a tympanotomy flap has been elevated, it is replaced. The auricle and posterior canal wall skin are repositioned. The postauricular incision is closed in two layers with 3-0 or 4-0 catgut and a 4-0 or 5-0 nylon suture. An absorbable cutaneous suture or a subcuticular stitch can be used if suture removal is expected to be difficult. The ear canal is packed with absorbable gelatin sponge, an expandable ear wick, or gauze strips. A mastoid compressive dressing is applied. Mittens can be placed on the hands of young children to prevent them from removing the dressing.

• FIGURE 4-9.

A facial recess approach to the chorda tympani nerve and the facial nerve canal.

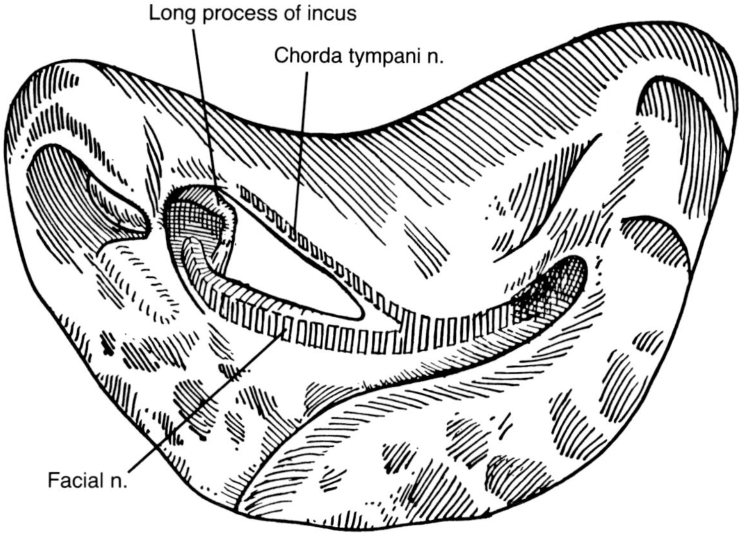

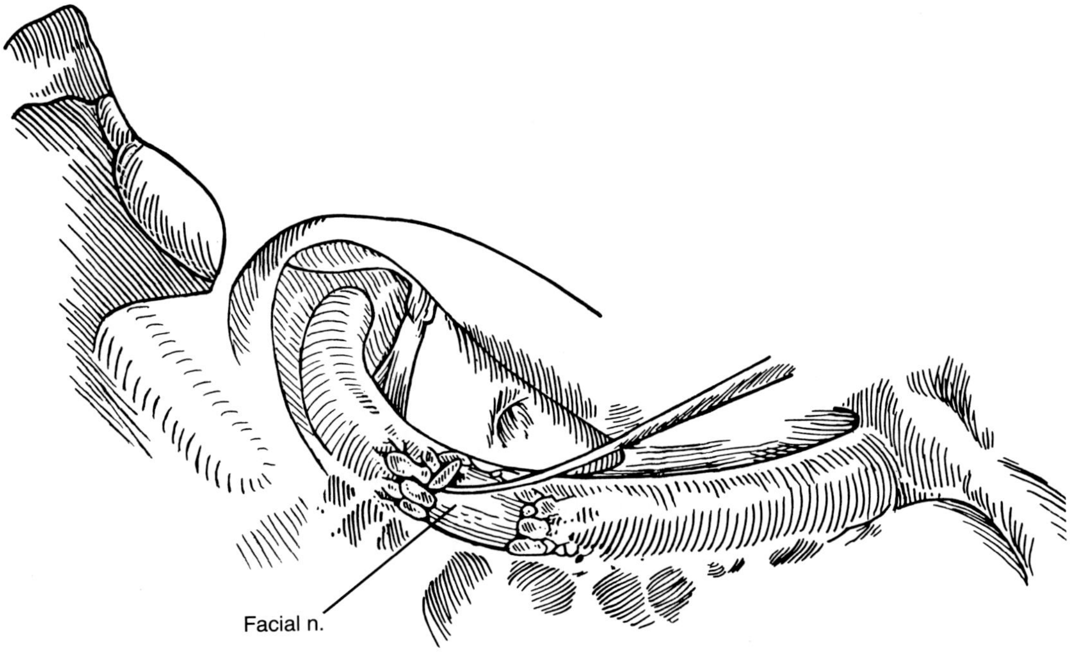

• FIGURE 4-10.

Bone fragments are lifted to expose the facial nerve.

Postoperative care

The mastoid dressing is reinforced for bloody drainage during the night and is changed or removed the next day.

If paralysis or paresis affects the orbicularis oculi muscle, artificial tears or eyedrops are used. The eyelid is closed manually while the patient is recumbent to prevent inadvertent corneal irritation.

The stitches and ear canal pack are removed in 5 to 7 days. If no denervation has occurred, recovery of facial muscle function should occur within 3 to 6 weeks. If compression has caused minimal or moderate denervation, recovery should take 4 to 12 weeks. If denervation is severe, recovery will take 8 to 12 weeks or longer.

INTRATEMPORAL FACIAL NERVE APPROXIMATION, SUTURING, REROUTING, AND GRAFTING

In cases of facial nerve laceration, the severed nerve endings must be exposed and approximated. Loss of less than 50% of the nerve fibers results in acceptable recovery, accompanied by midface contracture and synkinesis; this result is better than that produced by nerve grafting. Loss of 75% or more fibers results in an unacceptable recovery. Consequently, when avulsion of any more than 50% of the nerve's cross-section has occurred, intratemporal interposition nerve grafting or rerouting of the facial nerve with primary anastomosis is probably indicated, depending on the surgeon's clinical judgment. Possible nerve graft donor sites include the ipsilateral or contralateral great auricular nerve and the sural nerve. Choice of the donor site depends on the length of the defect, the size of the nerve, and the condition of the donor sites.[6]

Grafting is successful only if residual vitality of the entire neurovascular system exists. The proximal nerve and nuclei must be intact and functioning, the nerve distal to the dehiscence must be able to accept neural regeneration, and the facial muscles must be capable of contraction.[7]

Consequently, preoperative history concerning the cause and duration of the paralysis, CT or MRI imaging (or both) of the nerve and temporal bone, facial nerve excitability or electromyographic testing and, in cases with a delay of 1 year or more between onset and treatment, muscle biopsy may be necessary before deciding when and whether to operate and what technique to use. The skin and sensory function over the donor site must also be checked. If nonfunctional, the nerve may be fibrotic and unacceptable for grafting.[8]

Informed consent is extremely important. The patient and family must understand the various possible procedures, alternatives, risks, and complications. The surgeon must clearly articulate and make sure the patient or family or both understand that facial nerve regeneration occurs at a rate of 0.5 to 1 mm/day, that facial function will not be evident for at least 3 months, that improvement may take more than 12 months, and that recovery will not be total and is always associated with synkinesis.

Many current standards exist for both equipment and technique used in nerve repair. An operative microscope, a sharp blade (razor blade or 6500 Beaver Mini-Blade [R Beaver Inc, Waltham, MA]) for nerve transection, and the fewest nonreactive 9-0 or 10-0 monofilament sutures necessary to maintain coaptation are essential. Atraumatic technique is critical.[7,8]

The recipient nerve stump and nerve graft bed should be prepared or irrigated before graft harvesting. The graft, which should be long enough to preclude suture line tension, should be placed in position with no delay. Epineural suturing in the trunk seems more conducive to maximal nerve regeneration than perineural suturing does, possibly because it is less traumatic. When anastomosing nerves of different sizes, an epineural-perineural anastomosis may be indicated.

Nonstandard suggestions include cutting the nerve at a 45-degree instead of a 90-degree angle to increase surface exposure for healing (although the same number of neural tubules will still be present); reversing the graft orientation to facilitate neural ingrowth; and using tissue adhesives such as fibrin glue and laser welding.

Clipping of nonessential facial nerve branches to increase regeneration in the sutured branches in order to minimize synkinesis is controversial. Some believe that reinnervation of the zygomatic and buccal branches is most important for orbital and oral movement, particularly because return is rare in the frontal branch and poor in the marginal branch. Others, however, believe that the frontal and marginal branches are more important for good cosmesis because the zygomatic and buccal branches often recover secondary to cross-anastomosis or masseter neurotization. The advocates of these theories cut specific branches and clip or suture them with a nonabsorbable suture.[7–9]

Indications

- Facial nerve approximation is indicated in patients with an acute intratemporal facial nerve laceration with no separation, if the affected nerve endings can be approximated and will remain in apposition without other stabilization.

- Facial nerve suturing is indicated when there is an acute intratemporal facial nerve laceration with

  No separation, but the ends will not remain in an unsupported approximated position

  Minimal nerve ending separation, but the ends can be approximated with sutures without tension

- Facial nerve rerouting may be elected when the nerve ends are under tension after suturing or if there is a space of up to 1 cm between nerve endings in the fully developed person or correspondingly less space in a younger, less developed person. The advantage of successful rerouting is that only one suture line is needed, versus the two suture lines needed for nerve grafting. The disadvantages of rerouting include the limited length that can be gained, additional trauma to the nerve by the required circumferential exposure and elevation, interruption of the nerve's blood supply, loss of the facial canal as a stent, possible surgical damage to the ossicular chain with subsequent conductive hearing loss, and loss of the posterior bony canal wall. In children, in whom the mastoid segment of the facial nerve is shorter, the disadvantages of rerouting seem to outweigh the advantages.

- Interposition nerve grafting is indicated when direct approximation of the separated nerve is impossible or is possible only under tension. Compared with rerouting, interposition nerve grafting has the advantages of being less traumatic to the facial nerve and less disruptive to the middle ear anatomy and conductive mechanism. It has the disadvantages of necessitating both two suture lines and an additional surgical site. Nerve grafting is contraindicated in the presence of infection. Grafting in an open cavity is problematic because of lack of protection and possible contamination.

Anesthetic considerations

General endotracheal anesthesia is used; refer to the section on intratemporal bone facial nerve exploration or decompression.

Preparation

Prior to anesthesia, the ipsilateral and contralateral sides of the neck are tested for sensation. The patient is prepared as described in the section on intratemporal bone facial nerve exploration with or without decompression.

The neck, ear, and side of the face are prepared for possible great auricular nerve graft. The lower leg, ankle, and foot are prepared for possible sural nerve graft, as described in the section on extratemporal facial nerve suturing, rerouting, grafting, and nerve transfer.

Procedure

Simple mastoidectomy is always done, with or without exploratory tympanotomy. If necessary, a facial recess approach is attempted; if that approach is unsuccessful, a modified radical or radical mastoidectomy may then be necessary. Facial nerve exploration is done, exposing the nerve for several millimeters proximal and distal to the site of trauma. All bone fragments are carefully lifted from the nerve (see Fig. 4–10).

In a simple nerve laceration, when the severed edges are in approximation or can be positioned and maintained in approximation, sutures may not be necessary (Fig. 4–11). If the nerve edges will not lie in an approximated position, they are sutured with enough 9-0 or 10-0 monofilament nylon sutures in the epineurium to maintain coaptation.

For rerouting, the entire facial nerve must be exposed from the geniculate ganglion to the stylomastoid foramen. The posterior bony canal wall is removed. The nerve is elevated out of the facial canal and sutured with the fewest 9-0 or 10-0 monofilament nylon sutures needed to achieve coaptation.

A neofacial nerve canal can be drilled for nerve stability, but only if it will not cause additional injury to the ear. In patients with total ipsilateral sensorineural hearing loss, however, the ossicles can be removed, and additional space can be gained by removing the cochlea. This procedure is not done if cochlear implantation is an option.

For interposition grafting, the nerve is explored and exposed, using diamond burs for several millimeters proximal and distal to the avulsed or lacerated section. One half to two thirds of the circumference of the nerve must be exposed with drilling. Once the bony lining is thinned, it can be removed with picks and elevators (see Fig. 4–10). The ends of the nerve are freshened with the sharpest possible blade (razor blade or 6500 Beaver Mini-Blade) to expose healthy nerve. In delayed repairs and neuromas, the nerve endings are submitted for frozen section to confirm viable neural tissue.

The great auricular nerve (C2, C3) is the sensory branch of the cervical plexus that courses from medial to lateral around the posterior border of the sternocleidomastoid muscle (Erb's point). It ascends toward the inferior auricle and mastoid tip, on the lateral surface of the sternocleidomastoid muscle, and usually terminates in three branches (Fig. 4–12*A*).

The location of the great auricular nerve can be predicted by drawing a vertical line that bisects a straight line between the mastoid tip and the angle of the mandible (Fig. 4–12*B*).

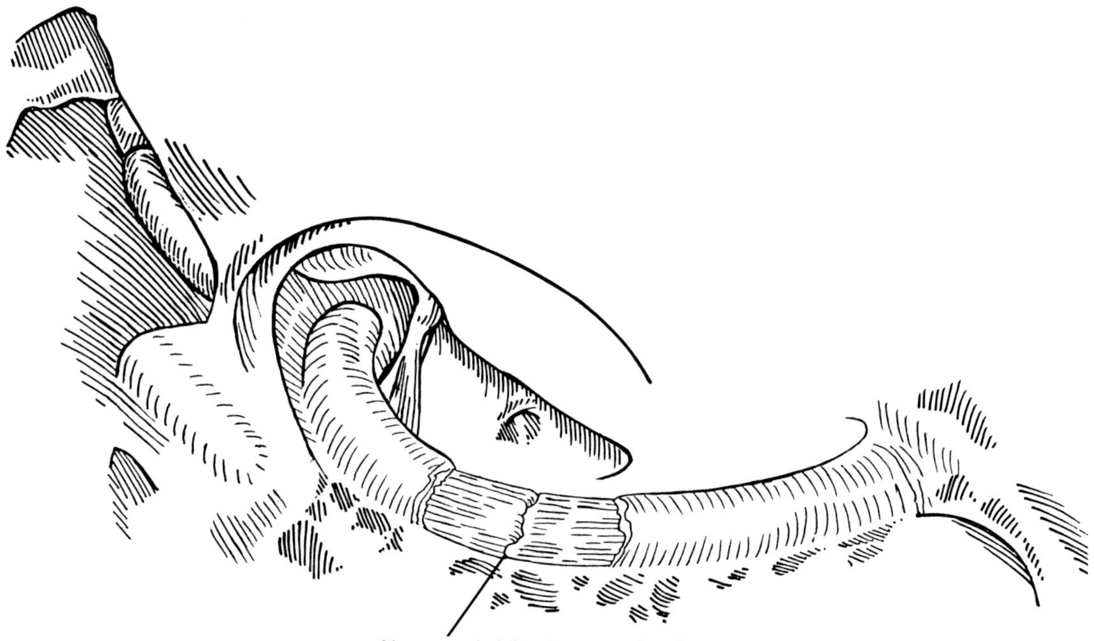

• **FIGURE 4-11.**

Facial canal exploration and exposure of facial nerve proximal and distal to a facial nerve laceration.

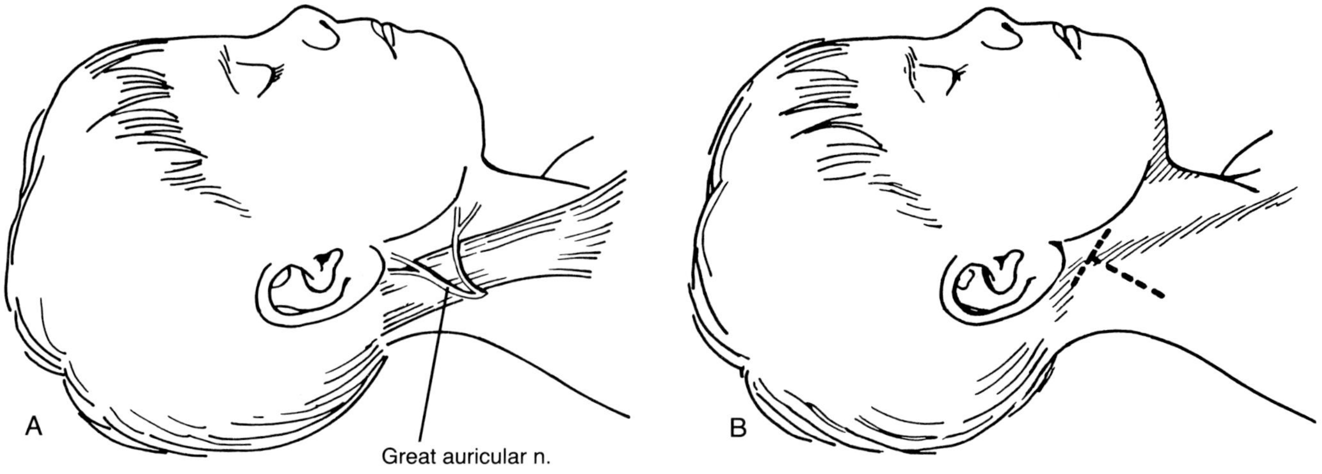

• **FIGURE 4-12.**

Prior to a great auricular nerve graft. *A*, Schematic drawing of great auricular nerve. *B*, The approximate position of the nerve is located by drawing a vertical line that bisects a straight line between the mastoid tip and the angle of the mandible.

The ipsilateral great auricular nerve is most desirable because it is in the surgical field and has the appropriate length and thickness. Viability of either the facial or donor nerve can be confirmed by frozen section. The contralateral great auricular nerve (C2, C3) or the sural nerve can also be used as a graft.

The postauricular incision can be continued onto the neck approximately 2 cm inferior to the mandible to expose the great auricular nerve. A sufficient length of nerve graft is obtained through elevation, sharp and blunt dissection, and sharp incision with a razor blade or 6500 Beaver Mini-Blade. The graft is interposed in the facial canal and may stay in position without suturing. One to three 9-0 or 10-0 nylon monofilament sutures in the epineurium will hold the graft in position (Fig. 4–13).

The postauricular incision is closed in two layers with 3-0 to 4-0 catgut and 4-0 to 5-0 nylon sutures. The neck skin can be approximated with staples. Antibiotic ointment is applied to the incision line. Fluffed gauze sponges and 4 × 4″ dressing gauze sponges are used as a pressure dressing. A mastoid, Barton, or nylon tubular net dressing can be applied for pressure.

Postoperative care

The dressing is reinforced for bloody drainage during the night and is changed or removed the next day.

Eyedrops or artificial tears are used, and the eyelid is closed manually while the patient is recumbent to prevent inadvertent corneal irritation.

The stitches and ear canal pack are removed in 5 to 7 days. The patient should notice the start of recovery in 4 to 6 months. Improvement in facial function may continue for 12 months or longer.

EXTRATEMPORAL BONE FACIAL NERVE PROCEDURES

SURGERY FOR PAROTID AND NONPAROTID GLAND DISEASES

Neoplastic disease is uncommon in the parotid area in children. Hemangiomas are more common than lymphangiomas. Pleomorphic adenoma is the most prevalent benign solid tumor. Of the malignant tumors, mucoepidermoid carcinoma is the most common, and adenocarcinoma is the next most common. Malignant parotid gland disease tends to occur later in childhood, although sarcomas can occur at an earlier age. Non-neoplastic disease is infrequent. First branchial cleft congenital anomalies are rare.[5,10–13]

The complete examination includes an accurate history and physical examination, radiographic studies, including CT or MRI (or both), with or without fine-needle aspiration biopsy. These tests are more difficult to do in younger children and may require sedation or general anesthesia. Because none of the tests can ensure an accurate diagnosis, as with adults, an excisional biopsy, consisting of superficial or total parotidectomy, is usually indicated for a nonresolving or enlarging growth. If possible, hemangiomas and lymphangiomas are left to regress spontaneously. Likewise, surgery for other suspected nonmalignant disease can be delayed until the child is well developed unless complications occur.[5,11–14]

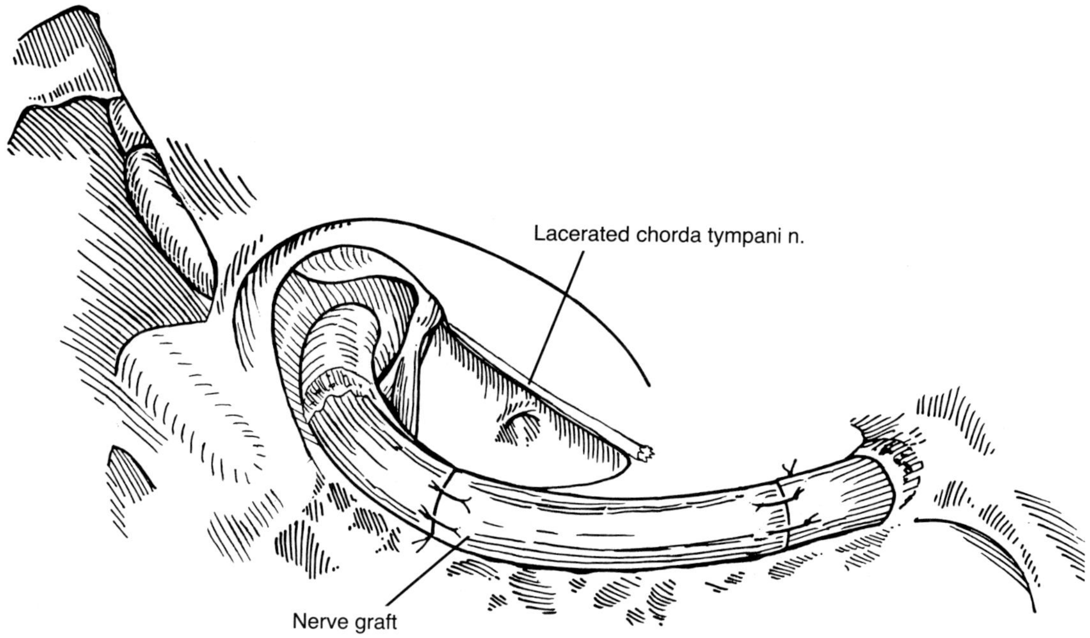

• FIGURE 4-13.

A nerve graft is in position in the facial canal.

Indications

- Parotidectomy for parotid gland cysts, neoplasms, and chronic parotitis
- Surgery for nonparotid neoplasms that invade or are contiguous with the parotid gland when the facial nerve is at risk during surgery
- First branchial cleft cysts and fistulas

Anesthetic considerations

General anesthesia is used; refer to the section on facial nerve exploration with or without decompression.

Nasotracheal intubation is used to increase the distance between the mastoid tip and the ascending ramus of the mandible and thus to facilitate location of the facial nerve trunk.

The anesthesiologist is positioned on the side of the operating table opposite the surgeon, inferior to the patient's contralateral shoulder, so that the entire head and both sides of the neck are available to the surgeon and surgical assistants (Fig. 4–14).

Preparation

The patient is placed in the supine position with the top of the head flush with the edge of the operating table and the body positioned closest to the side of the table at which the surgeon stands.

The head is turned away from the operating surgeon and toward the anesthesiologist so that the involved parotid is exposed. A rolled towel is placed underneath the shoulders to accentuate the operative field. The patient's hair is taped away from the surgical field with Hy tape (Hy Tape Surgical Products Corp., Yonkers, NY).

In patients with no facial paralysis, or in whom paralysis has been present for less than 72 hours, a nerve stimulator can be used to determine the approximate position of the facial nerve and its branches.

Nerve integrity monitor electrodes are placed in the orbicularis oculi and orbicularis oris muscles, connected to the unit, tested for function, and activated before surgery.

The proposed incision line is injected with a 1:100,000 epinephrine solution (0.1 ml of 1:1000 epinephrine in 10 ml of sterile saline) for increased vasoconstriction and improved visualization.

The entire side of the face, including the auricle and ear canal as well as the neck, is sterilized with a surgical preparation. The nasotracheal tube is covered with a towel so that when a 3M 1050 Steri-Drape is applied to the side of the face and neck, the drape does not attach to the endotracheal tube. Use of the plastic drape enables exposure of the chin, corner of the lips, nasofacial junction, eye, and forehead.

If a sural nerve graft is anticipated, the ipsilateral ankle, foot, and lower leg are prepared.

A thyroid or a split sheet is used to cover the patient and to drape the entire surgical field.

The scrub nurse stands next to the surgeon and in front of the back scrub table. Surgical loupes as well as the microscope should be available for the surgeon to facilitate location of and dissection along the nerve.

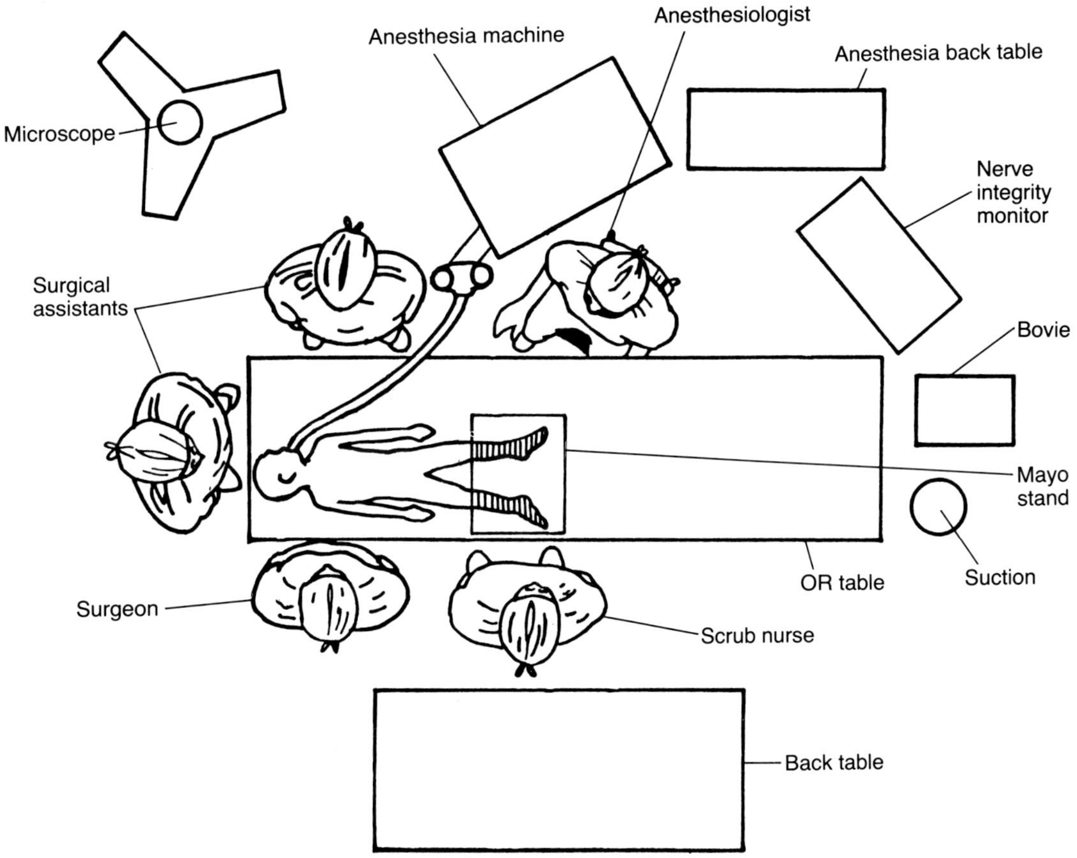

• FIGURE 4-14.

Operating room arrangement for a right ear extratemporal bone facial nerve procedure.

Procedure

The proposed preauricular incision is marked with a surgical marker. If it is curved posteriorly to conform to the anatomic indentation just superior or inferior (or both) to the tragus, the incision will be less noticeable postoperatively. The incision is continued just inferior to the earlobe and posteriorly, onto the mastoid process, and is then curved inferiorly and anteriorly about 2 cm inferior to the mandible rim, preferably within a skin crease (Fig. 4–15*A*).

In infants, in whom the mastoid tip has not yet developed, or in patients in whom the course of the nerve is considered to be anomalous, an upper neck incision is made 2 cm inferior to the rim of the mandible, curving onto the postauricular area. After the skin incision is made, the skin flap is elevated superiorly with sharp and blunt dissection until the facial nerve is located. If necessary, a more superior extension of the incision can be made after the facial nerve is located (Fig. 4–15*B*).[4]

The skin flap is elevated with sharp and blunt dissection to a point about 1 cm superior, anterior, inferior, and posterior to the parotid gland. Elevation is usually continued until the zygomatic arch, the buccal fat pad, the upper third of the neck, and the mastoid tip are exposed (Fig. 4–16).

The anterior border of the sternocleidomastoid muscle is identified. The great auricular nerve is located at the posterior border of the upper midportion of the sternocleidomastoid muscle and exposed superiorly until it branches just inferior to the auricle. The nerve is kept in position as long as possible. In smaller infants, transection of the great auricular nerve may not be necessary because the parotid gland is located more anteriorly than it is in older children and adults.[4]

• FIGURE 4-15.

A, Incision line for a parotidectomy. *B*, Incision line for a parotidectomy in an infant in whom the mastoid tip has not developed. The incision can be extended along the dotted lines as necessary, following the location of the facial nerve. (Adapted from Farrior JB and Santini H: Facial nerve identification in children. Otolaryngol Head Neck Surg 93:173–176, 1985.)

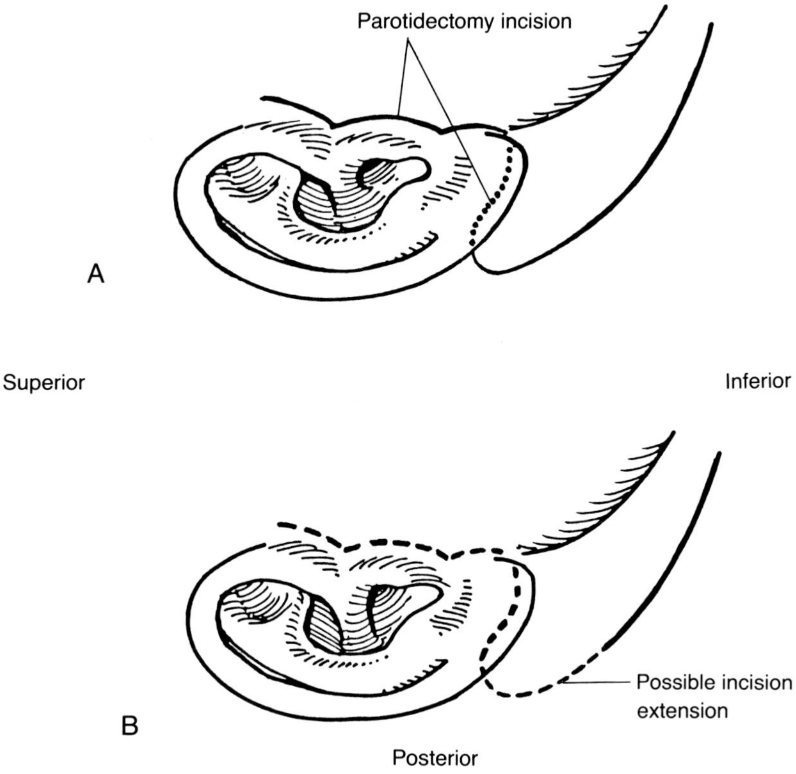

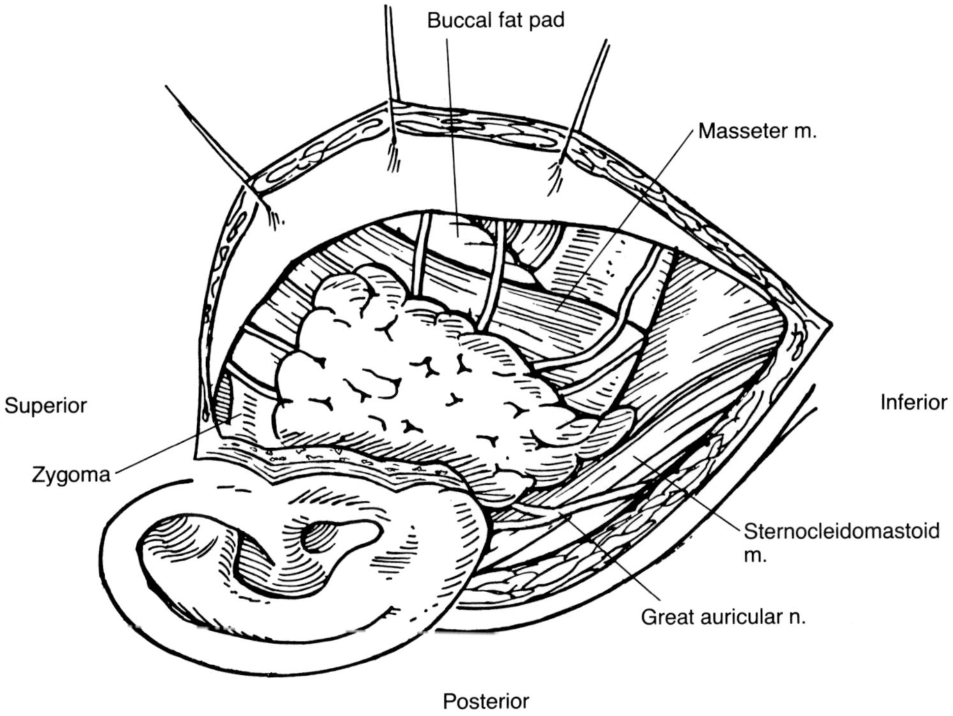

• FIGURE 4-16.

Elevation of parotidectomy skin flaps to expose the zygoma, buccal fat pad, masseter muscle, and sternocleidomastoid muscle.

The anterior border of the sternocleidomastoid muscle is dissected medially until the posterior belly of the digastric muscle is located (Fig. 4–17). The inferior border of the parotid gland is retracted superiorly, and the digastric muscle is followed to its origin, medial to the mastoid tip. Because the parotid gland is located more anteriorly in the infant, this dissection may suffice to locate the main trunk of the facial nerve (Fig. 4–18).[4]

The preauricular area is dissected medially along the external canal perichondrium. The parotid gland is retracted anteriorly. Sharp and blunt dissection is continued medially until the cartilaginous pointer is identified at the bony cartilaginous junction of the external auditory canal (Fig. 4–19).

This dissection plane is continued superiorly to the level of the zygomatic arch. The preauricular dissection is continued medially, both superior and inferior to the expected location of the facial nerve. This technique facilitates eventual visualization of the nerve by widening the surgical field. The facial nerve is located about 1 cm medial to the tympanomastoid suture line and cartilaginous pointer at the external auditory canal–bony cartilaginous junction. This area is separated with blunt dissection parallel to the expected course of the nerve. The main trunk of the nerve is located just anterior to the stylomastoid foramen (Fig. 4–20).

Bleeding is controlled throughout this portion of the surgery with clamps, 3-0 absorbable suture ties, bipolar cautery, a Shaw scalpel, or light pressure using small or large moist dissecting sponges.

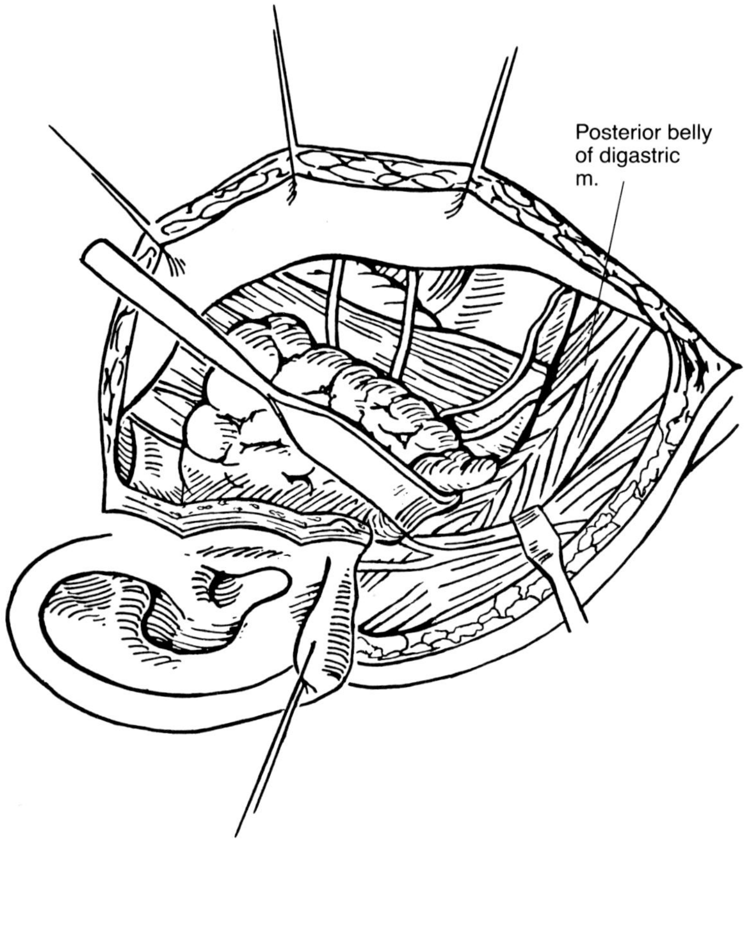

• FIGURE 4–17.

Retraction of the inferior parotid gland and the sternocleidomastoid muscle to locate the posterior belly of the digastric muscle.

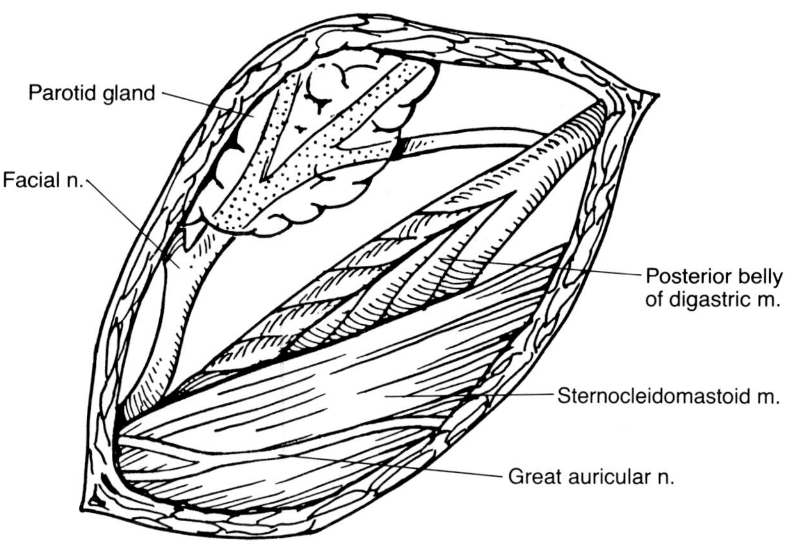

• FIGURE 4–18.

Location of the facial nerve in an infant with an anteriorly placed parotid gland. (Adapted from Farrior JB and Santini H: Facial nerve identification in children. Otolaryngol Head Neck Surg 93:173–176, 1985.)

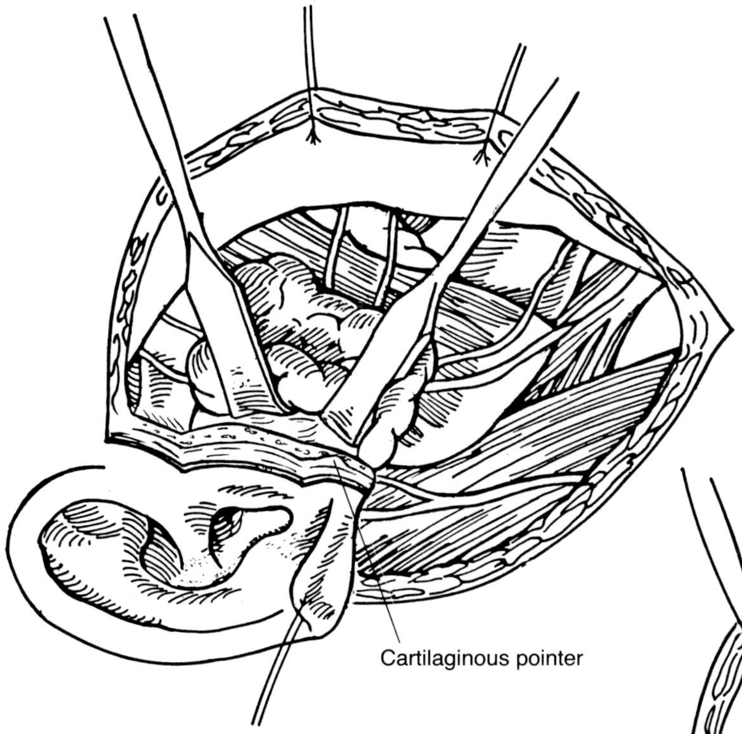

• FIGURE 4–19.

Retraction of the posterior border of the parotid gland anteriorly to dissect the external canal medially toward the cartilaginous pointer.

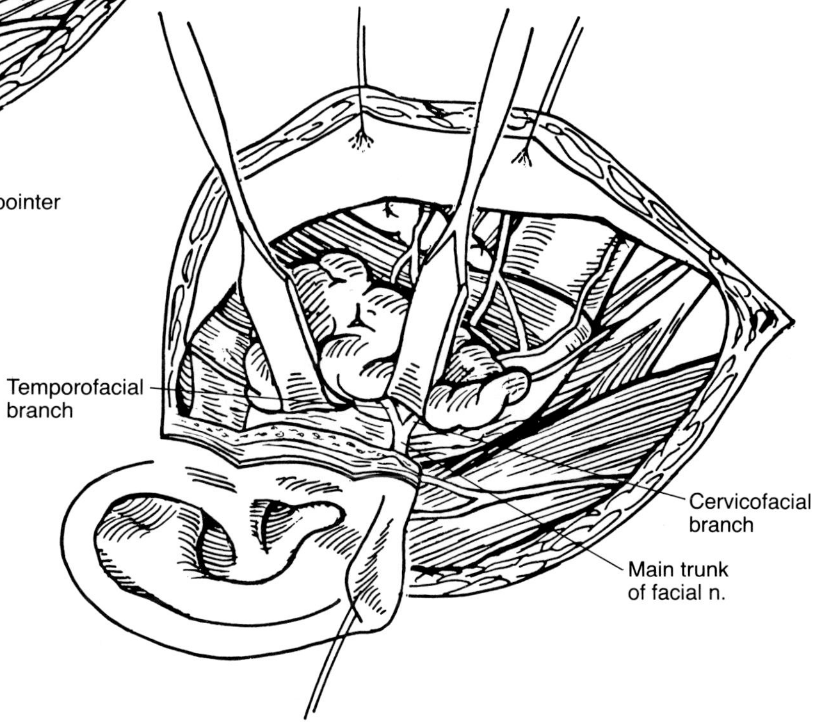

• FIGURE 4–20.

Exposure of the main trunk of the facial nerve and its temporofacial and cervicofacial divisions.

Once the main trunk has been identified, blunt dissection is continued anteriorly along the trunk until its bifurcation is located; the facial nerve is then identified conclusively and the parotid tissue lateral to the nerve can be incised with a Shaw scalpel or a No. 11, 12, or 15 blade. Dissection along the nerve can be facilitated initially with a fine hemostat such as a McCabe facial nerve dissector. Once the proper plane has been established, curved mosquito-type forceps and small Kelly clamps suffice. Each branch is dissected to a point distal to the parotid gland (Fig. 4–21).

The parotid gland between the branches is removed, if possible, with the pathologic specimen. As large a margin of normal parotid tissue as possible is included around any tumor or cyst.

If the main trunk cannot be identified or if it is incorporated in scar tissue or tumor, peripheral branches must be located and dissected in retrograde fashion to the main trunk in the following areas: the mandibular branch, the temporal branch, buccal branches, and the zygomatic branch. The mandibular branch, or ramus mandibulae, is located in the neck lateral to the facial vessels and just superior to the submandibular gland. In infants, this branch is frequently found in a more superior position, lateral to the mandible. In older children, if the mandibular branch is not located easily, the fascia of the submandibular gland can be incised and elevated superiorly along the posterior facial vein until the cervical or mandibular branch is identified. The temporal branch is usually found overlying or just superior to the zygomatic arch deep to the superficial fascia, about halfway between the anterior border of the auricle and the lateral bony orbital rim. A buccal branch can be found coursing near and parallel to the parotid duct about 1 to 1.5 cm inferior to the zygomatic arch. The zygomatic branch can often be identified between the superior anterior border of the parotid gland and the lateral inferior orbital rim. Rarely, in large neoplasms or with severe scarring resulting from prior surgeries or trauma, mastoidectomy is indicated, with facial nerve exploration to locate the nerve and follow it through the stylomastoid foramen.

If, after the superficial portion of the parotidectomy has been completed, the disease process is medial to the facial nerve, the nerve is elevated gently with sharp and blunt dissection. The main trunk and each of the cervicofacial branches are retracted with vascular loops to expose the underlying parotid tissue (Fig. 4–22).

The masseter muscle is located anteriorly and medially to expose and remove the tissue medial to the facial nerve. Dissection is begun in a plane lateral to the masseter fascia and is continued to the posterior border of the masseter muscle at the ascending ramus of the mandible.

A second dissection plane is begun on the mastoid tip inferior to the stylomastoid foramen and main trunk of the facial nerve. This plane is continued medially and is connected with a plane beginning on the bony canal superior to the facial nerve trunk.

The remaining parotid tissue, which may be in the parapharyngeal space, can be removed by advancing along the dissection planes. If necessary, to protect the facial nerve, this portion of the excision can be done in segments from between the branches of the nerve or superior or inferior to the main trunk and the superior or inferior branches of the nerve. When dissecting superior to the trunk and posterior to the frontal branch, care should be taken to avoid injuring the auriculotemporal branch of the third division of the trigeminal nerve. This branch lies near the superficial temporal artery between the auricle and the mandible.

With large paraphyngeal space tumors, anterior traction on the mandible often provides adequate additional operating space. If not, mandibular osteotomy and mandibular swing may be necessary to adequately visualize and access the site to facilitate tumor or parotid tissue removal.

• FIGURE 4-21.

Exposure of the zygomatic branch of the facial nerve with a curved hemostat before parotid tissue lateral to the nerve is severed.

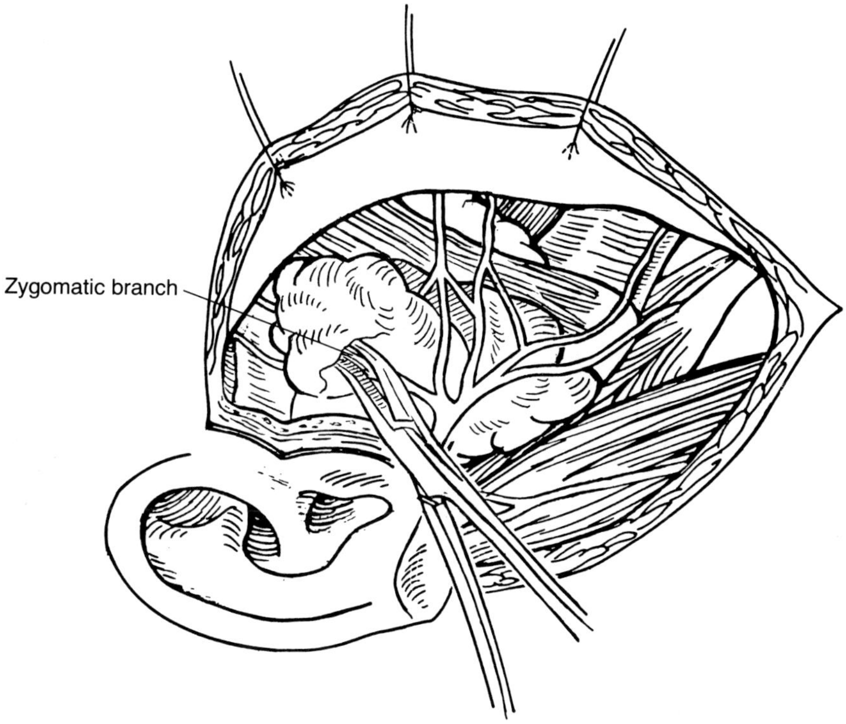

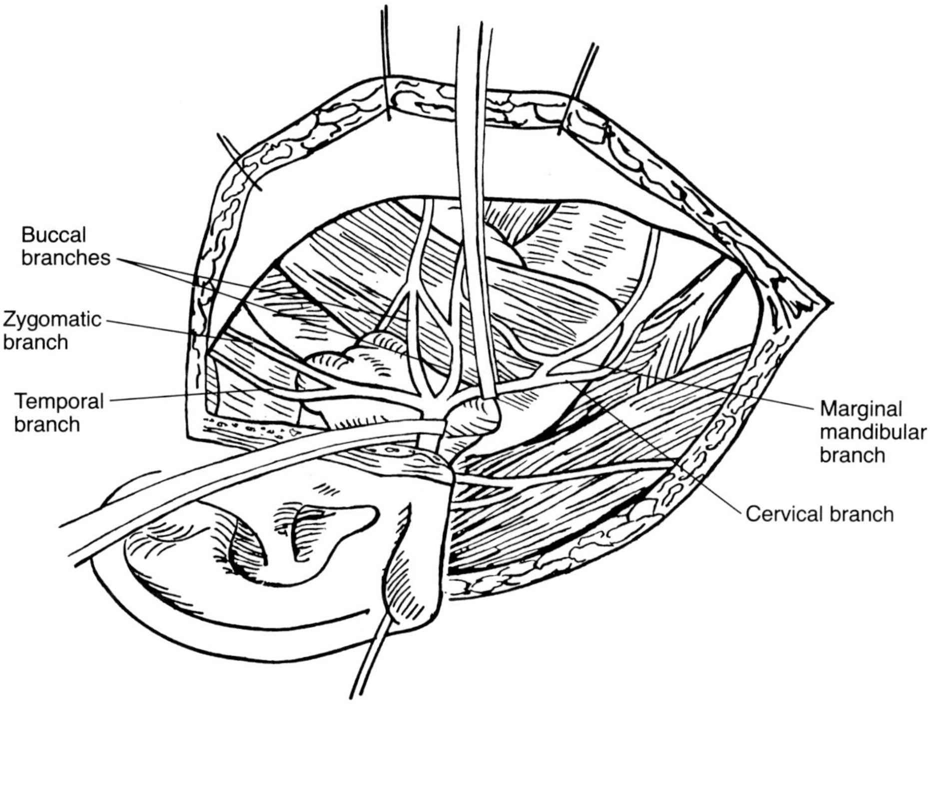

• FIGURE 4-22.

Retraction of the main trunk and cervicofacial branch of the facial nerve to expose the underlying parotid gland tissue.

The surgeon should minimize any contact with the facial nerve and its branches. Visualization, which is obscured by blood, can be improved by lightly touching the facial nerve with small and large moist dissecting sponges. Minimal pressure should be applied, and the nerve should not be rubbed or suctioned.

In most cases, knowledge of the anatomy of the facial nerve should obviate the need for a facial nerve stimulator, which can further traumatize the nerve. In revision surgery, post-traumatic exploration, and certain extensive neoplastic and infectious cases, however, judicious use of a facial nerve stimulator, at the lowest setting, may help to locate the nerve.

Once the pathologic specimen has been removed, the nerve is inspected to ensure that it is intact.

If the nerve is transected at the trunk or at the temporalis, zygomatic, or mandibular branches, it is reapproximated with the fewest 9-0 or 10-0 monofilament nylon sutures needed to achieve coaptation (Fig. 4–23). Anastomosis of severed buccal branches is usually unnecessary because of the rich interanastomosis of buccal branch nerve fibers.

The cervical branch is usually routinely sacrificed during parotidectomy and does not require repair because loss of function is minimal.

In cases in which a segment of the nerve is removed, an immediate interposition nerve graft can be sutured in place (Fig. 4–24). If a graft is not immediately desirable, the severed proximal and distal ends should be marked with nonabsorbable (nylon) sutures to facilitate localization at subsequent repair. Rather than using an interposition graft, less important branches may be severed and anastomosed to more valuable ones; for example, the buccal to the temporal or zygomatic branch, or the buccal or cervical to the mandibular branch (Fig. 4–25).[15]

The wound is irrigated with saline solution. The facial nerve is re-examined for continuity. A Penrose or vacuum drain is placed inferior to the trunk, posterior to the branches, and through either the inferior neck incision or a separate incision. The preauricular skin can be approximated with 3-0 to 4-0 catgut and 4-0 to 5-0 nylon sutures. The neck incision can be approximated with staples.

Antibiotic ointment is applied to the incision. Fluffed gauze sponges and 4 × 4″ dressing gauze sponges are used for a pressure dressing. Either a Barton or nylon tubular net dressing can be applied for pressure.

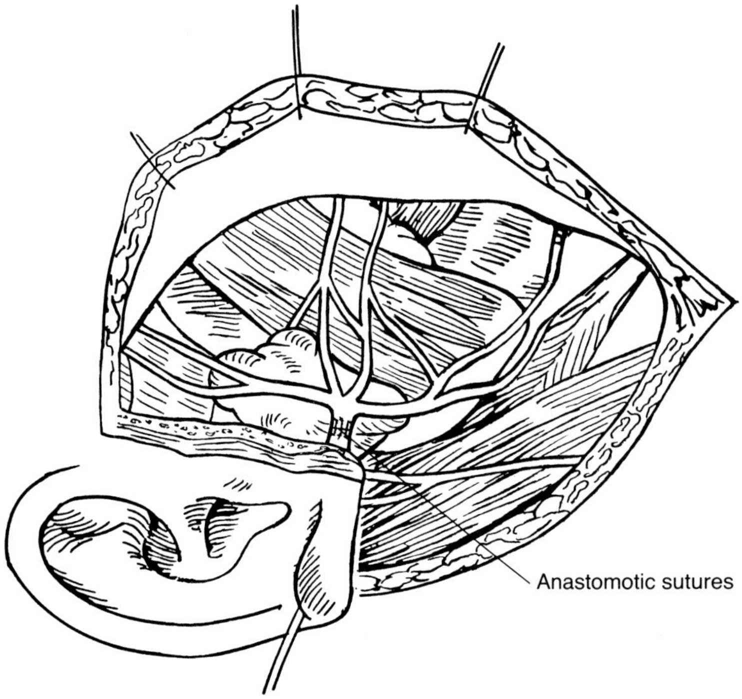

• FIGURE 4–23.

Sutured laceration of the main trunk of the facial nerve.

• FIGURE 4-24.

Interposition nerve grafts sutured into the zygomatic and marginal branch defects.

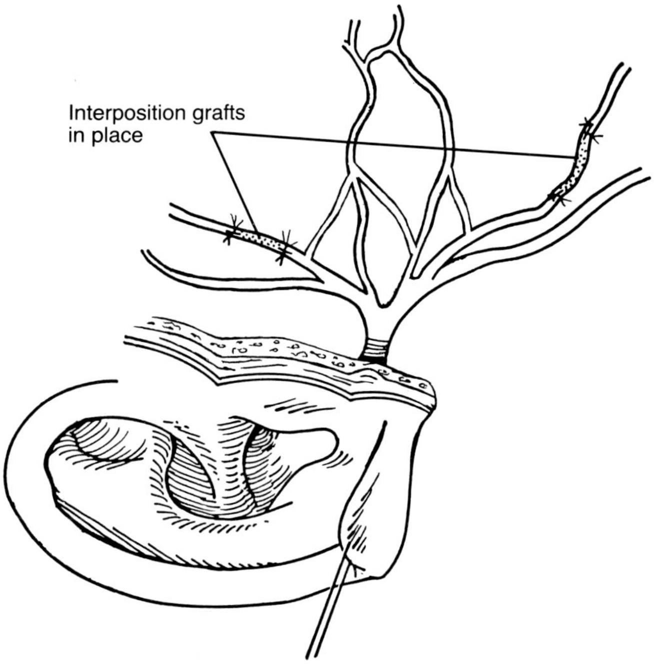

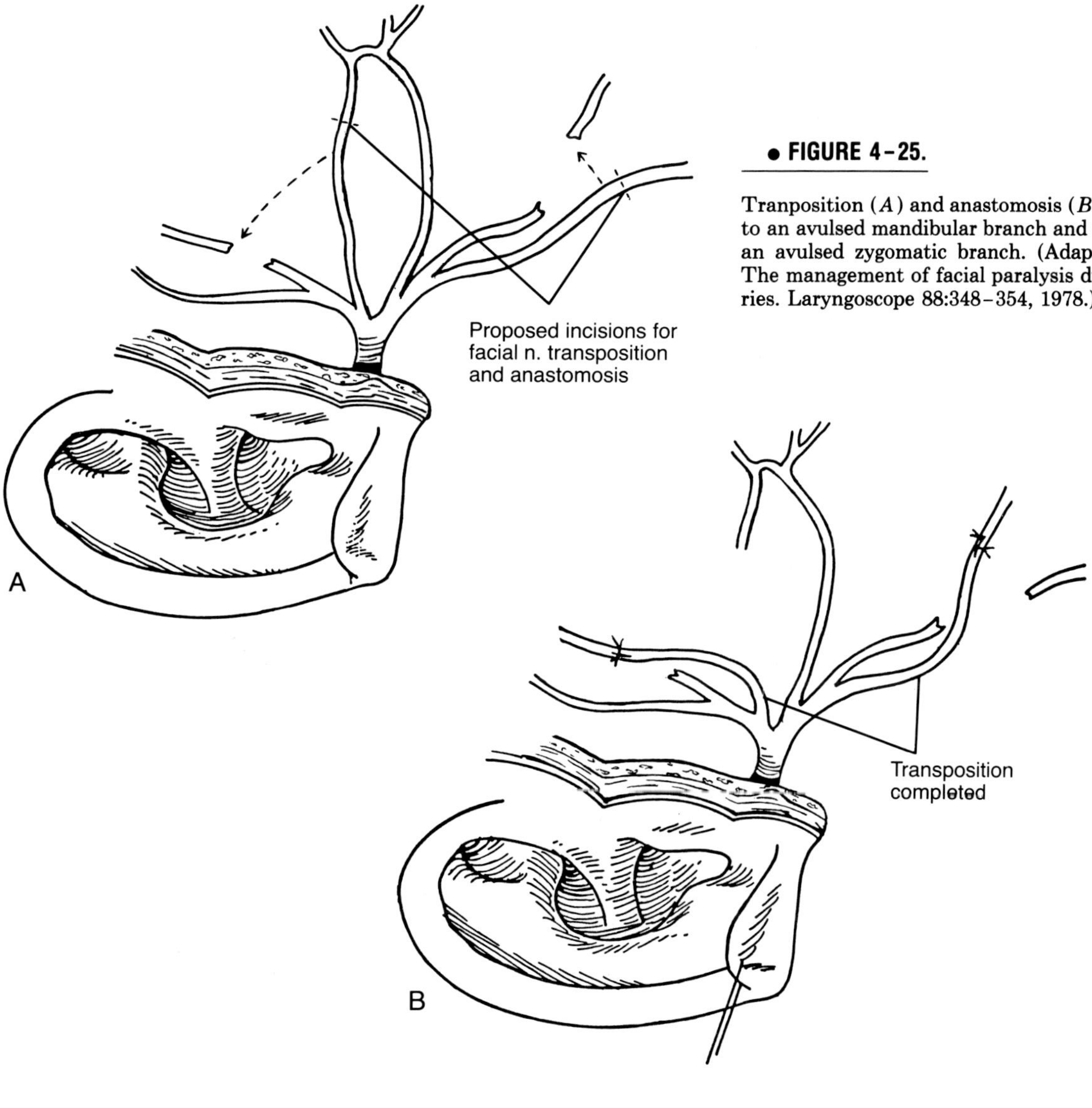

• FIGURE 4-25.

Tranposition (A) and anastomosis (B) of the cervical branch to an avulsed mandibular branch and of the buccal branch to an avulsed zygomatic branch. (Adapted from Tucker HM: The management of facial paralysis due to extracranial injuries. Laryngoscope 88:348-354, 1978.)

Postoperative care

Facial function is checked when the patient is awakened from anesthesia. If paresis or paralysis is present and the nerve was left intact, the patient should be observed. If paralysis is present immediately after surgery and was not present preoperatively, and if the status of the nerve was not checked, the nerve should be explored to establish continuity or repair any lacerations.

The patient is observed for development of a hematoma, seroma, salivary fistula, corneal irritation, or new facial paralysis. Gustatory sweating may be a late complication.

Artificial tears are used, and if the eye is affected by facial paresis or paralysis, the eyelid is closed before sleep. The dressing is reinforced overnight to absorb bloody drainage. The drain is removed on the first or second postoperative day, or when there is minimal or no drainage. The pressure dressing is applied for 4 to 7 days, and the sutures or staples are removed on the seventh postoperative day. If the nerve was intact at the end of surgery, any postoperative paresis should resolve in 4 to 6 weeks. If paralysis is present, recovery should begin within 3 months and should continue for 12 months.

SURGICAL EXPLORATION AND REPAIR AFTER EXTRATEMPORAL FACIAL NERVE TRAUMA

Penetrating wounds of the face may affect the main trunk of the facial nerve as well as any or all of its branches. Because the facial nerve injury may be part of more massive trauma, an assessment of the patient's airway and cardiovascular status is very important. Once the patient is stabilized, a neurologic evaluation, including an assessment of the facial nerve, is indicated.

The type of trauma and the duration of the paralysis are important. Differentiating partial from complete facial paralysis when facial edema, ecchymosis, or lacerations exist is difficult, particularly in an uncooperative patient.[7,8,16]

Any nerve branch lacerated anterior to the masseter muscle is usually too small to approximate; in addition, function often returns because of cross-anastomoses or neurotization.

A completely severed facial nerve continues to conduct impulses for about 72 hours.[6–8] Exploration of wounds within 72 hours can thus be facilitated by the use of nerve stimulation to help find the severed nerve branches. If the patient is evaluated after 72 hours the nerve stimulator will be of no help; however, exploration and repair should be done as soon as is feasible. Delay until scarring has matured facilitates dissection.[6–8] Nerve grafts should be performed before 18 months, by which time fibrosis of the neural tissues and subsequent atrophy of muscle fibers is sufficiently advanced to preclude grafting.

CT scans are appropriate when the temporal bone has been traumatized. MRI may help to locate the site of either nerve trunk or larger nerve branch injury.

Indications

- Immediate facial paralysis occurring after penetrating wounds anterior or inferior (or both) to the auricle and posterior to the anterior border of the masseter muscle (function of branches severed anterior to the masseter muscle usually returns spontaneously because of multiple facial nerve branch anastomoses)
- Immediate facial paralysis occurring after blunt trauma to the head and neck

Anesthetic considerations

General nasotracheal anesthesia is used; refer to the sections on intratemporal bone facial nerve exploration or decompression and surgery for parotid and nonparotid gland diseases.

Preparation

Preparations for possible parotidectomy, mastoidectomy with facial nerve exploration, and great auricular or sural nerve grafting are used; refer to the sections on intratemporal bone facial nerve exploration or decompression and surgery for parotid and nonparotid gland diseases.

A nerve integrity monitor, facial nerve stimulator, and microscope or surgical loupes should be available.

Procedure

For more peripheral cutaneous lacerations, with segmental paralysis, exploration of the wound and approximation of the severed nerve endings may be possible. In cases in which the lacerated peripheral branches cannot be located or approximated, in more proximal facial lacerations, in total facial nerve paralysis, and in cases involving blunt trauma with no external laceration, a parotidectomy approach must be taken to locate the facial nerve. As with the previously described procedures, in any surgical approach done within 72 hours of the onset of paralysis, the use of a facial nerve stimulator may facilitate location of the nerve. If the facial nerve trunk and its branches are found to be intact, or if the only lacerations are in the cervical or distal buccal branches, the nerve can be left as it is and the wounds can be cleaned, débrided, and sutured.

In acute cases, once a nerve laceration or avulsion is located, the nerve endings are mobilized and sutured with the fewest number of 9-0 or 10-0 monofilament nylon sutures necessary to achieve coaptation, if the ends can be approximated without tension. If this cannot be done, removal of underlying parotid tissue may enable approximation without suture line tension (Fig. 4–26*A* and *B*).[15]

When the laceration is situated at the stylomastoid foramen or is so posterior on the main trunk that suturing of the proximal stump is impossible, mastoidectomy with facial nerve exposure is necessary to locate and mobilize the proximal nerve for reapproximation or grafting (see Fig. 4–12).

In delayed cases, the nerve endings are mobilized, freshened with a razor blade or a 6500 Beaver Mini-Blade, and sutured with the fewest 9-0 or 10-0 monofilament nylon sutures needed to achieve coaptation (Fig. 4–27*A* to *C*). Removal of underlying parotid tissue sometimes enables approximation without suture line tension.

Interposition nerve grafting is necessary if the severed segments cannot be approximated or can be closed only under tension. This topic is covered in the section on extratemporal facial nerve grafting.

In cases in which immediate grafting is impossible or inadvisable (e.g., gross contamination, anesthetic complication), the severed proximal and distal ends should be tagged with nonabsorbable, nonreactive sutures (nylon) for easier localization at subsequent repair.

In delayed cases, a margin of nerve should be sent for frozen section to determine whether neural fibrosis has occurred. If this is the case, further nerve resection is needed until viable nerve tissue is located.

A Penrose or vacuum drain is placed inferior to the trunk and posterior to the branches of the nerve and is brought through either the inferior part of the incision or a separate incision. Any wound lacerations are then freshened, and these lacerations as well as the parotidectomy incision are approximated using 3-0 to 4-0 catgut subcutaneous sutures and 4-0 to 5-0 nylon cutaneous sutures. Antibiotic ointment is placed on the incision (or incisions). Fluffed and 4 × 4″ dressing gauze sponges are applied with either a Barton or nylon tubular net compression dressing.

Postoperative care

Postoperative care and nerve recovery time is the same as is discussed in the section on surgery for parotid and nonparotid gland diseases.

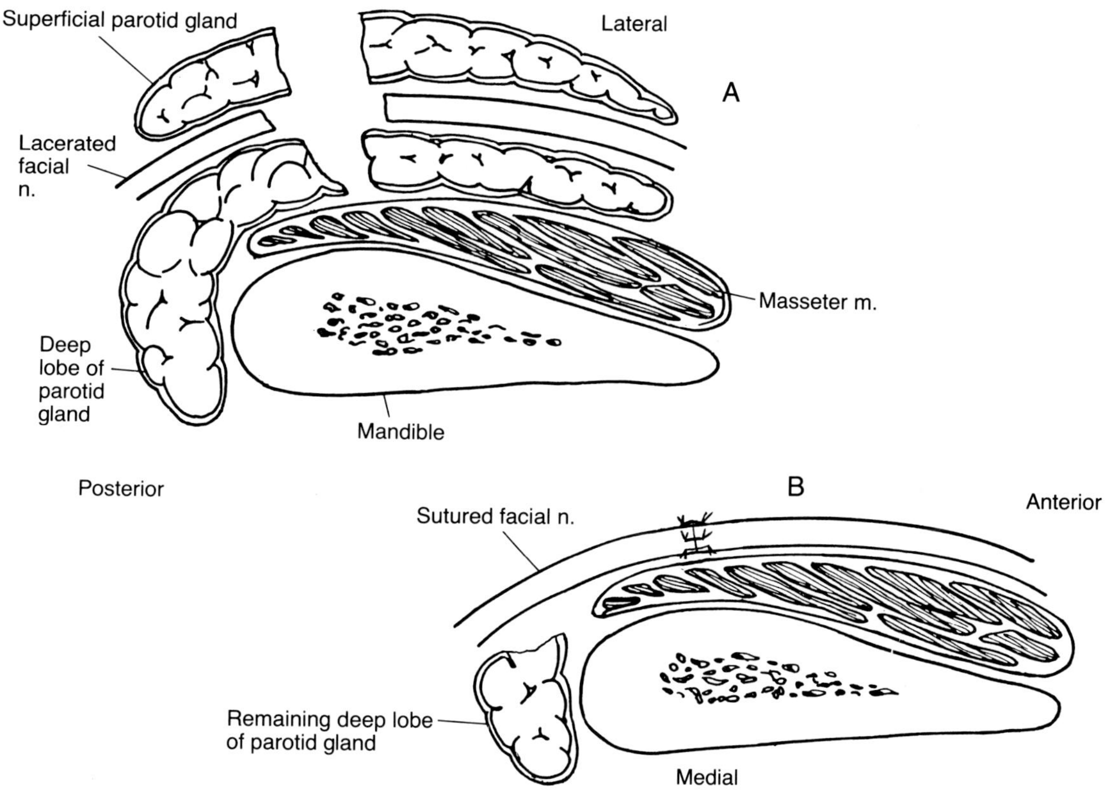

• FIGURE 4-26.

A, Avulsed parotid tissue and facial nerve. *B*, Removal of superficial and underlying parotid tissue to enable approximation of nerve branch ends after avulsion. (Adapted from Tucker HM: The management of facial paralysis due to extracranial injuries. Laryngoscope 88:348–354, 1978.)

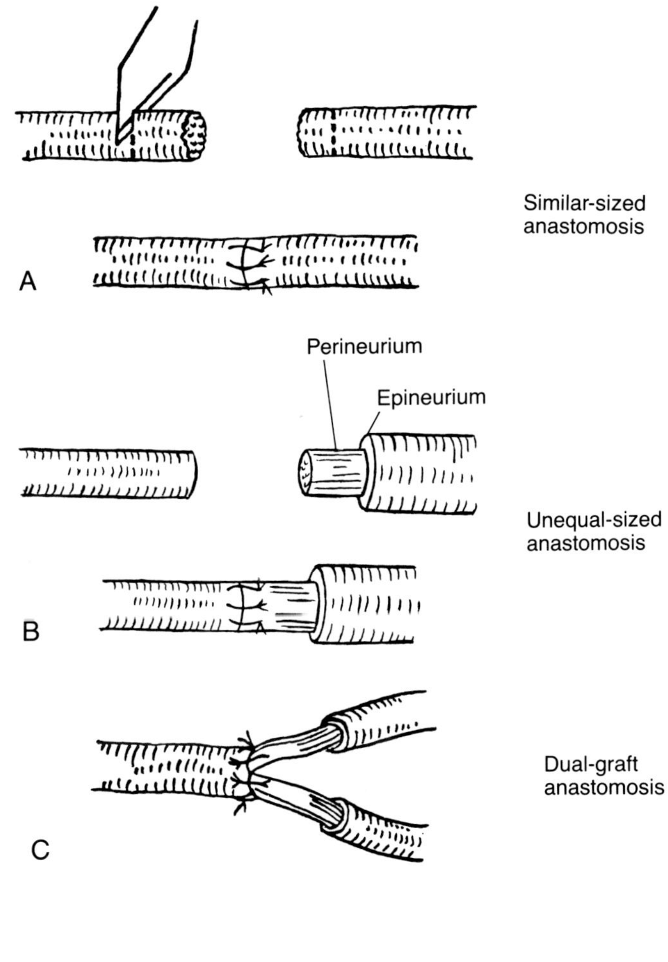

• FIGURE 4-27.

A, Similar-sized nerve and nerve graft ends cut at a 90-degree angle with a sharp blade and then sutured. *B*, When a smaller-diameter graft is needed, 5 mm of epineurium is stripped from the end and is sutured to the recipient nerve. *C*, Suturing of two nerve grafts of smaller diameter to a larger-diameter nerve trunk.

EXTRATEMPORAL FACIAL NERVE SUTURING, REROUTING, GRAFTING, AND NERVE TRANSFER

Extratemporal facial nerve rerouting or grafting is done when primary approximation of the nerve endings is impossible or cannot be done without tension. Extratemporal facial nerve rerouting is done by removal of the existing parotid gland to enable approximation without suture line tension.[6]

Nerve graft donor sites include the ipsilateral or contralateral great auricular nerve and the sural nerve, depending on the length of the defect, the size of the nerve, and the condition of the donor sites.

Various nerve transfers, predominantly the hypoglossal-facial (XII-VII) but also the cross-facial (VII-VII) and spinal accessory-facial (XI-VII), have been advocated. The simplest and least debilitating nerve transfer can be done by severing cervical or buccal branches and by approximating them to the distal stump of the mandibular, zygomatic, or temporal branches.[7–9,15]

Indications

- Approximation and suturing are indicated in any trunk or main branch laceration posterior to the anterior border of the masseter that can be done without tension.

- Rerouting of the extratemporal facial nerve is indicated if lacerated nerve segments cannot be approximated without tension and if there is residual parotid tissue, which, if removed, will enable approximation without tension.

- Interposition nerve grafting is indicated in any extratemporal facial nerve laceration in which primary approximation and suturing are not possible or, if they are achieved, in which the laceration is under tension or in which avulsion of any more than 50% of the nerve has occurred. Viable neural tissue must be present at the proximal and distal segment margins.

- Nerve transfer of a cervical or buccal branch is indicated when lacerations of mandibular, zygomatic, or temporal branches cannot be approximated without tension and a cervical or buccal branch is present in sufficient length and appropriate diameter for primary anastomosis without tension.

- Nerve transfer from another cranial nerve (XII, XI, or contralateral VII) may be indicated as a last resort in patients with a flaccid face, functioning distal nerve and neuromuscular junction, and no viable proximal nerve. An interposition nerve graft may be necessary to bridge the gap. Because of the additional cranial nerve deficit after nerve transfer, an extensive informed consent must be obtained.

Anesthetic considerations

General nasotracheal anesthesia is used; refer to the sections on intratemporal bone facial nerve exploration or decompression and surgery for parotid and non-parotid gland diseases.

Preparation

The preparations are the same as those for parotidectomy with or without intratemporal bone facial nerve exploration; refer to the sections on intratemporal bone facial nerve exploration or decompression and surgery for parotid and non-parotid gland diseases. If a sural nerve graft is anticipated, the lower leg, ankle, and foot are similarly prepared. A surgical glove is placed over the toes, and the foot and leg are draped with a sterile stockinette and placed on a sterile sheet. An extremity drape is used to cover the leg.

Procedure

Suturing and rerouting of the extratemporal facial nerve are described in the two previous sections on extratemporal bone facial nerve surgery.

Exposure and preparation of the proximal and distal facial nerve sites before nerve grafting are described in the four previous sections. The nerve graft is obtained from the ipsilateral or contralateral great auricular nerve or the sural nerve.

Before performing great auricular nerve grafting, the surgeon should test the skin of the neck for sensation in the area of the C2, C3 distribution on both the ipsilateral and the contralateral neck.

The cervical portion of a parotidectomy incision can be used to locate the great auricular nerve. Otherwise, a horizontal incision is made parallel to (or, preferably, in) a skin crease about 2 cm inferior to the mandibular margin, centered on the posterior border of the sternocleidomastoid muscle. One long incision or two smaller stairstep incisions can be made. Once isolated, the nerve can be dissected proximally toward its origin in the cervical plexus to gain up to 10 cm of additional length. The cervical incision can be approximated in two layers with 3-0 to 4-0 catgut sutures and 4-0 to 5-0 nylon sutures.

If the ipsilateral great auricular nerve is smaller than the severed branch of the facial nerve, the contralateral great auricular nerve or one or more fascicles of the sural nerve can be grafted as well (Fig. 4–28; see also Fig. 4–27).

Use of the great auricular nerve as a graft leaves a cutaneous sensory deficit over the mastoid process and auricle.

The sural nerve is formed by the junction of the communicating ramus of the lateral sural cutaneous nerve and the medial sural cutaneous nerve in the middle of the leg. The sural nerve is usually located just medial to the small saphenous vein and then continues inferiorly and curves anteriorly, inferior to the lateral malleolus, where it divides into several branches; it ends as the lateral dorsal cutaneous nerve. The sural nerve is easiest to locate just posterior to the lateral malleolus and next to the saphenous vein (Fig. 4–29).

• FIGURE 4-28.

Two grafts, or fascicles, are sutured to a facial nerve trunk larger in diameter than available donor grafts.

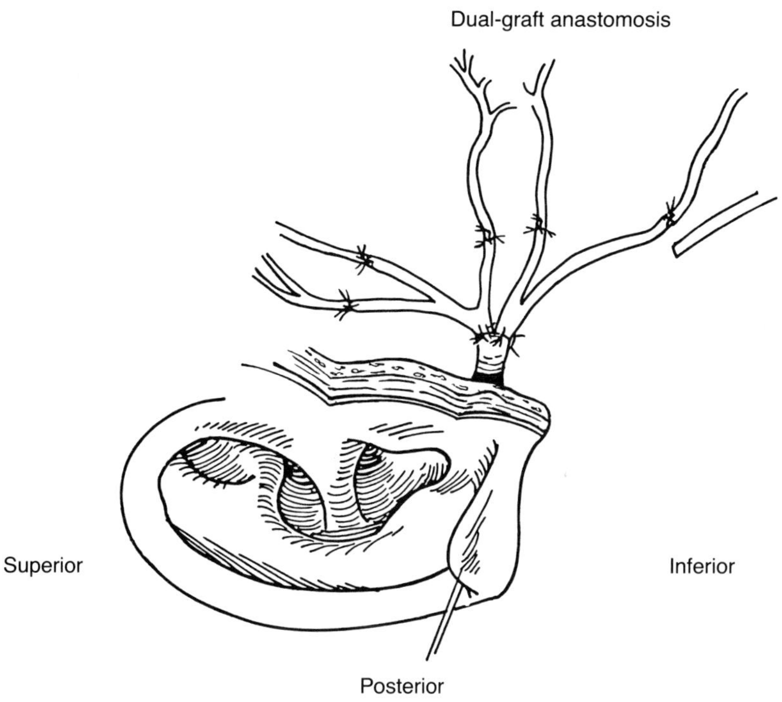

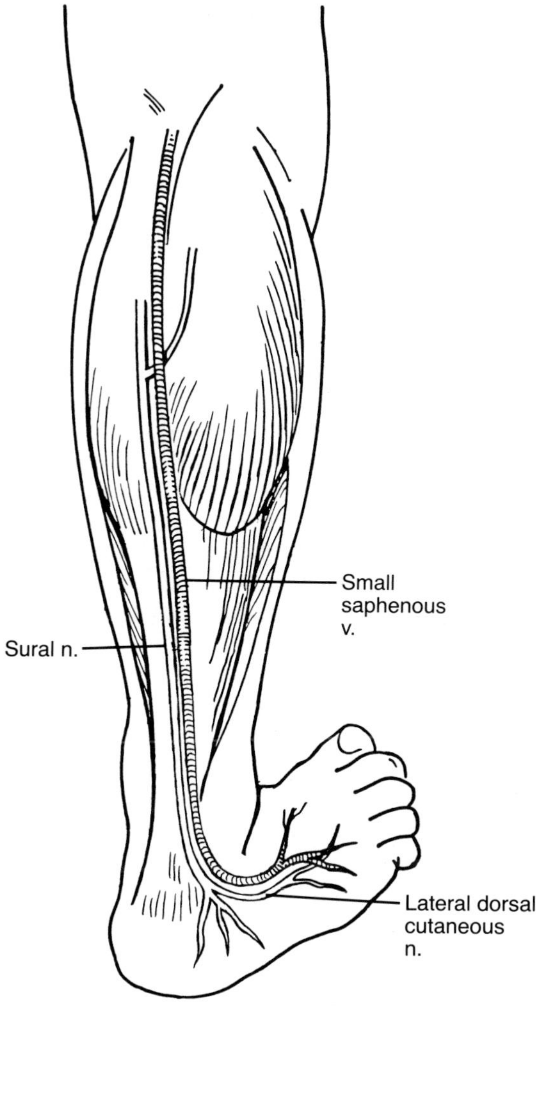

• FIGURE 4-29.

A schematic representation of the sural nerve, which is located adjacent to the saphenous vein in the lower leg.

The sural nerve can be exposed through a vertical incision that bisects the plane between the lateral malleolus and the Achilles tendon. The incision is then curved inferior to the lateral malleolus and onto the lateral aspect of the foot (Fig. 4–30*A*). An alternative, more cosmetically acceptable way to expose the sural nerve is to first make a horizontal incision at the level of and posterior to the lateral malleolus (Fig. 4–30*B*).

Lateral traction on the vein and the sural nerve reveals the nerve's superior and inferior course, enabling easier dissection. Horizontal incisions are then made at appropriate intervals to obtain a longer graft. As much as 35 cm of sural nerve, consisting of two to four fascicles, can be used.

The nerve graft should be obtained after the recipient site is prepared. If grafting is delayed after the nerve graft is obtained, the nerve should be placed in Ringer's lactate solution.

Similar to the cervical incision, the leg incision can be approximated in two layers with 3-0 to 4-0 catgut sutures and 4-0 to 5-0 nylon sutures.

Sacrifice of the sural nerve results in minimal sensory deficit. Although both incisions heal well, the stairstep incision is less conspicuous.

When ready for use, the graft is laid in position to determine the proper length. A slight excess should be taken to allow for contraction and to avoid tension on the suture lines. The ends are prepared by sharp razor blade incisions at a 45- to 90-degree angle. Epineurium may need to be stripped away from the nerve graft for about 5 mm if the diameter is too large. An appropriate number of 9-0 or 10-0 monofilament nylon sutures are used to approximate the perineurium of the graft to the epineurium of the nerve. Depending on the width of the proximal and distal nerve stump(s), either the entire nerve or one or more fascicles can be used.

For hypoglossal facial anastomosis, once the distal nerve stump has been located, the cervical portion of a parotidectomy incision is made. The hypoglossal nerve is found 1.5 cm superior to the carotid bifurcation, where it courses laterally to the internal and external carotid arteries, medially to the posterior belly of the digastric muscle. The nerve is dissected anteriorly as far as possible before transection to maximize its length. Interposition nerve grafts may be necessary for approximation without tension. Both the distal facial nerve segment and the hypoglossal stump are prepared for perineural or epineural anastomosis. The stump is sutured to the recipient facial nerve with an appropriate number of 9-0 or 10-0 monofilament nylon sutures (Fig. 4–31). Sacrifice of the hypoglossal nerve results in paralysis of the ipsilateral side of the tongue. Although facial function can be learned, ipsilateral facial contraction is initiated by swallowing.

The wound is irrigated with sterile saline. The skin incision is approximated with 3-0 or 4-0 catgut sutures and 4-0 or 5-0 nylon sutures. Staples can be used for the cervical portion of the incision. Antibiotic ointment is applied to the incision line. A compressive Barton or tubular net dressing or elastic tape is applied over fluffed and 4 × 4″ dressing gauze sponges to create pressure. After sural nerve grafting, a compressive leg dressing is applied using 4 × 4″ dressing gauze sponges and elastic tape.

Postoperative care

The facial and cervical dressing is reinforced overnight to absorb bloody drainage. The dressing is removed on the first or second postoperative day, and a fresh compressive dressing is applied and is left on for 4 to 7 days. The compressive leg dressing applied after sural nerve grafting is removed at 1 to 3 days. The leg and neck sutures or staples are removed at 7 to 10 days.

Recovery of facial function should begin within 4 to 6 months and should continue for at least 12 months.

• FIGURE 4-30.

The sural nerve can be identified through (*A*) a vertical incision that bisects the distance between the lateral malleolus and the Achilles tendon and curves inferiorly to gain additional length or branches or (*B*) a horizontal incision just posterior to the lateral malleolus with stair-step incisions above and below to gain additional length.

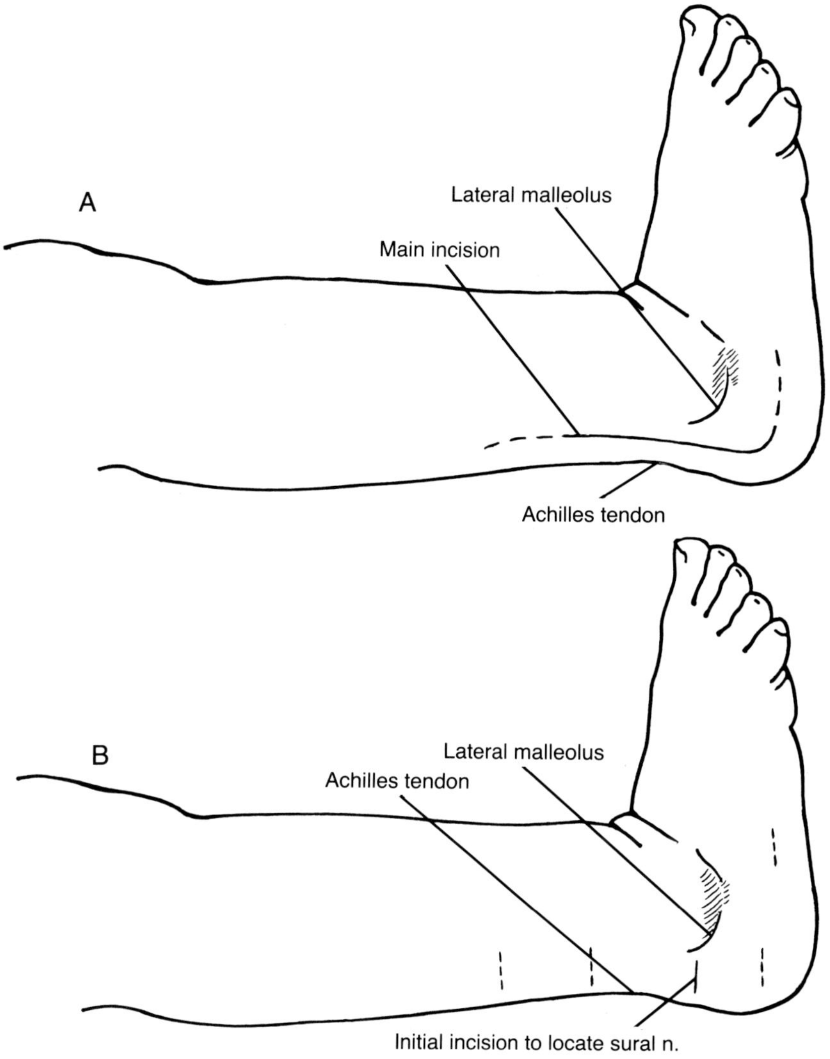

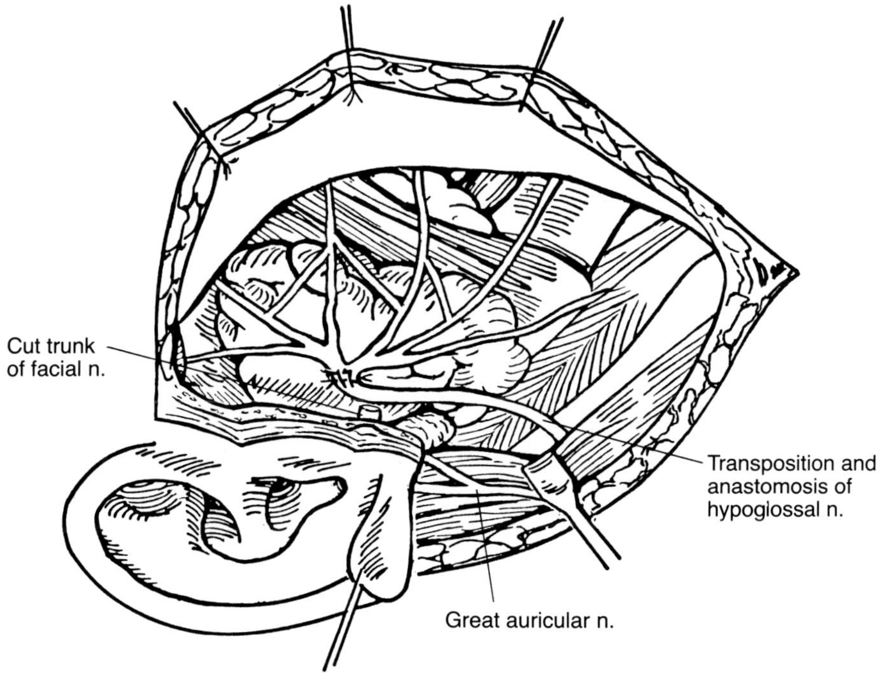

• FIGURE 4-31.

The hypoglossal nerve is transected and sutured onto a previously prepared distal facial nerve.

REFERENCES

1. Proctor B: The anatomy of the facial nerve. Otolaryngol Clin North Am 24:479–504, 1991.
2. Clemente CD (ed): Gray's Anatomy of the Human Body, 30th ed. Philadelphia, Lea & Febiger, 1985.
3. Hollinshead WH: Anatomy for Surgeons, 3rd ed. I: The Head and Neck. Philadelphia, Harper & Row, 1982.
4. Farrior JB and Santini H: Facial nerve identification in children. Otolaryngol Head Neck Surg 93:173–176, 1985.
5. May M: Facial paralysis in children. *In* Bluestone CD, Stool SE, and Arjona SK (eds): Pediatric Otolaryngology. Philadelphia, WB Saunders, 1983, pp 249–270.
6. Adkins WY and Osguthorpe JD: Management of trauma of the facial nerve. Otolaryngol Clin North Am 24:587–611, 1991.
7. Johns ME and Crumley RL: Facial nerve injury, repair, and rehabilitation. Washington, DC, American Academy of Otolaryngology, 1979. (Otorhinolaryngology Self-instructional Packages, 79200.)
8. Papel ID: Rehabilitation of the paralyzed face. Otolaryngol Clin North Am 24:727–738, 1991.
9. Fisch U and Lanser MJ: Facial nerve grafting. Otolaryngol Clin North Am 24:691–708, 1991.
10. Batsakis JG: Tumors of the Head and Neck: Clinical and Pathological Considerations, 2nd ed. Baltimore, Williams & Wilkins, 1979, pp 9–14, 64–66.
11. Gates GA: Diseases of the salivary glands. *In* Bluestone CD, Stool SE, and Arjona SK (eds): Pediatric Otolaryngology. Philadelphia, WB Saunders, 1983, pp 1023–1036.
12. McRae RG, Lee KJ, and Goertzen E: First branchial cleft anomalies and the facial nerve. Otolaryngol Head Neck Surg 91:197–202, 1983.
13. Schuller DE and McCabe BF: Salivary gland neoplasms in children. Otolaryngol Clin North Am 10:399–412, 1977.
14. Harris JP, Davidson TM, May M, and Fria T: Evaluation and treatment of congenital facial paralysis. Arch Otolaryngol 109:145–151, 1983.
15. Tucker HM: The management of facial paralysis due to extracranial injuries. Laryngoscope 88:348–354, 1978.
16. Olsson JE and Shagets FW: Blunt Trauma of the Temporal Bone, 2nd ed. Washington, DC, American Academy of Otolaryngology-Head and Neck Surgery, 1986. (Otorhinolaryngology Self-Instructional Package, 80386.)

ACKNOWLEDGMENTS

I thank Kedar K. Adour, M.D., Frederick M. Byl, M.D., and E. Lila Jordan, R.N., for helpful suggestions and for reviewing the manuscript. Jon Coulter provided the illustrations with the assistance of Juan Domingo. The Medical Editing Department of Kaiser Foundation Research Institute provided editorial assistance.

chapter

5

Surgery of the Ear Canal: Split-Thickness Skin Grafts and Surgical Correction of Atresia

SIMON C. PARISIER, M.D.
DAVID A. SEIDMAN, M.D.

PRINCIPLES OF EXTERNAL AUDITORY CANAL SURGERY

Inadequate attention to the external ear canal may result in the failure of an otherwise successful tympanomastoid operation. When performing ear surgery, a narrow canal or the presence of overhangs that prevent adequate exposure may compromise the desired results.

A common iatrogenic complication of operations involving the external ear canal is partial postoperative stenosis. Failure to provide good access to the mastoid recess following canal wall-down mastoidectomies, in which the mastoid cavity becomes marsupialized into the external ear canal, frequently results in problem ears that are difficult to take care of.

A narrow meatal opening defeats the self-cleaning mechanism of the external ear canal, leading to the "problem ear." An anatomic understanding of the ear canal with analysis and correction of the structures producing narrowing or obstruction allows for a systematic operative approach that surgically produces a patent meatus and canal.

Otologic surgery that involves the auditory canal is ideally performed when the skin is not inflamed and when any acute infectious processes have been controlled. Draining ears should be treated medically prior to surgery. As an office procedure, meticulous débridement of the ear canal is performed using an operating microscope and appropriate delicate instruments. Wax, retained keratin debris, and drainage fluid are eliminated to expose the underlying skin and eardrum remnant. Granulation tissue is removed and sent for pathologic examination. The resulting bleeding base is chemically cauterized. A culture of the ear canal may be obtained in selected refractory cases. Appropriate antifungal or antibiotic topical drops and systemic oral antibiotics are prescribed. The importance of preventing water from getting into the ear when bathing or swimming must be emphasized to the patient and family. Patients are instructed to plug the affected ear with either commercially available soft silicone plugs or petroleum-impregnated lamb's wool. Parents and patients are admonished not to use cotton-tipped applicators, which impact debris in the canal and irritate the skin. Occasionally, when a patient is unable to comply with the recommended instructions or is refractory to the treatment, hospitalization is recommended for intravenous antibiotic and intensive local therapy.

Most "wet" ears can be converted to a dry state in 4 to 6 weeks using the above recommendations. Surgery can be performed when the acute inflammatory ear process is quiescent. Occasionally, in spite of intensive therapy, suppuration persists. In these cases, the indicated ear surgery might be required, in spite of active drainage, in order to create a noninfected ear. Generally, surgery performed in an actively inflamed ear is accompanied by bleeding that makes visualization more difficult, compromising the surgical outcome. Also, in a small child, blood loss may be significant, requiring blood transfusions.

Audiometric evaluations should always be performed prior to surgery on an ear. The indications for obtaining radiographic imaging should be determined by the underlying existing clinical findings.

RECONSTRUCTION OF THE EXTERNAL EAR CANAL

Indications

Reconstruction of the external ear canal requires consideration of the two anatomic divisions—the lateral cartilaginous portion and the medial osseous tympanic bone—and their skin lining:

- Lateral cartilaginous portion

  Skin lining: contains hair follicles, sebaceous glands, dermal layer—thicker layer

  Perform meatoplasty by removing constricting cartilage from the anterior edge of the concha and by resecting cartilage that forms the floor of the canal. The skin lining is preserved.

- Medial osseous tympanic bone

  Skin lining: the lamina propria of the epidermis merges with the bony periosteum—thinner layer

  Develop pedicled canal wall skin flaps posteriorly and anteriorly. Expose bony overhangs, which are drilled away. Replace the meticulously preserved canal wall skin, maintaining an epidermis-lined canal. In cases in which canal wall skin is deficient, use a split-thickness skin graft to provide a stable epidermal canal lining.

Pertinent anatomy follows:

- In the tympanic part of the temporal bone: two prominent sutures, the anterior tympanosquamous suture (Fig. 5–1*a*) and the posterior tympanomastoid suture (Fig. 5–1*b*), may protrude, encroaching on the canal lumen. The anterior and inferior portions of the tympanic bone vary in bulk. When prominent, the canal lumen may be narrowed by these overhangs, which prevent visualization of the margin of the eardrum and of related pathologic changes. The suprameatal spine (Fig. 5–1*c*), when prominent and anteriorly oriented, can narrow the canal at the bony cartilaginous junction.
- The glenoid fossa is anterior to the ear canal.
- The mastoid bone and the air cell system are posterior to the ear canal.

Anesthetic considerations

General anesthesia is usually required for the pediatric population. Local anesthesia may be feasible for the adolescent for short procedures.

Preparation

Standard and routine drapings should be used, providing exposure of the ear; in some cases, facial nerve monitoring may be applicable. If facial nerve monitoring is used, muscle relaxants should be avoided.

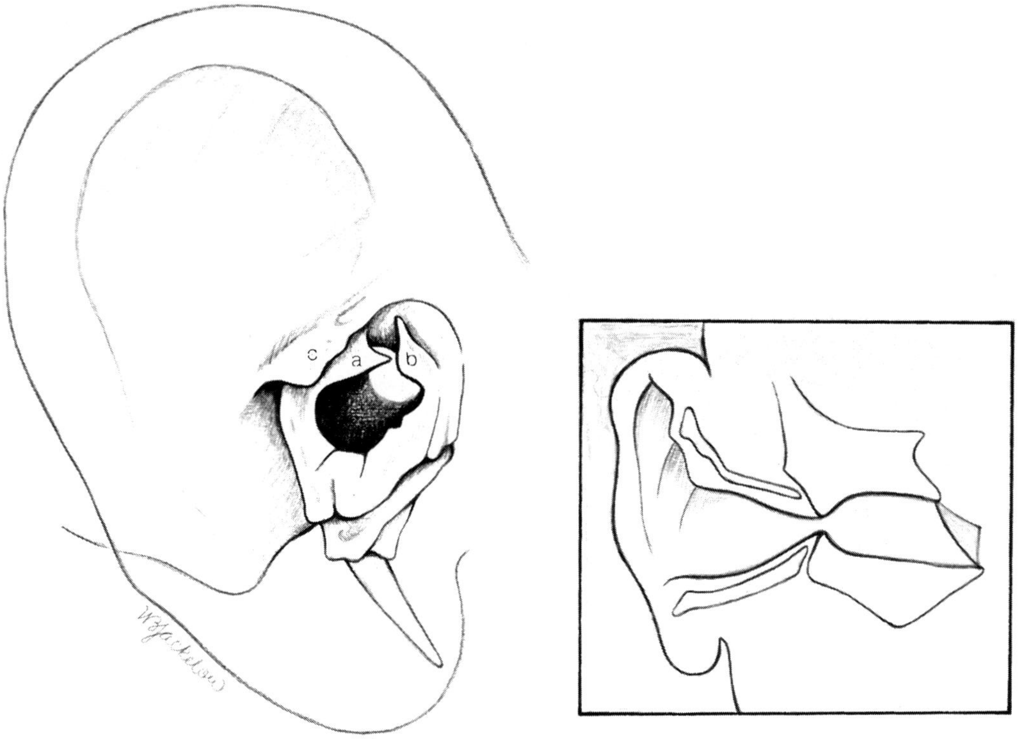

• **FIGURE 5-1.**

Tympanic portion of the temporal bone. (*a*) Anterior tympanosquamous suture, (*b*) posterior tympanomastoid suture, and (*c*) the suprameatal spine.

• TABLE 5-1.

ENDAURAL AND POSTAURICULAR APPROACHES

Endaural Approach

Advantages

This approach allows precise placement of ear canal incisions.
The approach facilitates the development of a rectangularly shaped, laterally based conchal-meatal-canal skin flap.
The pedicled flap promotes rapid healing, decreases granulation formation, and eliminates stenosis formation.

Limitations

Exposure is inadequate to eradicate disease in large pneumatized mastoids.
Resection of cartilage, especially from the canal floor, is technically difficult while preserving canal wall–meatal skin. This may hamper the construction of a large meatal opening.
The anterior sulcus area is more difficult to access, especially when there is a canal wall overhang.

Postauricular Approach

Advantages

Best exposure of extensively pneumatized mastoid bone is given.
Visualization of the anterior canal–tympanic membrane anterior sulcus is enhanced. The angle of vision obtained posteriorly is less obstructed than when working through an endaural approach.
This approach provides access that allows direct exposure of conchal and inferior canal cartilages from which the meatal and canal wall skin can be elevated with relative ease.
The approach facilitates harvesting two connective tissue grafts: first, areolar tissue and second, temporalis fascia. The fascia is used to graft the eardrum and, in canal wall-down mastoidectomies, the adjacent exposed bone. The areolar tissue is useful for resurfacing bone when a canal wall-down procedure has been performed, reducing healing that takes place by secondary intention.

Limitations

Imprecise placement of canal skin incisions results in possible loss of skin, delay in healing, and partial stenosis.
Additional surgical exposure and time are needed.

Procedure

The described approach is applicable for a wide variety of otologic procedures. It may be incorporated into tympanoplasties, both canal wall-up and wall-down mastoidectomies; exostoses; and acquired or congenital stenosis. The ear canal surgical method described combines endaural and postauricular approaches (Figs. 5–2 and 5–3). Table 5–1 lists the advantages and limitations of the endaural and postauricular approaches.

ENDAURAL APPROACH

• Inject the canal with 1:100,000 epinephrine. Using a 25-gauge needle, the injection is placed into the dermal portion of the ear canal where the last hair cells are located. Injecting into the osseous canal results in blebs and tears of the thin epidermis and should, therefore, be avoided. The bevel of the needle is directed so that it faces the bony surfaces. The fluid is injected using digital pressure, forcing the anesthetic to hydrodissect towards the eardrum. The canal is injected superiorly at 12 o'clock and inferiorly at 6 o'clock because the spread of the solution is confined by the tympanomastoid and tympanosquamous sutures. The skin is observed to blanch and thicken as the anesthetic is slowly injected.

• Through an ear speculum, using a stapes knife, a horizontal incision is made in the ear canal 2 to 3 mm lateral and parallel to the annulus. It extends from above the lateral process of the malleus (12 o'clock) to the floor of the external canal (6 o'clock) (Fig. 5–4).

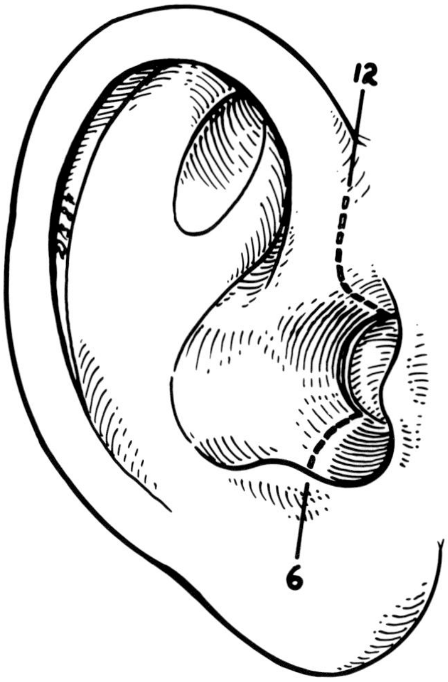

• FIGURE 5-2.

An endaural approach. (From Johnson JT, et al [eds]: American Academy of Otolaryngology—Instructional Courses, Vol 4. St Louis, MO, CV Mosby, 1991.)

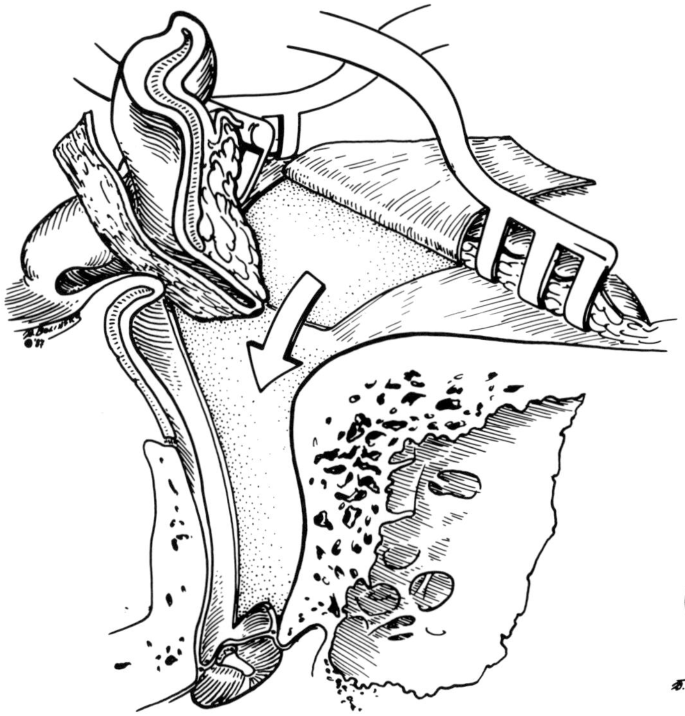

• FIGURE 5-3.

A postauricular approach. (From Johnson JT, et al [eds]: American Academy of Otolaryngology—Instructional Courses, Vol 4. St Louis, MO, CV Mosby, 1991.)

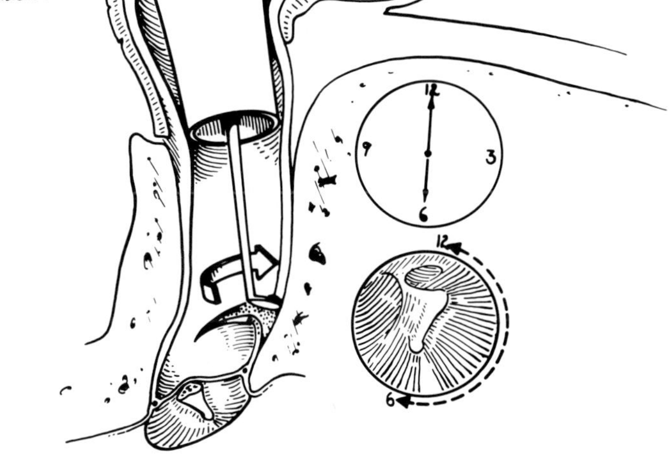

• FIGURE 5-4.

A horizontal incision is made using a stapes knife through an ear speculum. (From Johnson JT, et al [eds]: American Academy of Otolaryngology—Instructional Courses, Vol 4. St Louis, MO, CV Mosby, 1991.)

• The meatal opening is dilated widely using a Lempert endaural speculum (Fig. 5–5). Two vertical incisions are made using a needle point cautery to minimize bleeding that enhances visibility. The first is made superiorly in the notch between the tragus and the anterior root of the helix (12 o'clock) (Fig. 5–6). This incision is made in order to preserve a bridge of skin between it and the horizontal incision, ending 2 to 3 mm lateral to the initial tympanomeatal incision. This attachment serves to stabilize the skin. Working through this vertical incision, using a duckbill elevator, the superior and posterior canal wall skin is elevated off the underlying bone (Fig. 5–7). This undermining exposes the tympanosquamous suture anteriorly (Fig. 5–8), the canal bone, the suprameatal spine area and, if possible, the tympanomastoid suture posteriorly.

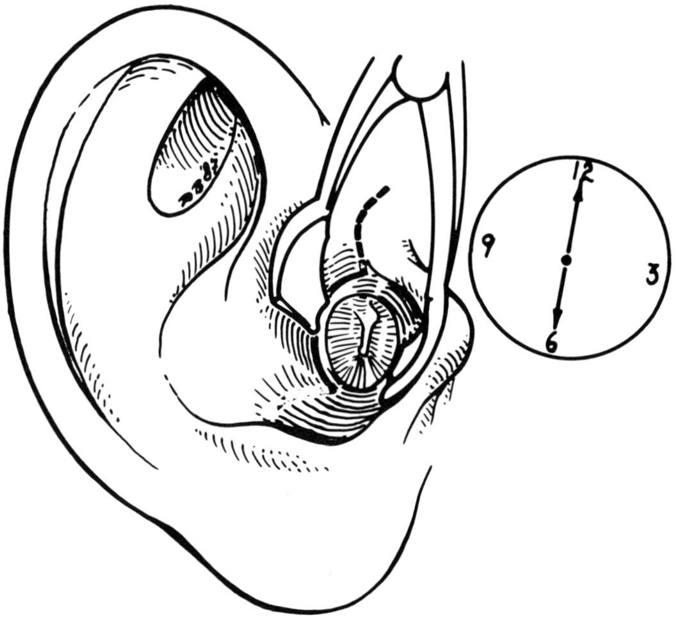

• FIGURE 5–5.

Dilatation of the meatal opening with a Lempert endaural speculum. (From Johnson JT, et al [eds]: American Academy of Otolaryngology—Instructional Courses, Vol 4. St Louis, MO, CV Mosby, 1991.)

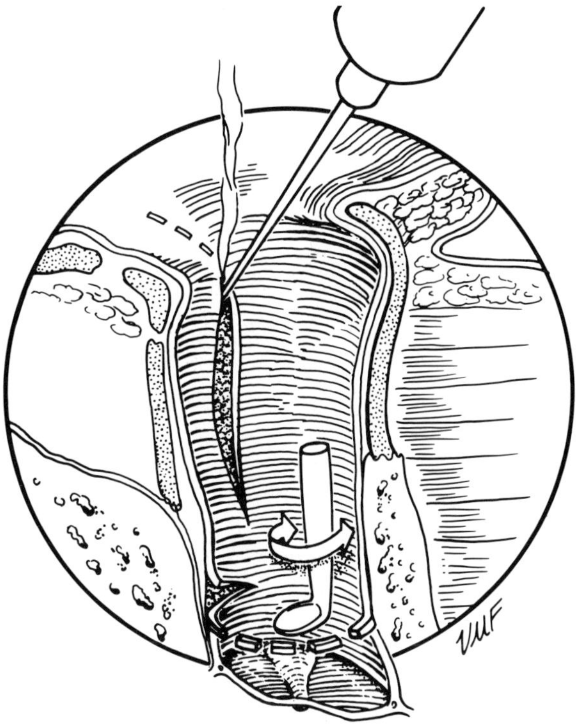

• FIGURE 5-6.

The first incision is made using a needle point cautery at the 12 o'clock position. (From Johnson JT, et al [eds]: American Academy of Otolaryngology—Instructional Courses, Vol 4. St Louis, MO, CV Mosby, 1991.)

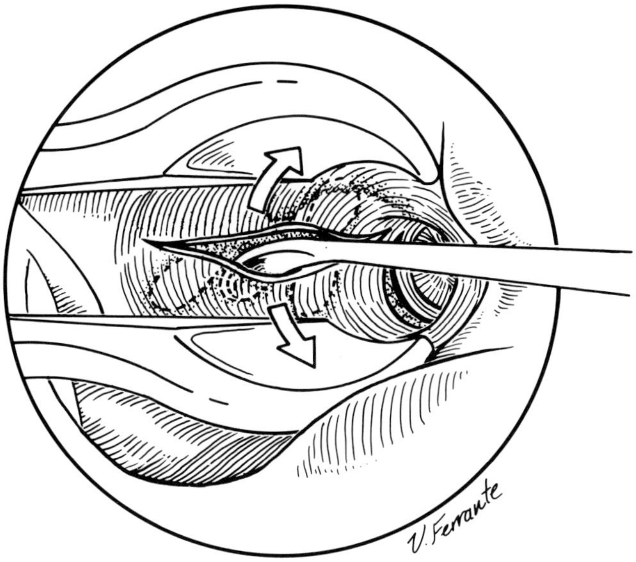

• FIGURE 5-7.

A duckbill elevator lifts the skin of the superior and posterior canal wall off the underlying bone. (From Johnson JT, et al [eds]: American Academy of Otolaryngology—Instructional Courses, Vol 4. St Louis, MO, CV Mosby, 1991.)

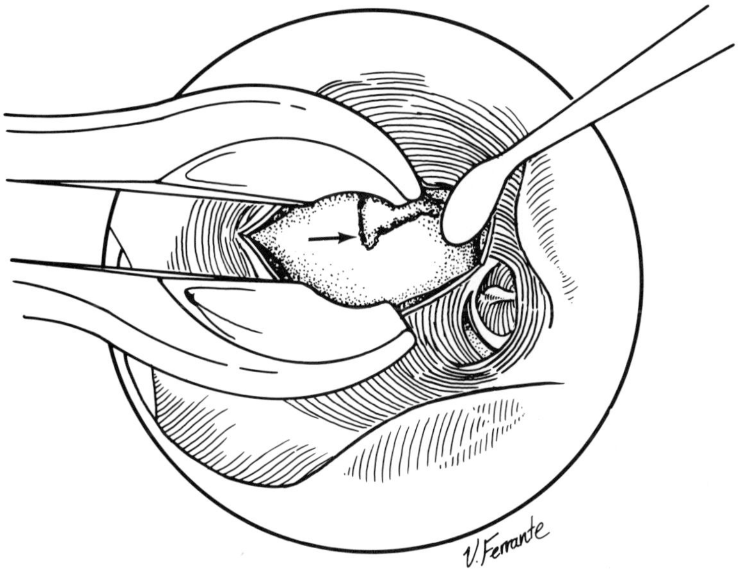

• FIGURE 5-8.

Undermining reveals a tympanosquamous suture (*arrow*). (From Johnson JT, et al [eds]: American Academy of Otolaryngology—Instructional Courses, Vol 4. St Louis, MO, CV Mosby, 1991.)

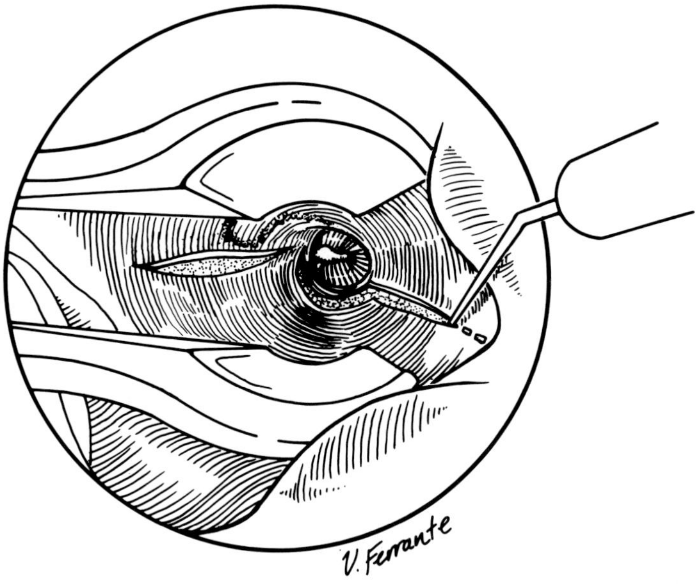

• FIGURE 5-9.

A second incision is made at the 6 o'clock position. (From Johnson JT, et al [eds]: American Academy of Otolaryngology—Instructional Courses, Vol 4. St Louis, MO, CV Mosby, 1991.)

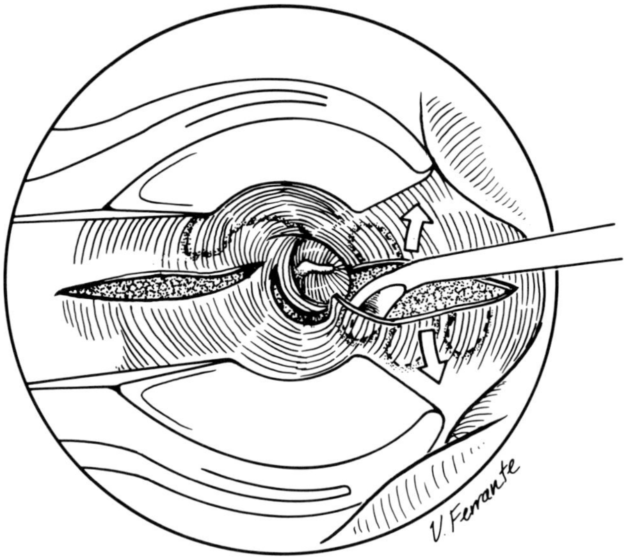

• FIGURE 5-10.

The skin of the inferior posterior canal wall is elevated. (From Johnson JT, et al [eds]: American Academy of Otolaryngology—Instructional Courses, Vol 4. St Louis, MO, CV Mosby, 1991.)

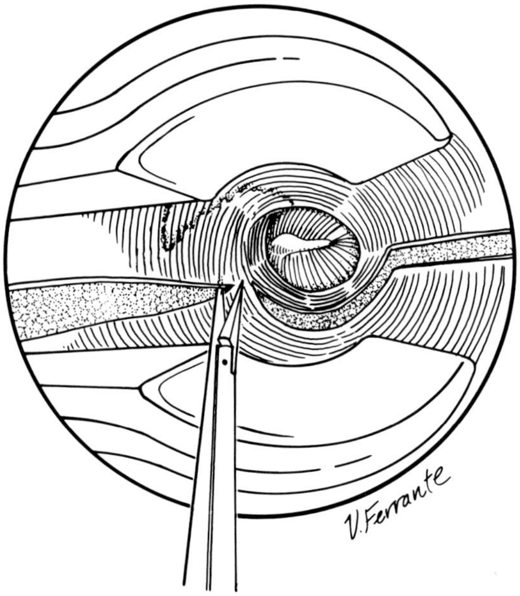

• FIGURE 5-11.

Preserved skin is cut with a Bellucci scissors to form the meatal canal skin flap. (From Johnson JT, et al [eds]: American Academy of Otolaryngology—Instructional Courses, Vol 4. St Louis, MO, CV Mosby, 1991.)

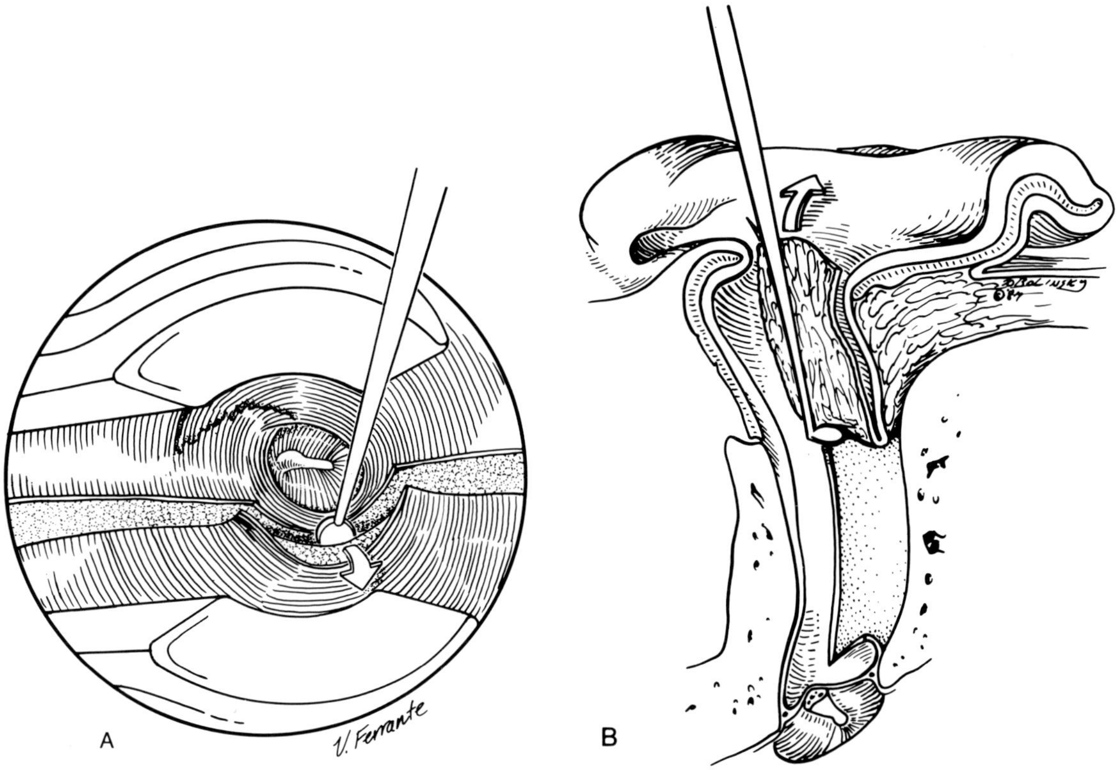

• FIGURE 5-12.

A and *B*, The flap is elevated out of the canal to the meatus. (From Johnson JT, et al [eds]: American Academy of Otolaryngology—Instructional Courses, Vol 4. St Louis, MO, CV Mosby, 1991.)

• In the same fashion as the previous step, an incision is made at the 6 o'clock position beginning at the horizontal incision and extending laterally to the conchal opening (Fig. 5-9).

• Using a duckbill elevator, the inferior posterior canal wall skin is dissected from the underlying bony canal (Fig. 5-10).

• The bridge of the skin superiorly that was preserved is now cut using Bellucci scissors, completing the mobilization of the rectangular meatal canal skin flap (Fig. 5-11).

• Elevate the rectangular skin flap retrograde out of the canal to the meatus (Fig. 5-12*A* and *B*). The meatal opening can be enlarged further by extending the vertical incisions into the conchal area and also by removing the underlying conchal and canal wall floor cartilages via the postauricular approach.

POSTAURICULAR APPROACH

The postauricular approach is done, and areolar tissue and temporalis fascia grafts are obtained.

- Make a skin incision using an electrocautery just posterior to the skin crease (Fig. 5–13). The dissection separating the tissues that connect the auricle to the scalp is facilitated by pulling the ear laterally, thus opening up the tissue planes. Cutting the auricularis muscle bundle mobilizes the auricle and facilitates visualization of the temporalis area.

- Areolar (prefascial connective tissue layer) and temporalis fascia grafts are obtained. The ear is retracted forward (Fig. 5–14).

  An areolar connective tissue graft is harvested. Make an incision through the thin areolar tissue (see Fig. 5–14 *inset*) parallel to the superior temporal line. Pick up the edge of the incised tissue (Fig. 5–15). Using a Freer elevator, dissect the areolar tissue that is being elevated from the temporalis fascia. Using a scissors (Fig. 5–16), excise the areolar tissue. Spread it out, and allow it to dry on a Teflon block for use as a graft to resurface bone when performing a canal wall-down mastoidectomy.

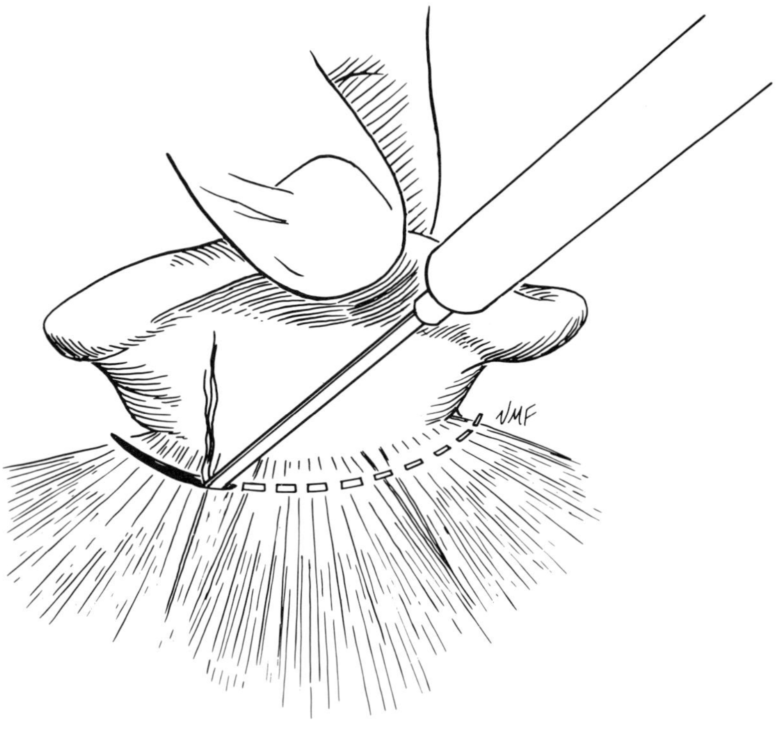

• FIGURE 5–13.

Using a postauricular approach, an incision is made using electrocautery. (From Johnson JT, et al [eds]: American Academy of Otolaryngology—Instructional Courses, Vol 4. St Louis, MO, CV Mosby, 1991.)

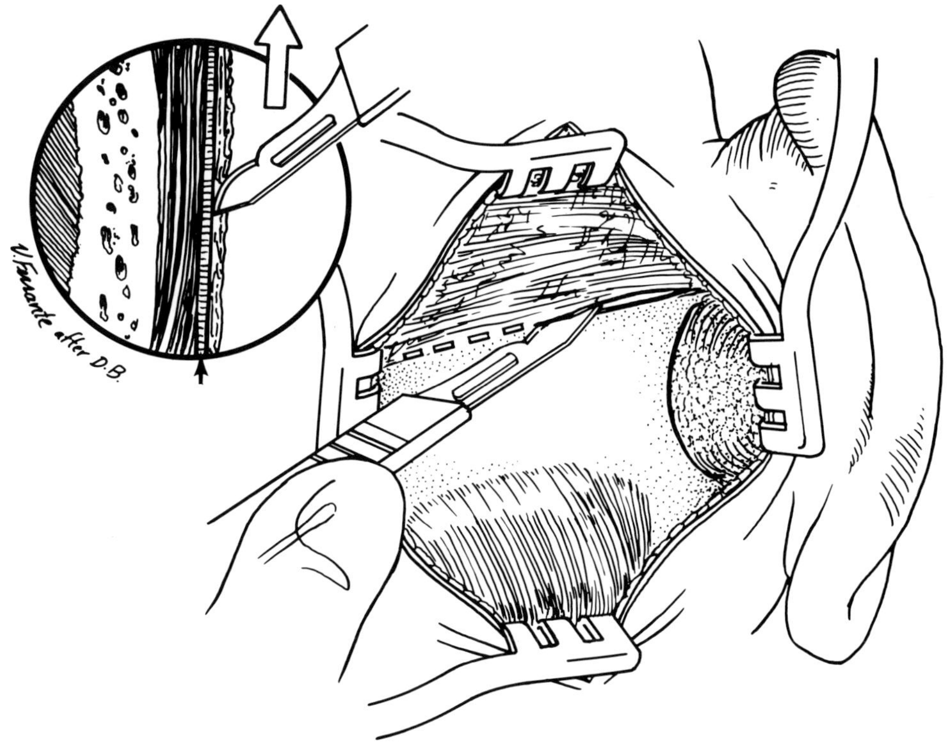

• FIGURE 5-14.

The ear is retracted forward, and an incision is made through the areolar tissue (*inset*). (From Johnson JT, et al [eds]: American Academy of Otolaryngology—Instructional Courses, Vol 4. St Louis, MO, CV Mosby, 1991.)

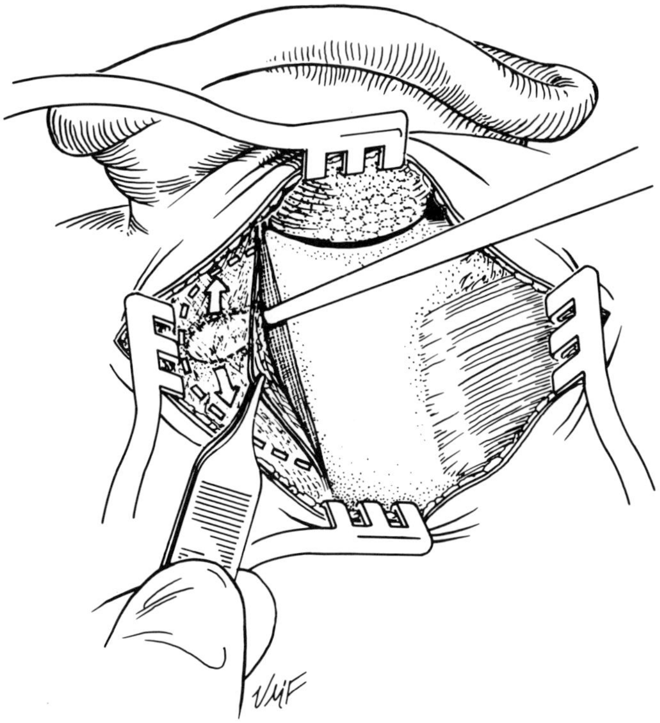

• FIGURE 5-15.

The incised tissue is lifted and dissected with a Freer elevator. (From Johnson JT, et al [eds]: American Academy of Otolaryngology—Instructional Courses, Vol 4. St Louis, MO, CV Mosby, 1991.)

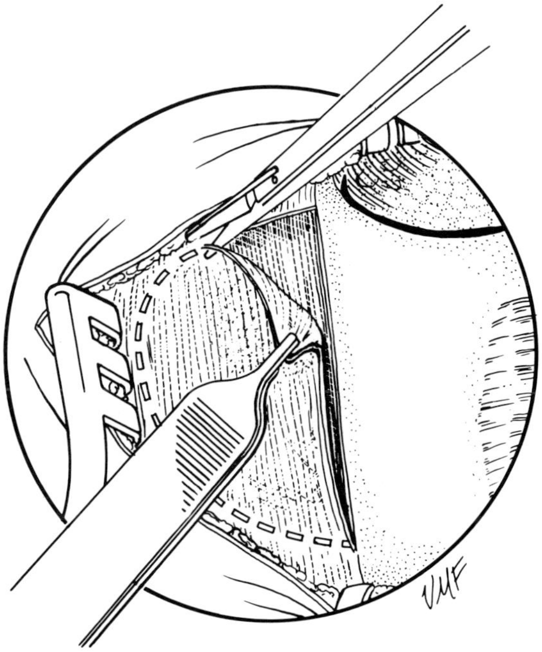

• FIGURE 5-16.

Areolar tissue is excised. (From Johnson JT, et al [eds]: American Academy of Otolaryngology—Instructional Courses, Vol 4. St Louis, MO, CV Mosby, 1991.)

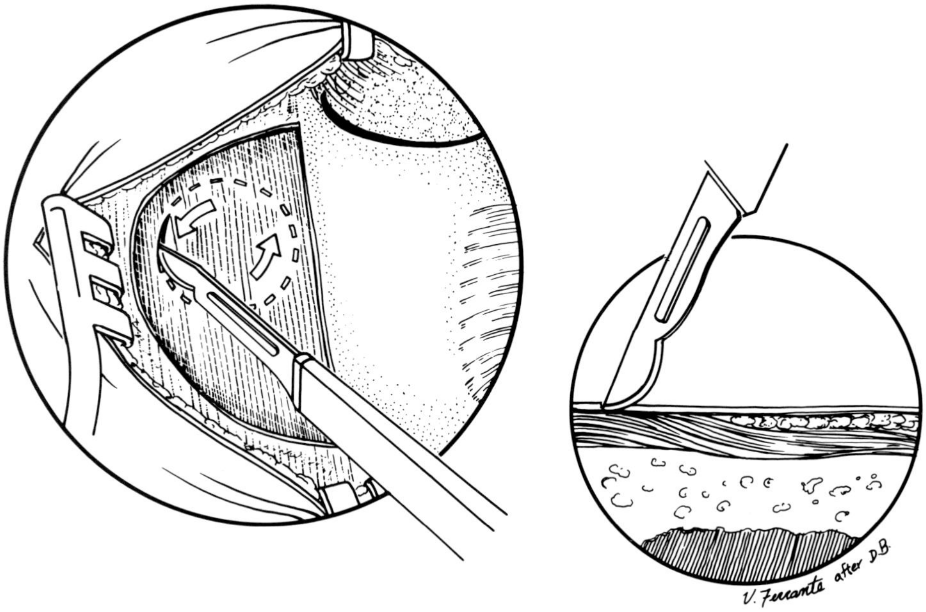

• FIGURE 5-17.

A temporalis fascia graft is obtained by making a circular incision through the fascial layer (*inset*). (From Johnson JT, et al [eds]: American Academy of Otolaryngology—Instructional Courses, Vol 4. St Louis, MO, CV Mosby, 1991.)

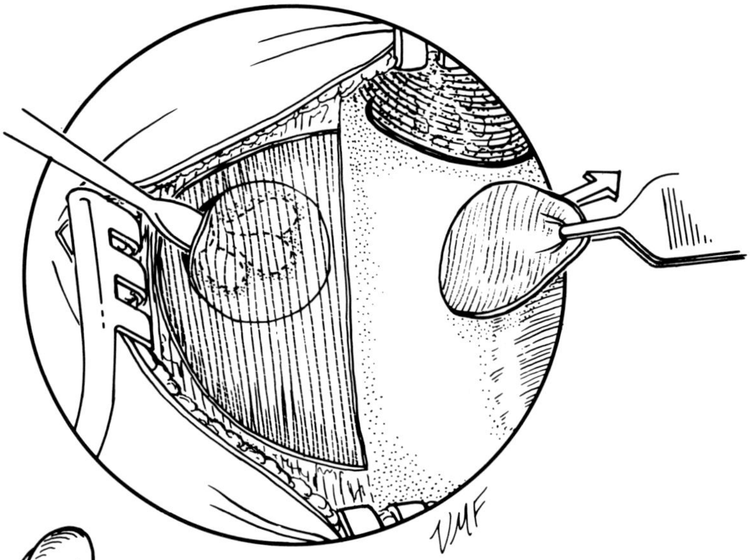

• FIGURE 5-18.

The graft is removed from the temporalis muscle. (From Johnson JT, et al [eds]: American Academy of Otolaryngology—Instructional Courses, Vol 4. St Louis, MO, CV Mosby, 1991.)

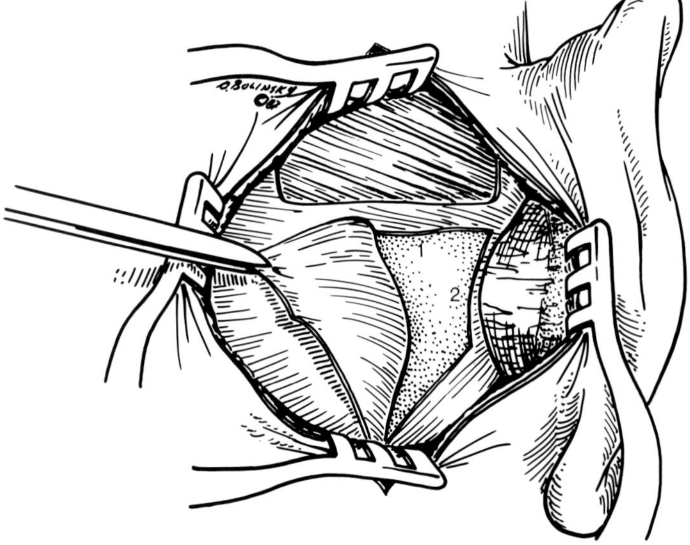

• FIGURE 5-19.

A T-shaped incision is made in the mastoid periosteum. The first incision (1) is made to the superior temporal line and is followed by another incision (2), which is made at a right angle to the mastoid tip. (From Johnson JT, et al [eds]: American Academy of Otolaryngology—Instructional Courses, Vol 4. St Louis, MO, CV Mosby, 1991.)

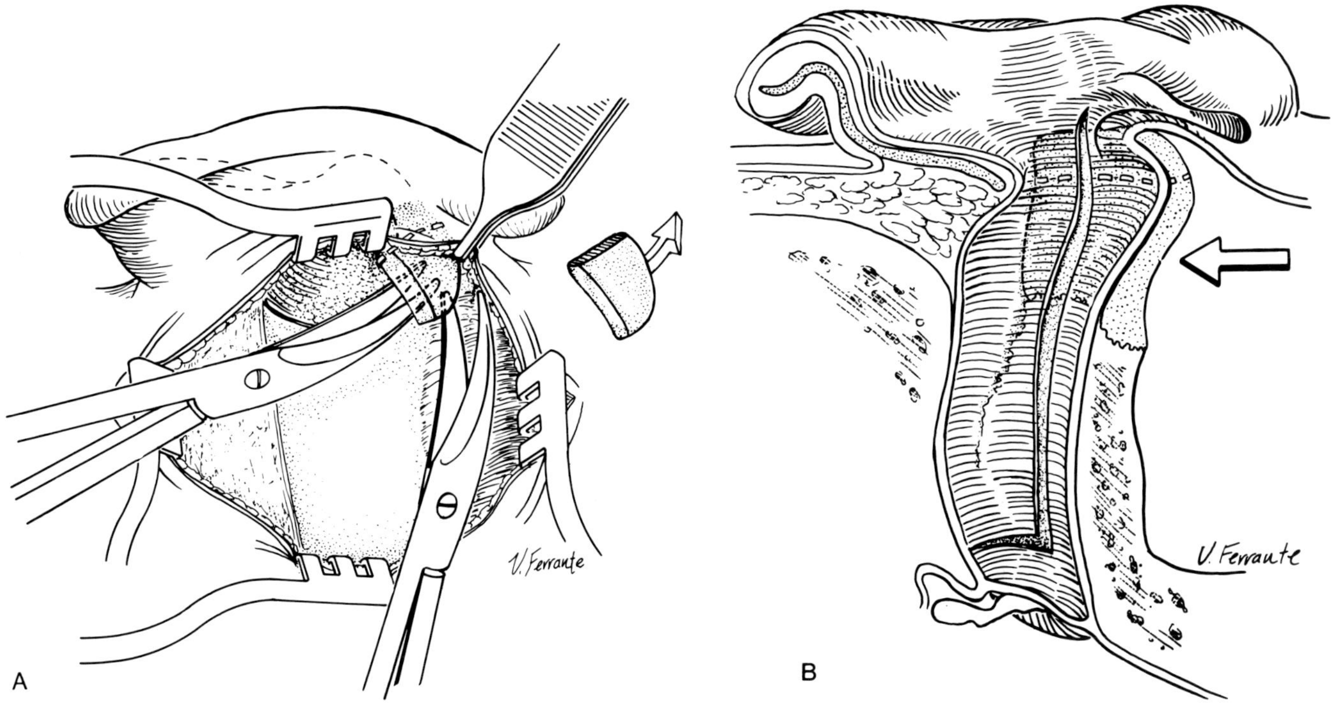

• FIGURE 5-20.

A, Cartilage is dissected from the floor of the canal in the tympanomastoid sulcus area and is removed from the remaining anterior attachment. (From Johnson JT, et al [eds]: American Academy of Otolaryngology—Instructional Courses, Vol 4. St Louis, MO, CV Mosby, 1991.) *B*, Space created from its removal (*arrow*) enables enlargement of the inferior portion of the cartilaginous canal.

The temporalis fascia graft is obtained by making a circular incision through the fascial layer (Fig. 5-17 *inset*). The size of the graft should be dictated by its purpose; for repair of a drum defect, a relatively small graft is harvested. When a canal wall-down mastoidectomy is performed, a larger segment is obtained both to graft the tympanic membrane and to cover exposed bone. The superior edge of the graft is grasped with a pickup and is bluntly freed off the temporalis muscle (Fig. 5-18).

• The mastoid periosteum is incised in a T-like fashion (Fig. 5-19). The first incision (1) is carried down to the superior temporal line. A second incision (2) is made at a right angle and is carried down to the mastoid tip. Using the Freer elevator and the electrocautery knife, the periosteum is elevated exposing the mastoid. This also allows the placement of large self-retaining retractors that enhances operative exposure.

• The cartilage of the floor of the canal in the tympanomastoid sulcus area is dissected and identified using Stevens scissors (Fig. 5-20*A*). This cartilage is known by parotid surgeons as "the pointer" and is used as a landmark for finding the facial nerve. The inferior canal wall skin is bluntly dissected from this cartilage. This facilitates the visualization of the previously made endaural inferior canal wall skin incision. The block of cartilage, freed from its adjacent connective tissue, is amputated from its remaining anterior attachment—the base of the tragal cartilage (Fig. 5-20*B* *arrow*). Its removal allows the inferior portion of the cartilaginous canal to be enlarged. It is set aside in saline and can be used in a variety of ways, such as for ossicular reconstruction, replacing a defective lateral epitympanic wall.

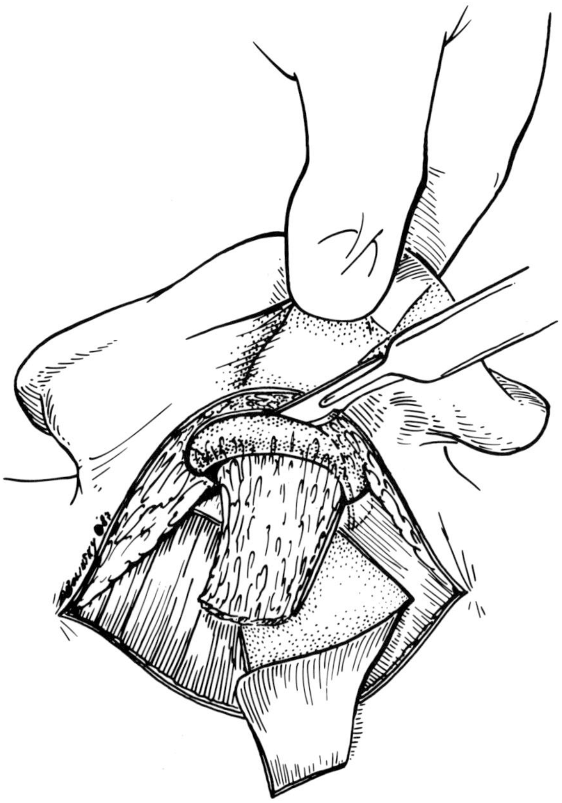

• FIGURE 5-21.

The conchal cartilage segment is excised. (From Johnson JT, et al [eds]: American Academy of Otolaryngology—Instructional Courses, Vol 4. St Louis, MO, CV Mosby, 1991.)

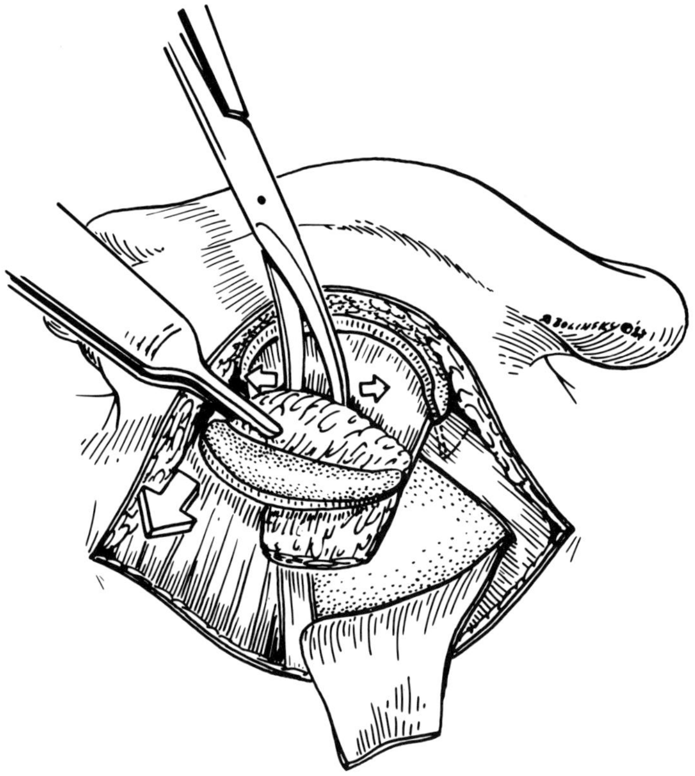

• FIGURE 5-22.

The tissue plane between the cartilage and the meatal skin is established. (From Johnson JT, et al [eds]: American Academy of Otolaryngology—Instructional Courses, Vol 4. St Louis, MO, CV Mosby, 1991.)

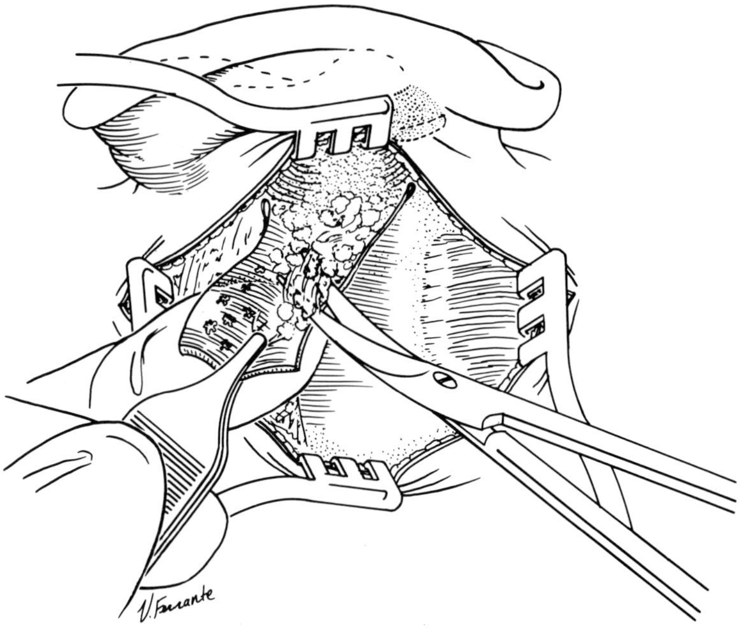

• FIGURE 5-23.

The conchal-based skin of the posterior meatal canal wall is debulked. (From Johnson JT, et al [eds]: American Academy of Otolaryngology—Instructional Courses, Vol 4. St Louis, MO, CV Mosby, 1991.)

• In order to complete the meatoplasty, a crescent-shaped segment of the anterior edge of the conchal cartilage is excised (Fig. 5-21). The auricle is held with the surgeon's thumb and index finger while the third or fourth finger is inserted into the lumen to dilate and stabilize the meatal opening. This facilitates the incision of the conchal cartilage and the development of a tissue plane between the cartilage and the meatal skin (Fig. 5-22).

• The mobilized, rectangular, conchal-based posterior meatal canal wall skin is debulked. The skin is grasped with a forceps and supported on a finger (Fig. 5-23), and a Stevens scissors is used to thin it until ceruminous glands are visible. This debulked flap is more pliable and easier to reposition into the canal, especially in cases where the canal wall has been preserved.

• An adequate meatus is approximately 1.5-2 cm in diameter. This meatus should easily admit the surgeon's index finger. If the meatus is too small, the vertical 12 and 6 o'clock incisions may be extended laterally into the concha, and additional soft tissue and cartilage may be resected (see the discussion of Figs. 5-19 and 5-20).

• The posterior bony canal and the tympanomastoid suture have been exposed during the earlier maneuvers. An incision is made through the anterior canal skin with a stapes knife parallel to the plane of the eardrum in the protruding area (Fig. 5–24*A*).

• The skin is raised in a retrograde fashion until the tympanic bone-cartilage junction (*arrow*) is reached (Fig. 5–24*B*).

• The skin is usually attached firmly at the tympanic bone-cartilage junction. The cartilage is separated from the rough bony surface using a duckbill elevator, thus mobilizing the skin and gaining adequate exposure of the entire tympanic ring (Fig. 5–25).

• The bony overhangs are removed with constant irrigation suction and drill (Fig. 5–26*A*). Removal of lateral position of the bony overhangs allows visualization of the more medial structures. The distal skin lining the anterior and inferior medial bony canal skin is elevated down toward the fibrous annulus (*arrow*). Great care is taken to preserve this skin that lines the anterior sulcus. Sponges are placed over the distal skin to protect it from the suctioning and drilling (Fig. 5–26*B*). The remaining bony overhangs are removed using diamond burs, which will not displace the protective sponges.

• Anteriorly, the overhang is thinned until it becomes translucent, thus allowing detection of the color of the periosteum of the glenoid, which can be appreciated through the intact layer of bone. Inferiorly, the floor of the canal is enlarged until the drum margin is visible. Posteriorly, when performing a procedure in which the canal is preserved, it is important not to enter the mastoid air cells. Prominent bony protuberances obscuring the drum margin are drilled away. Circumferential drilling of the tympanic bone is completed when the tympanic annulus and pars flaccida are clearly visible to permit adequate exposure for removal of pathology and to perform the necessary surgery.

• At the completion of the ear surgery, the anterior sulcus skin is repositioned and the area stented with Gelfoam (Fig. 5–27). It is critical to preserve the angle formed by the eardrum and canal wall skin in order to prevent blunting. The laterally raised anterior canal wall skin is replaced to resurface the bony canal.

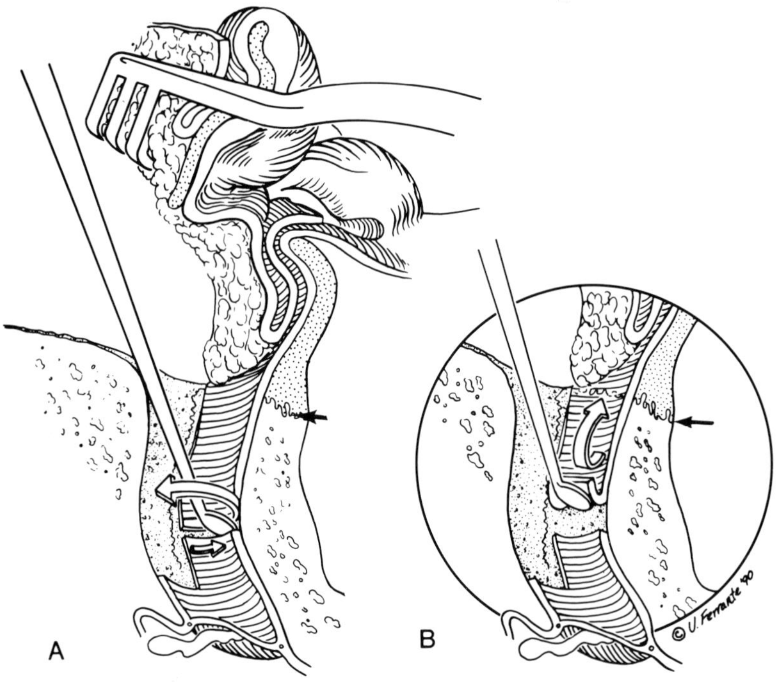

• FIGURE 5–24.

A, An incision is made through the anterior canal skin and is elevated (*B*) until the tympanic bone cartilage junction (*arrow*) is reached. (From Johnson JT, et al [eds]: American Academy of Otolaryngology—Instructional Courses, Vol 4. St Louis, MO, CV Mosby, 1991.)

• FIGURE 5-25.

A duckbill elevator separates the cartilage from the rough bony surface. (From Johnson JT, et al [eds]: American Academy of Otolaryngology—Instructional Courses, Vol 4. St Louis, MO, CV Mosby, 1991.)

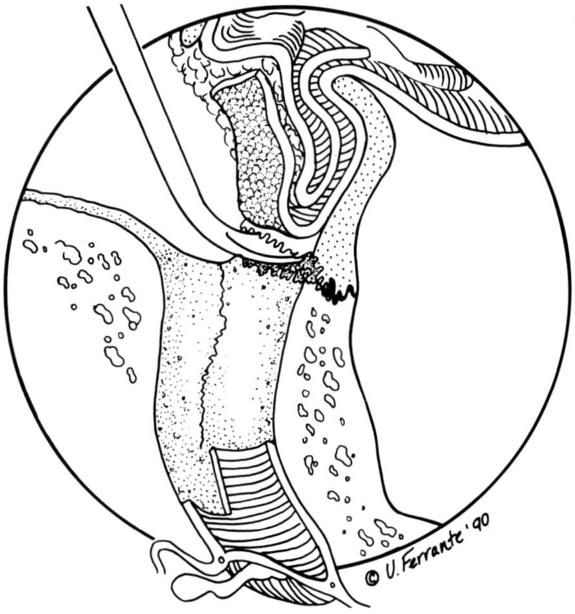

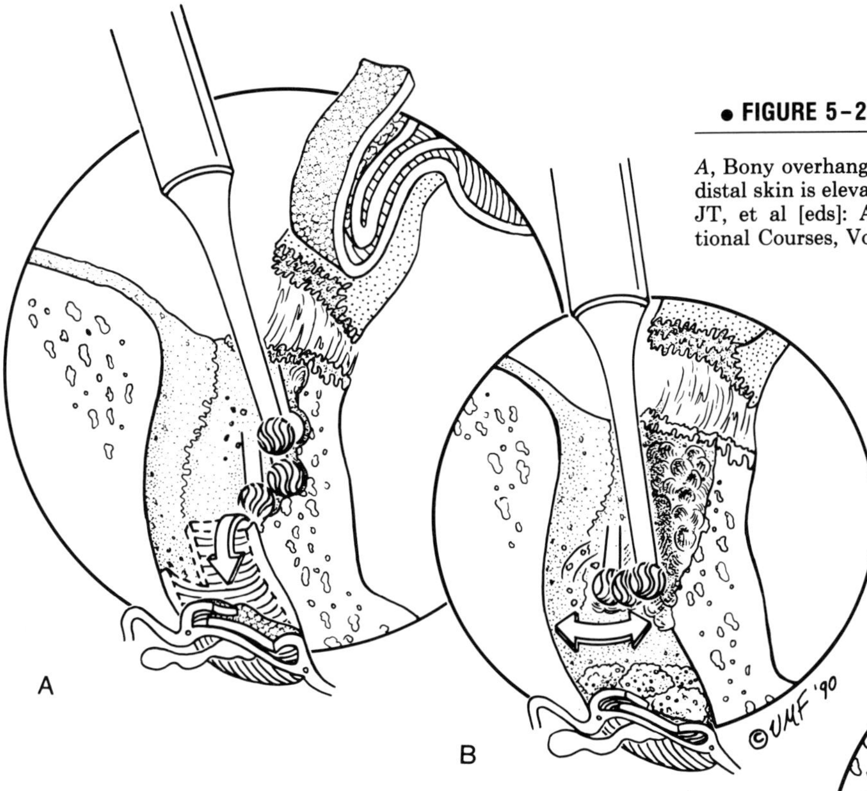

A

B

• FIGURE 5-26.

A, Bony overhangs are removed using suction and a drill while the distal skin is elevated and protected by sponges (*B*). (From Johnson JT, et al [eds]: American Academy of Otolaryngology—Instructional Courses, Vol 4. St Louis, MO, CV Mosby, 1991.)

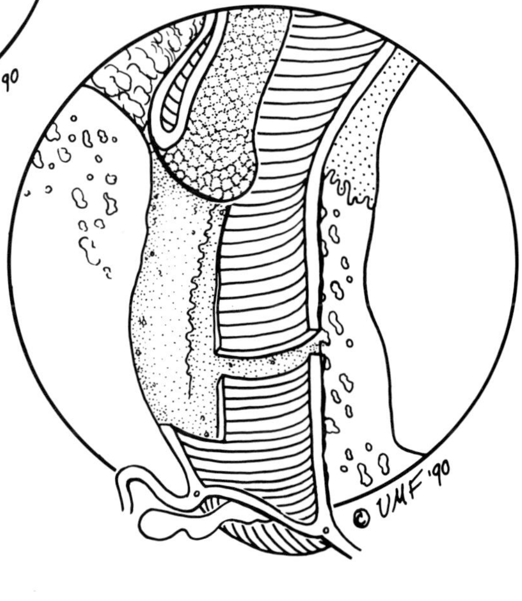

• FIGURE 5-27.

The anterior sulcus skin is repositioned, and the area is tinted with Gelfoam. (From Johnson JT, et al [eds]: American Academy of Otolaryngology—Instructional Courses, Vol 4. St Louis, MO, CV Mosby, 1991.)

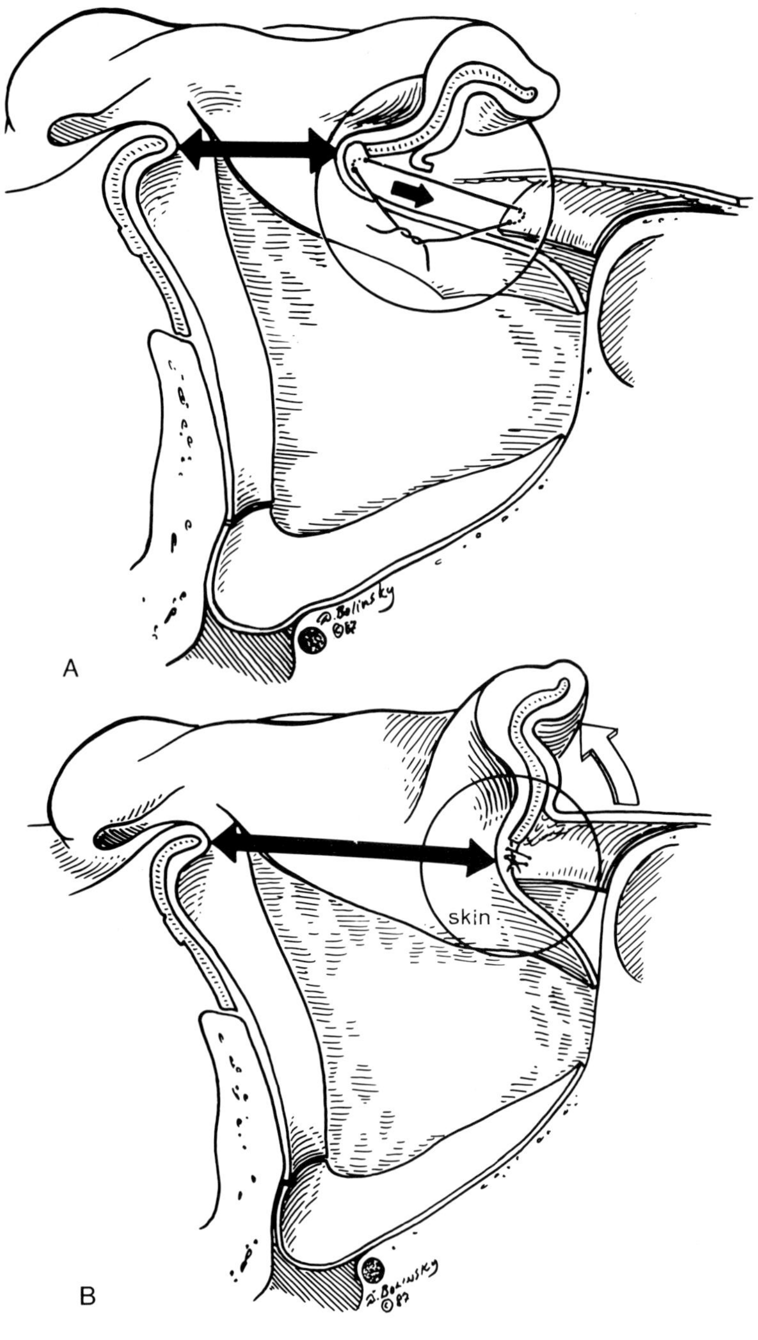

• FIGURE 5-28.

A, A suture is used to approximate connective tissue, resulting in enlargement and stabilization of the meatal openings (*B*). (From Johnson JT, et al [eds]: American Academy of Otolaryngology—Instructional Courses, Vol 4. St Louis, MO, CV Mosby, 1991.)

• The meatal opening is enlarged, the canal is packed, and the wound is closed after either a canal wall-up or a canal wall-down procedure.

Canal wall-down procedure:

The mastoid periosteum is turned into the posterior portion of the mastoid recess.

A 2-0 catgut suture is used to approximate the connective tissue in the area where conchal cartilage was excised to the mastoid periosteum (Fig. 5–28*A*). This enlarges and stabilizes the meatal opening (Fig. 5–28*B*).

The posterior canal wall skin is turned into the posterior mastoid recess. It serves as an epithelial pedicled flap to both resurface the posterior mastoid recess and enhance epidermization of the cavity. The cavity and ear canal

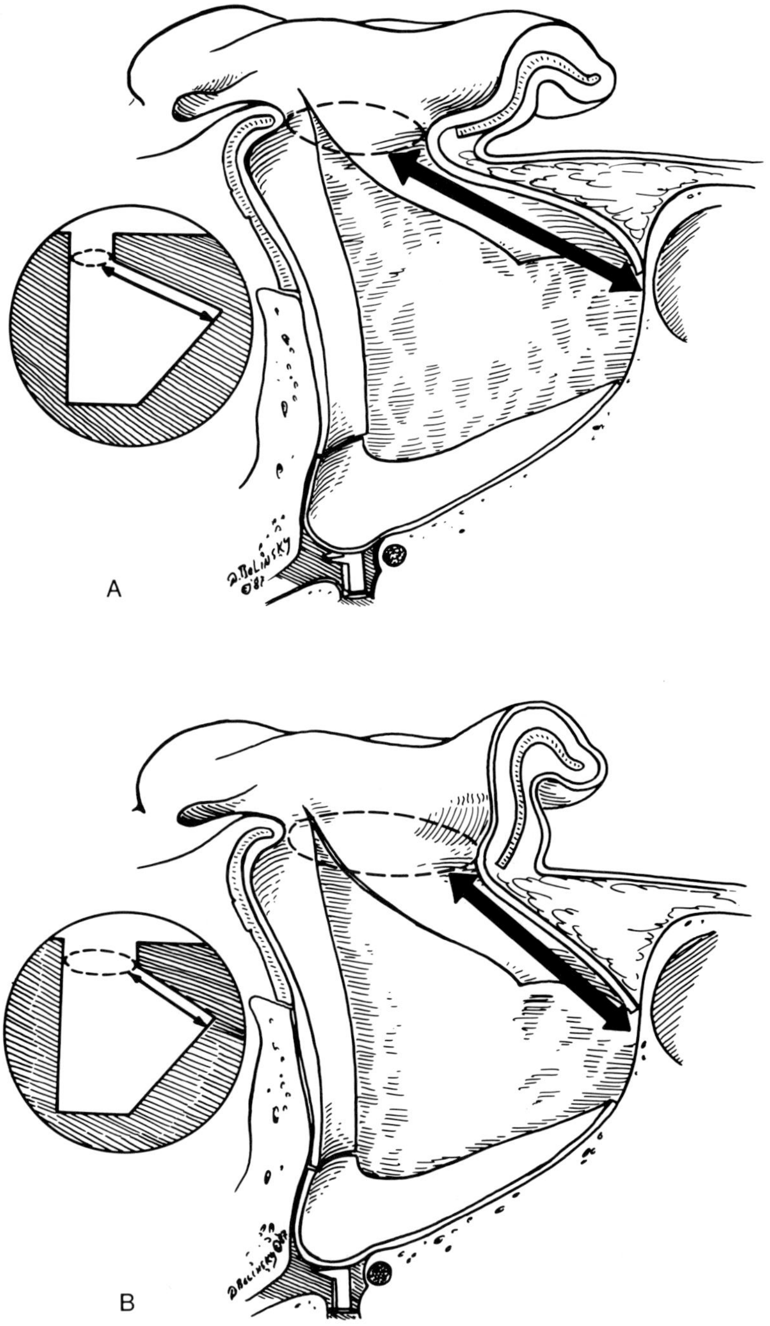

• FIGURE 5-29.

The size of the diameter of the meatal opening affects the size of the mastoid recess. *A*, A small diameter. *B*, A large diameter. (From Johnson JT, et al [eds]: American Academy of Otolaryngology—Instructional Courses, Vol 4. St Louis, MO, CV Mosby, 1991.)

are packed with absorbable gelatin (Gelfoam) to immobilize the temporalis fascia and areolar tissue grafts previously placed to resurface bony surfaces. Thin (0.001″) Silastic sheeting is positioned to line the partially Gelfoam-filled cavity and ear canal. Bismuth-impregnated petrolatum gauze strips (Xeroform) are packed within the Silastic-lined cavity.

The postauricular incision is closed. A Penrose drain is inserted for 24 hours, and a mastoid dressing is applied.

The diameter of the meatal opening affects the size of the mastoid recess. When the meatus is small, the area to the sinodural angle becomes longer and the cavity becomes larger (Fig. 5-29*A*). A large meatus reduces the area to the sinodural angle, and consequently the mastoid cavity is smaller (Fig. 5-29*B*).

Canal wall-up procedure:

Reapproximate the mastoid periosteum to the temporalis fascia with 4-0 catgut sutures.

Place a 2-0 suture through the connective tissue in the area where the crescent of conchal cartilage had been excised. Approximate this surface to the edge of the repositioned mastoid periosteum that enlarges the meatal opening.

Working endaurally, turn the conchal-based posterior canal wall–meatal skin flap into the canal to resurface the posterior canal wall. The meatal opening has been stabilized by the previously placed suture.

Pack the canal. Thin (0.001″) Silastic sheeting is used to line the canal, serving as a nonadherent dressing that prevents ingrowth of granulation tissue, which may occur when cloth is used. The lumen is packed with absorbable gelatin sponges (Gelfoam) and bismuth-impregnated petrolatum gauze strips (Xeroform).

The postauricular incision is closed. A Penrose drain is inserted for 24 hours, and a mastoid dressing is applied.

Postoperative care

The mastoid dressing is no longer required after 72 hours. After its removal, an aqueous suspension of antibiotic eardrops to be used three times a day is prescribed. The nonadherent Silastic sheeting within which the gauze strip packing had been placed is removed after 10 to 14 days. If properly inserted, this packing eliminates pain or bleeding when the gauze is removed. Topical eardrops are continued until the Gelfoam has either dissolved or been removed and the ear lining is healed.

SKIN GRAFTING THE EXTERNAL AUDITORY CANAL

The purpose of skin grafting is to restore epithelial lining to the external auditory canal using a combination of pedicled canal wall–meatal skin, and thin split-thickness skin grafts are used to resurface canals in which normal ear skin is deficient to ensure a stable, patent lumen.

Indications

Ear canal atresia or stenosis, congenital or acquired, is an indication.

- Post-traumatic
- As a consequence of auricular canal resections for neoplasms
- Iatrogenic
- Removal of exostoses
- Other

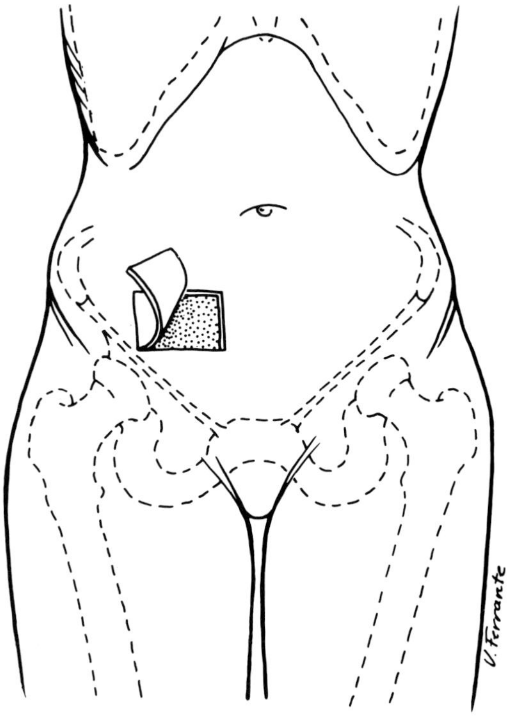

• **FIGURE 5-30.**

The lower abdomen skin graft site.

Preparation

The lower abdomen should be draped appropriately.

EQUIPMENT

- Dermatome
- Silicone sheeting 0.001″
- Benzoin-type adhesive
- Absorbable gelatin sponge
- Bismuth-impregnated petrolatum gauze strips (Xeroform)
- 5-0 plain gut suture

Procedure

• Take a thin, split-thickness skin graft, approximately 6 × 2 cm from the lower abdomen. Harvest the graft from an area between the inguinal crease and the umbilicus. This site is easily hidden by a bikini-style bathing suit (Fig. 5-30).

• Dress the donor site with Xeroform and an occlusive dressing for a few days. Then remove the dressing and have patient take a daily bath in a half-filled tub (avoid getting the ear wet). The Xeroform will peel off spontaneously, and the skin will heal in about 10 days.

- Unfurl silicone sheeting by placing smooth clamps at each corner to avoid curling (Fig. 5–31*A*).
- Apply benzoin adhesive to thin silicone sheeting. Allow this to dry and become sticky (Fig. 5–31*B*).
- Apply the epidermal side of the skin graft to the adhesive side of the silicone sheeting to form a composite graft (Fig. 5–31*C*).
- The dermal surface of the skin graft can now be applied to the raw bony surface of the canal.
- Trim the composite skin-silicone graft to appropriate measurements (Fig. 5–32*A*).
- Cut slits at the end of the graft so as to overlap the temporalis fascia, which has been used to construct the tympanic membrane (Fig. 5–32*B* and *C*).
- Slide the graft into the canal with the slit end medially (Fig. 5–33*A*).
- Place the graft over the reconstructed tympanic membrane (Fig. 5–33*B*).
- The lateral end may be sutured into the concha.
- Pack the canal.

    Place pieces of Gelfoam into the composite graft carefully.

    Pack it snugly. Use artificial sponges to suction the Gelfoam, thus compacting it into the canal and ensuring that the skin grafts become apposed to the bony surfaces (Fig. 5–34).

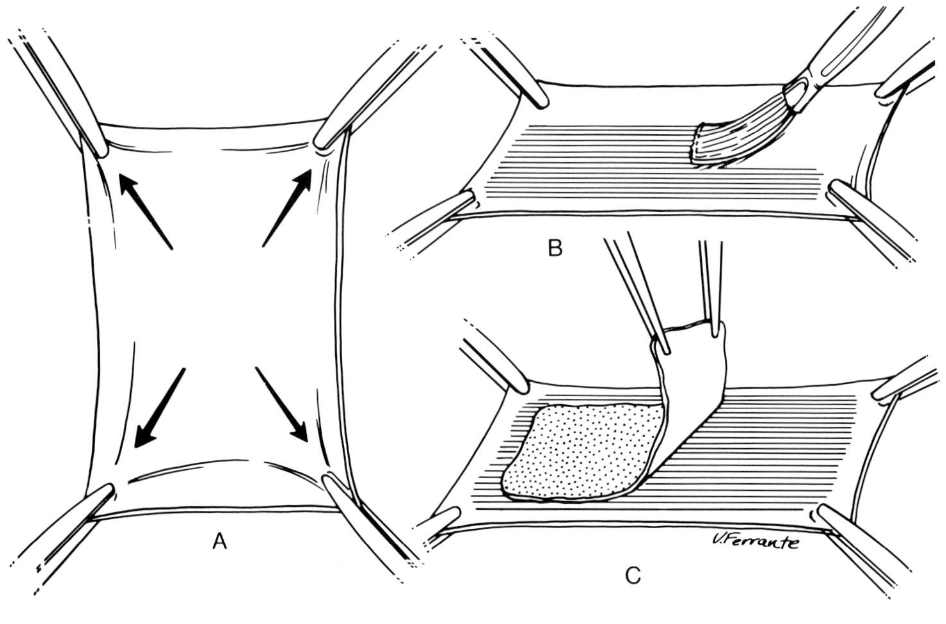

• FIGURE 5–31.

Silicone sheeting is unfurled (*A*) and treated with benzoin adhesive (*B*) before a skin graft is applied to it (*C*).

• FIGURE 5-32.

The skin-silicone graft is trimmed (*A*), and slits are cut (*B* and *C*) in order to overlap the temporalis fascia.

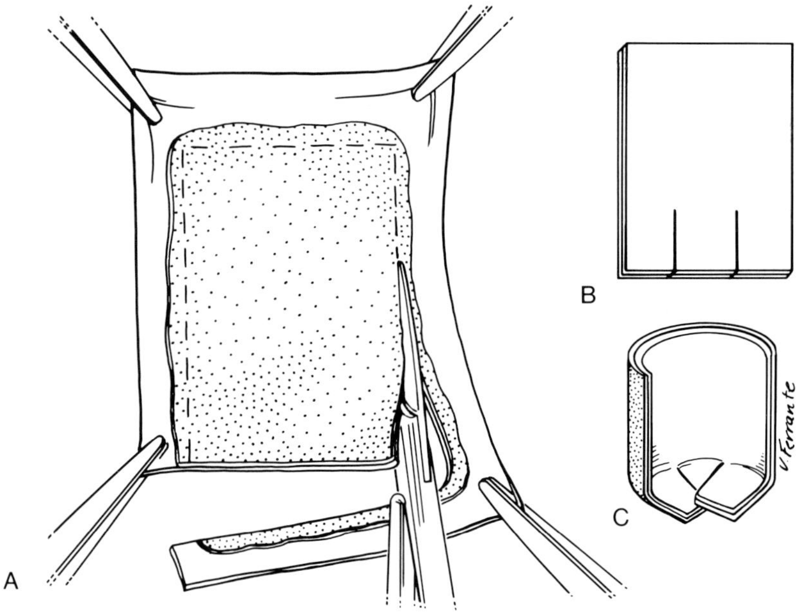

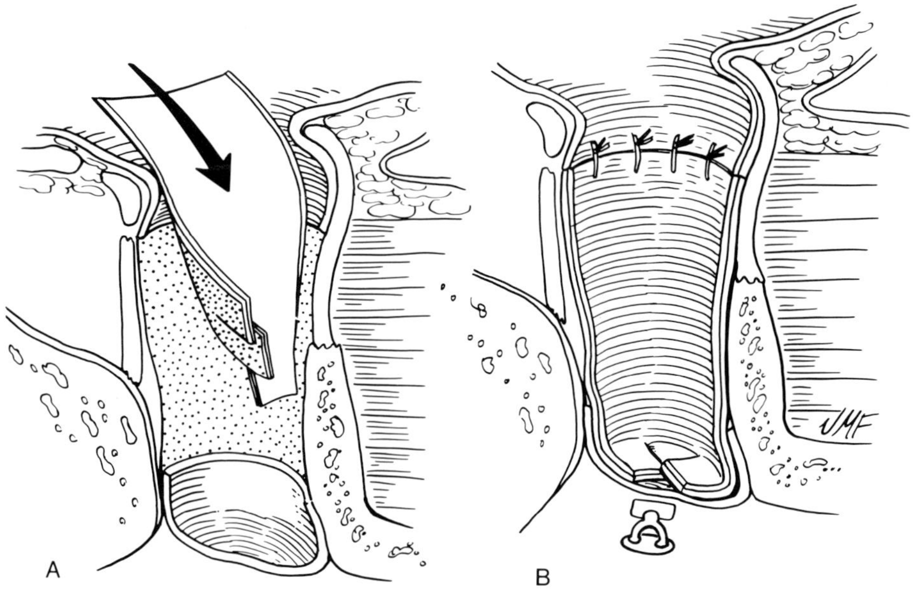

• FIGURE 5-33.

The graft is positioned into the canal (*A*) and is placed over the reconstructed tympanic membrane (*B*).

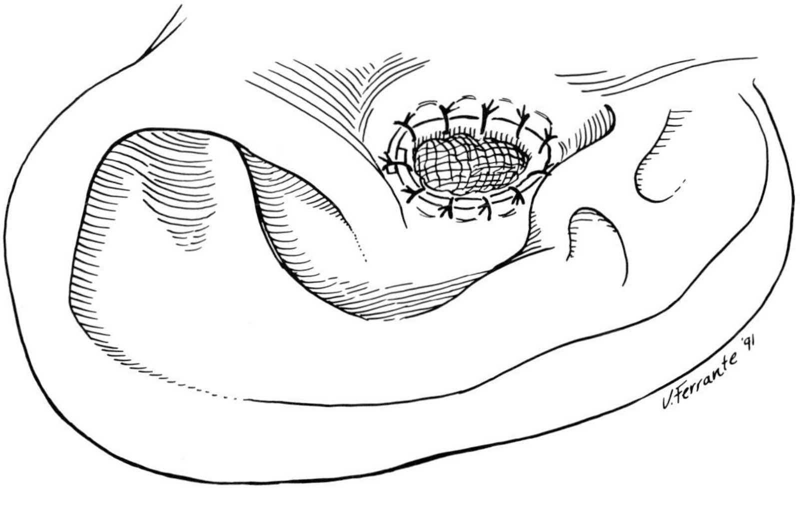

• FIGURE 5-34.

Artificial sponges are used to suction Gelfoam and ensure that grafts become apposed to bony surfaces.

Postoperative care

- The patient should avoid getting water into the canal for at least 3 months and possibly as a routine.
- Grafted skin is not as hardy as normal external canal skin; it does not migrate laterally and has no pilosebaceous cerumen glands.
- The patient may be allowed to swim 6 months after the surgery, but usually with ear protection (i.e., silicone disposable ear plugs).
- Clean the ear of accumulated keratin debris as required, usually during office visits every 6 months.
- Grafted bony ear canals are more likely to develop external otitis.

CONGENITAL AURAL ATRESIA

- If the atresia is bilateral, the child is fitted with a bone-conductive hearing aid at the earliest age possible. Canal reconstruction can be performed when the child is 4 to 5 years of age.
- If atresia is unilateral, reconstruction is elective. The surgery may be deferred until the patient is able to decide whether to undergo the operative procedure.
- Congenitally stenotic canals may be more urgent to repair because debris and keratin may collect, forming a cholesteatoma.
- Controversy exists regarding the order of correction when atresia is accompanied by microtia. The auricular reconstruction must be delayed until approximately 6 years of age. This allows for growth of the costochondral cartilage, which must be well enough developed to permit the sculpting of the auricular cartilaginous scaffold. Generally, the initial procedures to reconstruct the auricle precede the surgery for atresia. The presence of scar tissue and compromised vascularity that occurs when the atresia repair precedes the auricular surgery compromises the cosmetic results.
- Realistic expectations of hearing outcome need to be discussed with the family.

Indications

Because atresias are associated with temporal bone and other organ system developmental abnormalities, it is essential that potential accompanying disorders be investigated before attempting correction of the atresia.

- Middle ear: hypoplastic or absent tympanic cavity; anomalous course of the facial nerve; aeration of the middle ear and mastoid; carotid and jugular bulb anomalies

- Inner ear: dysplasia of the cochlea, vestibular structures, and auditory canal

- History of other associated anatomic or developmental entities. Malformations of other organ systems that develop synchronously with the ear, such as the genitourinary tract, should be investigated.

The following examinations are required to assess a candidate for atresia repair:

- Computed tomography (CT) (both axial and coronal views of the temporal bone) is mandatory. Three-dimensional CT scanning offers excellent information, such as the relation of the atretic plate to the tegmen and the glenoid fossa.

  The radiographic examination should demonstrate the following: the course of the facial nerve, the thickness and form of the atretic plate, the extent of the external canal development, pneumatization of the mastoid, the degree of development of the ossicles, inner ear structures, size and aeration of the middle ear cleft, and the presence of possible cholesteatoma in ears with stenotic canals.

- Assessment of hearing in both ears, even if one appears normal, is essential. Auditory brain stem–evoked potential testing in newborns is helpful in assessing auditory acuity. Subsequently, complete audiometric evaluation must be obtained to detect the possible presence of a significant neurosensory component that could not be corrected surgically.

Contraindications for correction of atresia are as follows:

- A significant neurosensory hearing loss/inner ear malformation

- Limited middle ear–mastoid pneumatization or a significantly hypoplastic middle ear cleft

- Anomalous facial nerve or aberrant major vascular structure

- Middle cranial fossa tegmen sagging, which would restrict anatomic access to the middle ear cleft.

Procedure

Continuous facial nerve monitoring, though not essential, may be helpful in avoiding iatrogenic injury to the facial nerve, which may have an anomalous course in the temporal bone.

- A skin incision is made posterior to the rudimentary or the reconstructed auricle (Fig. 5–35). Palpation of the temporomandibular joint may help to orient the surgeon in the patient with an aberrant, low-set, deformed auricle. The incision is carried down to the temporalis fascia, and a graft is obtained to reconstruct the eardrum.

- The periosteum is incised in a T-like fashion as described earlier (Fig. 5–36). The mastoid cortex is exposed, and the glenoid fossa is identified (Fig. 5–37). Occasionally, a rudimentary imperforate tympanic ring or a cribrose area (*circle*) is present. Alternatively, there may be no marks identifying where the canal should have developed. The level of the middle cranial fossa (cranium) roughly corresponds to the superior temporal line (*dashed line*).

- A canal is created by drilling between the glenoid fossa and the tegmen plate (see Fig. 5–37). In some cases, a core of dense bone represents the obliterated external canal. Occasionally, the atresia plate is pneumatized. To avoid entering the mastoid air cells, the surgeon should attempt to drill a circular canal-like opening toward the middle ear cleft (Fig. 5–38).

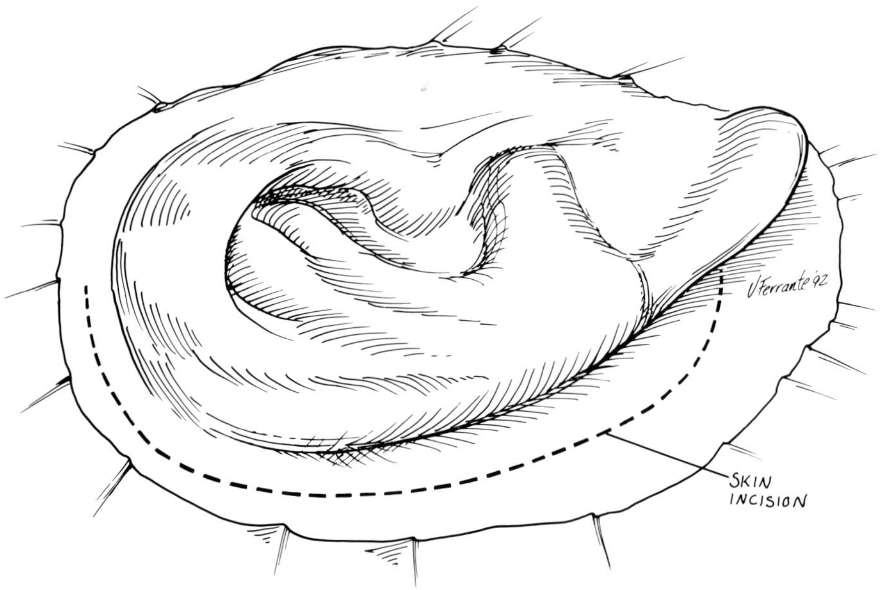

• FIGURE 5–35.

A skin incision is made posterior to the reconstructed auricle.

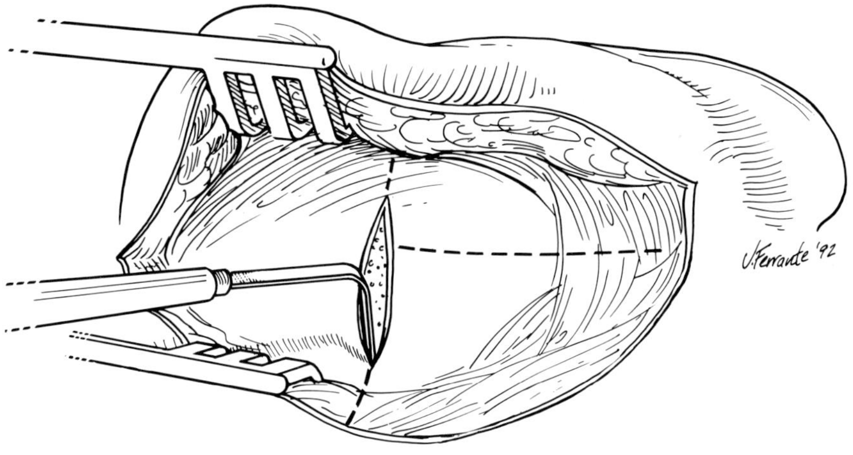

• FIGURE 5-36.

A T-shaped incision is made on the periosteum.

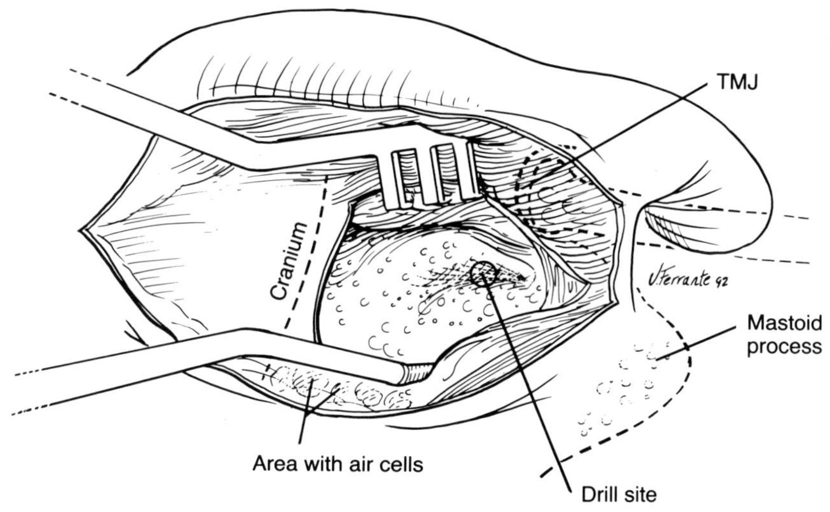

• FIGURE 5-37.

The mastoid cortex is exposed. The superior temporal line (*dashed line*) approximates the level of the tegmen. Drilling is begun in the rudimentary tympanic bone (*circle*).

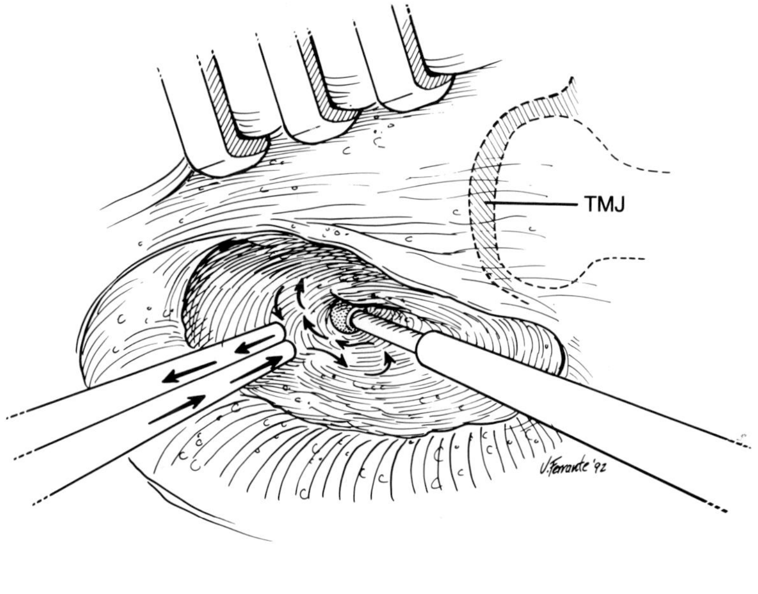

• FIGURE 5-38.

A circular canal-like opening is made with a drill.

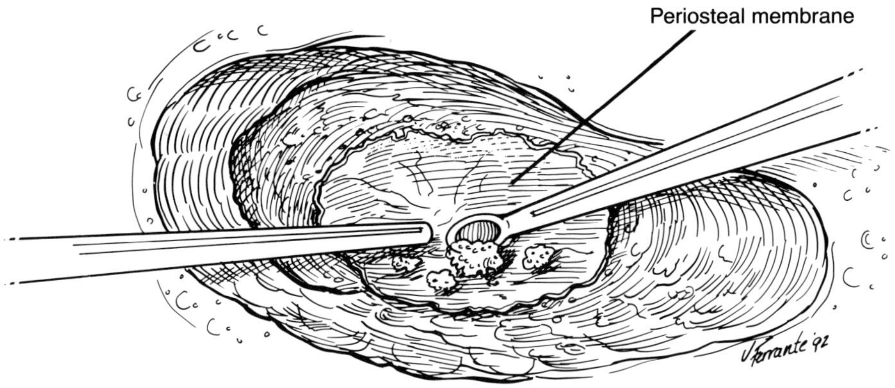

• FIGURE 5-39.

Dense periosteal membrane.

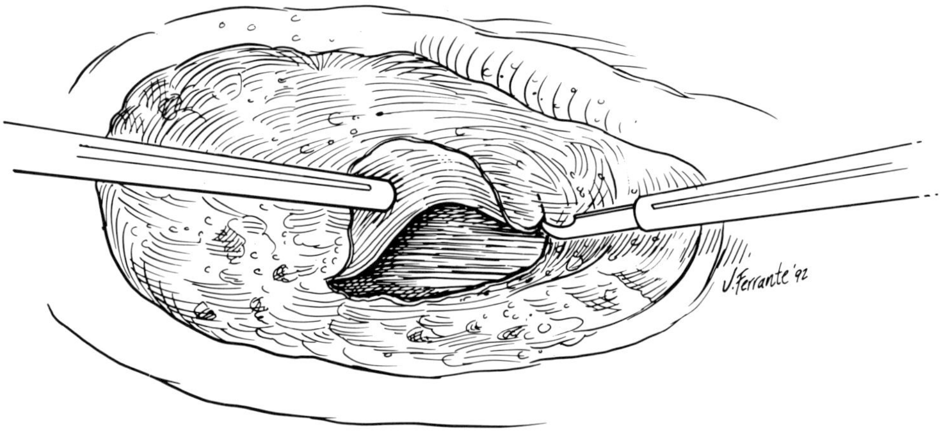

• FIGURE 5-40.

The middle ear is entered after an incision of the periosteal membrane has been made.

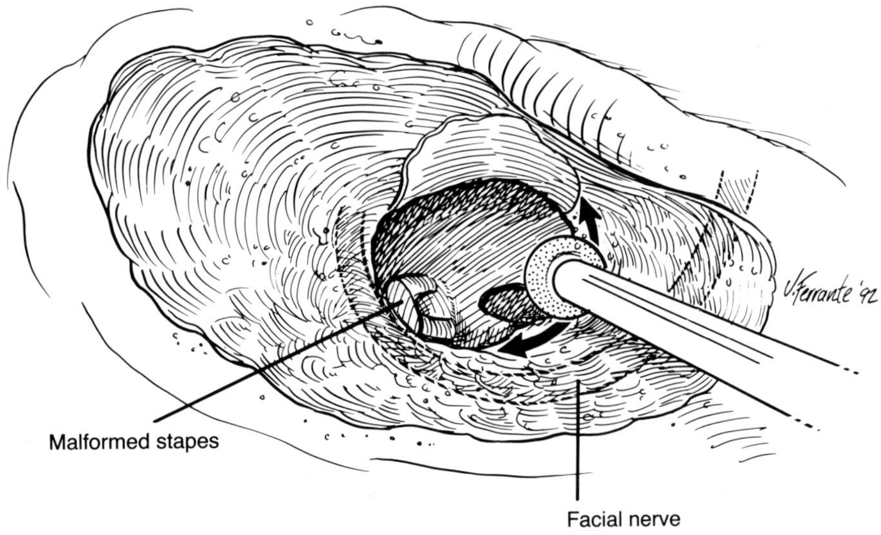

• FIGURE 5-41.

A round window niche.

• FIGURE 5-42.

A, Bone dust paté is used to plug air cells. *B*, Sheehy bone paté collector.

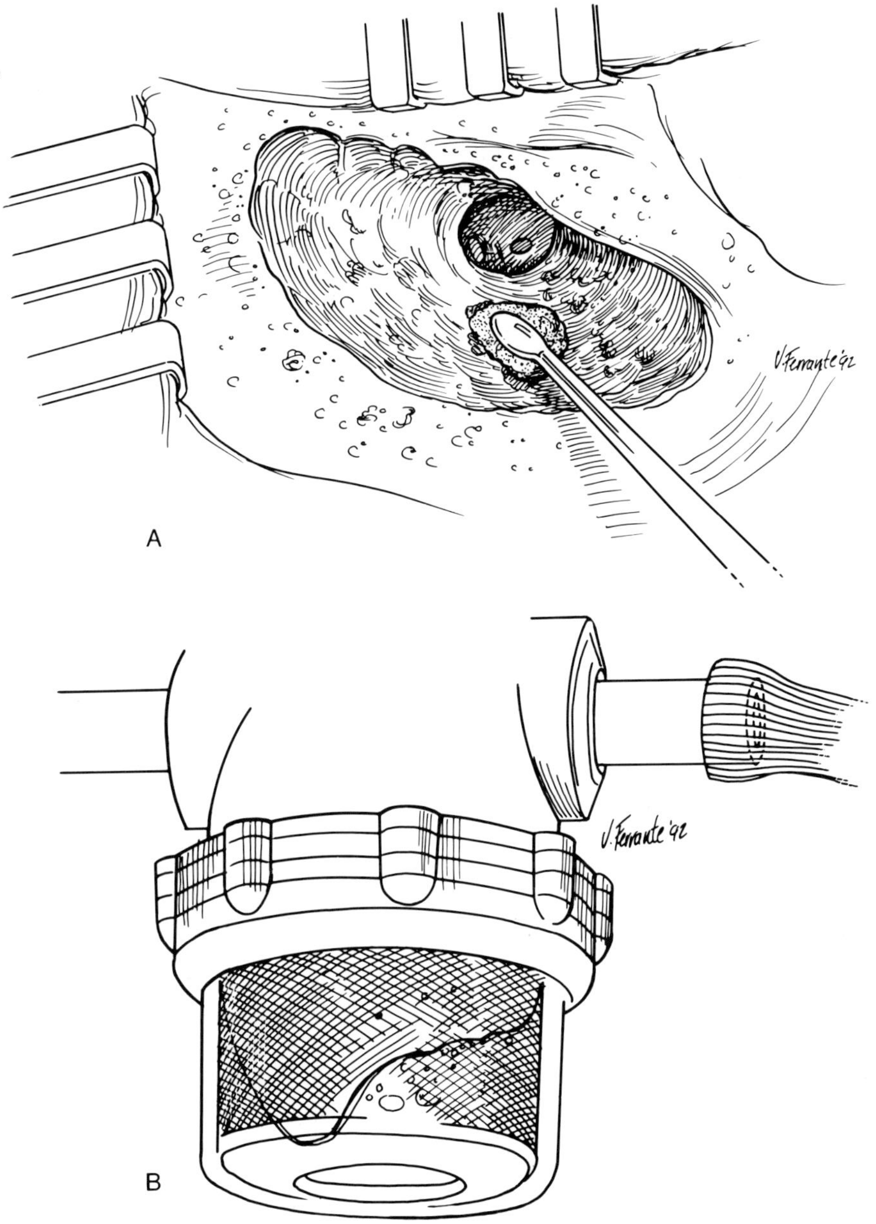

• Frequently, a dense periosteal membrane is identified at the medial end of the atresia plate (Fig. 5-39). In these malformed ears, the deformed maleus and incus are frequently fused into a single bony mass that is attached to the atresia plate. This ossicular mass may be continuous with a mobile stapes. Consequently, it is important not to inadvertently drill on these ossicles, which become mobilized when the atresia plate is removed. In order to avoid this vibratory inner ear injury, the atresia plate should be thinned down to an eggshell, translucent thickness, which is then curetted away from the periosteal membrane.

• The periosteal membrane is then incised, and the middle ear is entered (Fig. 5-40). An opening that is similar in dimension to a normal tympanic membrane must be made. Frequently, while the opening is enlarged posteriorly, the vertical portion of the facial nerve is identified. It is desirable though not always possible to identify the round window niche (Fig. 5-41). Occasionally, a forward-lying facial nerve prevents this.

• If air cells have been entered, they can be plugged using bone dust paté (Fig. 5-42*A*) collected in the Sheehy bone paté collector (Fig. 5-42*B*).

- An ossicular reconstruction is performed when the chain is not continuous. The observation of a round window reflex may be helpful in deciding if the chain is intact (Fig. 5–43). Silastic sheeting is used to prevent bony fixation of the reconstructed ossicles.

- A temporalis fascia graft is inserted as an underlay medial to the endosteal membrane, which can frequently be preserved (Fig. 5–44).

- A meatal opening is created. An anteriorly based pedicle flap using the imperforate skin from the conchal area is elevated from the underlying cartilage or connective tissue (Fig. 5–45*A*).

- The flap is debulked, removing cartilage and connective tissue (Fig. 5–45*B*). A rectangular full-thickness flap is created.

- The flap is rotated into the canal and is sutured anteriorly (*arrows*) to the soft tissue in the area of the glenoid fossa. This provides a vascular pedicled skin graft to resurface the lateral half of the anterior canal (Fig. 5–46). The remainder of the canal is resurfaced using thin split-thickness skin–Silastic sheeting grafts. (See the previous Section on skin grafting.) Slits are made in the Silastic-skin composites so that they drape onto the temporalis fascia graft. Gelfoam is packed snugly into the lumen.

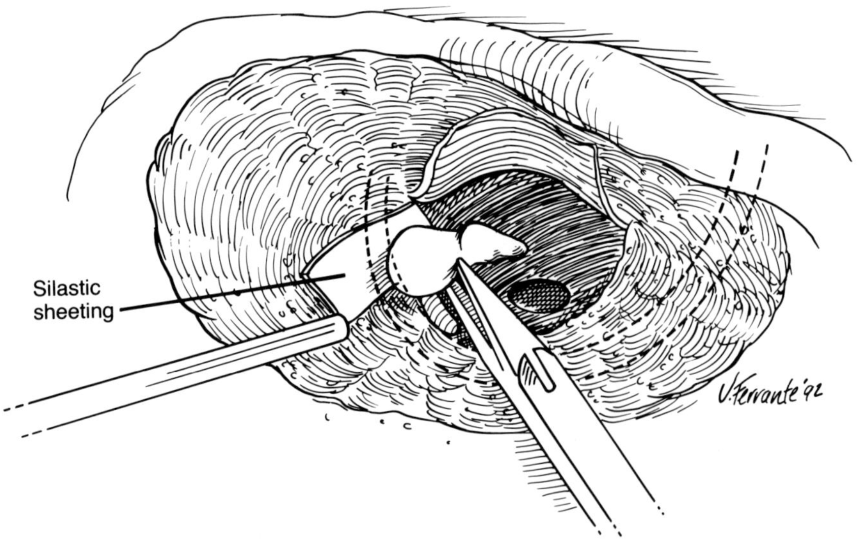

• FIGURE 5–43.

Silastic sheeting prevents bony fixation of the reconstructed ossicles.

• FIGURE 5-44.

A temporalis fascia graft is inserted medial to the endosteal flap (*arrow*).

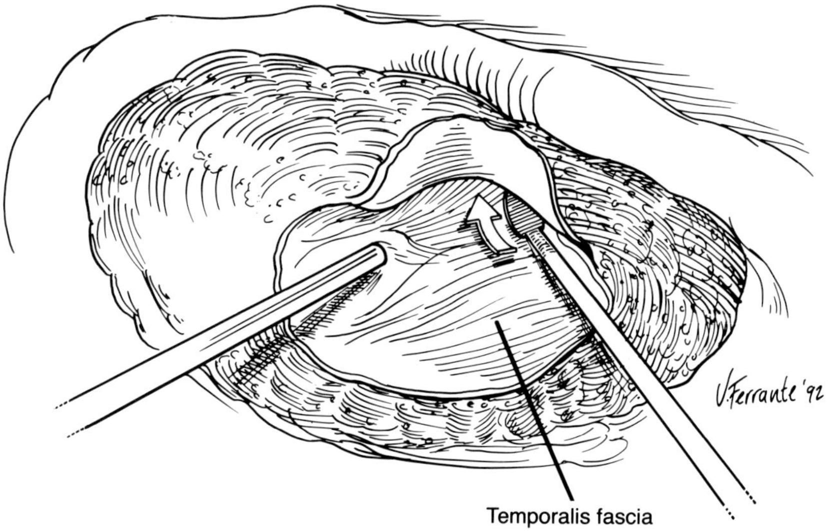

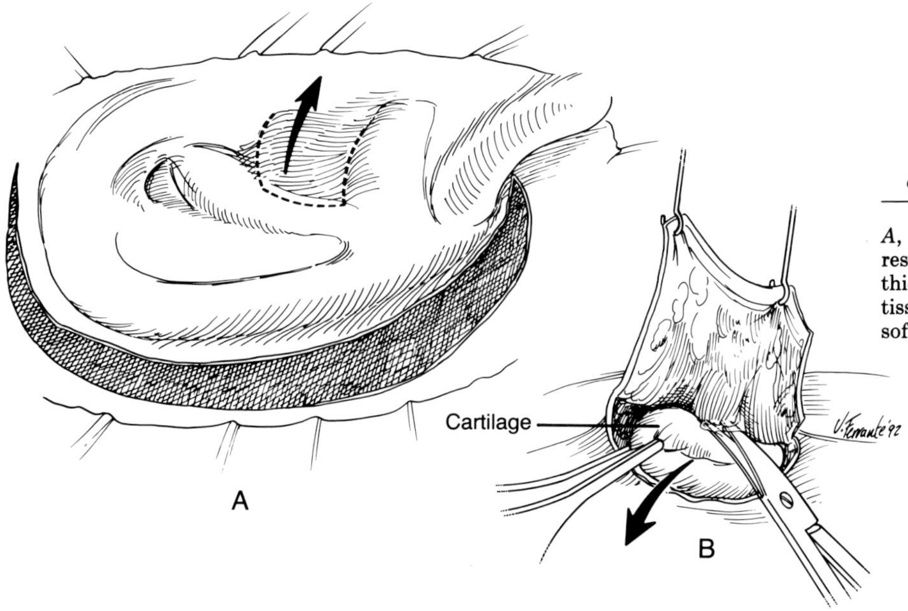

• FIGURE 5-45.

A, The flap is elevated (*arrow*) and debulked, resulting in the creation of a rectangular full-thickness flap. *B*, Cartilage and/or connective tissue is excised (*arrow*) to create a lumen in the soft tissue atresia.

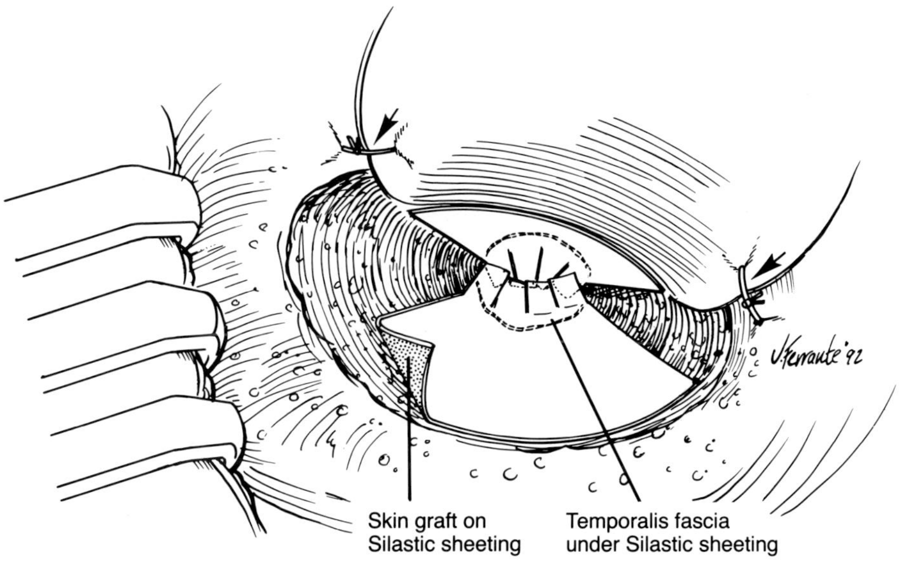

• FIGURE 5-46.

The lateral half of the anterior canal is resurfaced with a skin graft.

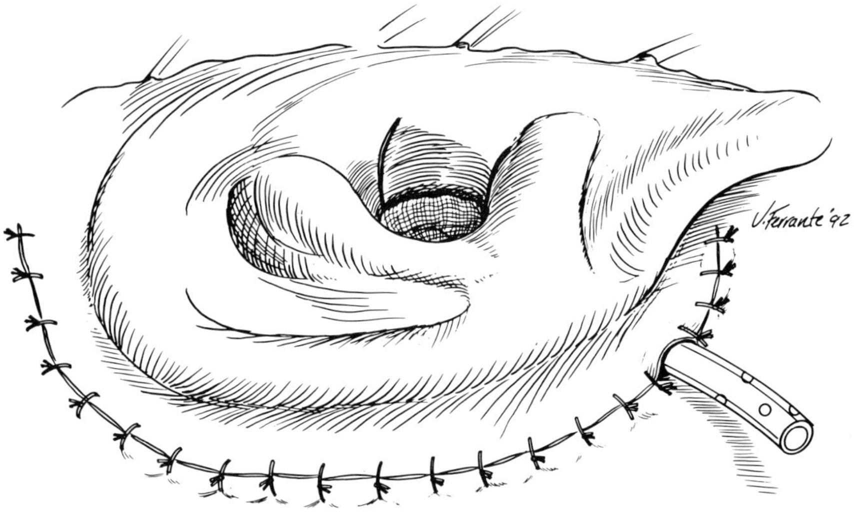

• FIGURE 5–47.

A Penrose drain.

• The postauricular incision is closed with either removable or absorbable subcuticular sutures. A Penrose drain is inserted for 24 hours (Fig. 5–47).

Postoperative care

See postoperative care for ear canal atresia or stenosis.

BIBLIOGRAPHY

Andrews JC, Anzai Y, Mankovich NJ, et al: Three-dimensional CT scan reconstruction for the assessment of congenital aural atresia. Am J Otol 13(3):236–240, 1992.

Beck DL and Benecke JE: Intraoperative facial nerve monitoring—technical aspects. Otolaryngol Head Neck Surg 102(23):270–272, 1990.

Bellucci RJ: Tympanoplasty, the malleus, stapes wire and total defect skin graft. Laryngoscope 76:1439–1458, 1966.

Bellucci RJ: Congenital malformations of the ear. Otolaryngol Clin North Am 14:95–124, 1981.

Bellucci RJ and Converse JM: The problem of congenital auricular malformation. Trans Am Acad Ophthalmol Otolaryngol 64:840, 1960.

Curtin HD: Congenital malformations of the ear. Otolaryngol Clin North Am 21(2):317–335, 1988.

Jahrsdoerfer RA: Congenital atresia of the ear. Laryngoscope 88(Suppl. 13):1, 1978.

Jahrsdoerfer RA, Yeakley JW, Hall JW, et al: High resolution CT scanning and auditory brainstem response in congenital aural atresia: Patient selection and surgical correction. Otolaryngol Head Neck Surg 93:292–298, 1985.

Lambert PR: Major congenital malformations: Surgical management and results. Ann Otol Rhinol Laryngol 97:641–649, 1988.

Leonetti JP, Matz GJ, Smith PG, and Beck DL: Facial nerve monitoring in otologic surgery: Clinical indications and intraoperative technique. Ann Otol Rhinol Laryngol 99:911–918, 1990.

Molony TR and De La Cruz A: Surgical approaches to congenital atresia of the external auditory canal. Otolaryngol Head Neck Surg 103(6):991–1001, 1990.

chapter

6

Perilymphatic Fistula

JAMES S. REILLY, M.D.

Perilymphatic fistulas (PLFs) are well-recognized abnormal communications between the inner ear and the middle ear. These channels permit spontaneous leaks of CSF (cerebrospinal fluid) into the middle ear and mastoid air cell system. Either trauma or a congenital weakness can cause the defect in the temporal bone. Many leaks are intermittent and are observed only after head trauma or middle ear surgery. However, spontaneous ruptures of the round or oval window membranes can also occur in infants and children from minor exertion, causing subtle clinical signs.

Symptoms are variable and are not always specific. Any child with an unexplained progression of hearing loss should be investigated thoroughly. The burden of the diagnosis rests with the parents, the physicians, and the audiologists. Careful monitoring appears to have the potential for stabilization of hearing. The vigilance of the physicians is essential to initiate surgical exploration and confirmation of the diagnosis. (See also Chapter 3.)

Indications

Noted clinical markers of PLF include radiographic evidence of malformations of the temporal bone or asymmetric fluctuations and decreases in hearing.

The radiographic evaluation is best completed with computed tomographic (CT) evaluation of the temporal bone using both the axial and coronal planes. CT images should be at 1.5-mm sections and programmed to enhance bony detail. The images must be thoroughly evaluated by radiologists who are well versed in temporal bone anatomy. Subtle malformations of the cochlea and semicircular canals have been documented. The most obvious abnormalities include complete aplasia or hypoplasia of the cochlea or labyrinth. More subtle changes including undersized and underdeveloped structures have recently been documented. These structures are associated with sensorineural hearing loss.

Diagnosis is based on audiometric and radiographic data. The careful monitoring of hearing to show progression of the hearing loss is the most important clinical sign.

The type and degree of hearing loss experienced by children are variable. Patterns vary from severe to mild. In children with mild hearing loss, the lower frequencies appear to be more at risk for fluctuations.

Careful observation and monitoring of children with hearing loss suggests a prevalence of perilymphatic fistula in approximately 6% of children.

Anesthetic considerations

The procedure is performed under general anesthesia. The ear is prepared and draped in the usual manner.

Procedure

- Using a transcanal approach and a tympanomeatal flap, the middle ear is exposed (Fig. 6–1*A*).
- The chorda tympani nerve must be mobilized and/or the posterior superior canal curetted (Fig. 6–1*B*).
- Adequate visualization of the oval and round windows is obtained, and each window is observed closely for at least 60 seconds (Fig. 6–1*C*).
- Spontaneous appearance of clear fluid must be documented. Suctioning of clear fluid and observation of reaccumulation are critical.
- When there is not clear visual evidence of the presence of PLF, the child is repositioned in a Trendelenburg position (head down). The anesthesiologist can sustain hyperinflated breaths (Valsalva maneuver) for three sequential periods of 30 seconds, each through the endotracheal tube.
- The mucosa around the oval and round window is carefully denuded with a pick. This area is then packed with small pieces of temporalis muscle, as illustrated (Fig. 6–1*D*).
- Absorbable gelatin sponge is placed over the area, which is packed with muscle to prevent any leakage, and the tympanic membrane is replaced.
- Antibiotic ointment is placed in the ear canal to protect the incisions during healing.

Postoperative care

- The child is discharged and is given a prescription for an oral antibiotic to be taken for 2 weeks.
- A repeat audiogram is obtained between 4 and 6 weeks after surgery, and the ear canal should be well healed.
- Follow-up audiograms are performed at 3-month intervals for the first year and at 6-month intervals for the second year.

Series to date have shown that hearing is stabilized in approximately 69% of patients. Improvement in hearing occurs in a limited fashion in approximately 15%. Deterioration appears to occur despite this surgery in approximately 15%.

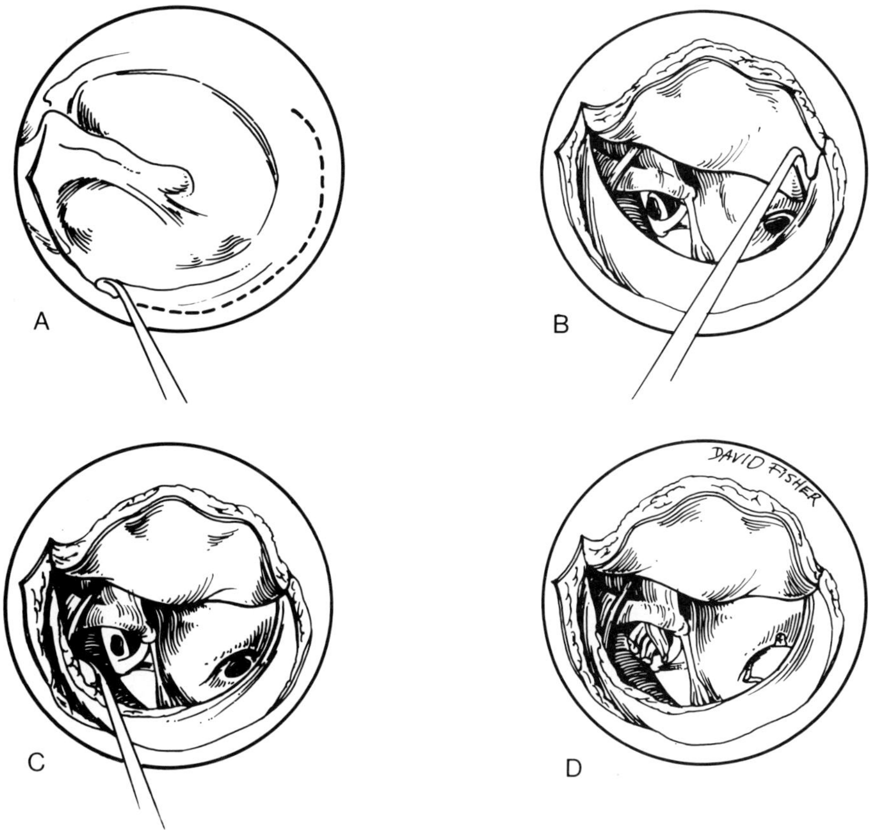

• FIGURE 6–1.

A to *D*, Surgical treatment of perilymphatic fistula.

BIBLIOGRAPHY

Althous S: Perilymphatic fistulas. Laryngoscope 91:538, 1981.

Reilly JS: Congenital perilymphatic fistula—a prospective study in infants and children. Laryngoscope 99:393, 1989.

Reilly JS and Kenna MA: Congenital perilymphatic fistula: An overlooked diagnosis? Am J Otol 10:6 496, 1989.

Seltzer S and McCabe B: Perilymph fistula—the Iowa experience. Laryngoscope 94:37, 1986.

chapter

7

Endoscopy of the Nose and Nasopharynx

GLENN C. ISAACSON, M.D.

Anterior rhinoscopy should be a part of the routine pediatric otolaryngology physical examination of every child.

Indications

Endoscopic examination of the posterior nose, middle meatus, and nasopharynx is useful for evaluating several types of problems.

- Nasal obstruction
  - Septal deviation
  - Nasal polyposis
  - Allergic rhinitis
  - Sinusitis/rhinitis
  - Nasal or choanal stenosis
  - Adenoid hypertrophy
  - Tumor
- Epistaxis
  - Sinusitis
  - Vascular abnormality
  - Tumor
- Otitis media
  - Adenoiditis
  - Tumor
- Headache
  - Sinusitis
  - Sinus ostial obstruction
- Speech disorders
  - Velopharyngeal function
  - Adenoid hypertrophy

Anesthetic considerations

Vasoconstriction and topical anesthesia are achieved using *very short* sprays from a forced air atomizer. We prefer to use 2% ephedrine and 2% tetracaine. These agents are toxic, and a 1-second spray in each naris is all that is needed. Rigid posterior endoscopy and rigid nasopharyngoscopy often require general anesthesia in young children.

Preparation

Lap restraint, as described for ear examination, is usually sufficient for anterior rhinoscopy and flexible nasopharyngoscopy. Papoosing may be preferable in infants. (Note that flexible *laryngoscopy* of infants is not recommended in the office setting because of the risk of protracted laryngospasm.)

Procedure

Anterior rhinoscopy with an otoscope gives an excellent view of the nasal vestibule, septum, and turbinates. To remove intranasal foreign bodies in uncooperative children, a headlight or an operating microscope provides better illumination and leaves the hands free to work (Fig. 7–1*A* to *E*).

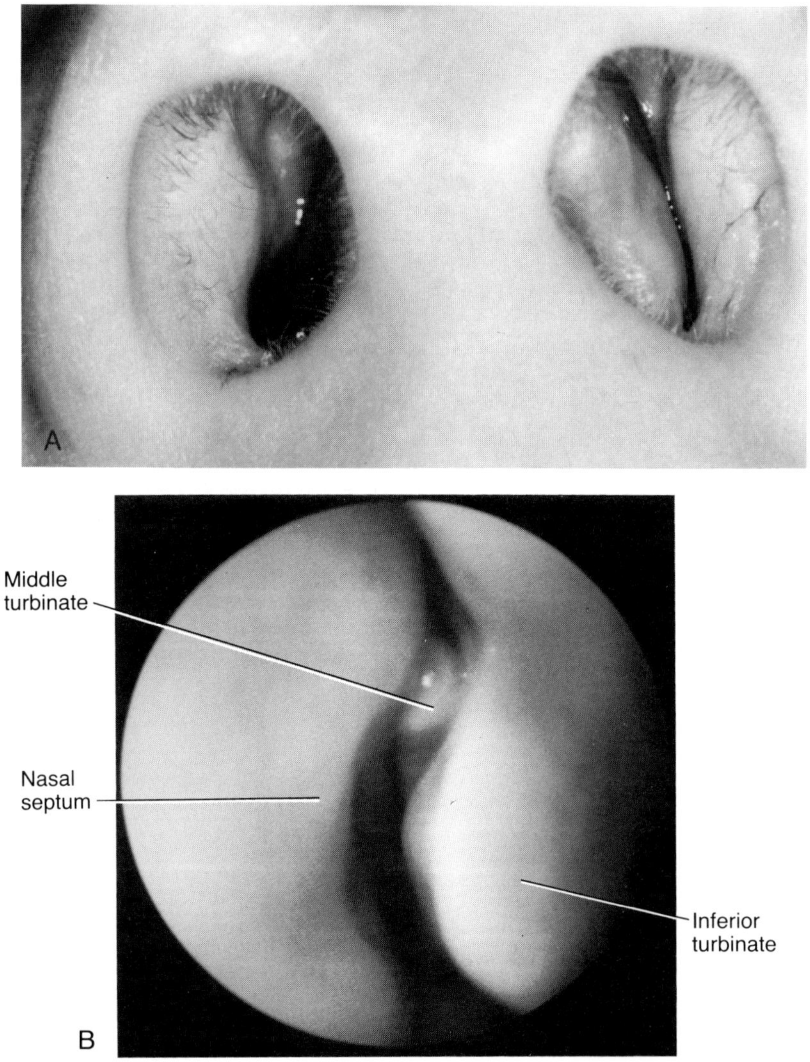

• FIGURE 7–1.

A, Anterior rhinoscopy—a caudal nasal septal deflection. *B*, Anterior rhinoscopy—a newborn's nose.

Illustration continued on following page

• FIGURE 7–1. *(continued)*

C, Anterior rhinoscopy—a child's nose. *D*, Anterior rhinoscopy—purulence in the middle meatus. *E*, Anterior rhinoscopy—a middle meatus polyp in cystic fibrosis.

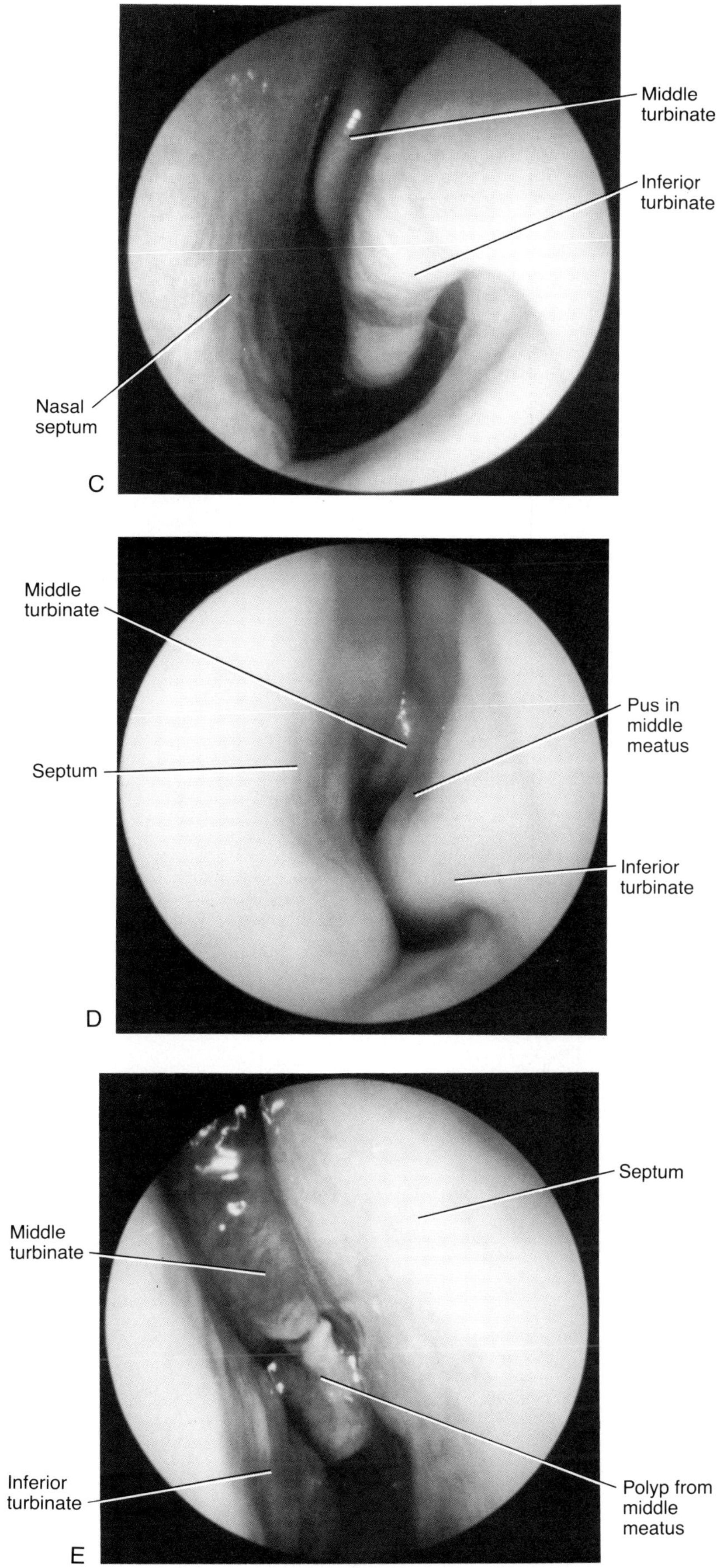

Rigid endoscopy with a 0-degree, 4-mm telescope gives the clearest view of all portions of the nose and nasopharynx and is the best instrument for intranasal photography and for inspection of post-surgical sinus cavities (Fig. 7–2). Posterior rhinoscopy requires much cooperation and may be impractical in the office for young children (Fig. 7–3*A* to *C*). When inspecting the middle meatus or eustachian tube, a 30-degree, 4-mm or 2.8-mm telescope may be helpful but is more difficult to maneuver.

Flexible rhinoscopy and nasopharyngoscopy allow visualization of the middle meatus, posterior nasal cavity, nasopharynx, and eustachian tube orifices. Assessment of the dynamics of velopharyngeal function during phonation and swallowing requires a flexible instrument.

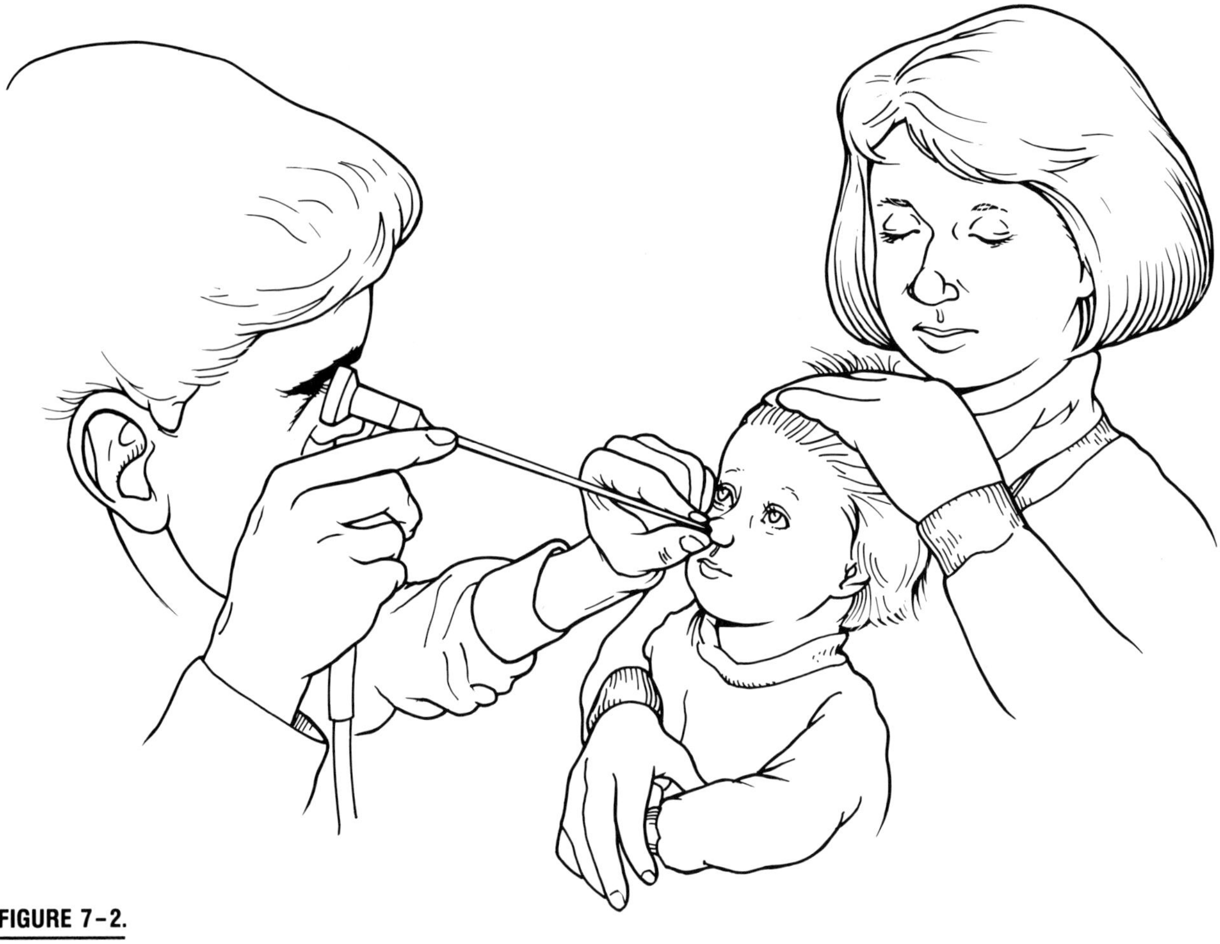

• FIGURE 7–2.

Rigid rhinoscopy—the shaft of the telescope rests on the thumb of the nondominant hand. This allows the hand and telescope to move in concert with minor head movements, avoiding injury.

• FIGURE 7-3.

A, Posterior rhinoscopy—choanal stenosis. *B*, Posterior rhinoscopy—enlarged, nonobstructing adenoids. (Courtesy of Richard M. Rosenfeld, M.D.) *C*, Posterior rhinoscopy—normal nasopharynx and eustachian tube. (From Yanagisawa E, Isaacson G, Kmucha ST, and Hirokawa R: Video nasopharyngoscopy: A comparison of fiberscopic, telescopic, and microscopic documentation. Ann Otol Rhinol Laryngol 98:19, 1989.)

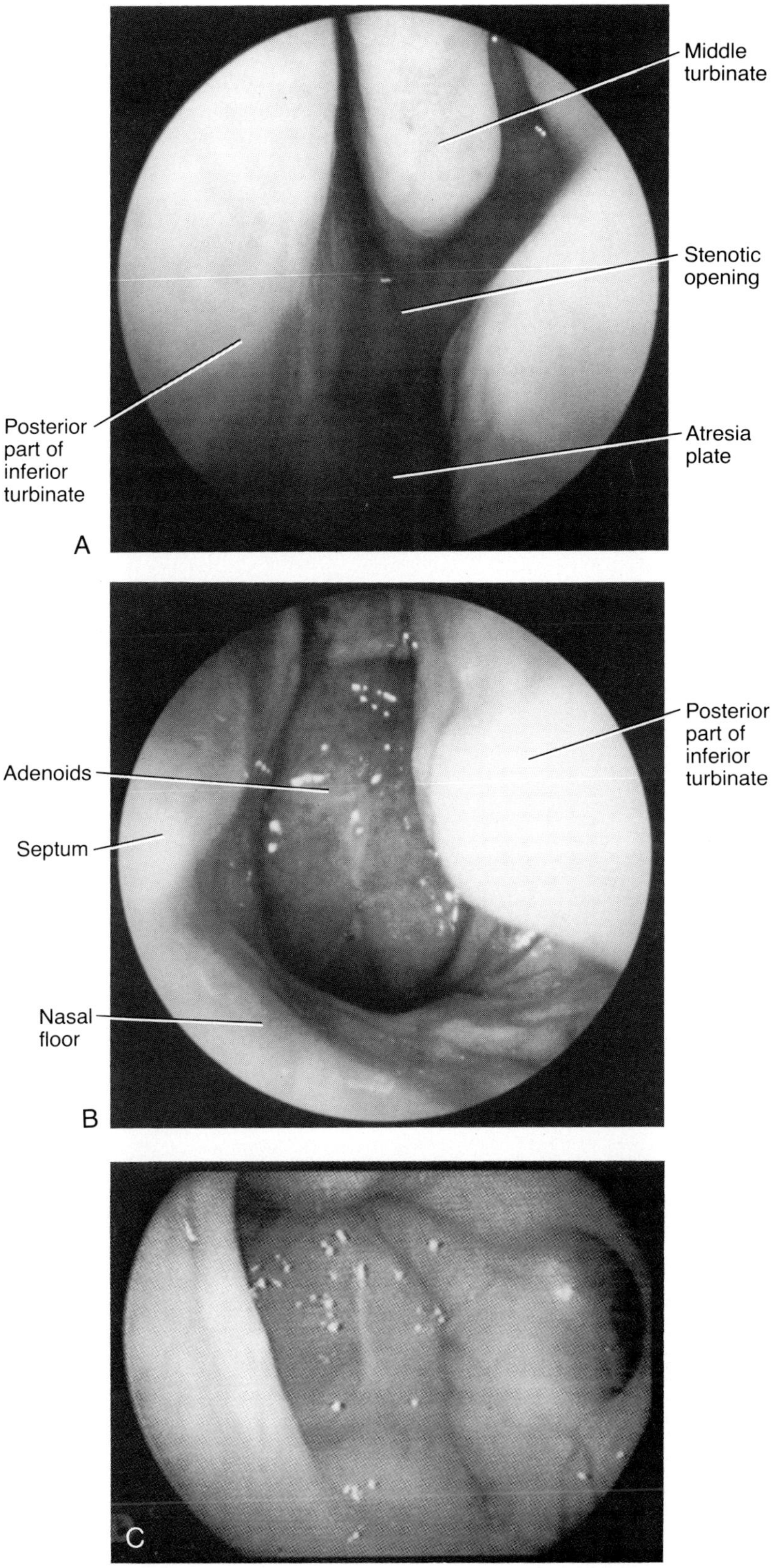

BIBLIOGRAPHY

Chait DH and Lotz WK: Successful pediatric examinations using nasoendoscopy. Laryngoscope 101:1016–1018, 1991.

Yanagisawa E, Isaacson G, Kmucha ST, and Hirokawa R: Video nasopharyngoscopy: A comparison of fiberscopic, telescopic and microscopic documentation. Ann Otol Rhinol Laryngol 98:15–20, 1989.

chapter

8

Cochlear Implants

NOEL L. COHEN, M.D.

Cochlear implants are designed for patients with bilateral profound to total deafness, who derive little or no benefit from amplification. Whereas most adult patients who have received cochlear implants lost their hearing subsequent to the acquisition of speech, there is a smaller population of congenitally or prelinguistically deafened adults who have received cochlear implants. The results, in general, are better for the postlinguistically deafened adults.

There is more experience with congenitally hearing handicapped and prelinguistically deafened children than with postlinguistically deafened children. Although the results to date do not indicate quite as great an improvement in the former group as in the latter, this may, at least in part, be due to the relatively short experience with cochlear implants in children. It is reasonable to assume that, as the child matures, uses the implant, and participates in rehabilitation and education, performance will improve.

Cochlear implants may be single-channel, multichannel, intracochlear, or extracochlear. In theory, a multichannel implant offers advantages over the single-channel implant, because the cochlea is organized tonotopically. An extracochlear device offers, at least in theory, the opportunity of stimulating the eighth nerve without direct damage to the cochlea. These devices are, however, more difficult to design and to place than are the intracochlear multichannel electrodes and have failed to gain much popularity. Comparative studies have demonstrated superior performance of multichannel over single-channel devices. At the time of this writing, only one device is available in the United States for use in children: the Nucleus 22 electrode cochlear implant. Although no longer available commercially, the 3M/House single-channel implant has also been used for both adults and children in the United States and abroad.

Indications

- Designed for patients with bilateral profound to total deafness who derive little help from amplification

Anesthetic considerations

General anesthesia is used.

Preparation

SURGICAL TECHNIQUE

The operation is performed in the conventional otologic position, with perioperative antibiotics being started in the operating room and continued until the drain is removed.

The surgical technique for children is similar to that for adults, with the size of the skull, lack of mastoid development, and thin nature of the scalp and skull forming the critical differences.

POSITIONING THE IMPLANT

Sufficient hair is shaved from the side of the head in order to allow draping around the periphery of the incision. The dummy device is placed on the side of the head, and its position is marked in ink (Fig. 8–1*A*). The device should be slightly behind the edge of the auricle, with the anterior edge at or slightly above the canthomeatal line. The posterior part of the device is angled 30 to 45 degrees above the horizontal. After the position of the device and the proposed center of the well are marked (Fig. 8–1*B*), an incision is marked on the skin. A variation of the inferiorly based inverted "U," which has a short posterior arm that causes it to resemble a question mark, is used (Fig. 8–1*C*).

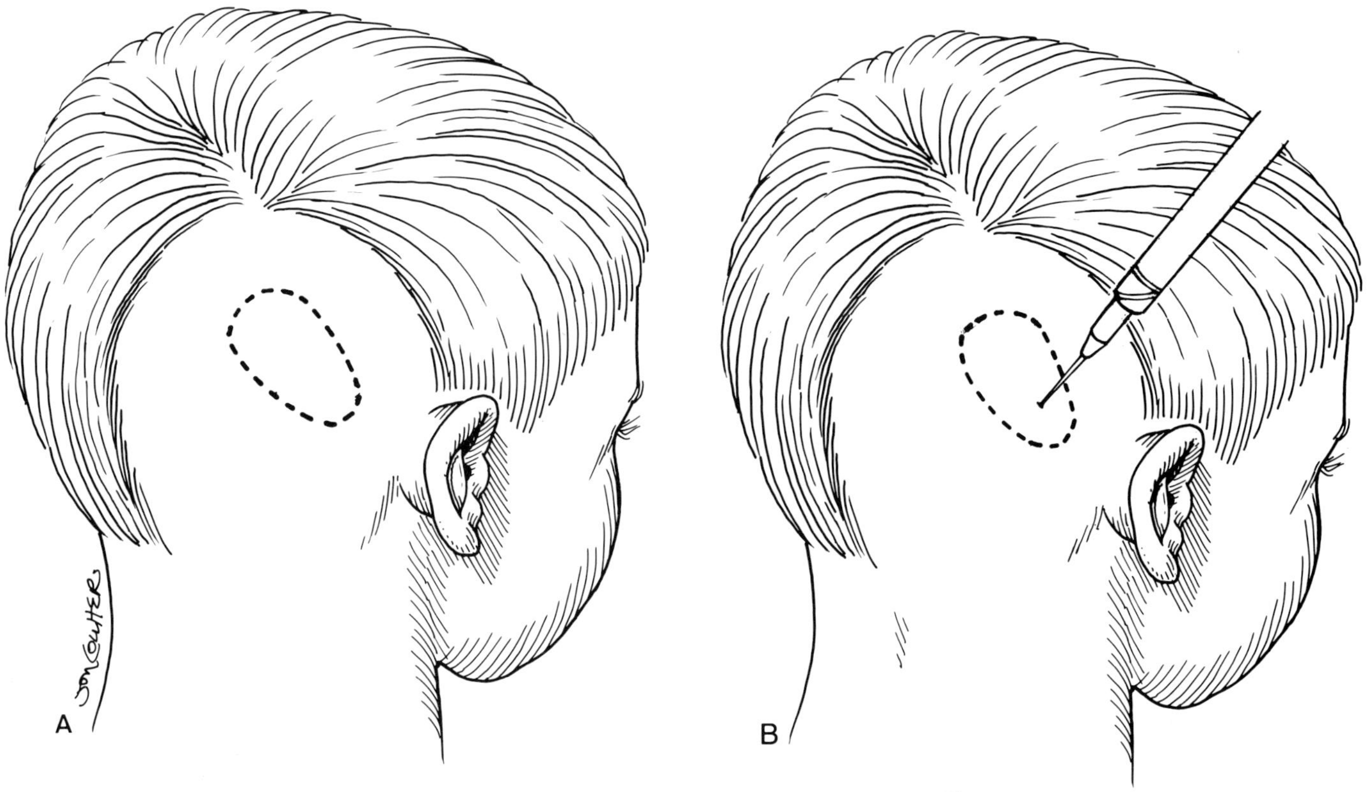

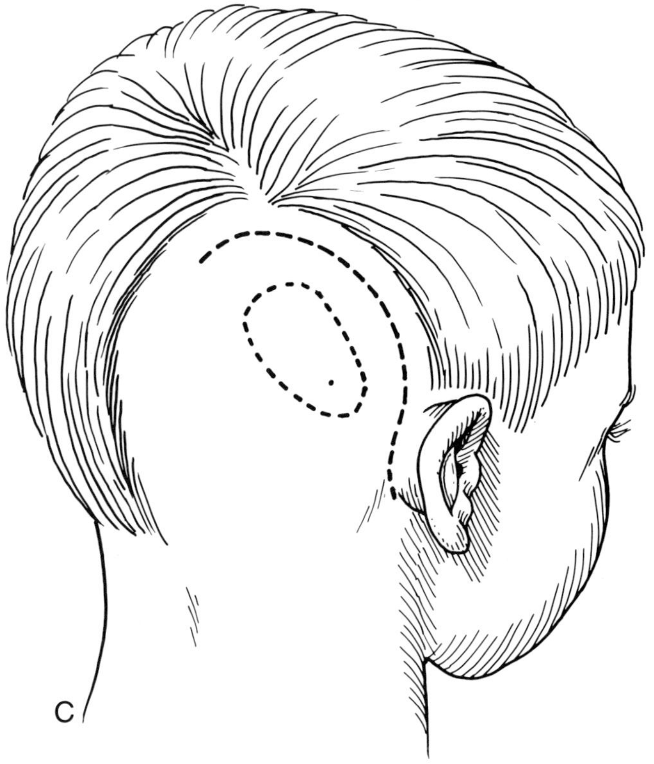

• FIGURE 8-1.

A, The implant is positioned on the side of the head. *B*, A needle with methylene blue is inserted to the bone, marking the center of the well. *C*, The incision is then marked. (Redrawn from Cochlear Corporation: Surgical Procedure Manual. Englewood, CO, Cochlear Corporation, 1987.)

PLANNING THE FLAP

The incision begins in the postauricular sulcus near the mastoid tip, ascends to the attachment of the auricle, and then in a curved fashion extends posteriorly and superiorly, allowing at least 15 mm around the position of the implant, after which a short, curved vertical posterior arm descends only far enough to allow reflection of the flap sufficient for the drilling of the well and the mastoidectomy.

Procedure

INCISION

The skin is then prepared with an organic iodine solution and thoroughly draped. The center of the proposed well is marked by dipping a 22-gauge needle in methylene blue and depositing a droplet of methylene blue on the surface of the bone. The line of the incision is infiltrated with 1:200,000 epinephrine, following which the incision is made with the cutting current. In the older child, the flap is elevated deep to the galea, allowing the pericranium to remain in place. In the younger child, the pericranium and posteroinferior temporalis muscle are elevated with the flap (Fig. 8–2).

The pericranium is elevated in all directions, leaving bare bone under the position of the implant. An anteriorly based pericranial flap is elevated to cover the proximal electrode when the incision is closed. Nontraumatic barbless fish-hooks are used to gently retract the flap interiorly. The flap should be kept moist with gauze sponges throughout the procedure.

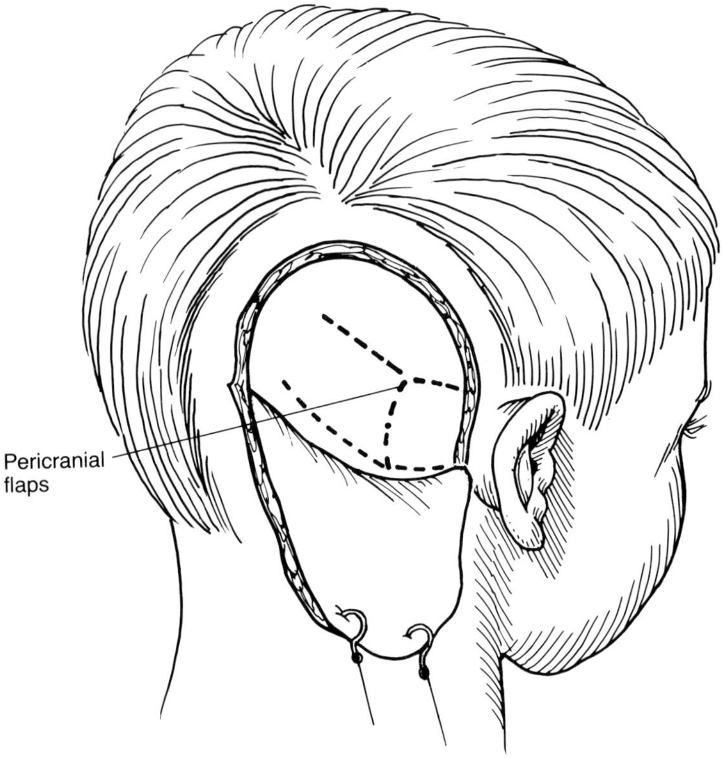

• FIGURE 8–2.

The flaps are elevated. (Redrawn from Cochlear Corporation: Surgical Procedure Manual. Englewood, CO, Cochlear Corporation, 1987.)

CREATING THE WELL

A well is then created for the electronics package. Drilling is begun with cutting burs (Fig. 8–3*A*) and is then finished with diamond burs (Fig. 8–3*B*). A special milling bur may be used to achieve a flat floor and vertical sides for the well. The metal die is used to ensure the proper size (Fig. 8–3*C*). In the case of small children, it is necessary to drill down to the dura or to create an island of bone by thinning the floor of the well and by then cutting around the periphery with a small diamond bur (Fig. 8–3*D*).

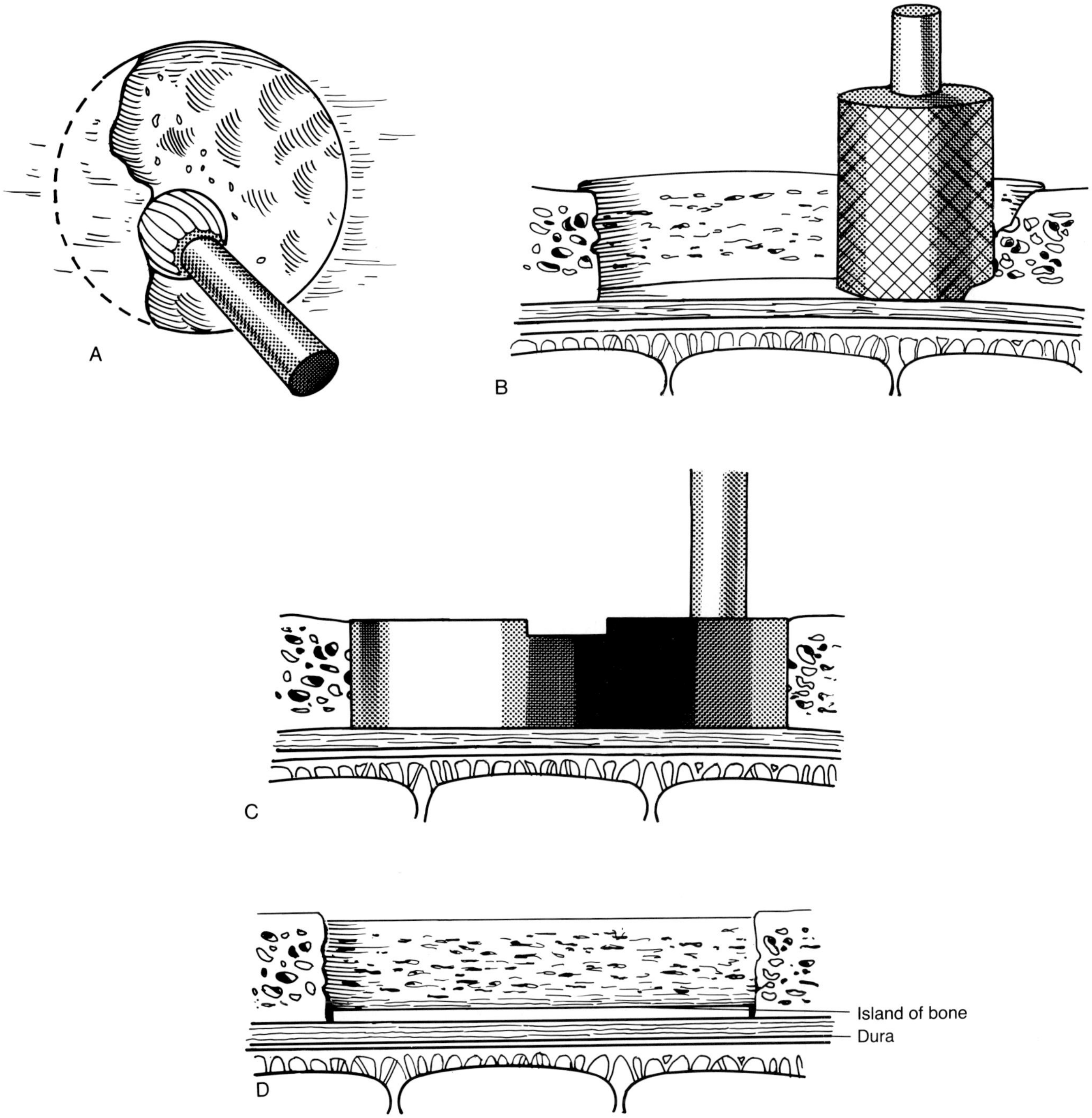

• FIGURE 8–3.

A to *D*, A well is created for the implant.

Illustration continued on following page

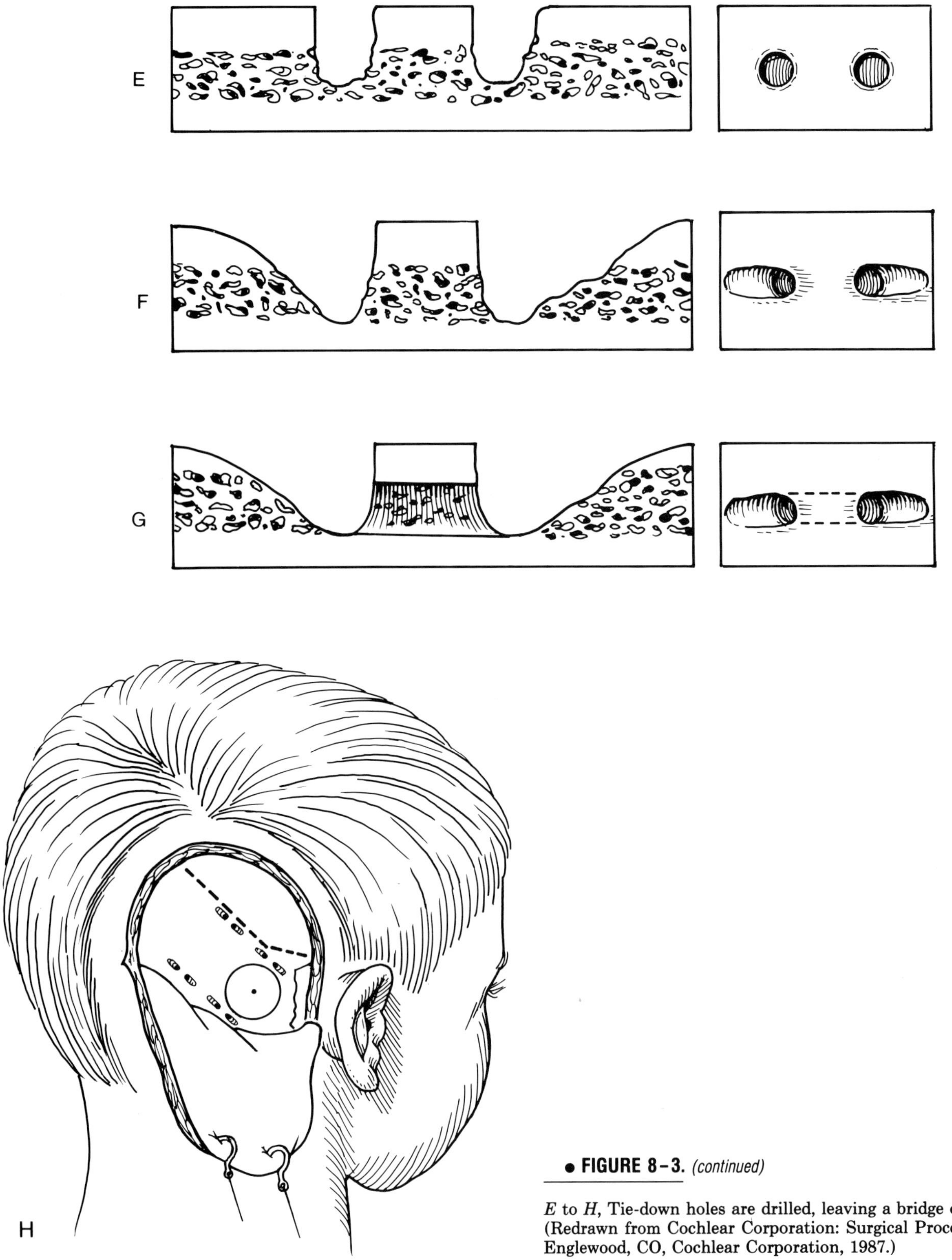

• FIGURE 8-3. *(continued)*

E to *H*, Tie-down holes are drilled, leaving a bridge of bone intact. (Redrawn from Cochlear Corporation: Surgical Procedure Manual. Englewood, CO, Cochlear Corporation, 1987.)

TIE-DOWN HOLES

Four holes are then drilled above and below the anterior and posterior parts of the receiver-stimulator. These are cut with a 3-mm bur, creating a series of grooves that are then connected with a 2-mm diamond bur, leaving a bridge of bone intact (Fig. 8–3*E* to *H*).

MASTOIDECTOMY

The mastoidectomy is performed in conventional fashion, keeping in mind the lack of development of the mastoid tip in a small child and the fact that the object of the mastoidectomy is to approach the facial recess. It is, therefore, not necessary to create an extensive cavity below the area of the antrum. The posterior and superior edges of the cavity should not be saucerized but should be allowed to overhang in order to attach the proximal electrode (Fig. 8–4).

Sufficient bone is removed to visualize the lateral semicircular canal and short process of the incus. Using a medium-sized cutting bur, a groove is created between the anterior edge of the stimulator well and the posterior margin of the mastoid cavity. This groove should point in the direction of the facial recess; it should be wide; and it should have rounded corners (see Fig. 8–4).

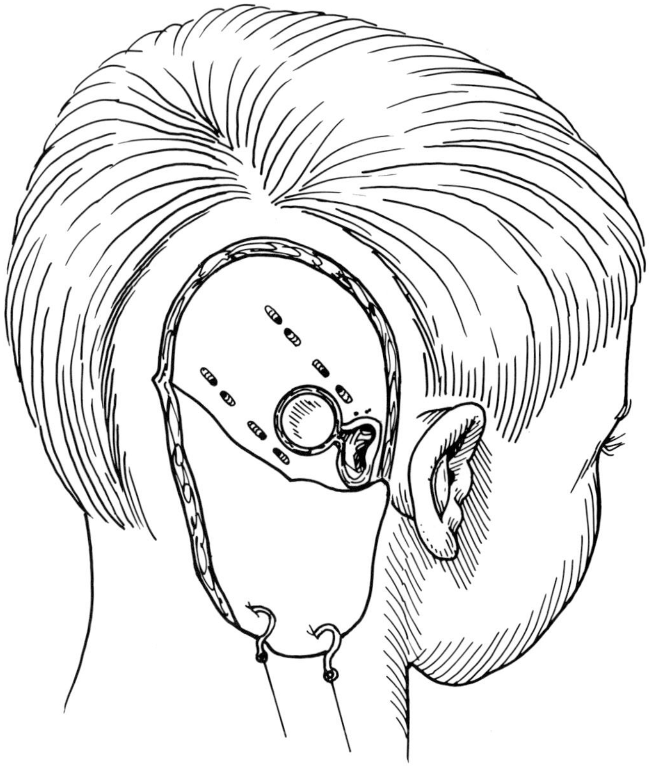

• **FIGURE 8–4.**

Mastoidectomy. A groove is created leading toward the facial recess. (Redrawn from Cochlear Corporation: Surgical Procedure Manual. Englewood, CO, Cochlear Corporation, 1987.)

FACIAL RECESS

The facial recess is a triangular space bounded posteriorly by the upper vertical portion of the facial nerve, superiorly by the short process of the incus, and anteriorly by the chorda tympani nerve (Fig. 8–5). This space must be opened adequately for visualization of the round window area and the electrode placement (Fig. 8–6).

Drilling is begun by exenterating mastoid cells and by thinning the posterior canal wall. This is important to allow visualization from the lateral to the medial parts of the posterior mesotympanum. The facial nerve is then identified in its vertical segment, but bone is allowed to remain on the nerve. Drilling is begun superiorly, where the triangular facial recess is widest. The chorda tympani nerve is identified and can usually be spared. The tympanic membrane annular ligament should always be spared. It is important not to perforate the posterior canal wall.

Often, a cell tract may lead through the facial recess into the middle ear. As the bone is removed, care should be taken not to allow the rotating shaft of the bur to rub against the posterior wall of the facial recesses, since this might cause heating of the bone and edema of the underlying facial nerve.

Once the facial recess is opened superiorly, the area of the oval window can usually be identified. The facial recess is then gradually opened inferiorly in order to visualize the round window (see Fig. 8–6). It is occasionally necessary to sacrifice the chorda tympani in order to visualize the round window. The round window is never more than 3 mm from the inferior border of the oval window. Care should be taken not to mistake the hypotympanic air cell for the round window niche (Fig. 8–7). There may be membranous adhesions over the round window niche; these can be removed for better visualization. Pumping the stapes and looking for a round window reflex may also be of assistance. The shape of the cochlea deep to the promontory should be understood (Fig. 8–8).

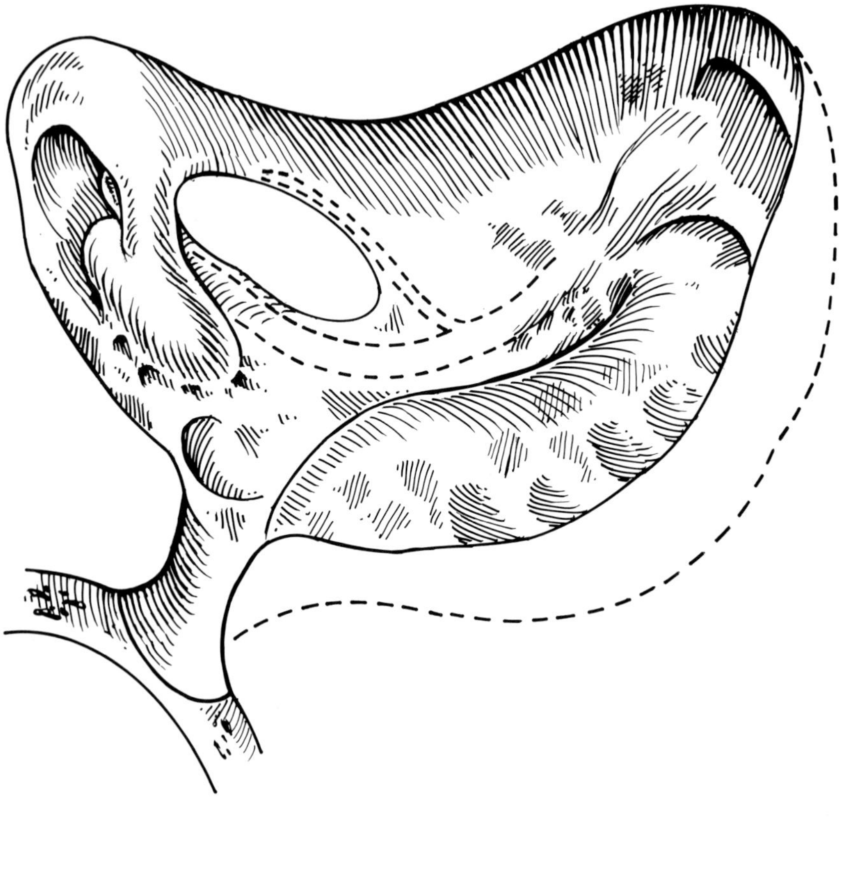

• FIGURE 8–5.

Mastoidectomy and facial recess. (Redrawn from Cochlear Corporation: Surgical Procedure Manual. Englewood, CO, Cochlear Corporation, 1987.)

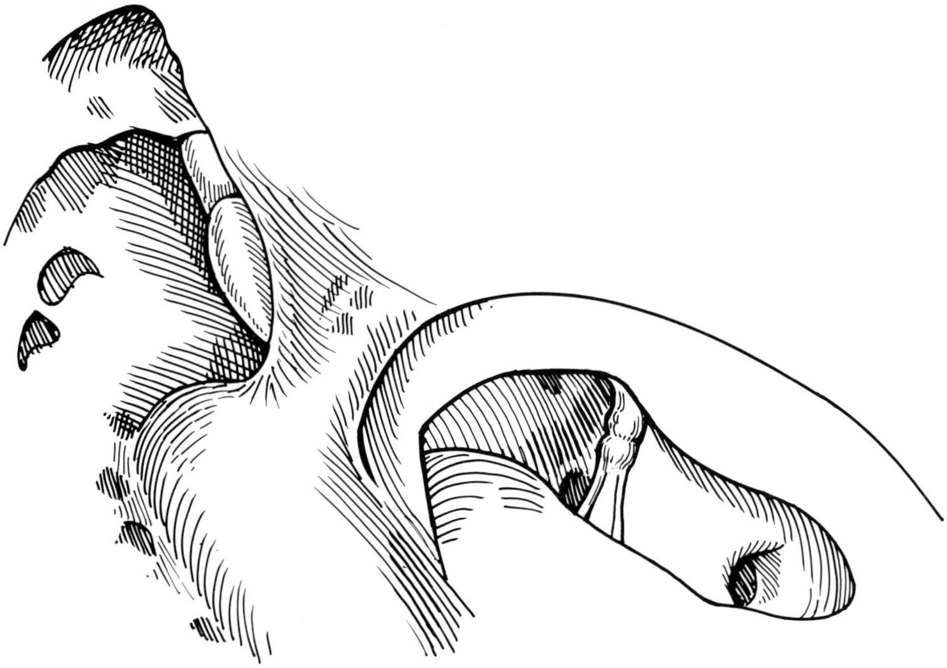

• **FIGURE 8-6.**

The facial recess is opened. (Redrawn from Cochlear Corporation: Surgical Procedure Manual. Englewood, CO, Cochlear Corporation, 1987.)

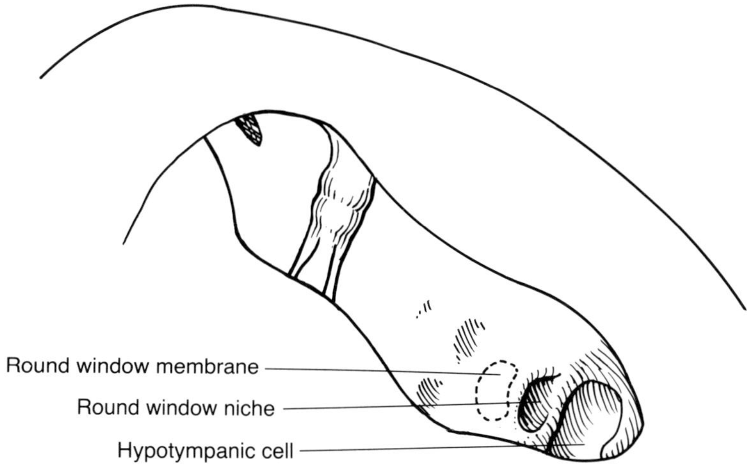

• **FIGURE 8-7.**

The appearance of a round window niche and a hypotympanic cell. (Redrawn from Cochlear Corporation: Surgical Procedure Manual. Englewood, CO, Cochlear Corporation, 1987.)

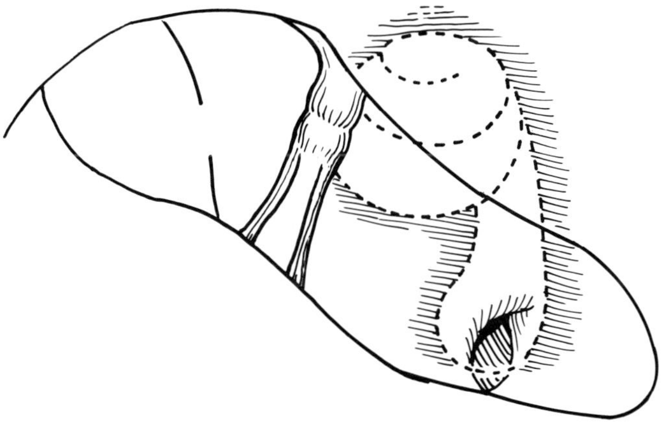

• **FIGURE 8-8.**

The cochlea is viewed through a round window membrane. (Redrawn from Cochlear Corporation: Surgical Procedure Manual. Englewood, CO, Cochlear Corporation, 1987.)

COCHLEOSTOMY

The scala tympani of the cochlea may be opened either by taking down the round window membrane or by direct cochleostomy immediately anterior and inferior to the round window. We prefer the latter, but the round window membrane approach is also acceptable. If that is the route chosen, bone should be drilled away from the inferior margin of the round window membrane to allow easier access past the "hook" area (Fig. 8–9*A*).

The direct cochleostomy is performed immediately anterior to the round window niche using a 1-mm diamond bur (Fig. 8–9*B*). It should be remembered that the scala tympani is aligned in a lateral to medial position, more or less parallel with the thinned posterior canal wall. When the bone over the scala tympani is thinned, the white endosteum is visualized. This should be removed with right-angled picks or stapes footplate instruments to avoid drilling directly into the scala tympani, with resultant trauma and deposition of bone dust (Fig. 8–9*C*). The cochleostomy should be more than adequate for the introduction of the electrode array, which measures 0.6 mm at its maximum diameter. If necessary, proximal bony obstruction may be perforated with a 0.75-mm bur, or fibrous tissue or osteoid may be removed with picks (Fig. 8–9*D*).

When the CT scan shows an obstruction of the cochlea, the surgeon should be prepared to drill out the scala tympani to a sufficient depth to allow electrode insertion. Accordingly, a small drill, capable of being passed through the facial recess and drilling at least 7 mm into the scala tympani, should always be available in the operating room at the beginning of surgery. If a free lumen cannot be located, drilling should continue in the axis of the scala tympani for up to 8 mm in order to allow partial electrode placement. Care must be taken not to traumatize the internal carotid artery, which is located just anterior to the junction of the pars inferior and the pars ascendens of the scala tympani.

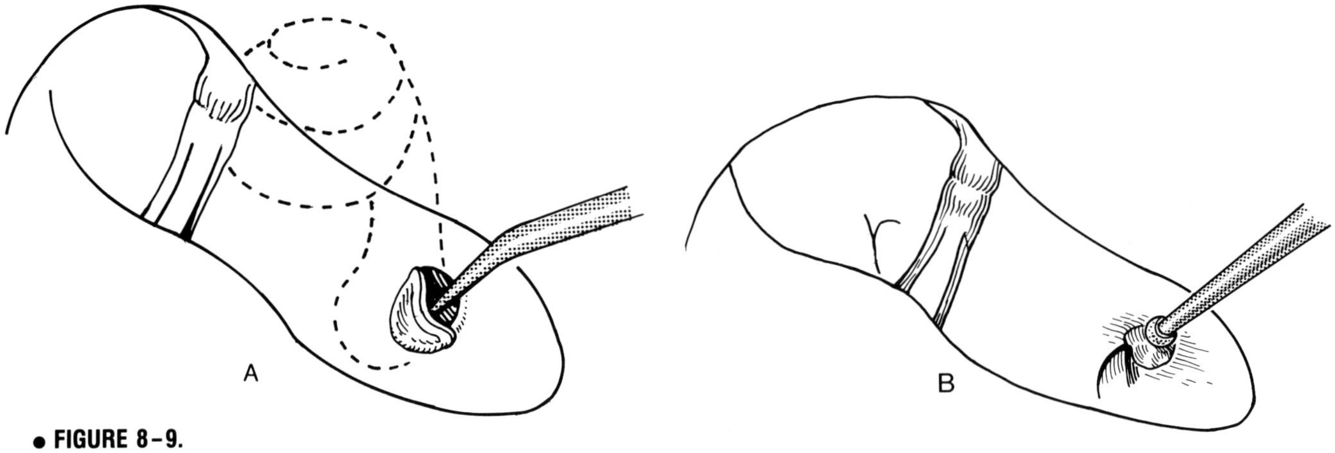

• FIGURE 8–9.

A, Opening of the scala tympani using the round window membrane approach. *B*, Anteroinferior fenestration (cochleostomy).

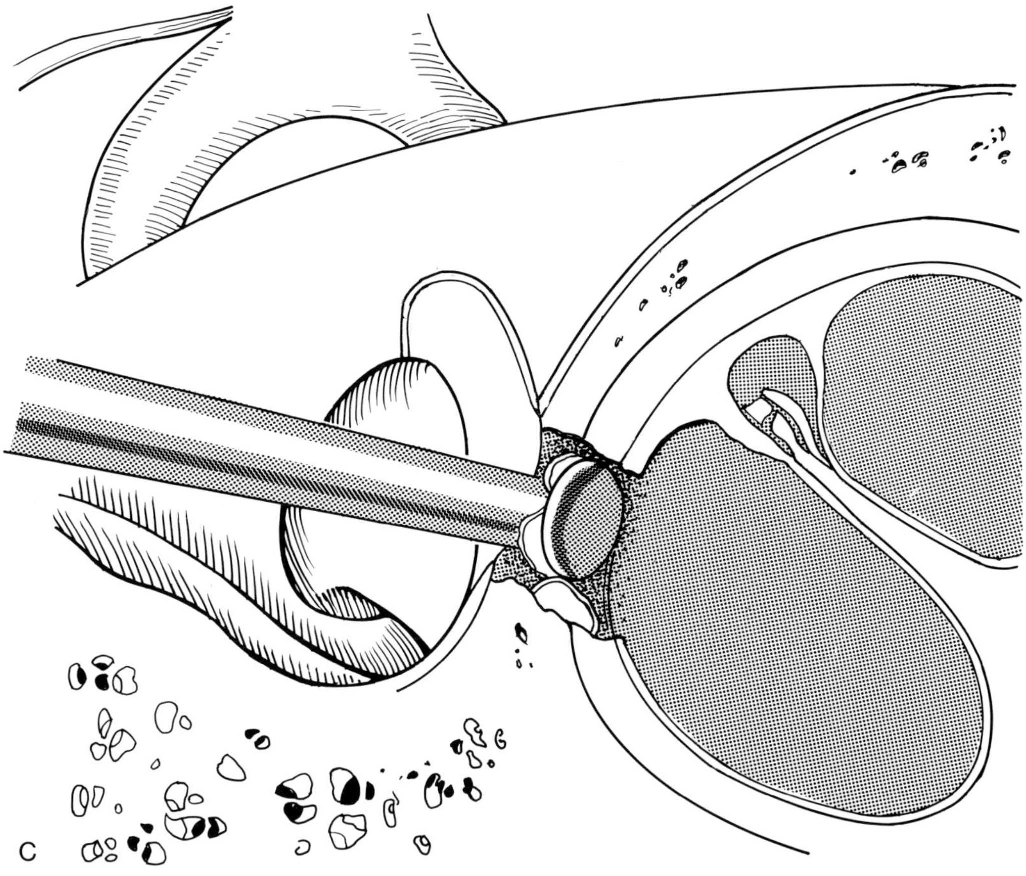

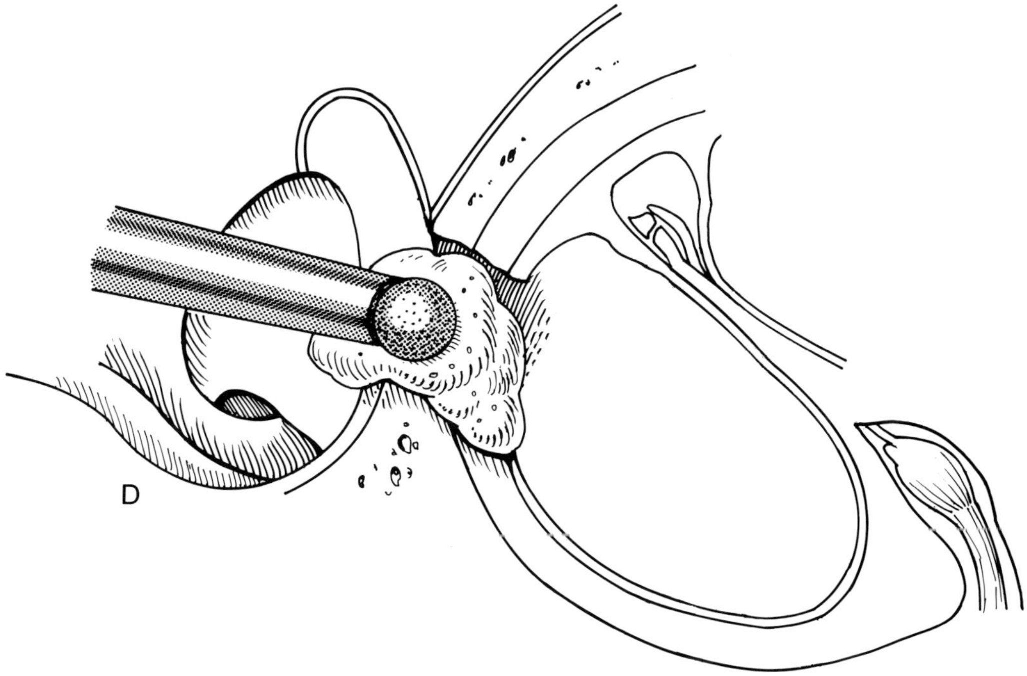

• FIGURE 8-9. *(continued)*

C, Removal of bone debris. *D*, Drilling through bony obstruction. (Redrawn from Cochlear Corporation: Surgical Procedure Manual. Englewood, CO, Cochlear Corporation, 1987.)

ELECTRODE INSERTION

The electrode is inserted into the scala tympani using either the specially designed claws or other atraumatic instruments (Fig. 8–10*A*). The receiver-stimulator is grasped in the surgeon's nondominant hand, and the tip of the electrode array is presented to the cochleostomy. It is then guided in with the claws or a stapes crimper. Ordinary alligator forceps should not be used, because they are potentially damaging. The electrode array usually advances easily, with steady pressure from both hands. If it appears to impact, the electrode should be withdrawn one or two rings, rotated 90 degrees or more (counterclockwise for the right ear and clockwise for the left ear) in order to disimpact the tip of the electrode array, and then gently reinserted (Fig. 8–10*B*). If the electrode array appears to buckle, force should never be used; the surgeon should be satisfied with a partial insertion.

SECURING THE IMPLANT

Once the electrode has been inserted, the receiver-stimulator is placed in the well. It is then sutured down with the nonabsorbable material, taking care that the knot is at the edge of the implant rather than over its center (Fig. 8–11).

We prefer a 2-0 Tevdek. The proximal electrode may then be tied in place with the special Dacron mesh. Soft tissue is packed around the cochleostomy as well as in the facial recess. The wound is then thoroughly irrigated.

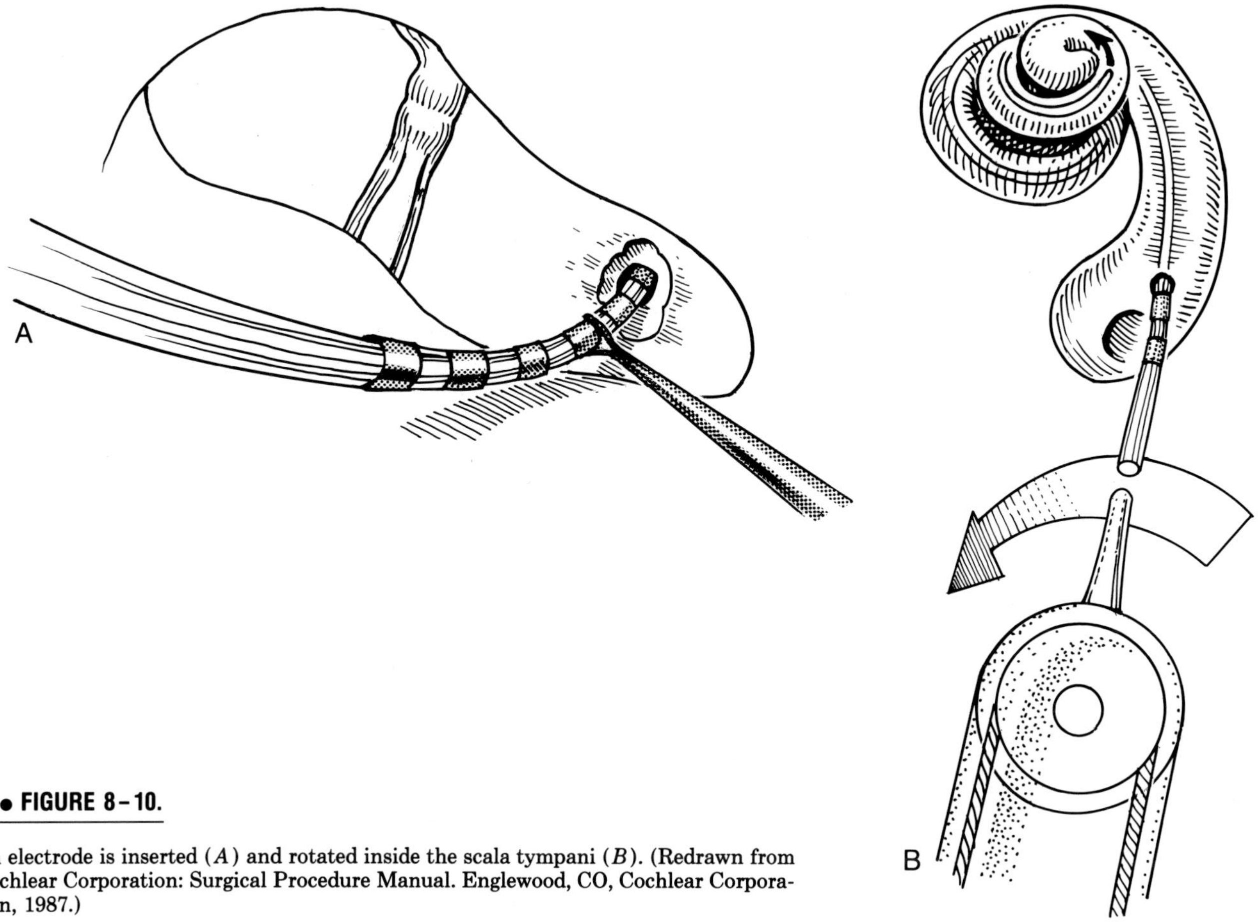

• FIGURE 8-10.

An electrode is inserted (*A*) and rotated inside the scala tympani (*B*). (Redrawn from Cochlear Corporation: Surgical Procedure Manual. Englewood, CO, Cochlear Corporation, 1987.)

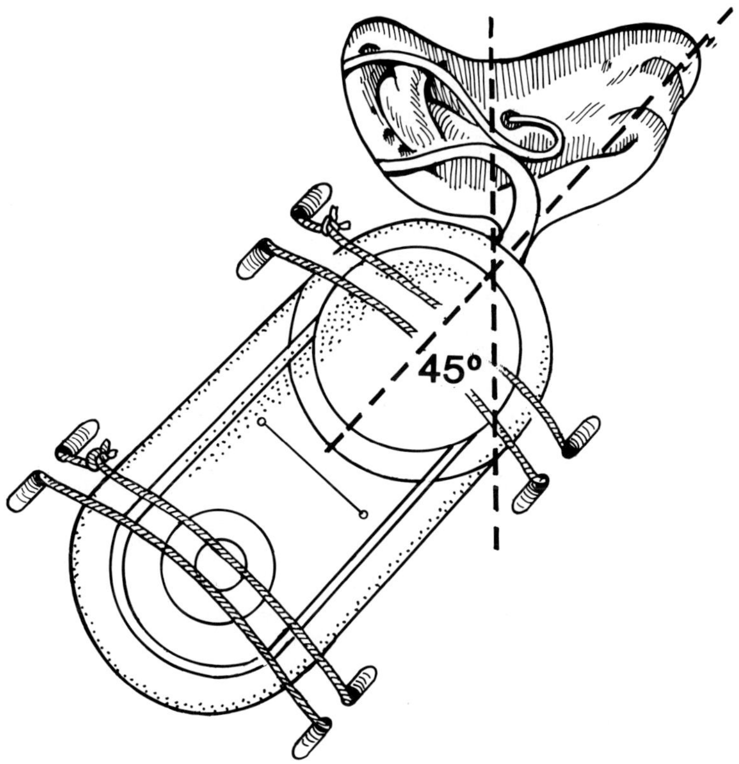

• FIGURE 8-11.

Fixation of the implant and electrode. (Redrawn from Cochlear Corporation: Surgical Procedure Manual. Englewood, CO, Cochlear Corporation, 1987.)

CLOSURE

The anteriorly based pericranial flap is sutured over the proximal electrode lead with absorbable sutures. A self-contained suction drain is then placed under the flap, proportionate to the size of the child. This is generally brought out through a stab wound posteriorly and inferiorly. The incision is then closed in layers with staples or, in the case of the very small anxious child, subcuticular sutures and tape strips (Fig. 8–12). A gentle mastoid dressing is applied.

X-RAY

It is strongly advised that an intraoperative x-ray be taken to verify electrode position while the patient is still asleep. To accomplish this, the patient's head is straightened on the table, either before or after application of the dressing. A single anteroposterior transorbital view (slightly over-penetrated) is taken (Fig. 8–13). If the electrode is placed incorrectly or compressed, this should be discovered in the operating room rather than 4 weeks later when the child is found to be nonstimulable.

Postoperative care/complications

POSTOPERATIVE CARE

The drain can usually be removed in 24 to 36 hours. Antibiotics are then discontinued, and the dressing is removed. Staples are generally removed in 10 days. No specific aftercare is necessary.

PRECAUTIONS

Ventilation tubes should not be placed in an ear that has received a cochlear implant. Certain sports are probably better avoided after cochlear implant surgery: these include soccer, wrestling, and rugby. It is advisable that children engaging in contact sports always wear protective head gear.

Magnetic resonance imaging must be avoided due to the presence of the magnet, but there is no contraindication to CT scanning. A monopolar cautery should never be used in the vicinity of the cochlear implant or where the implant lies between the active electrodes and the ground electrodes. Other forms of radiant energy (e.g., diathermy) should also be avoided.

COMPLICATIONS

As with all types of surgery there are, inevitably, complications. In more than 756 children implanted in the United States with the Nucleus device, there have been no deaths or life-threatening surgical complications. The complication rate is lower than that for a comparable group of adults and can probably be lowered further by modifications of surgical techniques (Table 8–1). We defined major complications as those that required rehospitalization of the child for either surgery or intravenous antibiotic treatment. Minor complications were handled in an outpatient setting.

The most common major complication had to do with flaps, many of which could probably have been avoided. The displacement of a cochlear implant electrode could also have been detected by an intraoperative x-ray and the electrode replaced. Some complications are, however, unavoidable. Of seven cases of a facial palsy, six cases came on immediately after surgery, and one was delayed for more than 1 month postoperatively. Most of these were probably caused by direct surgical trauma or by thermal injury.

• FIGURE 8-12.

The incision is closed. (Redrawn from Cochlear Corporation: Surgical Procedure Manual. Englewood, CO, Cochlear Corporation, 1987.)

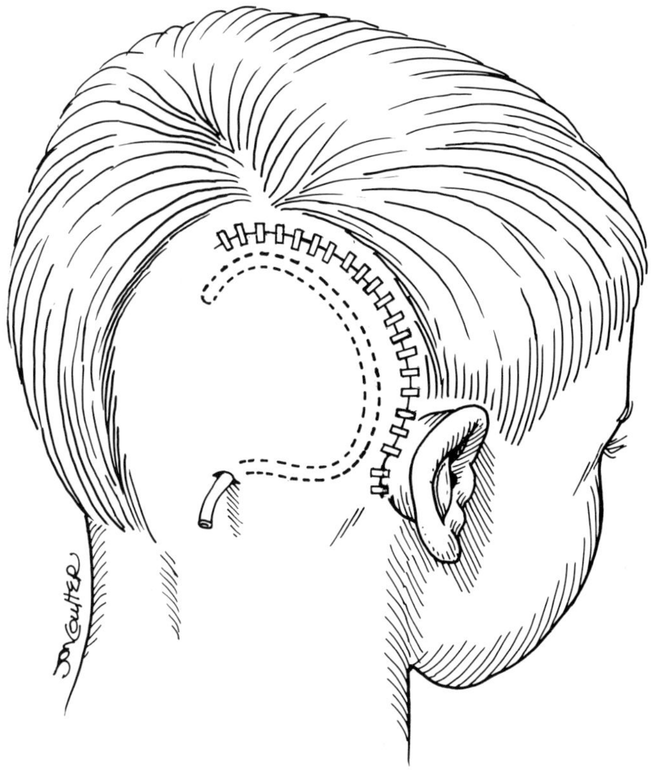

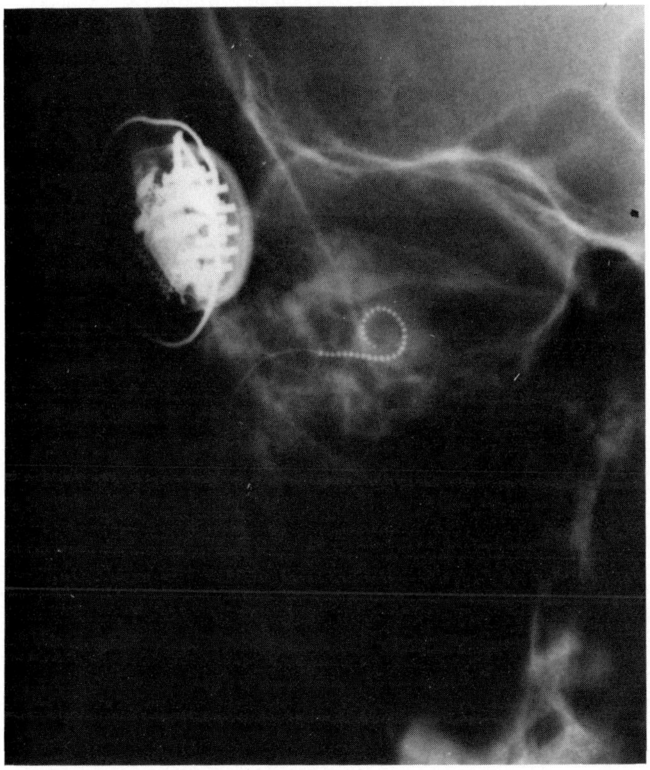

• FIGURE 8-13.

An intraoperative radiograph is taken to verify the position of the electrode.

• TABLE 8-1.

COMPLICATIONS IN ADULTS VERSUS CHILDREN FOLLOWING IMPLANTATION OF THE NUCLEUS DEVICE

	Adult (No. = 1995) (%)	Child (No. = 756) (%)
Life threatening	0.1	0
Flap	3.46	1.85
VII Palsy	0.65	0.93
Hypotympanic electrode	0.80	0.79
Compressed/kinked electrode	0.85	0.3
Delayed electrode migration	1.00	0.53
Gusher	0.05	0.53
R/S migration	0.20	0.13
R/S extrusion	1.30	0.13
Device failure (Mini 22)	1.08	1.81

The minor complications were resolved without the patient requiring hospitalization and did not significantly increase the morbidity of the procedure.

This complication rate compares favorably with the complications in operations on 1995 adults using the same device (see Table 8-1).

Finally, although there have been concerns about the possibility of an increased incidence of otitis media in children who have received cochlear implants, as well as the complications caused by the presence of the implant or the loss of an implant secondary to otitis media, none of these problems has occurred. There is no increased incidence of otitis media in the ears of children who have received cochlear implants, nor have there been any complications of otitis media as a result of the implants.

In summary, cochlear implant surgery in children can be accomplished satisfactorily in the overwhelming majority of properly selected candidates. The surgery requires some modifications from the adult technique, but the complication rate is not greater. In the short term, there appears not to have been a deleterious effect on the middle or inner ear as a consequence of implantation of either a single- or a multichannel cochlear implant in children.

BIBLIOGRAPHY

American Academy of Otolaryngology—Head and Neck Surgery Subcommittee on Cochlear Implants with Kveton J and Balkany TL. Status of cochlear implantation in children. J Pediatr 118:1-17, 1991.

Bielamowicz SA, Coker MJ, Jenkins HA, and Igarashi M: Surgical dimensions of the facial recess in adults and children. Arch Otolaryngol Head Neck Surg 114:534-537, 1988.

Clark GM, Franz BK-H, Pyman BC, et al: Nucleus 22 channel cochlear implant system surgical procedure manual. Englewood, CO, Cochlear Corporation, 1987.

Clark GM, Cohen NL, and Shepherd RK: Surgical and safety considerations of multichannel cochlear implants in children. Ear Hear 12(4):15S-24S, 1991.

Cohen NL and Hoffman RA: Complications of cochlear implant surgery in adults and children. Ann Otol Rhinol Laryngol 100:708-711, 1991.

Cohen NL and Hoffman RA: Complications of cochlear implant surgery. *In* Eisele DW (ed): Complications in Head and Neck Surgery. St Louis, Mosby-Year Book, 1993, pp 722-729.

Cohen NL, Waltzman SB, Fisher SG, el al: A prospective, randomized study of cochlear implants. N Engl J Med 328:233-237, 1993.

Rosenberg RA, Cohen NL, and Reede DL: Radiographic imaging for the cochlear implant. Ann Otol Rhinol Laryngol 96:300-304, 1987.

Webb RL, Pyman BC, Evanz BK-H, and Clark GM: The surgery of cochlear implantation. *In* Clark GM, Tong YC, and Patrick JF (eds): Cochlear Implants. London, Churchill Livingstone, 1990.

Webb RL, Lehnhardt E, Clark GM, et al: Surgical complications with the cochlear multiple-channel intracochlear implant: Experience at Hannover and Melbourne. Ann Otol Rhinol Laryngol 100:131-136, 1991.

chapter

9

Epistaxis

SCOTT C. MANNING, M.D.
BRADLEY MARPLE, M.D.

Local factors are responsible for most cases of pediatric epistaxis. Trauma to the anterior septum from digital manipulation, nose rubbing ("allergic salute"), or blunt injury are the most common predisposing factors. Allergic, viral, and bacterial rhinitis commonly contribute via mucosal irritation, crusting, and increased vascularity. In most areas, pediatric epistaxis is more common in winter because of the combination of dry air and more frequent upper respiratory infections. Unilateral epistaxis and nasal obstruction in a young child should prompt a careful examination for a foreign body. Less common in the pediatric population, obstruction from septal deviation or polyps may create focal areas of mucosal drying and ulceration. Rarely, vascular tumors, such as rhabdomyosarcomas in young children or angiofibromas in adolescent boys, may be responsible for dramatic, difficult-to-control epistaxis. Appropriate radiographic evaluation, such as computed tomography, is indicated when tumors are suspected.

Systemic diseases can contribute to epistaxis via effects on blood clotting and blood pressure. Primary coagulopathies, such as the hemophilias, are usually recognized by way of the history; however, von Willebrand's disease may occasionally present as epistaxis in the absence of a prior history of bleeding. The onset of recurrent epistaxis around puberty, combined with the family history of nosebleeds or recurrent gastrointestinal hemorrhage, should arouse suspicion for hereditary hemorrhagic telangiectasis (Osler-Weber-Rendu disease).

Note:

- Direct vessel ligation is rarely necessary as a treatment for pediatric epistaxis.
- In cases of extremely refractory epistaxis, especially in patients with primary or acquired coagulopathies, selective embolization of involved vessels can be used with success by experienced interventional radiologists.

ANTERIOR EPISTAXIS

The most common site of nasal bleeding in children is the anterior septum, where several terminal branches of both the internal and external carotid systems come together under a thin, delicate mucosa. Kiesselbach's plexus or Little's area is also the part of the nose that is most likely to be adversely affected by trauma and dry air (Fig. 9–1).

LOCAL CAUTERY

Indications

- Identified focal bleeding site on the anterior septum
- Bleeding unresolved with 5 minutes of local pressure via nose pinching

Anesthetic considerations

- Use topical anesthesia and vasoconstriction with 4% cocaine solution via spray or cotton application (or with a Xylocaine/oxymetazoline combination).

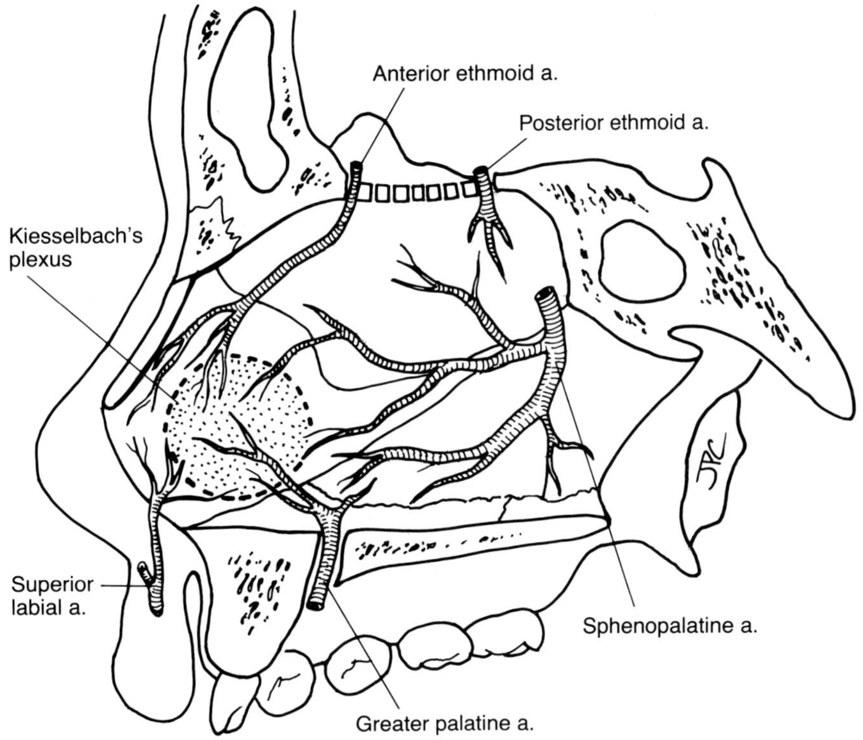

• FIGURE 9-1.

Arteries supplying the nasal septum. (Modified from Culbertson MC and Manning SC: Epistaxis. *In* Bluestone CD and Stool SE [eds]: Pediatric Otolaryngology, 2nd ed. Philadelphia, WB Saunders, 1990, p 673.)

- Carefully inspect the nasal cavity with a headlight and speculum, microscope, otoscope, or rigid endoscope.

Preparation

- Remove all blood and clots by gentle blowing and suctioning.

Procedure

- Limited cautery of the bleeding site with an electrocautery or silver nitrate
- Application of antibiotic ointment to the cautery site

ANTERIOR PACKING

Indications

- Failure of local cautery
- Diffuse mucosal bleeding sites
- Coagulopathy

Anesthetic considerations

- Use topical anesthesia and vasoconstriction with 4% cocaine solution via spray or cotton application (or with a Xylocaine/oxymetazoline combination).
- Carefully inspect the nasal cavity with a headlight and speculum, microscope, otoscope, or rigid endoscope.

Preparation

- Remove all blood and clots by gentle blowing and suctioning.

Procedure

- From the inferior to the superior, place small strips of absorbable packing (oxidized cellose or gelatin sponge) coated with small amounts of antibiotic ointment.
- Alternatively, layer ointment-coated gauze or cotton strips from the inferior to the superior (this method may cause further mucosal irritation when the gauze is removed).

Postoperative care/complications

Following successful management of routine anterior septal bleeding, preventive measures include humidification with topical nasal saline and/or room humidifiers and application of petroleum-based ointments to the distal septum. Steroid-containing ointments can be used for up to 2 weeks to more rapidly control inflamed vessels in the distal septum.

General management of suspected allergic rhinitis can help prevent recurrent epistaxis by reducing trauma from facial rubbing and by reducing mucosal inflammation in general.

Embolization of bleeding nasal vessels can rarely lead to ischemic tissue complications; the most common reported serious complication of selective embolization is facial nerve weakness, which is usually transient.

SUPERIOR EPISTAXIS

Superior epistaxis usually involves terminal branches of the anterior or posterior ethmoid arteries, which are themselves branches of the ophthalmic arteries from the internal carotid system. The anterior ethmoidal artery supplies the anterior third of the lateral nasal wall and adjacent septum, whereas the posterior ethmoidal artery supplies the superior turbinate, posterior superior lateral nasal wall, and septum. These arteries have taken on more significance with the advent of endoscopic sinus surgery.

ANTERIOR PACKING

- As previously described

ENDOSCOPIC GUIDED CAUTERY

Indications

- Failure of anterior packing
- Cooperative patient

Anesthetic considerations

- Use topical anesthesia and vasoconstriction with 4% cocaine solution via spray or cotton application (or with a Xylocaine/oxymetazoline combination).
- Carefully inspect the nasal cavity with a headlight and speculum, microscope, otoscope, or rigid endoscope.

Preparation

- Remove all blood and clots by gentle blowing and suctioning.

Procedure

- Carefully visualize the bleeding site with an endoscope in a cooperative patient — young children may require general anesthesia (Fig. 9–2).
- Nasal septoplasty may be necessary to allow an endoscopic view of the bleeding areas around septal deviations.
- Focal cautery of the bleeding site is done with an insulated "sinus" cautery or suction cautery.
- Apply antibiotic-coated absorbable gelatin sponge or oxidized cellulose.

Postoperative care/complications

For unusual severe superior bleeding episodes requiring bilateral nasal packing, patients should be admitted to the hospital, if they are not already hospitalized. These patients should be monitored with an oxygen saturation monitor for development of hypoxia, especially during sleep. They may require supplemental oxygen. Nasal packs themselves can cause tissue injury to nasal septal mucosa, and bleeding may therefore recur when packs are removed, especially with systemic coagulopathies. Nasal packs can also result in ischemic injury to the nasal ala or columella, and special care can be taken to avoid applying significant pressure to these areas when placing nasal packs.

Embolization of bleeding nasal vessels can rarely lead to ischemic tissue complications; the most common reported serious complication of selective embolization is facial nerve weakness, which is usually transient.

POSTERIOR EPISTAXIS

Posterior epistaxis usually involves terminal branches of the sphenopalatine artery. This artery arises from the internal maxillary artery and enters the nose just posterior to the posterior inferior tip of the middle turbinate. A medial branch supplies much of the septum, while a lateral branch supplies the inferior and middle turbinates (Fig. 9–3). This has also become more important with endoscopic sinus surgery, and not infrequently the medial branch of the sphenopalatine artery is injured as it crosses the anterior inferior face of the sphenoid sinus.

ANTERIOR-POSTERIOR PACKING

Indications

- Relatively rare in children — identified posterior (sphenopalatine area) bleed
- May occur with facial fractures or severe coagulopathies or as a consequence of sinus surgery

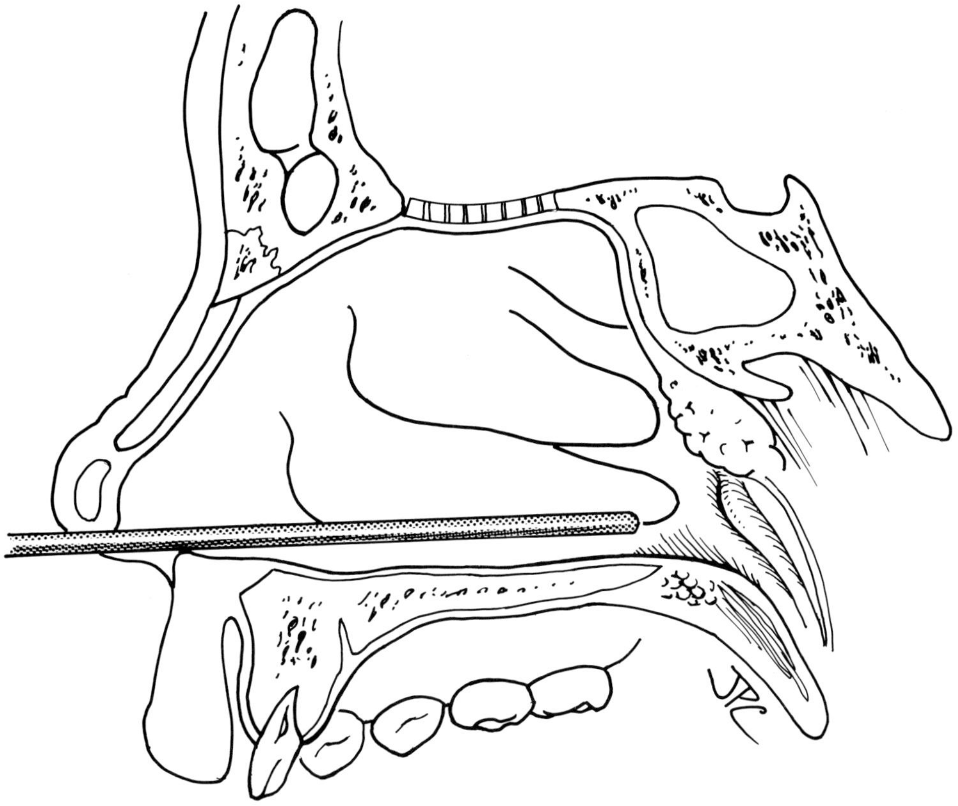

• **FIGURE 9–2.**

Demonstration of the rigid endoscope used to visualize the posterior nasal cavity.

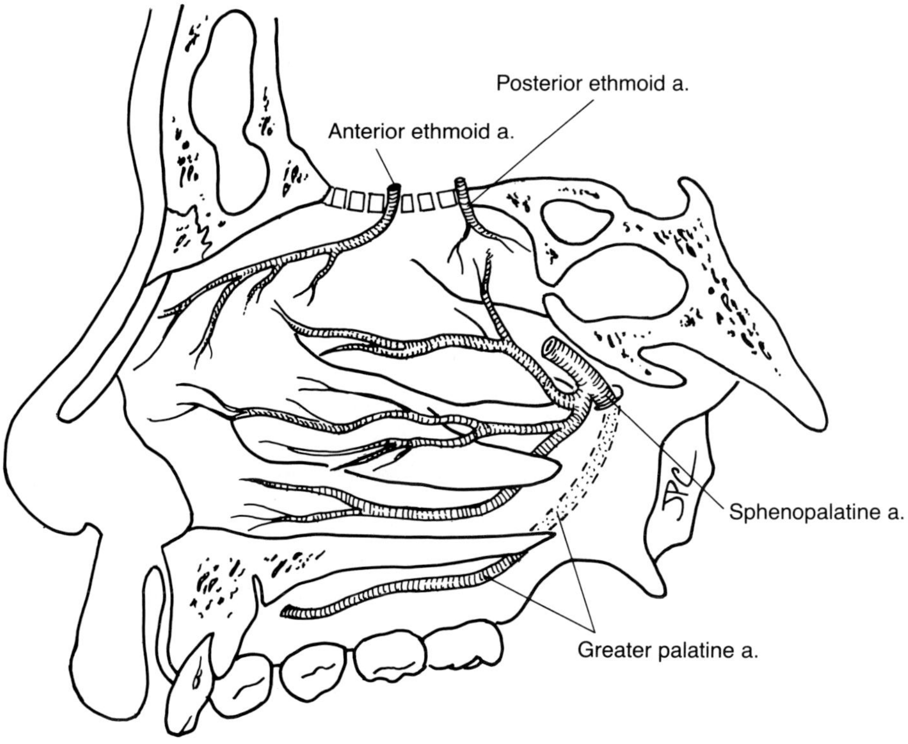

• **FIGURE 9–3.**

Arteries supplying the lateral nasal wall. (Modified from Culbertson MC and Manning SC: Epistaxis. *In* Bluestone CD and Stool SE [eds]: Pediatric Otolaryngology, 2nd ed. Philadelphia, WB Saunders, 1990, p 673.)

Anesthetic considerations

- Use topical anesthesia and vasoconstriction with 4% cocaine solution via spray or cotton application (or with a Xylocaine/oxymetazoline combination).
- Carefully inspect the nasal cavity with a headlight and speculum, microscope, otoscope, or rigid endoscope.

Preparation

- Remove all blood and clots by gentle blowing and suctioning.

Procedure

- Manufactured nasal balloons may be placed in the nasal cavity and inflated as per instructions (Fig. 9–4).
- A posterior pack can be fashioned from a 15-ml urinary catheter.

  Cut a 1- to 2-cm length segment of endotracheal tube of a size that will slide over the urinary catheter back to the insufflation ports.

  Place the urinary catheter through the nose so that its tip is visualized just beyond the soft palate on oral examination.

  Inflate the balloon with 5 to 10 ml of sterile saline.

  Place an anterior nasal pack around the catheter with either gauze or absorbable hemostatic material.

  Slide the "sleeve" forward so that it fits within the nostril and puts pressure against the anterior pack.

  Put tension on the posterior balloon by pulling the catheter forward while placing counter-traction against the sleeve.

  Add further saline to the posterior balloon as necessary to stop all bleeding.

  Fix the catheter in place by placing a C clamp or other type of clamp on the catheter just in front of the sleeve.
- Gauze packs (Fig. 9–5) can be utilized.

  Fix a gauze pack to a catheter passed through the nose and retrieved through the mouth.

  Pull the gauze pack, via a suture, firmly against the posterior choanal opening.

  Place an anterior nasal layered gauze pack and fix the posterior pack suture to a soft rubber or gauze bolster outside the nares.

  In young children it may be advisable to use absorbable packing, as surgical gauze may adhere and can be difficult to remove in the uncooperative child.
- An endoscopic-guided direct cautery can be attempted, as described for superior epistaxis.

Postoperative care/complications

For unusual severe posterior bleeding episodes requiring bilateral nasal packing, patients should be admitted to the hospital, if they are not already hospitalized.

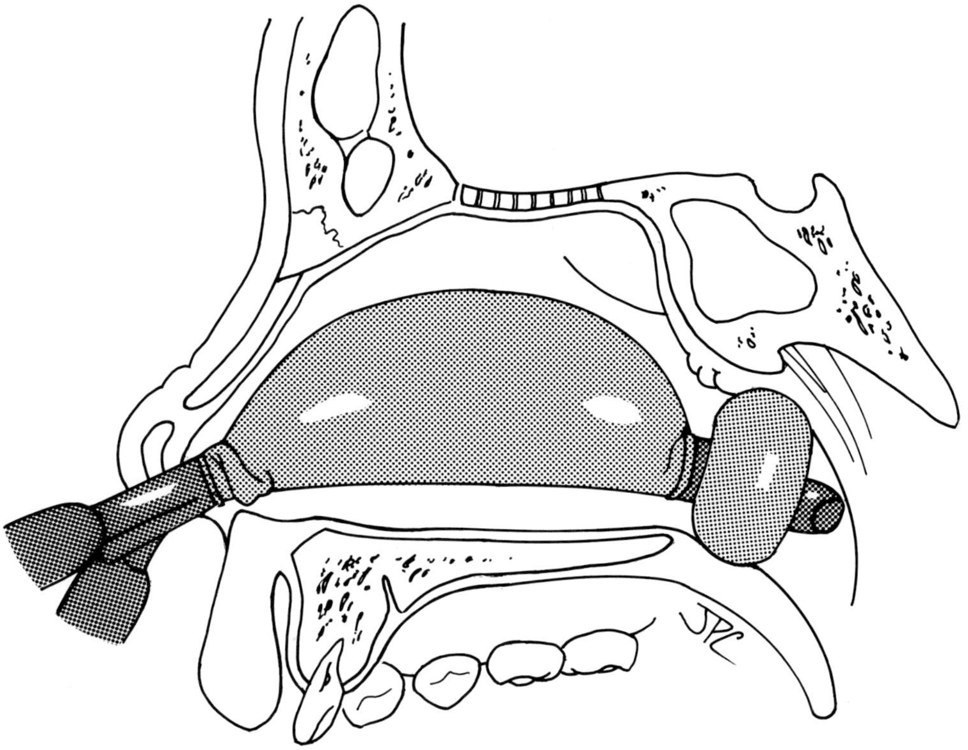

• FIGURE 9–4.

Demonstration of a manufactured epistaxis balloon. The posterior balloon in the nasopharynx provides an anchor for the anterior balloon to apply pressure to the posterior nasal cavity.

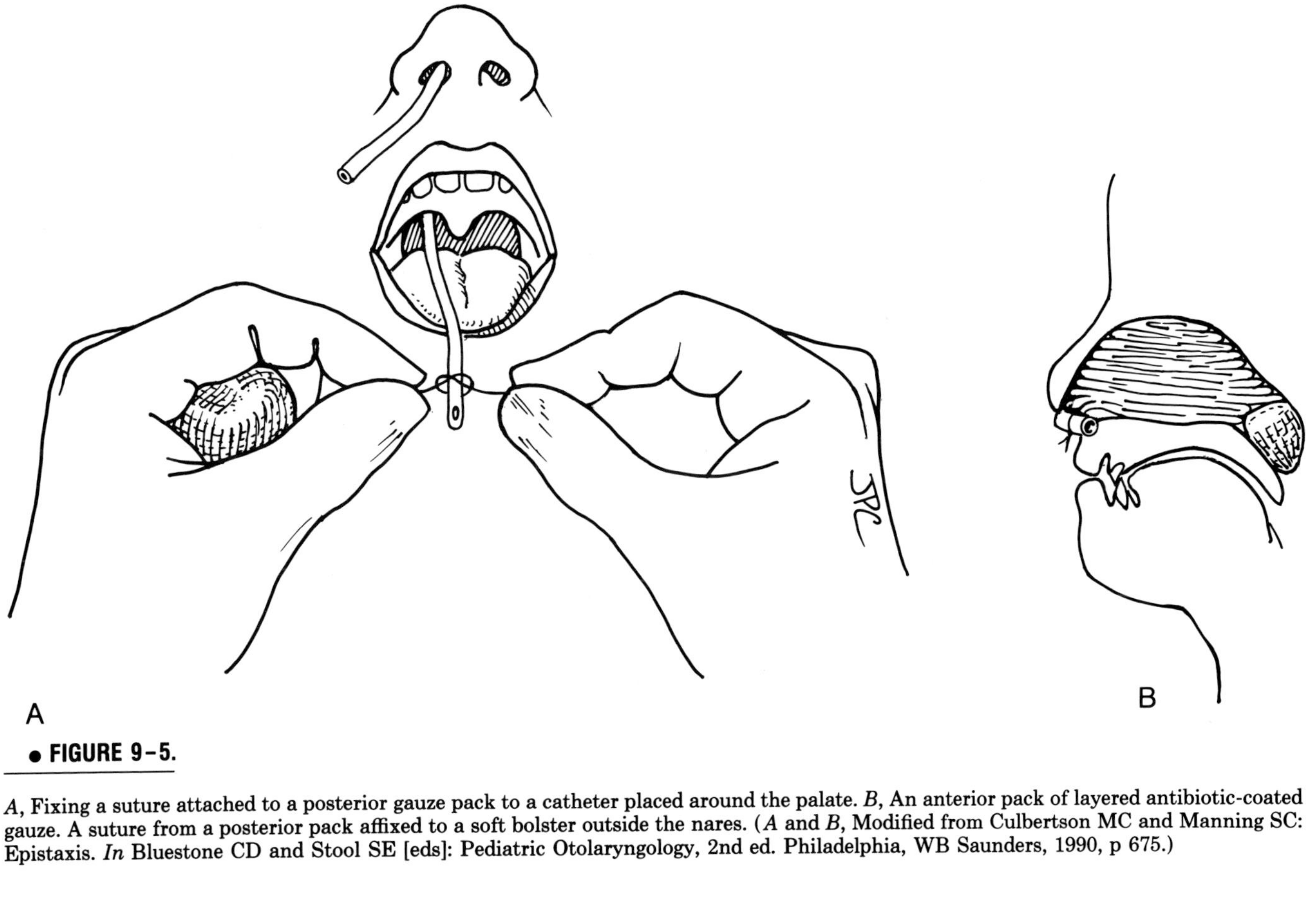

A

B

• FIGURE 9–5.

A, Fixing a suture attached to a posterior gauze pack to a catheter placed around the palate. *B*, An anterior pack of layered antibiotic-coated gauze. A suture from a posterior pack affixed to a soft bolster outside the nares. (*A* and *B*, Modified from Culbertson MC and Manning SC: Epistaxis. *In* Bluestone CD and Stool SE [eds]: Pediatric Otolaryngology, 2nd ed. Philadelphia, WB Saunders, 1990, p 675.)

These patients should be monitored with an oxygen saturation monitor for development of hypoxia, especially during sleep. They may require supplemental oxygen. Nasal packs themselves can cause tissue injury to nasal septal mucosa, and bleeding may therefore recur when packs are removed, especially with systemic coagulopathies. Nasal packs can also result in ischemic injury to the nasal ala or columella, and special care can be taken to avoid applying significant pressure to these areas when placing nasal packs.

Embolization of bleeding nasal vessels can rarely lead to ischemic tissue complications; the most common reported serious complication of selective embolization is facial nerve weakness, which is usually transient.

chapter

10

Plastic and Reconstructive Surgery

CHARLES W. GROSS, M.D.

The field of pediatric facial plastic and reconstructive surgery is extensive and complicated. This chapter highlights the areas of particular practical importance to the pediatric otolaryngologist.

Pediatric facial plastic and reconstructive surgery primarily concerns traumatic and developmental problems. Trauma is the greatest cause of morbidity and mortality and is probably the most important illness of childhood. The ABCs of trauma are critical in the evaluation and care of the injured child.

- Airway: The small size of the pediatric airway is the reason even a small amount of edema or other compromise produces a significant degree of airway obstruction. Blood, vomitus, teeth, posterior tongue displacement, and foreign material are frequent causes of obstruction. Endotracheal intubation or tracheostomy should be used liberally in children who have sustained trauma. Early placement of the nasogastric tube often prevents further vomiting with subsequent pharyngeal obstruction or aspiration.

- Blood loss: The blood volume of children is proportionately equal to that of adults. However, because of the small size of children, small amounts of blood loss may be quite significant. For example, in a 5-lb infant, 35 ml of blood loss is equivalent to 1 liter of blood loss in an adult. Infants may rapidly slip into shock without the gradual fall in blood pressure that is seen in older children and adults. The traumatized infant and young child may be hypovolemic without significant external loss, especially if there is bleeding into the chest, abdomen, or limbs.

- Circulation and body heat: In addition to blood replacement, body fluid replacement and prevention of body heat loss are of great importance. Because of these factors and also the small physiologic reserve, inattention and inadequate treatment may allow the child's condition to deteriorate rapidly as a result of hypothermia, particularly in the infant. Fluid and blood for replacement should be warmed prior to administration. As a general rule, infants tolerate mild underhydration better than overhydration.

The child who sustained trauma to the face, head, and neck must be evaluated thoroughly to rule out systemic injuries, especially cervical spine injuries. Both the detailed history and physical examination are essential for evaluating and planning repairs. For example, approximately 40% of children who sustain severe facial trauma will have a skull fracture, and approximately 25% will have aspiration or other pulmonary complications. In addition, the battered child syndrome should be suspected. Because of the aforementioned small physiologic reserve, there may be a shorter course from health to illness to death; consequently, timely evaluation and treatment are of particular importance.

In assessing and timing the repair of injuries, it should be remembered that cellular activity is greater in children. Tissues have a tendency to require earlier treatment and to heal faster. The greater metabolic activity can lead to better molding of defects or to exaggeration of the deformity, depending on the circumstances. Edema generally resolves more quickly the younger the child. Although a thorough physical examination is desired prior to beginning treatment, often after the child is stabilized, a definitive examination of the facial and head and neck structures must await general anesthesia. It is most important to pay particular attention to the suture lines, particularly when injuries to the facial skeleton are suspected. A thorough examination of the head and neck area in the injured child should be carried out before treatment begins.

Photographic documentation is encouraged for good medical records, for documentation for possible financial or legal purposes, and for physician training.

SOFT TISSUE INJURIES (Table 10-1)

Some sedation, if appropriate, is beneficial during both evaluation and treatment of less extensive injuries. Extensive injuries are best treated in the operating room under general anesthesia. Precise primary repair of injuries often alleviates the necessity for later revisions.

Indications

CONTUSIONS

Contusions are treated by immobilization, elevation, and evacuation of a hematoma, if present.

ABRASIONS

Abrasions generally require cleaning, immobilization, good generalized wound care, and occasionally skin grafting.

• TABLE 10-1.

PEDIATRIC SOFT-TISSUE REPAIR

General Principles
Ensure early aseptic repair.
Conserve tissue with minimal débridement.
Thoroughly explore the depth of the wound.
Remove all foreign material—scrub the wound or even acutely dermabraid it if necessary.
Handle the tissue gently.
Accurately repair individual tissue layers, but use buried sutures only if necessary (to decrease chance of infection)
Wound Care
Keep the wound clean and dry.
Use discretion in application of dressings.
Remove sutures early—use adhesive strips to reinforce the repair after suture removal.

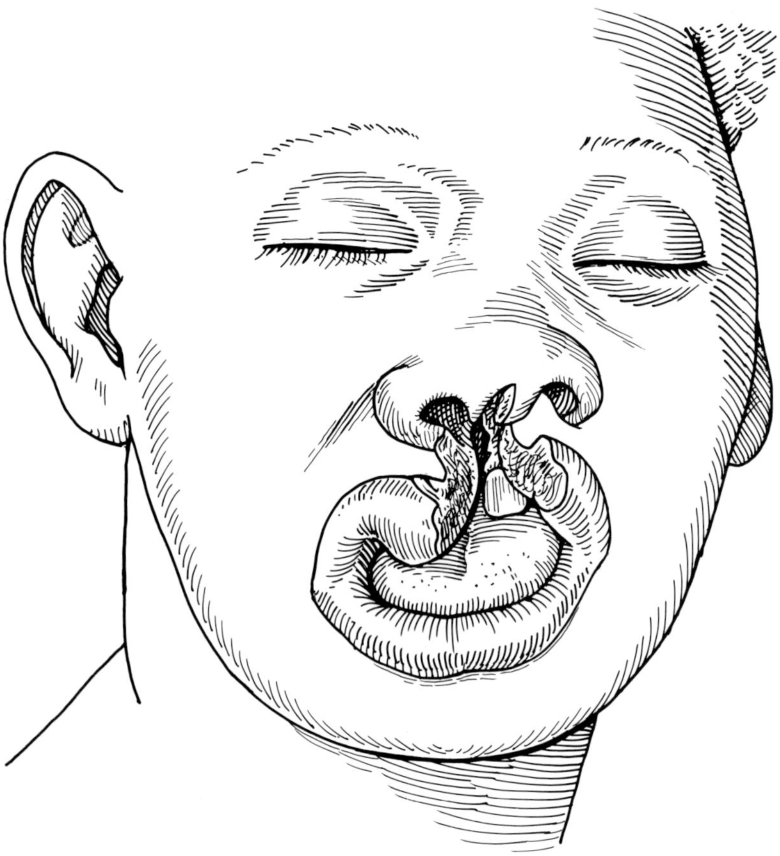

• FIGURE 10-1.

The patient sustained a gunshot wound to the face that divided the upper lip, the columella, and a portion of the hard palate, giving the appearance of a great deal of tissue loss.

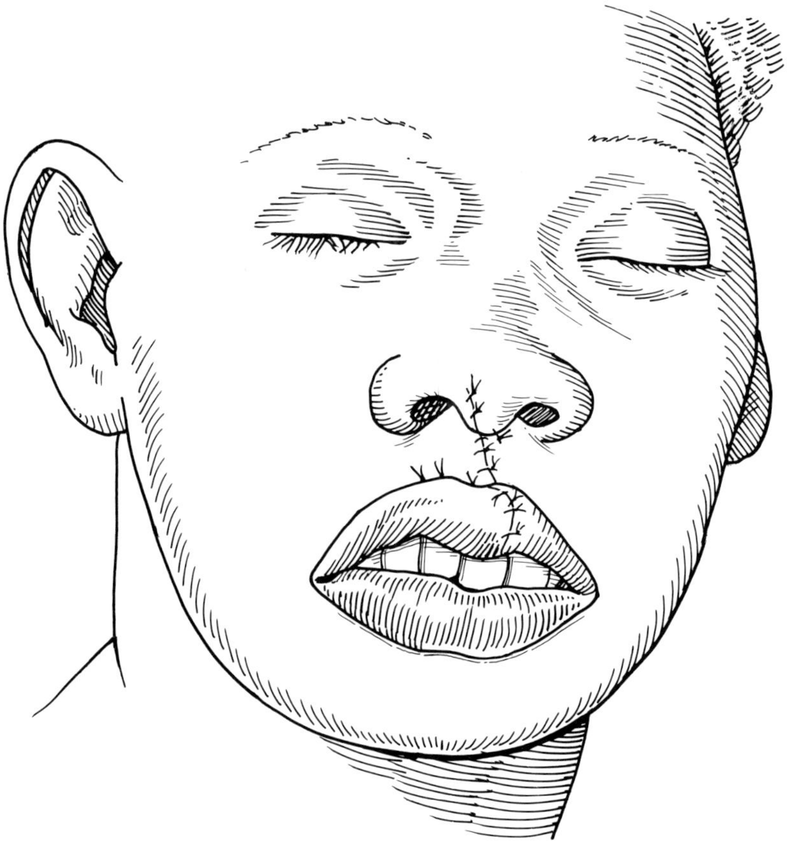

• FIGURE 10-2.

The patient is shown very shortly after repair that required no tissue replacement. The patient will now have scar revision.

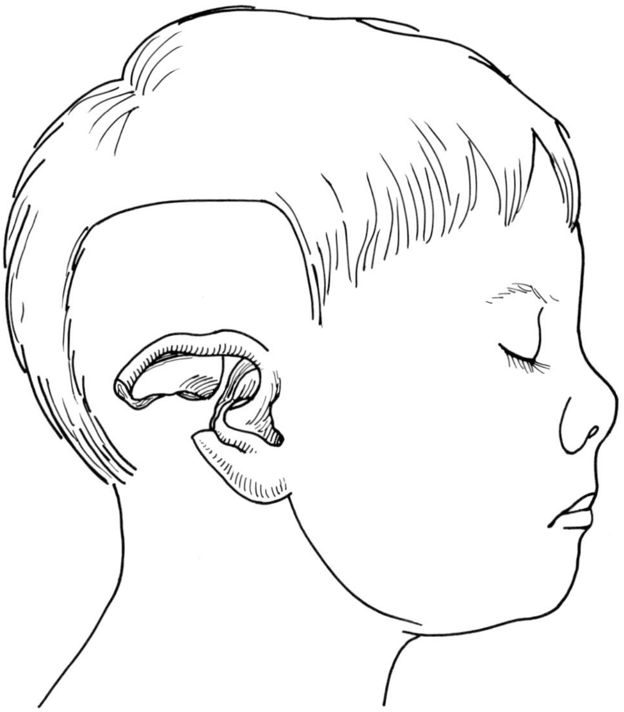

• **FIGURE 10-3.**

A patient who was in an automobile accident had a severe laceration of the ear with near-avulsion of the large portion of the auricle.

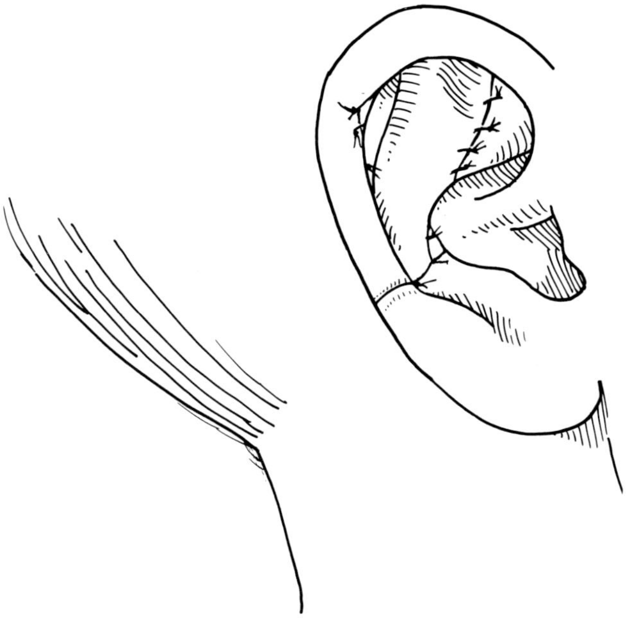

• **FIGURE 10-4.**

The same patient as shown in Figure 10-3, 2 weeks after repair with tissue surviving.

AVULSIONS

Avulsions are seldom of such degree that they require extensive grafting and reconstructive procedures. If such treatment is required, the techniques similar to those outlined in standard textbooks on the subject are employed. The standard local flaps for reconstruction are used in children as for adults; the major modification is that owing to the lessened elasticity of the child's skin, modifications in design must be applied. New studies have shown that, in general, grafts tend to grow in response to tissue demands. Injuries crossing the lips, nose, or eyelids give the appearance of significant tissue loss but will frequently prove not to be so as repair ensues (Figs. 10-1 and 10-2).

Tissue subtotally avulsed in the head and neck area, with only minor pedicles of attachment retaining, often survives because blood supply to the head and neck area is so abundant (Figs. 10-3 and 10-4).

LACERATIONS

Principles of repair and handling damaged tissue:

- Instruments used should cause minimal damage to the tissues.
- Preoperative planning results in minimal tissue manipulation.
- Traction sutures may help to avoid tissue necrosis and undue scarring and to facilitate closure of larger defects.
- Tissue undermining is used to reduce tension on the suture lines. However, generally less undermining is needed in children than in adults (Fig. 10–5).
- When possible, sutures should approximate tissue with minimal tension, thus avoiding wide scarring and tissue ischemia.
- Incisions, when necessary, should not cross basic aesthetic units or facial landmarks. This applies to the repair of traumatized tissue as well as to elective excision of lesions in the head and neck (Figs. 10–6, 10–7, 10–8, and 10–9).
- In hair-bearing areas, the incision should be parallel to the follicles to minimize follicular loss.
- Blood supply is generally good in the head and neck areas, usually allowing minimal débridement and good healing.
- Trapdoor lacerations are converted to elliptical defects by excision, if possible. If not, they may be closed in layers and revised later.
- Scalp injuries require specialized closure because the galea is relatively inelastic. The galea is closed in a separate layer after utilizing relaxing incisions if necessary. The other layers of the scalp are closed in a single layer using heavy sutures, taking large bites on both sides of the wound. These sutures are left in place for approximately 2 weeks.

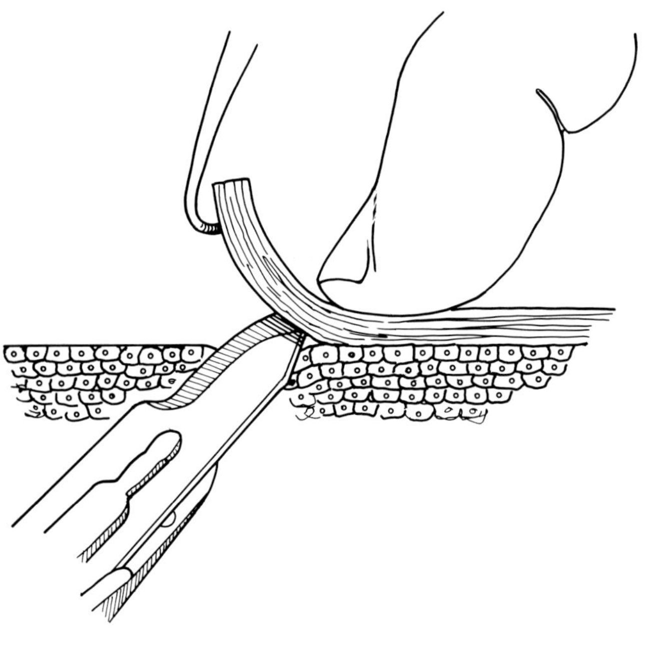

• FIGURE 10–5.

Tissue undermining is done sharply and conservatively in children. (Modified from Cook TA. Basic Soft Tissue Surgery. McGaw Park, IL, Baxter Healthcare Corp., 1988. Modified with permission of the American Academy of Facial Plastic and Reconstructive Surgery.)

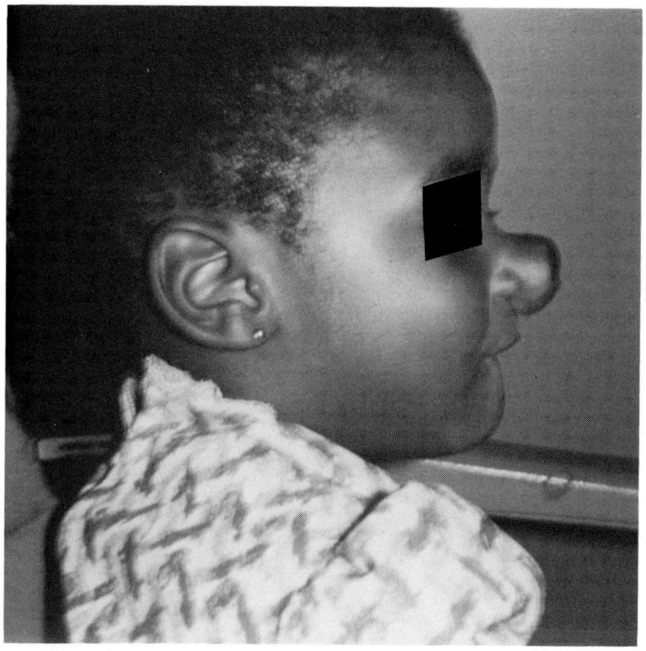

• FIGURE 10-6.

A child with Cyrano de Bergerac hemangioma of the tip of the nose, which gave a unsightly appearance and bled easily.

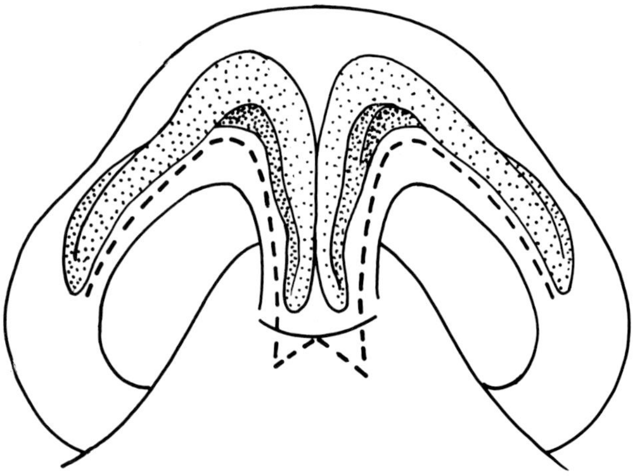

• FIGURE 10-7.

Surgical exposure is achieved with a modified open rhinoplasty incision, avoiding a nasal dorsal incision.

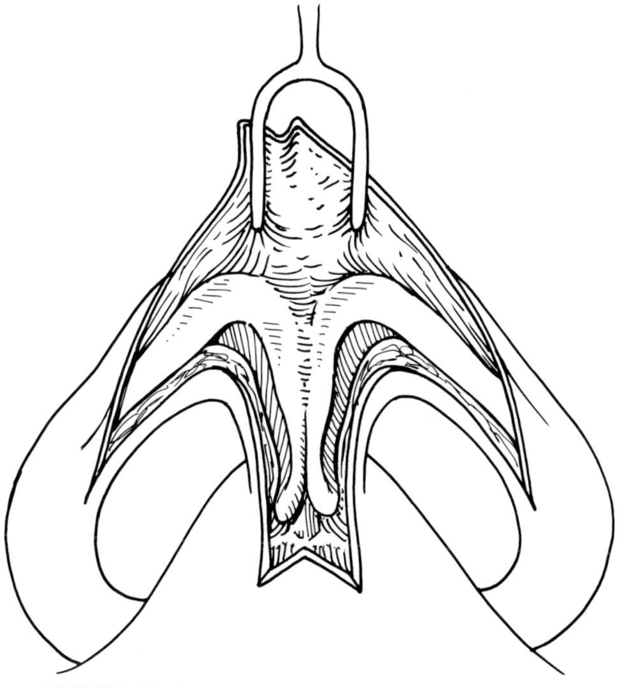

• FIGURE 10-8.

The nasal skin is elevated for exposure of the tip and dorsal area.

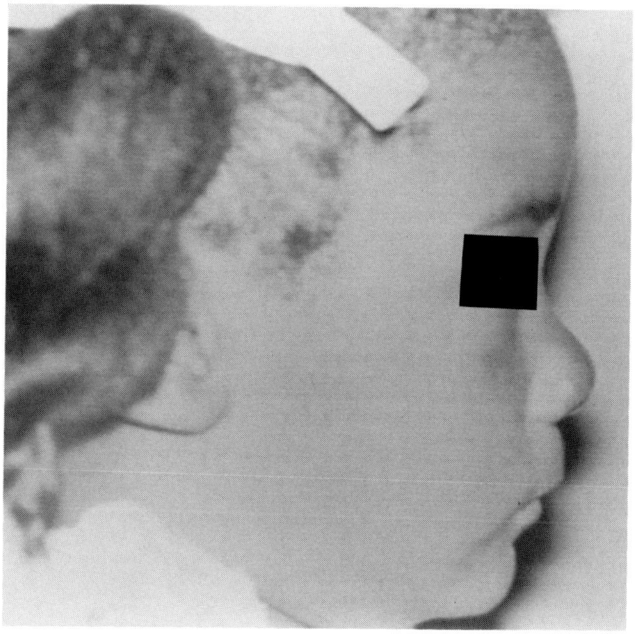

• FIGURE 10-9.

The patient shown in Figure 10-6, $2\frac{1}{2}$ years after the excision.

Anesthetic considerations

A variety of anesthesia techniques are available. Options include topical measures (tetracaine 0.5%, adrenaline 1:2000, cocaine 11.8%, applied directly to the wound for 10 to 20 minutes prior to closure[1]) and local measures (lidocaine with or without epinephrine is the usual choice) with or without general anesthesia. The choice generally depends on the patient's ability to cooperate, the length of the procedure, and the difficulty of the repair. General anesthesia is used in repairing facial injuries, because the advantage of precise technique outweighs the inconvenience and cost considerations. When local anesthesia is used, it may be used with topical anesthesia or with general anesthesia, as well as alone. If it is used alone, injection is usually in a field block technique to prevent distortion; if the wound is not unduly large, the injection can be placed through the edges of the laceration.

CLOSURE OF LACERATIONS

Preparation

The wound is generally sterilized with the standard surgical preparation. In the repair of a contaminated wound, meticulous cleansing is necessary, often requiring the use of a scrub brush after anesthesia. By doing so, foreign body tattooing and wound infection may be avoided. Tissue conservation is paramount, and only obviously necrotic tissue should be débrided. Ragged skin edges, however, may be conservatively removed to facilitate better closure (Figs. 10–10 and 10–11).

INSTRUMENTATION

- Small skin hooks
- Needle driver
- Razorblade breaker
- Appropriate needle holder
- Fine tissue forceps (e.g., Brown-Adison or toothed ophthalmic)
- Scalpels with No. 10, No. 11, and No. 15 blades
- Needlepoint cautery
- Fine tissue scissors
- Suture scissors
- Magnifying loops (optional)
- Absorbable and nonabsorbable sutures

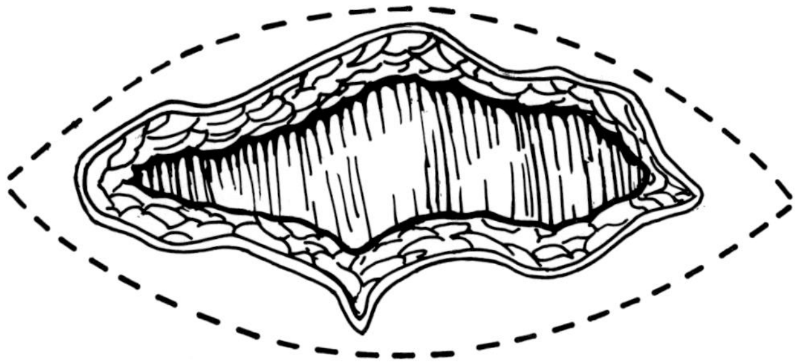

• **FIGURE 10-10.**

Closure of a beveled laceration will be more precise if the laceration is converted to a perpendicular defect. (Modified from Burget GC: Surgical Restoration of the Nose. St. Louis, BC Decker, 1989, pp 405–406.)

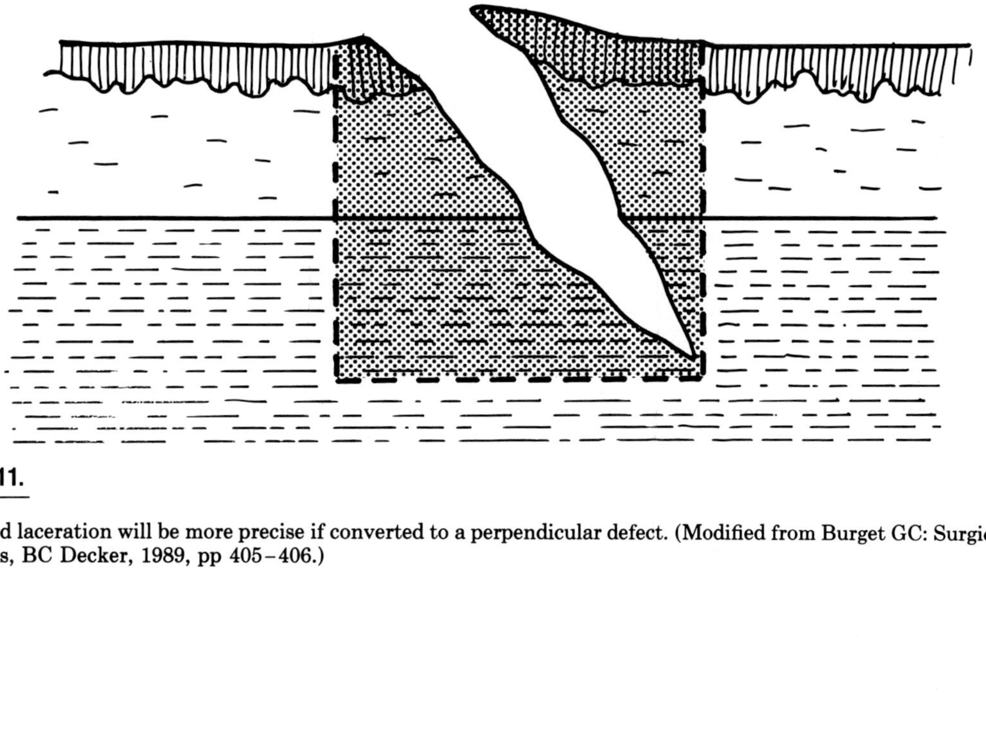

• **FIGURE 10-11.**

Closure of a beveled laceration will be more precise if converted to a perpendicular defect. (Modified from Burget GC: Surgical Restoration of the Nose. St. Louis, BC Decker, 1989, pp 405–406.)

• TABLE 10-2.

ABSORBABLE AND NONABSORBABLE SUTURES*

Type	Strength	Half-life	Reactivity	Throws Required	Comment
Absorbable:					
Gut	±3.3	5–20 days	++++	3–4	Low knot security until moist; nonuniform, can fray
Collagen	±3.3	5–20 days	++++	3–4	Low knot security until moist
Dexon	6	10 days	++	3–4	Half-life pH-dependent
Vicryl	6	10 days	++	4–5	Half-life pH dependent
Polydiaxone (PDS)	±4	4.5 wk	+	4–5	New, promising monofilament
Nonabsorbable:					
Silk	3	$\frac{1}{2}$–1 yr	+++	3–4	Inconsistent strength
Cotton	≤3	>1 yr	+++	2–3	Drags, cuts tissue
Dacron	4	—	+++	2–3	Rough surface causes capillary action
Coated Dacron	4	—	+++	4–5	Coatings may fragment
Nylon monofilament	3.6	$\frac{1}{2}$–1 yr	+	5	Can fracture
Nylon braided	4	≤1 yr	++	3–4	Dead spaces
Polypropylene	3.5	—	+	5+	Can fracture
Stainless steel	9.5	—	+	2–3	Poor handling

*From Cook TA: Basic Soft Tissue Surgery. McGaw Park, IL, Baxter Healthcare Corp., 1988. With permission of the American Academy of Facial Plastic and Reconstructive Surgery.

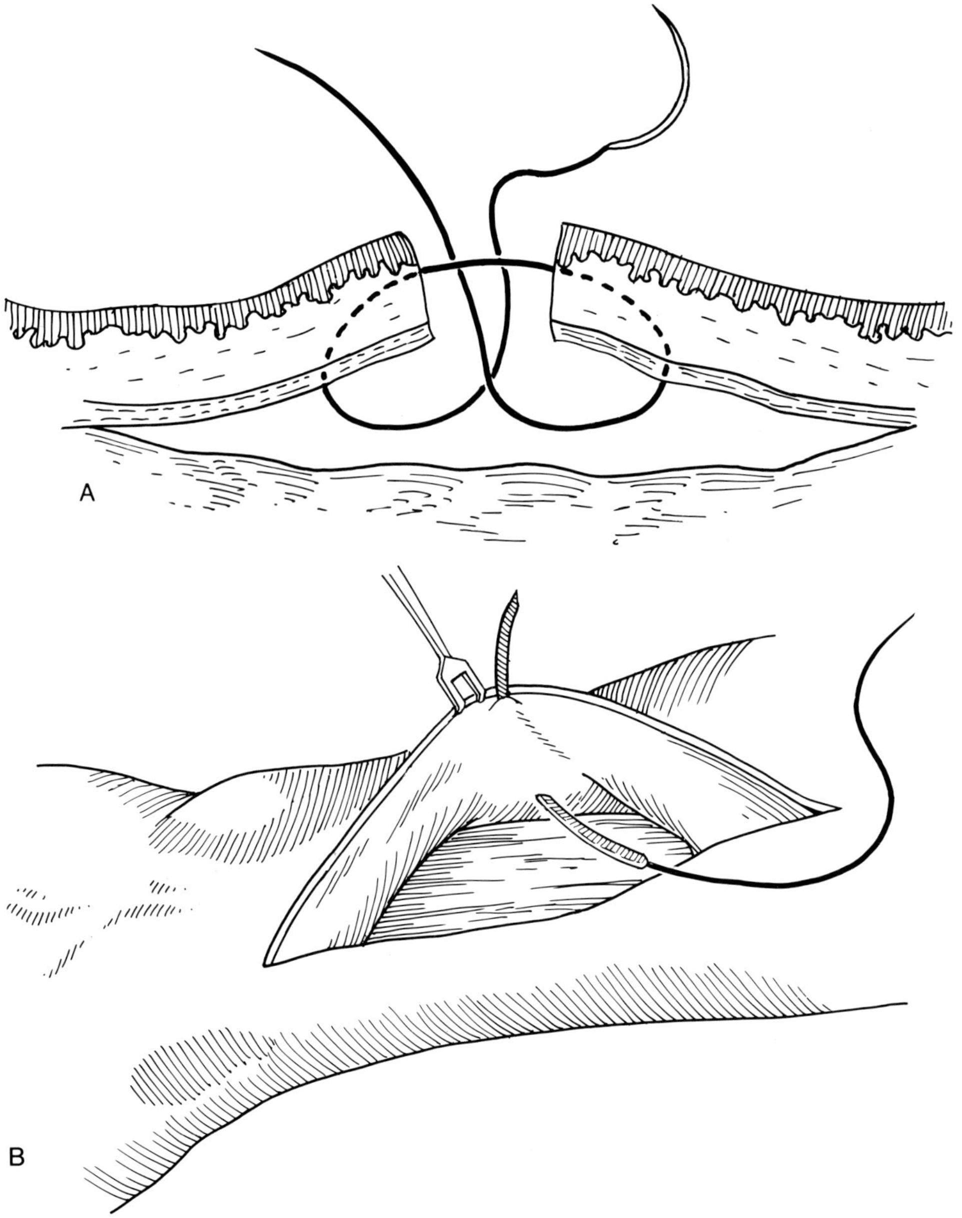

• FIGURE 10-12.

A to *D*, Closing the subdermal layer further approximating deep tissues and slightly everting the epidermis. A modified Halsted suture is shown. This is an excellent skin closure suture for children with a buried knot. Care must be given to take equal bites of tissue on each side, and these bites must be aligned precisely to provide smooth, accurate wound closure. (*C* modified from Cook TA. Basic Soft Tissue Surgery. McGaw Park, IL, Baxter Healthcare Corp., 1988. Modified with permission of the American Academy of Facial Plastic and Reconstructive Surgery.)

• **FIGURE 10–12.** *(continued)*

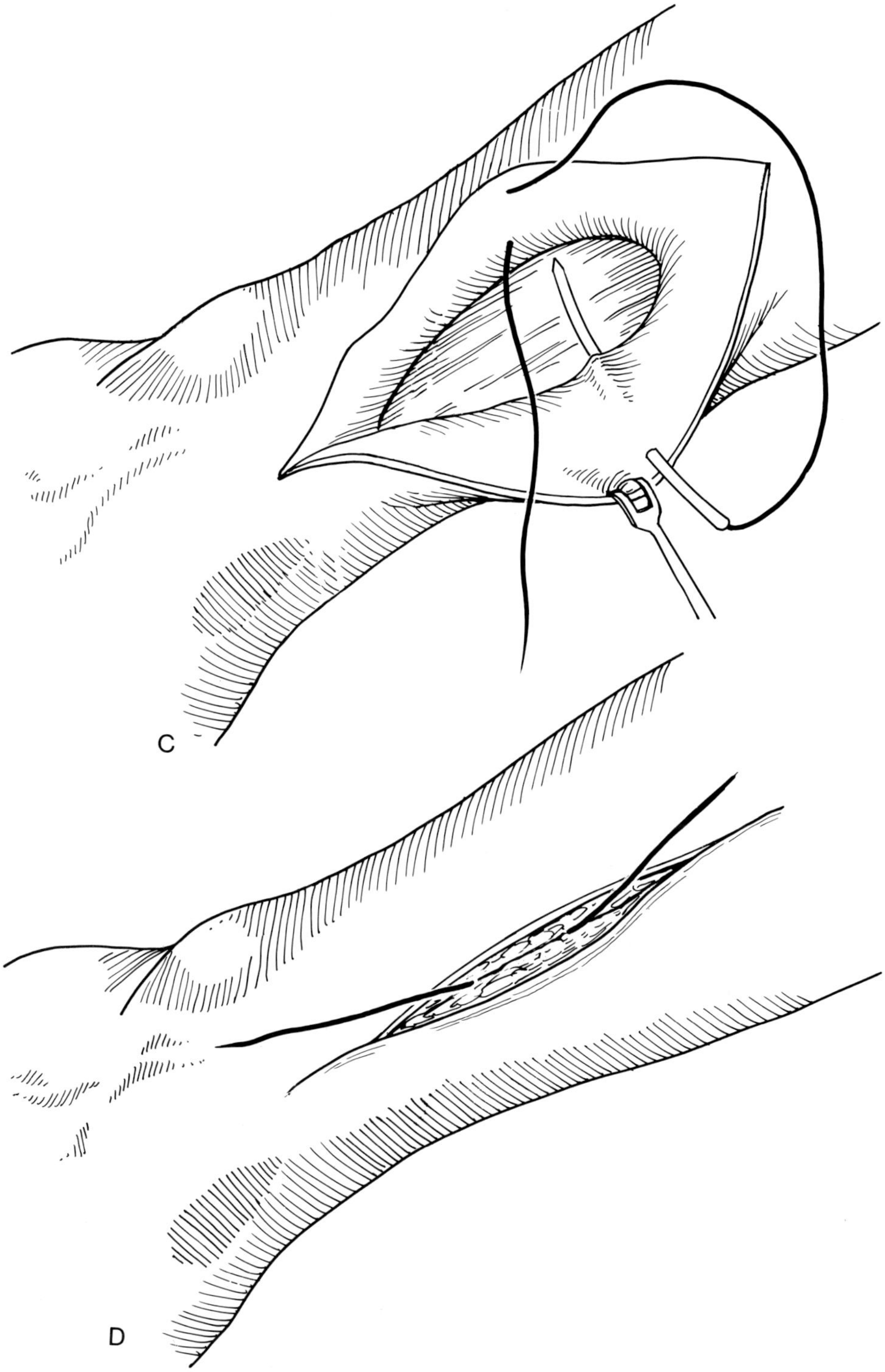

C

D

Procedure

SUTURING TECHNIQUES (Table 10–2)

After the wound is surgically sterilized, hemostasis is achieved prior to wound closure. Layered closure is employed in most circumstances, the number of layers depending on the depth of the injury, the number of tissue layers involved, and wound tension. Absorbable sutures are usually used in an inverted, interrupted fashion to close the deep layers, obliterating dead space, accurately realigning tissue planes, and relieving wound tension, especially at the more superficial aspects (Fig. 10–12).

Careful attention to this aspect of wound closure contributes to reduced scar formation much more than the actual skin closure itself. Skin sutures may or may not be used. If the interrupted subcutaneous suture has produced sufficient closure, antitension taping may be all that is necessary to support the repair. If skin sutures are used they are removed in 3 to 5 days, and antitension taping is then applied for 1 week.

In addition to the usual skin sutures, a 5-0 mild chromic suture may be used in sensitive areas to avoid the need for suture removal (Fig. 10–13).

Staples are not usually used for wound closure in children.

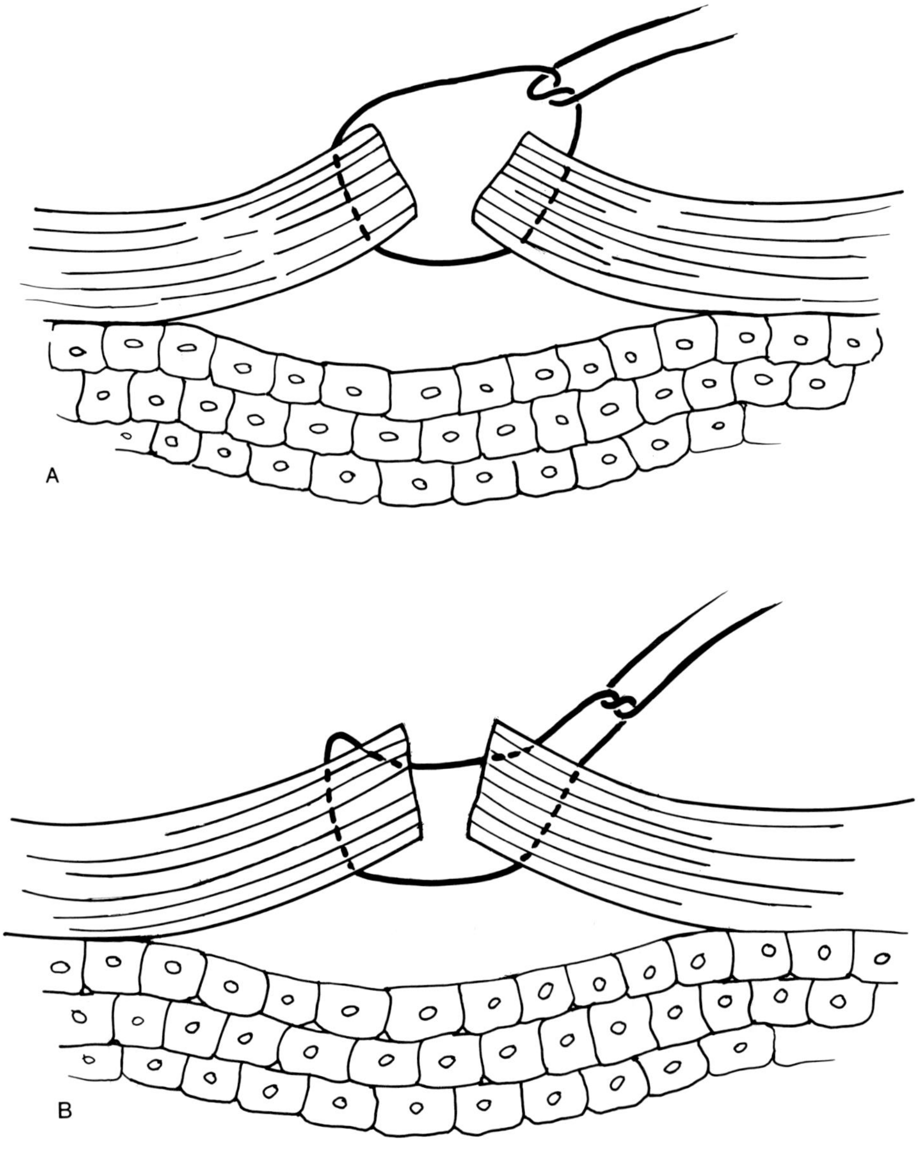

• FIGURE 10–13.

A, A simple suture for wound closure. Note that equal tissue bites are taken on each side. (Modified from Cook TA. Basic Soft Tissue Surgery. McGaw Park, IL, Baxter Healthcare Corp., 1988. Modified with permission of the American Academy of Facial Plastic and Reconstructive Surgery.) *B*, A vertical mattress suture. This suture is used when a simple suture will not resolve improper eversion of the skin edge. (Modified from Cook TA. Basic Soft Tissue Surgery. McGaw Park, IL, Baxter Healthcare Corp., 1988. Modified with permission of the American Academy of Facial Plastic and Reconstructive Surgery.)

• FIGURE 10-13. *(continued)*

C, A running subcuticular suture may be used to hold (not bring together) skin edges in approximation for short distances, avoiding suture skin marks. *D*, wound closed.

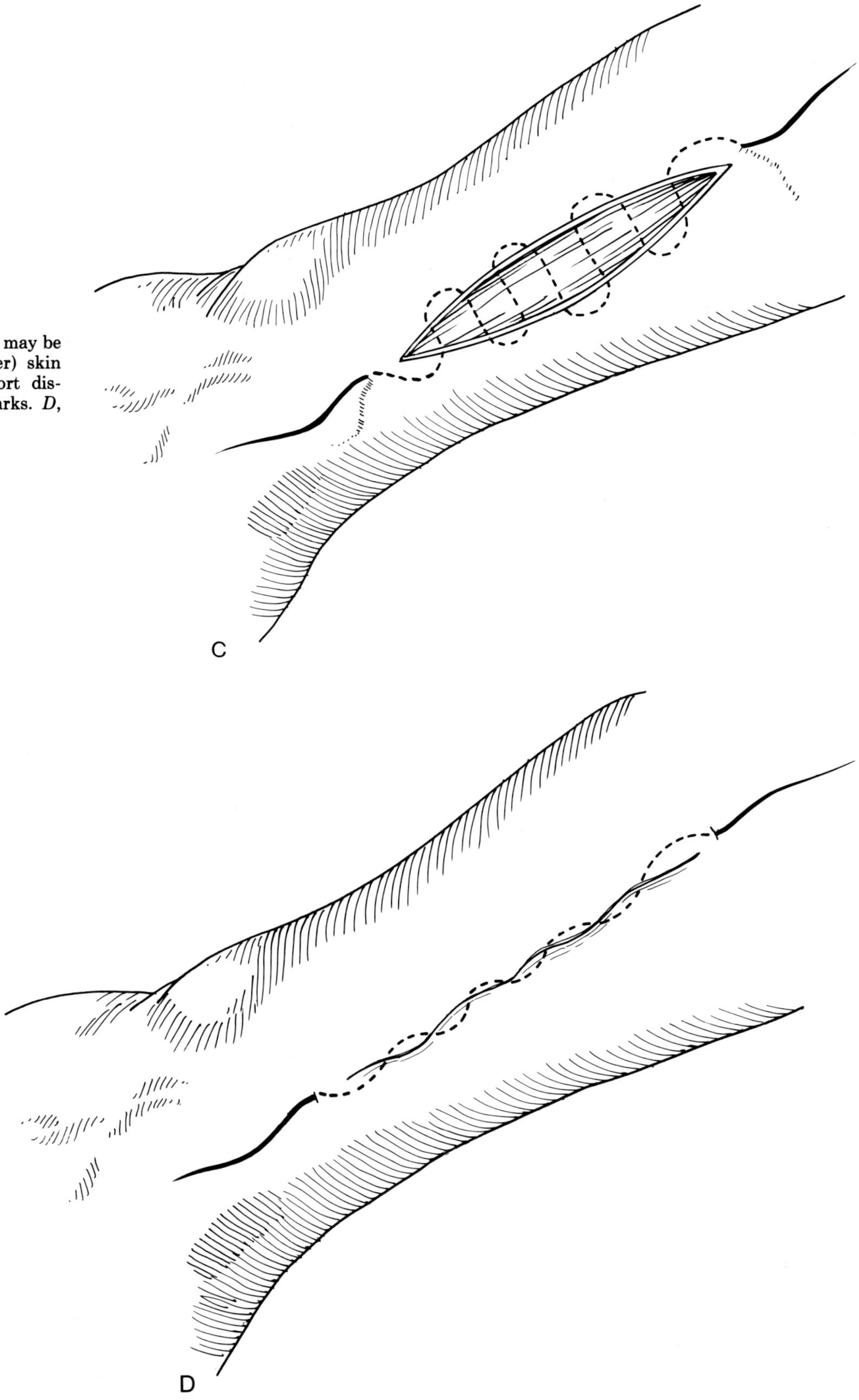

Postoperative care/complications

Patients and their families are counseled concerning the following:

- The wound usually requires 6 to 12 months to achieve its final results. Children's wounds remain erythematous and elevated for several months. This in itself does not indicate a future bad result.

- Revision is usually not considered until after at least 18 months. By this time erythema has usually subsided, and the wound is fully stabilized. If wounds are still changing at this time, revision should be delayed.

- Sun exposure may cause hyperpigmentation of scar tissue. Liberal use of sunblocks is advised after any trauma to the head and neck.

- Keloid formation may occur and require intralesional steroid injections or scar revision.

- When revising scars, do not excise normal uninvolved skin. Approximately 1 mm of scar tissue should be left. Large scars may be excised in successive stages. Skin over a keloid or other large scar may be used as a full-thickness graft over the defect without inducing further keloid or scarring. When revising scars, skin tension may be alleviated by changing the direction of the tension (e.g., deep Z-plasty), by using grafts (full-thickness or pedicle), or by using tension-relieving sutures, which are especially beneficial when placed in fascia or other "strong" tissue. Many initially unacceptable scars in children often spontaneously involute over a period of time.

Z-Plasty

Knowledge of the principles and application of Z-plasty is an essential part of facial plastic surgery. It requires the application of the aforementioned soft tissue techniques to form two adjacent flaps, which are then realigned geometrically in the proper fashion. Z-plasty may be employed singularly or in a multiple fashion (Fig. 10–14*A*).

Halving techniques are employed liberally in the repair of lacerations (Fig. 10–14*B*).

Z-plasty has multiple applications in facial plastic surgery, among which are

- Lengthening the scar to release a contracture
- Breaking up a straight-line scar
- Changing the direction of a scar from an unfavorable to a more favorable one
- Repositioning of the canthi or oral commissure
- Repairing a stenotic nostril or tracheostoma
- Repairing a stenosis of the nasopharynx or pharynx[2,3]

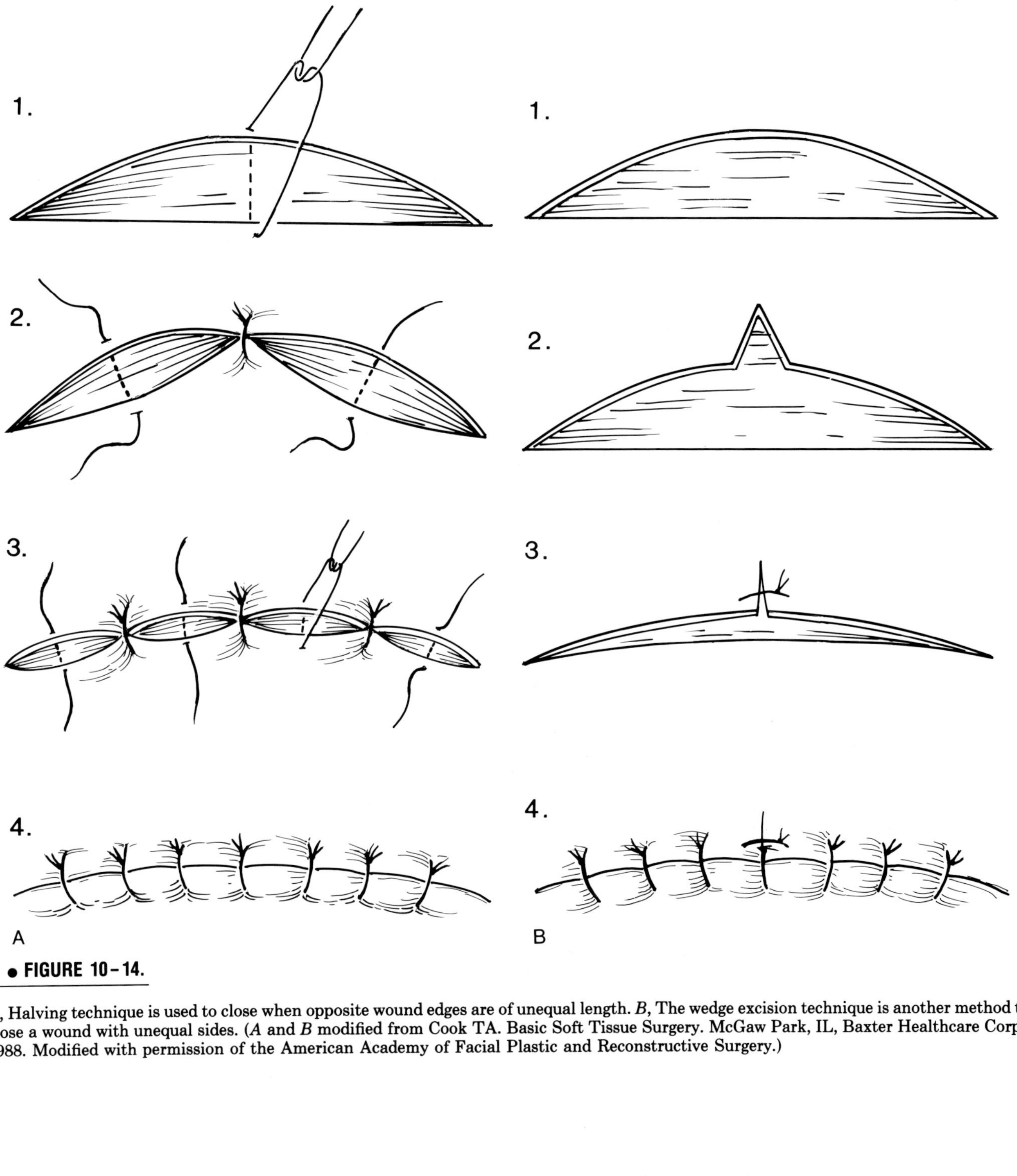

• **FIGURE 10-14.**

A, Halving technique is used to close when opposite wound edges are of unequal length. *B*, The wedge excision technique is another method to close a wound with unequal sides. (*A* and *B* modified from Cook TA. Basic Soft Tissue Surgery. McGaw Park, IL, Baxter Healthcare Corp., 1988. Modified with permission of the American Academy of Facial Plastic and Reconstructive Surgery.)

Facial Nerve Injuries

The anatomic course of facial nerves is complex but is well known to most otolaryngologists. In any extensive injury to the face, an evaluation of facial nerve function is mandatory. Facial nerve injuries should be recognized and, when possible, treated immediately. A few helpful points follow:

- In the unconscious patient, rubbing the sternum or pinching the nose may cause grimacing, which may reveal facial asymmetries.
- Children have excellent facial tone and, therefore, should be assessed supine as well as upright to reduce the tendency for the eye to close spontaneously.
- Injuries medial to a line drawn from the medial canthus of the eye to the lateral oral commissure do not require facial nerve repair because of anastomotic innervation and primary healing.
- The nerve should be assessed prior to any injection of local anesthesia.
- Assessment of extensive wounds often necessitates identification of the proximal and distal segments of the injured nerve away from the actual site of trauma. If this occurs, the operating microscope and magnifying loops are often useful for locating as well as repairing the damaged nerve.
- If the facial nerve is not identified in the wound, other approaches may be used to locate it. The standard parotidectomy incision, locating the pes anserinus, then following the nerve to the wound edge is a secure method of finding the proximal stump. Occasionally, it will be necessary to locate the nerve in the mastoid and follow it peripherally. The distal stump may be located by finding the branches of the facial nerve just anterior to the parotid gland and then by following these posteriorly. The nerve stimulator may be helpful in locating these distal elements.
- Reanastomosis of the facial nerve segments should be performed with 10-0 nylon sutures on a tapered needle with the sutures passing through the epineurium only. If the ends of the severed facial nerves are contused, they should be freshened with a sharp scalpel to provide best results after reanastomosis (Fig. 10–15).
- Reanastomosis must be under no tension. Deep sutures in adjacent tissue may be used to relieve tension.
- A nerve interposition cable graft is preferable to repair of the nerve under tension at the anastomotic site. (Greater auricular and sural nerves are generally the preferred donors.)
- In grossly contaminated wounds or in those in which further tissue loss from the injury is expected (e.g., a gunshot wound), it is preferable to tag the identified nerve endings with the suture and repair the nerve at a time when the wound is suitable for repair.
- The facial nerve grows at approximately 3 mm/day, and studies have shown that repair should probably be done within the first 21 days.

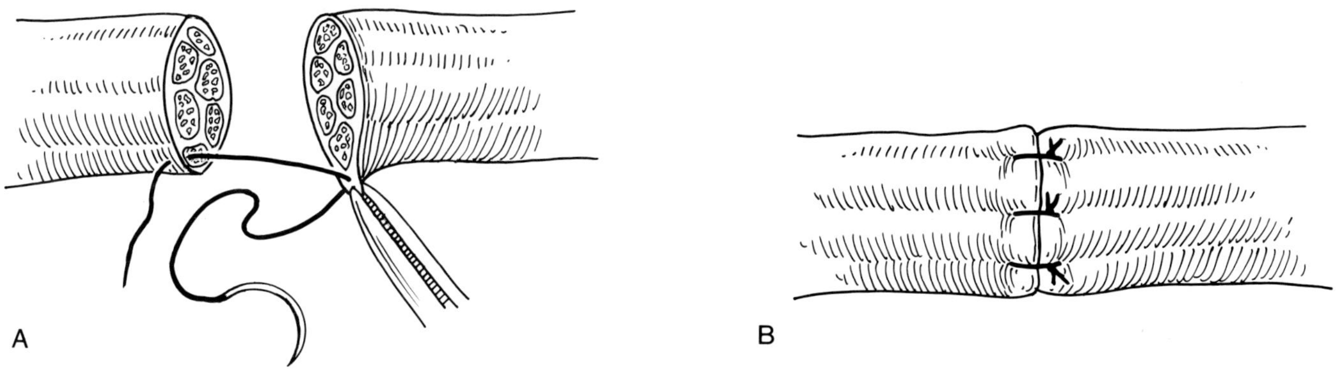

• FIGURE 10–15.

Reanastomosis of the facial nerve segments. *A*, Suture placed. *B*, Wound closed.

Parotid Duct Lacerations

The parotid duct exits the parotid gland and enters the mouth at approximately the second molar. Cheek lacerations may involve the duct, causing possible salivary cutaneous fistulas if they are not recognized and treated appropriately. Also, unrepaired ducts may result in cystic formations.

The lacerated duct ends should be identified in the laceration by applying pressure on the parotid gland, which will cause saliva to flow from the duct. The distal end may be identified by passing a lacrimal probe through the intraoral puncta. The duct is repaired over a No. 90 polyethylene tube stent with fine absorbable sutures. The stent is left in place for 2 to 3 weeks. Suturing the stent to the buccal mucosa with permanent suture will keep it in place for this time (Fig. 10–16).

If the distal end of the duct is severely damaged, the proximal duct may be reimplanted directly into the cheek mucosa.

Salivary cutaneous leaks may persist from the wound for quite some time, even with adequate duct repair. These leaks usually resolve spontaneously; however, clean pressure bandages and an occasional cautery of the fistula tract may be helpful.

Eyebrow Lacerations

Principles of repair include the following:

- Do not shave eyebrows.
- Save all viable tissues.
- Any incision for débridement should parallel the hair follicles.
- Eyebrow reconstruction may be accomplished by using free scalp grafts or an arterial flap based on the superficial temporal artery.

Eyelid Lacerations (Fig. 10–17)

- If the patient is old enough and can cooperate, an adequate eye examination should be performed. This should include acuity checks using a Snelling chart; an evaluation of the range of extraocular motion; an evaluation of pupillary action; and an evaluation of the anterior chamber for hyphema.
- If fat is in the wound, the orbital septum has been violated and an ophthalmology consultation is necessary to evaluate for globe and other injuries.
- In full-thickness injuries to the eyelid, tissue loss usually appears greater than it truly is, owing to the orbicularis oculi pull.
- It is important to line up the gray and white lines of the lid margin to avoid notching. This may be done by using fine silk sutures and magnifying loops.
- Alignment of medial and lateral canthi is critical to regain pretraumatic eye symmetry. If the canthi are avulsed from bony segments, they should be reattached using permanent sutures. If there are bony attachments to the displaced canthi, they need to be anatomically reduced.

• FIGURE 10–16.

Parotid duct repair.

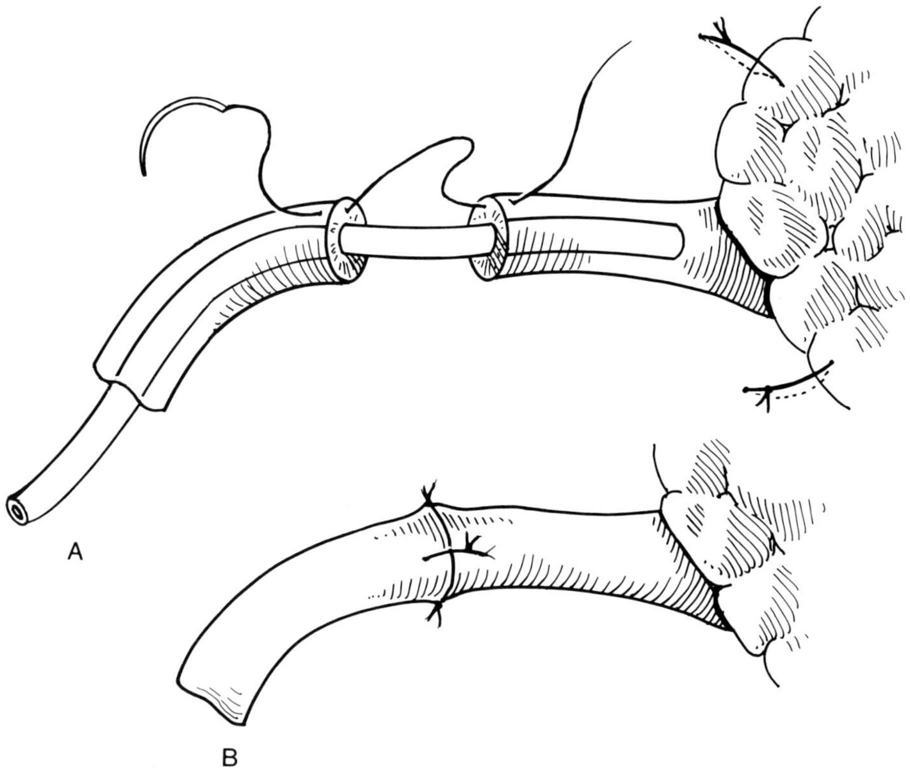

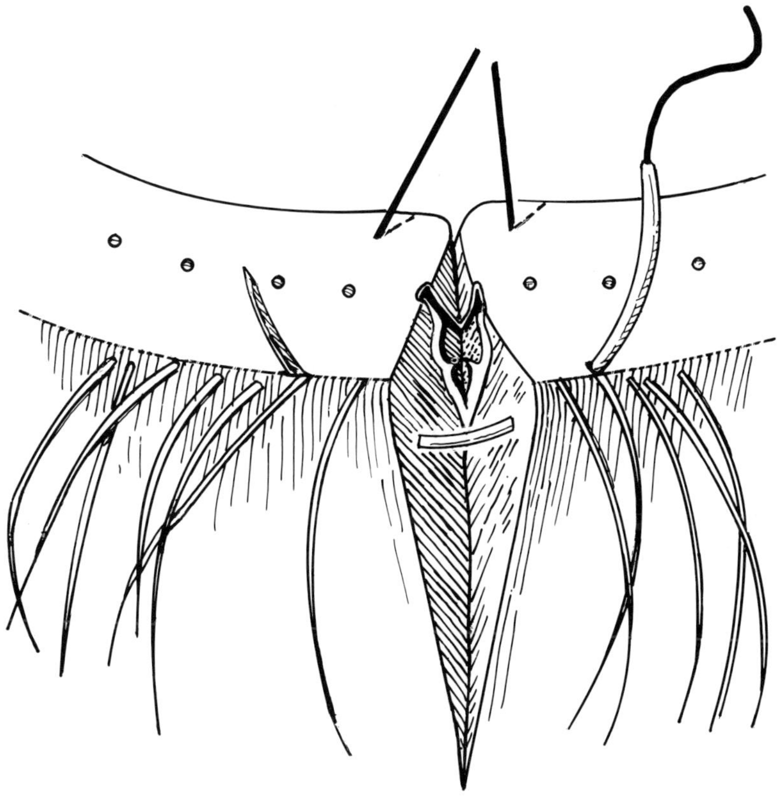

• FIGURE 10–17.

Eyelid closure aligning gray and white lines before proceeding with the remainder of closure.

Lip Lacerations

Injuries may be minor, such as a small intraoral lip laceration caused from incisor penetration. This type of injury heals well without surgical closure and with good oral hygiene.

In lacerations involving the full thickness of the lip, the key to successful repair is to accurately reapproximate the white line of the vermillion border and to perform adequate muscle repair to avoid notching (Fig. 10–18).

- Avoid overinjection of local anesthesia that distorts the white line–vermillion distinctions.
- Before local anesthetic is injected, mark the white line–vermillion border with either a marker or a scratch from a suture needle.
- Use key-tacking sutures to approximate the vermillion lines; then, use fine suture to obtain the best anatomic realignment.
- Prior to cutaneous repair, reapproximate the deep muscle layers with heavy absorbable sutures to the point of slight overcorrection.
- Accurately reapproximate the skin with skin sutures; however, loosely approximate the mucosa with absorbable interrupted sutures.
- Avulsion injuries up to 25% of the length of the lip may be closed primarily with a W-plasty or the V-closure technique. Larger avulsions require more complicated closures.
- Oral commissure repair should be achieved with maximal tissue sparing, because this is a difficult area to reconstruct. It is preferable to save badly damaged tissue, even if viability is marginal, rather than to sacrifice such tissue.

Ear Lacerations

After the nose, the auricles are the most frequently involved element in head and neck trauma. Simple lacerations and abrasions are managed in the usual manner. Hematomas must be evacuated aseptically. Through-and-through mattress sutures over a small bolster will prevent a recurrence. A mastoid dressing may also be required. Exposed auricular cartilage must be covered at the time of repair either by tissue advancement or by conservative cartilage resection. Cartilage may be buried under the postauricular skin if there is insufficient auricular skin to cover the cartilage. As previously stated, subtotally avulsed portions of the auricle will often survive owing to excellent blood supply (see Figs. 10–3 and 10–4). Survival is enhanced by accurate repair, careful cleaning, and gentle handling of the tissue. The details of repair of injuries to the auricle are the same as for the lip, nose, and preauricular areas.[2]

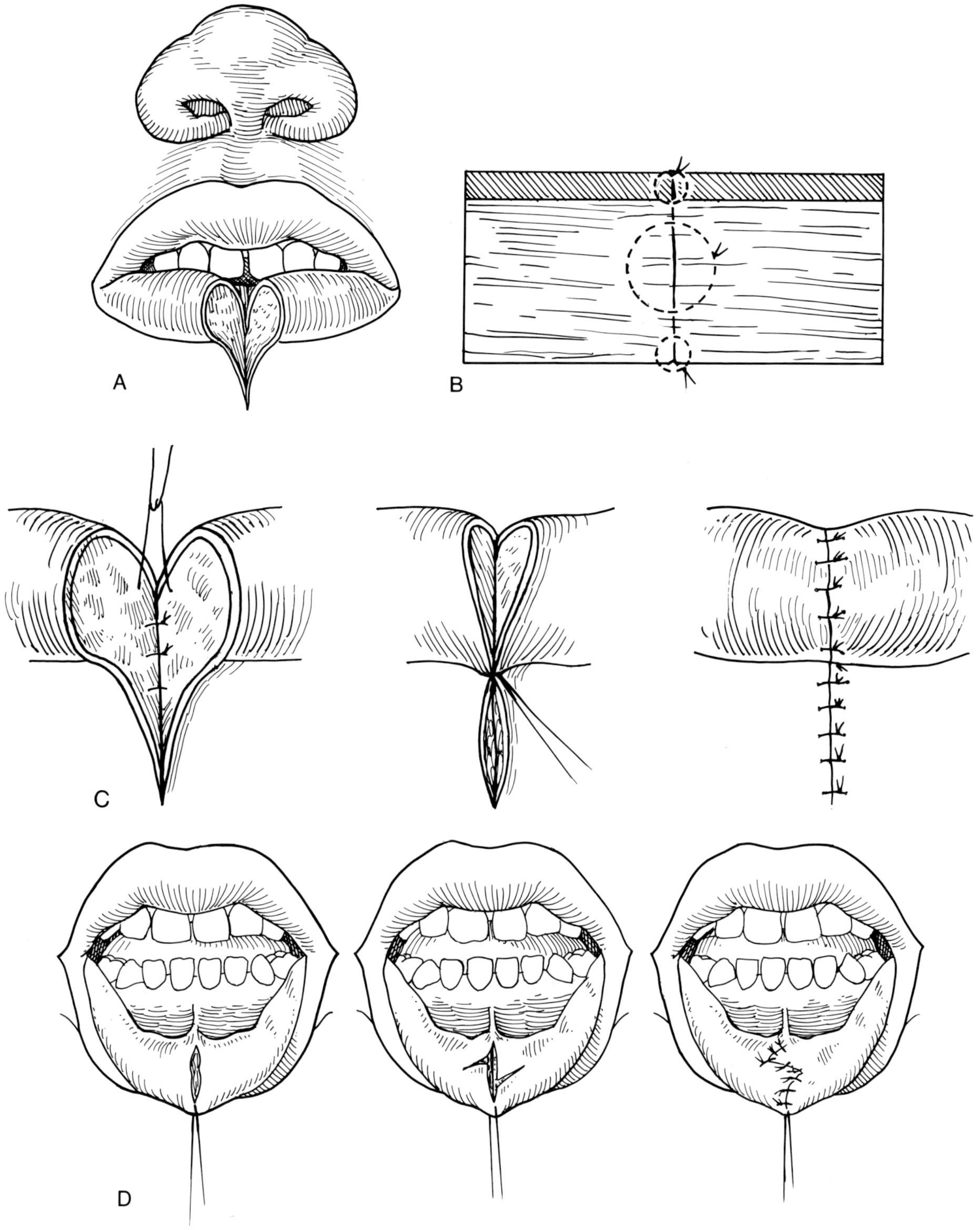

• FIGURE 10–18.

Surgical repair of lip lacerations. *A*, Simple through-and-through lip laceration. *B*, Schematic of 3-layer closure. *C*, Layered closure illustrating the importance of the vermillion border suture. *D*, Z-plasty closure of the mucosal surface to permit contracture.

Nose Lacerations

Repair of soft tissue injuries and tissue losses of the nose requires a higher degree of skill than that of the other soft tissues of the face because of the importance of the appearance of the nose and the adherence of skin to underlying tissues. As a general rule, as with injuries of the lips and eyelids in through-and-through injuries, tissue loss is less than is apparent. Assessment of soft tissue trauma and tissue losses of the nose must be done systematically to appreciate the tissue elements involved in the defect in order that each element may be repaired individually. Mucosal losses usually do not need to be replaced because the mucosa will often regenerate if packing and stenting measures are employed. Skin losses are repaired by adjacent flaps.

Small alar defects are repaired with composite auricular grafts. However, in repairs too extensive to utilize these techniques, we have found the methods proposed by Burget to be useful.[4–7]

In addition to obvious tissue losses, trauma to the nose frequently results in septal hematomas that must be recognized and treated appropriately, as septal hematoma with subsequent abscess and cartilage necrosis will result in saddle nose deformities, which require reconstructive procedures (Fig. 10–19).

PEDIATRIC FACIAL SKELETAL TRAUMA

Bony facial trauma in children is usually secondary to accidental injuries (particularly automotive), assault, or child abuse. Although child abuse constitutes the smallest segment, detection is imperative because undetected child abuse almost always leaves the child susceptible to further abuse. If abuse is suspected, it is the physician's responsibility to involve appropriate social services and authorities.

The details of trauma care are beyond the scope of this chapter. As mentioned earlier, a complete evaluation of the patient is necessary. Injuries severe enough to result in fracture of facial bones, especially midface fractures, are associated with a high incidence of other injuries. For example, in the series by McCoy and associates,[8] facial fractures are associated with skull fractures 40% of the time. Treatment of neurologic, cardiothoracic, and abdominal injuries obviously takes precedence over treatment of facial injuries, unless trauma embarrasses the airway. Pediatric injuries of the facial skeleton differ from similar injuries in adults in the following aspects:

- Evaluation should proceed in an orderly fashion after airway, hemorrhage, and circulation problems have been attended to. In the evaluation, a computed tomography (CT) scan is often necessary for the accurate diagnosis of facial fractures in children because conventional radiologic studies are often inadequate.

- There is a low incidence of fracture in children, because bones are more flexible. Greenstick fractures are common and may or may not require treatment.

- The presence of unerupted teeth and/or mixed dentition may complicate the treatment. Also, treatment may lead to a higher risk of dental injury.

- Early repair is necessary because of the rapid healing. Injuries and repair may have unknown effects on growth centers.

- Unsatisfactory treatment or unwarranted intervention may lead to progressive deformities and long-term disabilities.

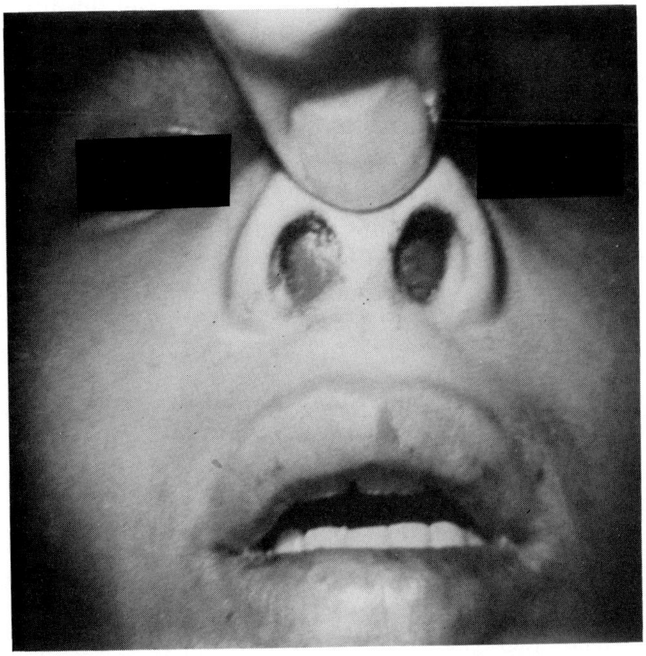

• **FIGURE 10-19.**

Septal hematoma in an 8-year-old girl who sustained trauma to the nose while she was playing. There was no other injury.

NASAL FRACTURES

Nasal fractures are the most frequent facial fractures in both children and adults. Key considerations are as follows:

- Isolated injury
- Diagnosis of elements in site of involvement
- Age of the patient
- Early versus delayed treatment
- Open versus closed reduction

The nasal bones in the child are relatively small and are separated in the midline by an open suture. The nasal bones are formed on the surface of the cartilaginous nasal capsule, and in children there is a large overlap between the upper lateral cartilage of the nasal bones.[9] These cartilages may become detached from the undersurface of the nasal bone and collapse into the nasal fossa. The area between the upper lateral cartilages and the nasal bone is a common site for hematoma formation. Because nasal bones have a midline separation, the open-book type of fracture with the nasal bones overriding the frontal process of the maxilla is commonly seen in children, although it is not usually seen in adults. Treatment of nasal fractures in children may be under local or general anesthesia, although general anesthesia is more frequently employed. The reduction techniques are similar to those of an adult, although the septum is more frequently involved in children than in adults. The possibility of septal hematoma is more likely. Nasal fractures in children heal rapidly; however, there is frequently overgrowth in the area of fracture, and a hypertrophic callus may form with resultant widening of the nose or secondary deformity.

MANDIBULAR FRACTURES

The mandible is the second most frequently fractured facial bone in children. The site of fractures and treatment vary greatly according to age, as shown in Figure 10–20, which shows the distribution of fracture sites in 73 patients with mandibular fractures.

The sites of these fractures are affected greatly by the state of dentition, because fractures commonly occur through developing tooth buds. Operative treatment is infrequently required in children. When operative treatment is required, wiring or plating should be as close to the inferior border of the mandible as possible to avoid tooth buds. The panorex x-ray is useful in evaluating mandibular fractures.

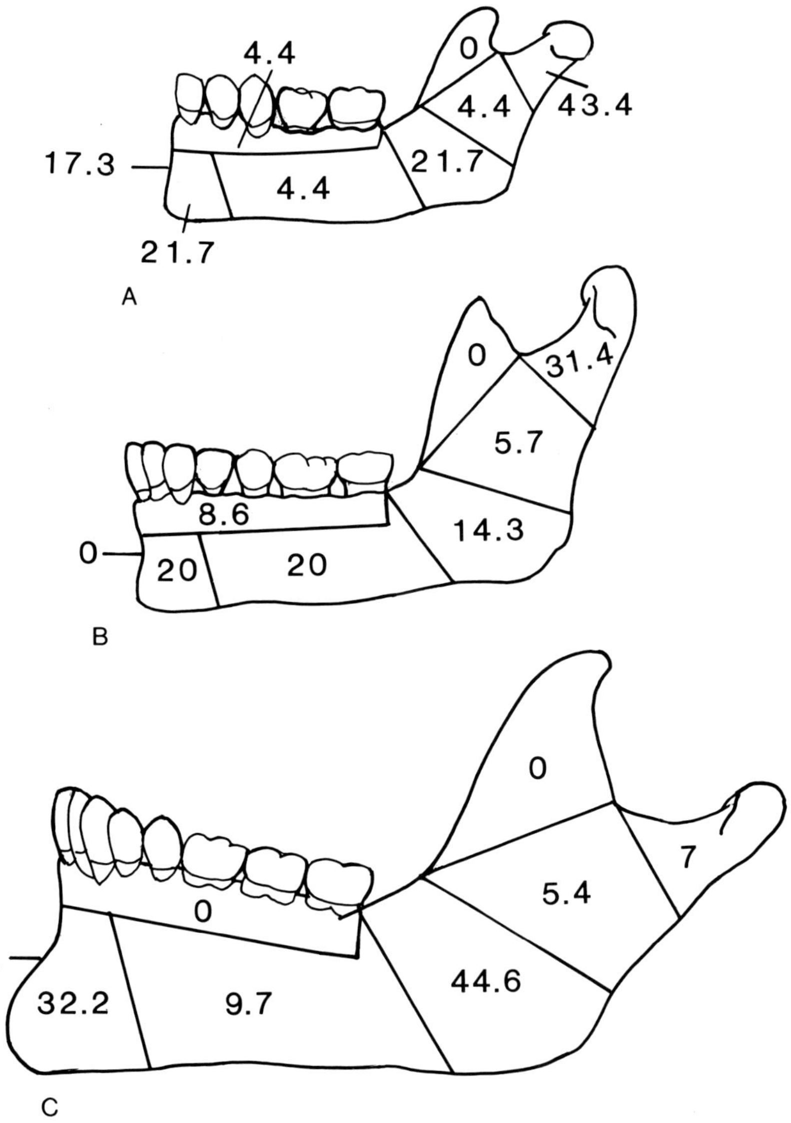

• FIGURE 10-20.

Distribution of mandibular fractures in 73 patients. *A*, Ages from birth to 6 (15 patients). *B*, Ages from 7 to 12 (24 patients). *C*, Ages from 13 to 18 (34 patients).

SUBCONDYLAR FRACTURES

Subcondylar fractures are the most common site of mandibular fractures in children through 12 years of age but are less common after this time. These fractures frequently lead to mandibular asymmetry, which is often due to late growth abnormalities.[10]

Unilateral subcondylar fractures rarely require operative treatment and seldom require intermaxillary fixation. Generally, a liquid diet for 2 weeks followed by soft diet for another 2 weeks is adequate. If the malocclusion does not begin to resolve in the first few days after fracture, a loosely placed Barton-type bandage will reduce the necessity for intermaxillary fixation. If intermaxillary fixation is required, 2 weeks of fixation is usually sufficient.

Mandibular splints and intermaxillary fixation are the primary methods of interventional treatment.

MAXILLARY FRACTURES

The principles of maxillary fracture treatment are very similar in adults and children, and such fractures should usually be treated within 10 days after injury, if possible. Because of the small size and soft quality of the bones, interosseous wiring is used more frequently than plating in children who require operative intervention.

ZYGOMATIC COMPLEX AND ORBITAL FRACTURES

These fractures are very unusual in children younger than 10 years of age due to the lack of extensive pneumatization of the maxilla. However, when these do occur, the principles of treatment are similar to those used in adults.

REFERENCES

1. Gross CW and Gurucharri MJ: Pediatric facial plastic surgery. *In* Myers E, Bluestone C, Brachman D, and Krause C (eds): Advances in Otolaryngology—Head and Neck Surgery, Vol 3. Chicago, Year Book Medical Publishers, 1989.
2. Gross CW: Soft tissue injuries of the lips, nose, ears and preauricular area. Otolaryngol Clin North Am 2:265–302, 1969.
3. Gross CW and Harris AS: Relief of stricture in the cervical esophagus by Z-plasty technique. Laryngoscope 81:658–672, 1971.
4. Burget GC: Surgical restoration of the nose. Curr Ther Plastic Reconstr Surg 1:400–412, 1989.
5. Burget GC: The subunit principle in nasal reconstruction. Plastic Reconstr Surg 76:239–247, 1985.
6. Burget GC and Menick FJ: Nasal reconstruction: Seeking a fourth dimension. Plastic Reconstr Surg 78:145–157, 1986.
7. Burget GC: Aesthetic restoration of the nose. Clin Plast Surg 12(3):463–480, 1985.
8. McCoy FJ, Chandler RA, and Crow ML: Facial fractures in children. Plast Reconstr Surg 37:209, 1966.
9. Gross CW and Johnson CQ: Nasal fractures. *In* English GM (ed): Plastic and Reconstructive Surgery of the Head and Neck. Vol IV. Philadelphia, JB Lippincott, 1989.
10. Kaban LB: Facial fractures in children. *In* Healy EB (ed): Common Problems in Pediatric Otolaryngology. Chicago, Year Book Medical Publishers, 1990, pp 237–250.

chapter

11

Congenital Malformations of the Nose and Paranasal Sinuses

MARGARET A. KENNA, M.D.

Congenital malformations of the nose and paranasal sinuses are very uncommon but extremely important because neonates are obligate nose breathers. When these malformations are associated with significant nasal obstruction, recognition and repair or bypass of the obstruction often must be undertaken in the delivery room or during the first few hours or days of life.

TYPES OF MALFORMATIONS

The most common midline nasal malformation is nasal septal deviation, either embryologic or traumatic (secondary to birth). A severely deviated nasal septum is occasionally noted at birth, most commonly as a result of birth trauma. Most of these deviations represent displacement of the cartilaginous septum from the maxillary crest and can be reduced in a closed fashion under local anesthesia. Most septal deviations, however, are not noticed or are not significantly symptomatic at birth and therefore are not usually diagnosed until months or years later. The traditional approach to septal deviations in children has always been conservative because of concern that the nasal septum may play a significant role in growth of the midface. If the septal deviation is causing severe obstructive symptoms, however, limited repair should be considered, with the knowledge that revision may be needed when the child reaches adolescence or young adulthood.

Another malformation, which is frequently overlooked, is pyriform aperture stenosis—either unilateral or bilateral. A bilateral form can cause significant nasal obstruction. Because pyriform aperture stenosis is very uncommon, it is often overlooked, and the child remains symptomatic. The diagnosis can be made using an axial computed tomography (CT) scan of the nasal cavity. Brown and associates suggested that the narrowing is a result of overgrowth of maxillary ossification at the area of the nasal process of the maxilla.[1] Repair is successful using either a transnasal approach or a sublabial approach, with placement of stents for several weeks to allow for healing.[1,2]

Many congenital nasal malformations can be loosely grouped by their embryology.[3,4] Dermoids, gliomas, and encephaloceles all may result from abnormal closure of the foramen cecum; gliomas and encephaloceles probably form at 2 to 3 weeks of embryonic life, and dermoids most likely form at 2 to 3 months. All three anomalies may have either a connection (stalk) or an actual extension to the central nervous system (CNS) and can present either externally or intranasally. Dermoids, which contain mesodermal elements, are the most common congenital midline nasal mass and may contain hair follicles, sebaceous glands, and sweat glands, whereas gliomas and encephaloceles contain neural tissue. Teratomas comprise elements of all three embryonic layers and can occur anywhere in the midline. CT scanning is important to help determine whether these lesions have any intracranial extension and should always be performed preoperatively.[5] If there is any question of an intracranial extension, neurosurgical consultation should be obtained prior to surgical intervention. Magnetic resonance imaging (MRI) may further clarify abnormal soft tissue elements, aiding in the presurgical diagnosis and in the planning of the surgical approach.

Complete agenesis of the nose, nasal clefting, nasal dysplasia, proboscis lateralis, and polyrhinia are rare defects that can occur with other abnormalities of the head and neck area. Median facial anomalies may frequently be associated with holoprosencephaly, mandating (if possible) a complete evaluation of the CNS before undertaking any major surgical intervention.

Choanal atresia is present in approximately 1:7000 live births, with a female to male ratio of 2:1 and a unilateral to bilateral ratio of 2:1. Eighty to 90% of atresias contain bone.[6] Embryologically, choanal atresia probably results from nonrupture of the nasobuccal membrane, with a defect in the region of the nasal and palatal processes surrounding the nasobuccal membrane leading to the associated findings of an accentuated arch of the hard palate, a medial location of the lateral and posterior nasal walls, and thickening of the vomer.[7] Especially in bilateral cases, choanal atresia is associated at least 50% of the time with other congenital anomalies, the most common being CHARGE association: C—coloboma (ocular); H—heart defects; A—atresia choanae; R—retarded postnatal growth, developmental, and/or CNS anomalies; G—genital hypoplasia; and E—ear deformities, hearing loss.[8] The child often has respiratory distress at birth if atresia is bilateral, requiring the use of a McGovern nipple, oral airway, orogastric tube, intubation, or tracheotomy. Definitive repair of atresia can occur any time after the airway is secure and other anomalies have been evaluated. Unilateral atresia is often not very symptomatic at birth, and repair can usually be undertaken when the child is older. Transnasal, transseptal, transantral, and transpalatal approaches have all been used for the repair of choanal atresia, with the transpalatal and transnasal approaches being most commonly used. Access by Le Fort I osteotomy has been described for use in the adult; this approach would not be appropriate for use in an infant or a child.[9]

Abnormalities of the paranasal sinuses are not usually of concern at birth, and there is a certain amount of normal variation in sinus shape and size. The advent of CT scanning revealed that maxillary sinus hypoplasia is not uncommon, and there are many other variants, including abnormalities of the bony turbinates. Additionally, approximately 5% of the population does not have significant frontal sinus development.[10]

DIAGNOSIS OF CONGENITAL MALFORMATIONS

Diagnosis of congenital nasal malformations is by physical examination and nasal endoscopy, with confirmation by CT scanning.[5,6] MRI, as a method of examination, may further define soft tissue abnormalities. If the lesion is causing life-threatening airway obstruction, either repair or bypass must be undertaken early in the child's life. If the child is critically ill or if other malformations are suspected, bypass of the obstruction may be the best solution until all other abnormalities have been defined.

SURGICAL APPROACHES

A few basic surgical approaches can be used for the correction of most congenital malformations of the nose. The transpalatal approach for the repair of choanal atresia could also be used for a transsphenoidal encephalocele or for a well-defined nasopharyngeal lesion.[11] A lateral rhinotomy can be used to approach some intranasal dermoids, gliomas, and encephaloceles. The incision for the sublabial transseptal approach to choanal atresia can also be used for the correction of pyriform aperture stenosis.[6,12] The external rhinoplasty approach, although not described here, should be considered for dermoids or for other lesions involving the anterior nasal septum or columella.

A description of these surgical approaches and the transnasal approach for choanal atresia follows. All procedures are performed under general anesthesia, with prior control of the airway by endotracheal tube or tracheotomy. Continued nasal obstruction after these surgical procedures is common, and in the obligate nose-breathing neonate constant attention to the airway must be maintained even after repair is done. Also, because there are many variations of every surgical approach, the reader is advised to consult the references for further details and information.

TRANSNASAL REPAIR OF CHOANAL ATRESIA

Indications

- This technique is best suited to the primary repair of membranous or very thin bony atresias.
- Bilateral atresia usually presents as airway distress at or shortly after birth, and therefore repair or bypass must occur almost immediately.
- Unilateral atresia may not be significantly symptomatic at birth, and repair can be undertaken later in childhood.
- If atresia consists of thick bone, transpalatal rather than transnasal repair may need to be considered.

Anesthetic considerations

This procedure should be performed under general anesthesia with prior control of the airway (usually by endotracheal [ET] tube, occasionally via tracheostomy). Topical vasoconstriction should be used if the child's overall medical condition allows. Gauze packs should be placed in the nasopharynx to prevent blood from being swallowed or aspirated.

Preparation

The use of an operating microscope with a 300-mm lens greatly facilitates visualization. An infant nasal speculum or a Lempert aural speculum is used to visualize the nasal cavity (Fig. 11–1).

Procedure

Multiple approaches to making an opening in the choanae through the atretic area can be used. The most precise is illustrated in Figure 11–2. The mucosa on the anterior face of the atretic area is incised vertically, with medial and lateral flap development. If the atresia is only membranous, this incision may open the choanae and no further removal is needed. If bone is present, however, it can be removed using one of several methods.

• FIGURE 11-1.

A nasal speculum exposing the posterior choana atresia mucosa.

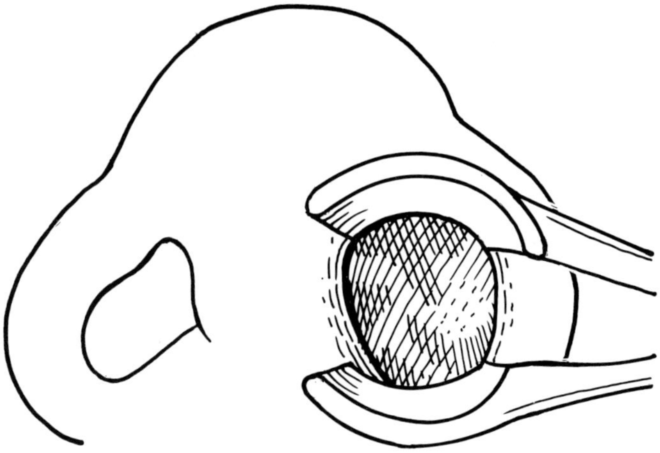

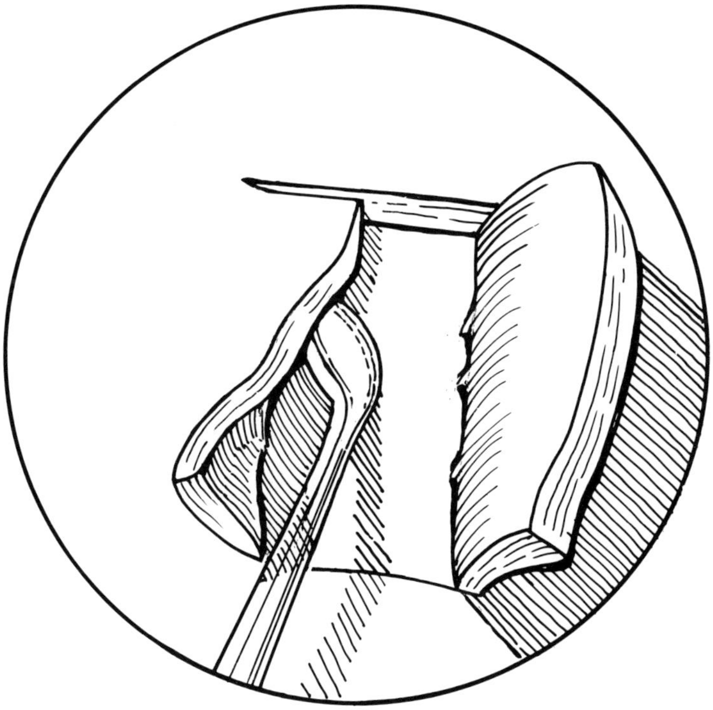

• FIGURE 11-2.

The anterior mucosa is incised vertically with a medial and lateral flap elevation.

Bone removal has also been accomplished with mastoid curettes, the CO_2 laser, or transnasal puncture.[13–17] Many advocates of transnasal puncture do not make the intranasal incisions, and the procedure is done with a finger in the nasopharynx, both to detect successful puncture and to prevent damage to the posterior nasopharynx and skull base structures. Transnasal puncture is most appropriate for membranous atresias, and stenting should still be used. In addition, the use of nasal endoscopes in four patients to aid in surgical repair of choanal atresia has been demonstrated.[18]

Figure 11–3 *A* and *B* illustrates bone removal using a cutting bur. In many of these children, the vomer is very thick posteriorly; therefore, removal of bone inferiorly and medially to include the posterior vomer is crucial to achieve a permanent correction.

Figure 11–4 illustrates an incision of the posterior mucosa horizontally to create superior and inferior flaps. If possible, after bone removal the mucosal flaps should be folded and advanced as shown.

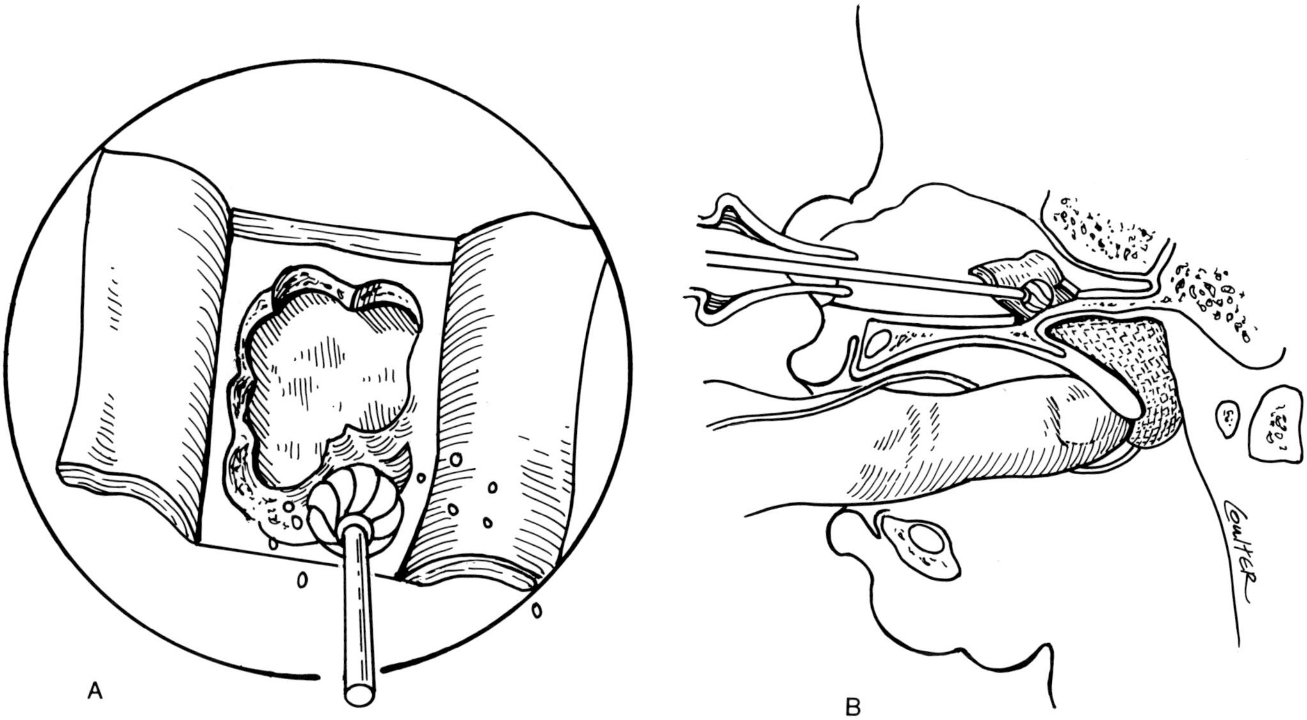

• **FIGURE 11-3.**

A and *B*, Removal of atretic bone inferiorly and medially.

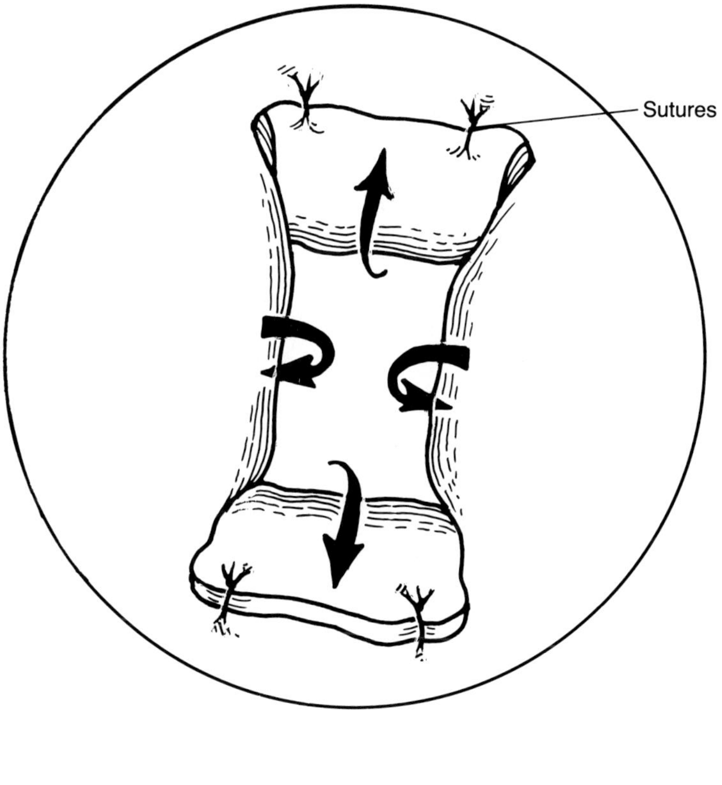

• **FIGURE 11-4.**

Folding of mucosal flaps anteriorly (superior and inferior flaps) and posteriorly (medial and lateral flaps) (*arrows*).

A stent through the posterior choanae holds the flaps in place and keeps the choanae open (Fig. 11–5). Multiple materials have been used for stenting, but a No. 3.5 or 4.0 ET tube is most commonly used, is readily accessible in the operating room, and is easily shaped and trimmed. If the choanal atresia is bilateral, a single ET tube can be utilized. This tube should be bent into a U shape, and an opening should be made posteriorly in the part of the tube that loops around the vomer. The opening should face the nasopharynx and should be large enough to allow easy passage of suction catheters through both sides of the ET tube anteriorly into the nasopharynx (Fig. 11–6 *A* and *B*). The anterior portion of the ET tube should be sutured to the membranous septum with a single stitch (Fig. 11–7).

Other methods of securing the stent anteriorly include use of a suture placed through the nasal spine or placement of the anterior suture through a "washer" placed anterior to the columella, so that the stent is not actually sutured to the child.[19, 20] In most cases, the anterior ends of the stent should be trimmed so that they lie just inside the nares; if a washer is used, the stents will protrude through the nasal opening and beyond the columella.

Occasionally, use of a single stent (unilateral atresia) or two stents (bilateral atresia) may be desirable for the nasopharynx that is especially narrow. The use of a single or double stent may aid in suctioning and maintain the patency of the nasopharynx end of the tubes. The stents will extend through the posterior choanae and curve down into the nasopharynx behind the soft palate. Complications with this type of stent include regurgitation of oral feedings through the tubes.

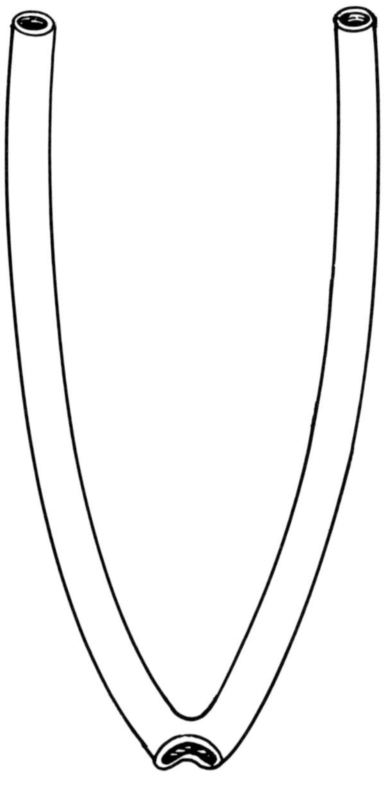

• **FIGURE 11–5.**

A stent made from flexible endotracheal tube is used to keep the posterior choanae open bilaterally.

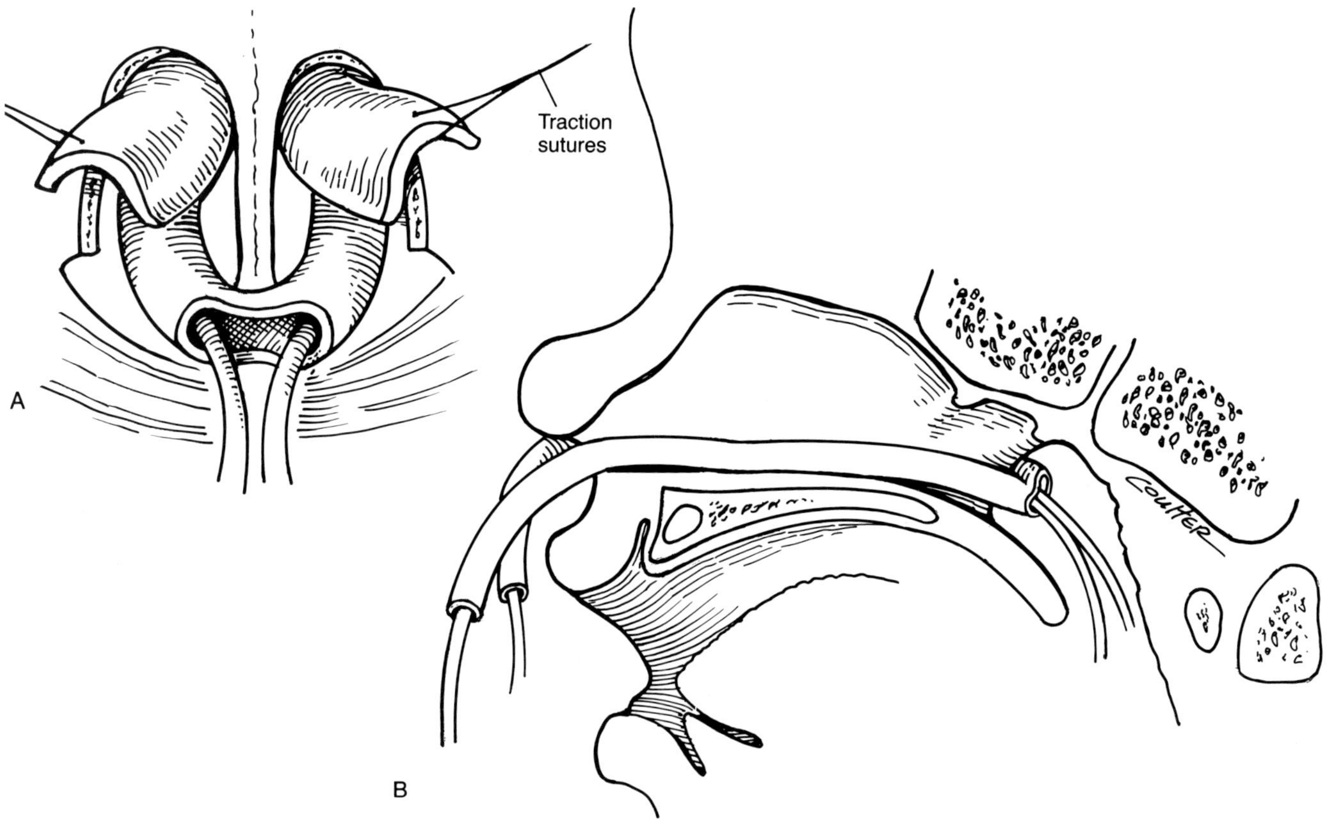

• **FIGURE 11-6.**

A, The stent as it appears in the nasopharynx. Suction catheters are shown coming through the posterior opening in the stent. Sutures are on mucosal flaps, which are partially held in place (an out-of-the choanal opening) with the stent. *B*, A stent is used to keep the choanae open bilaterally. The stent passes behind the vomer, and suction catheters can be passed from the anterior to the posterior into the nasopharynx.

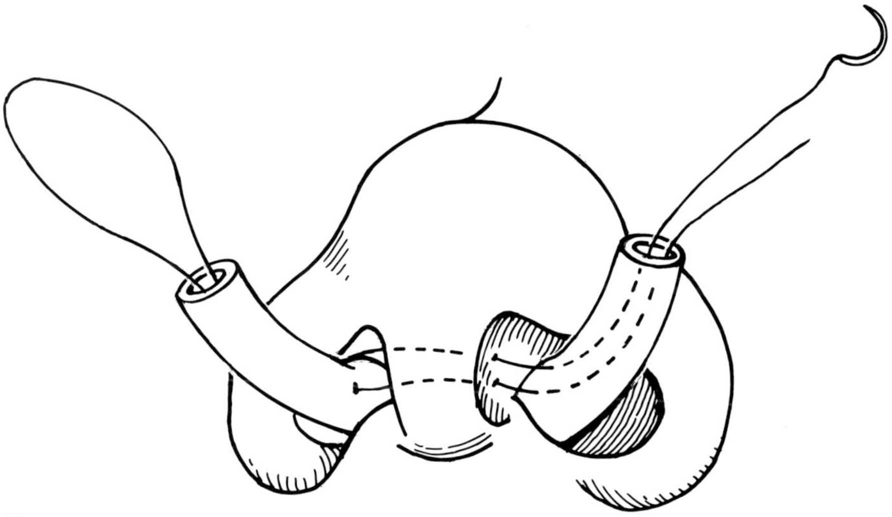

• **FIGURE 11-7.**

The anterior ends of the stent are shown coming out through the nares. Several methods of fastening the stents anteriorly can be utilized. In this illustration, a suture is being passed from medially inside the stent through the cartilaginous septum to the medial portion of the contralateral stent and then back again. This keeps the stent firmly in place but allows for unimpeded passage of the suction catheter.

Postoperative care/complications

Meticulous attention to the stents is necessary to prevent plugging and displacement. Soft catheters are used for suctioning every few hours, and normal saline can be used for irrigation of the stents to dislodge crusts and secretions. Attention should also be paid to the area of fixation of the stents (i.e., nasal septum, columella, nasal spine) to prevent erosion and permanent scarring.

The major problem with the transnasal approach for choanal atresia repair is inadequate visualization. A deviated nasal septum, large turbinates, or simply the small size of the nose can make it difficult or impossible to see the posterior area adequately to allow for sufficient bone removal. Also, although making the incisions in the mucosa seems easy, in practice the creation and maintenance of these flaps can be very difficult. If the puncture method is used, it is difficult to remove enough bone inferiorly and medially, which may result in a higher incidence of restenosis.

Possible complications of the transnasal approach include cerebrospinal fluid (CSF) leak, meningitis, pressure necrosis of anterior nares or columella (when the stent is fixed anteriorly), plugging of the indwelling stents, and displacement of the stents. Granulation tissue may develop around the stents, especially in the posterior choanae, and may need to be removed.

TRANSPALATAL REPAIR OF CHOANAL ATRESIA

Indications

The transpalatal repair of choanal atresia, although a "bigger" operation than transnasal repair, has many possible advantages. These include wider surgical exposure, improved access to the posterior vomer, ability to preserve mucosal flaps, decreased stenting time, creation of larger initial openings, and decreased incidence of restenosis. Transpalatal repair is indicated for bony choanal atresia and for "re-do" procedures in which restenosis has occurred. If the baby is otherwise medically stable, the transpalatal procedure can be performed as early as the first few days of life, or at any time thereafter when transpalatal repair is appropriate.

Anesthetic considerations

This procedure should be performed under general anesthesia with the airway secured by an endotracheal or tracheotomy tube. The palate should be injected for hemostasis; $\frac{1}{2}$% lidocaine with 1:200,000 epinephrine works in the neonate. The anesthesiologist should be consulted prior to injection of the palate so that the appropriateness of the drugs and the dosages is verified.

Preparation

The operating microscope with the 300-mm lens should be used, especially in infants and young children. The Dingman mouth gag provides excellent exposure of the palate and posterior pharynx.

Procedure

Numerous incisions are used in Figure 11–8. The stippled area represents atresia. Both the Owens and Steinzeug incisions allow for maximal exposure of the superior lateral nasal wall, which may need to be drilled for maximum posterior choanal size. The incision starts behind the maxillary tuberosity and is carried medially to the alveolar ridge to the canine region; the Owens incision then continues to the nasopalatine foramen. A similar incision is made on the other side. The incision must leave enough mucosa so that closure can be accomplished. The mucoperiosteal flaps are elevated posteriorly to the edge of the hard palate, and care must be taken to preserve the neurovascular bundle coming out of the greater palatine foramen. This bundle should remain within the flap as it is elevated (Fig. 11–9 *A* and *B*). If a further length of the flap is needed, the posteromedial wall of the greater palatine foramen and canal can be removed to give more length to the greater palatine artery, while the tensor veli palatini can be sectioned or the hamulus of the pterygoid bone fractured. Sectioning of the tensor veli palatini, however, may result in eustachian tube dysfunction and otitis media. Fortunately, these additional techniques are rarely necessary, especially if choanal atresia is the primary lesion being repaired.

With elevation of the flap from the hard palate (Fig. 11–10), the soft palate retracts posteriorly and superiorly, exposing the posterior edge of the hard palate and the nasopharynx. An incision along the edge of the hard palate may be required to release the soft palate and allow retraction.

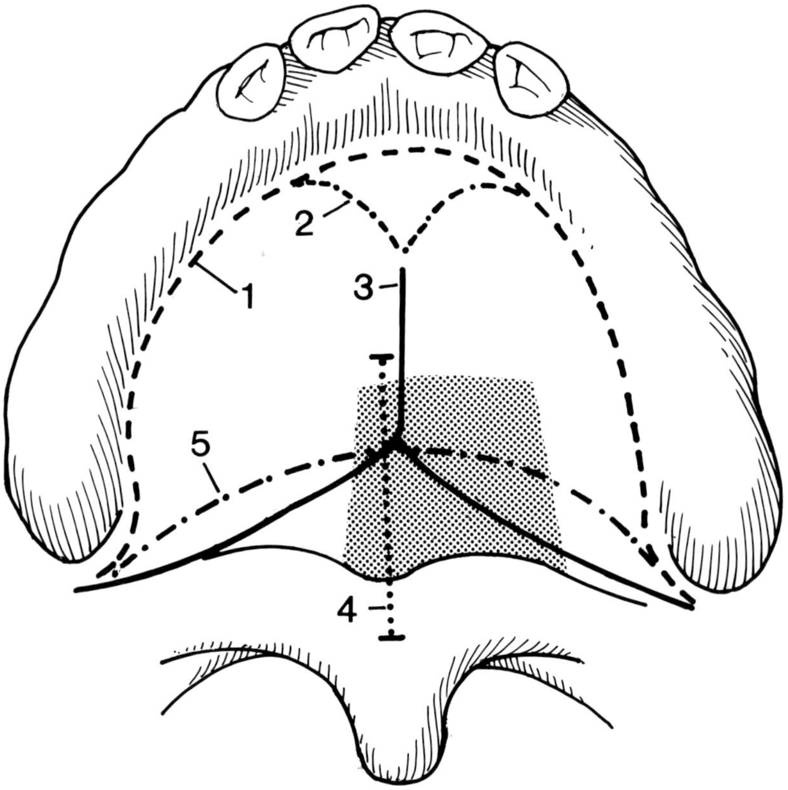

• FIGURE 11–8.

Incisions used in the transpalatal approach. (1 = Steinzeug; 2 = Owens; 3 = Wilson; 4 = Brunk; and 5 = Ruddy.)

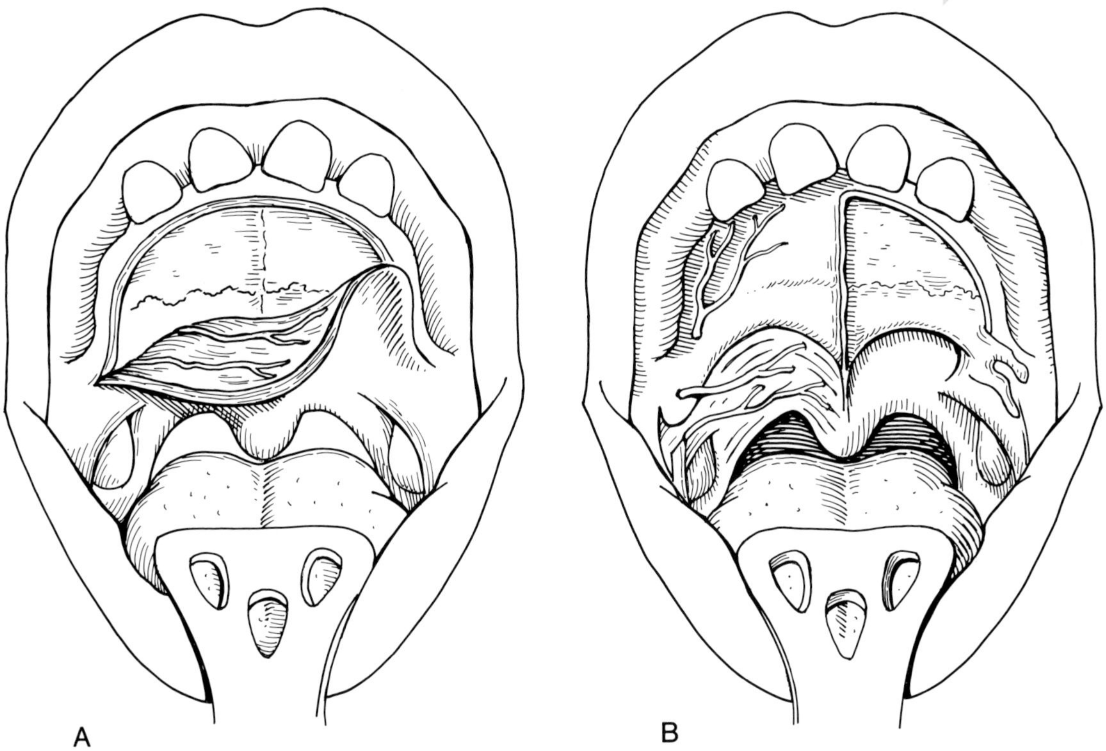

• **FIGURE 11–9.**

A and *B*, The greater palatine vessels are shown. (From Loré JM: An Atlas of Head and Neck Surgery, 2nd ed. Philadelphia, WB Saunders, 1973, p 153.)

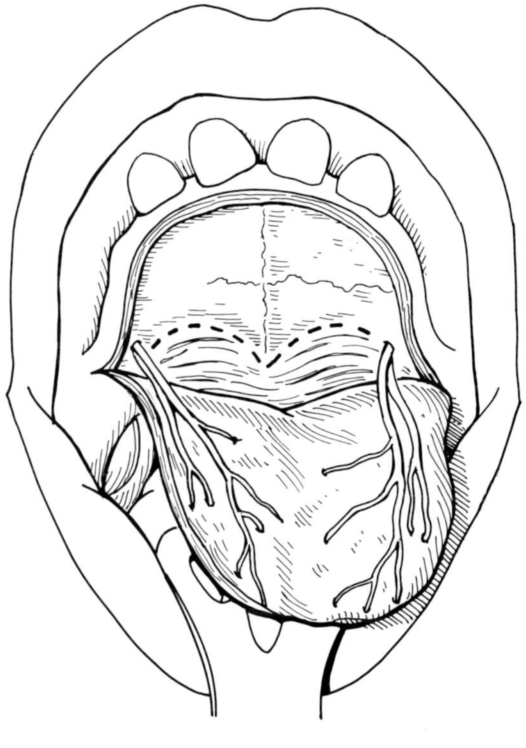

• **FIGURE 11–10.**

The mucoperiosteal flap has been elevated. Dashed lines indicate the incision between the hard and soft palates.

The nasal mucosa is elevated from the nasal surface of the hard palate, and then the posterior edge of the hard palate is removed using a cutting bur or a Kerrison punch. The area to be outlined is shown in Figure 11–11. Bone and abnormal soft tissue should be removed to the roof of the nasal cavity if possible. The posterior portion of the hard palate, vomer, and bony septum should be thinned or removed for adequate choanal size (Fig. 11–12). Finally, bone removal laterally between the lateral nasal wall, maxillary sinus, and pterygopalatine fossa may be needed for increased choanal size. Every attempt should be made to preserve nasal mucosa, which is then used to line the new choanal opening (Fig. 11–13).

When removal of atresia and any additional bone is completed, it should be possible to pass at least a No. 14 French catheter through the opening (in a newborn) without difficulty. Male urethral sounds of various sizes work well to determine the final dimensions of the choanae.

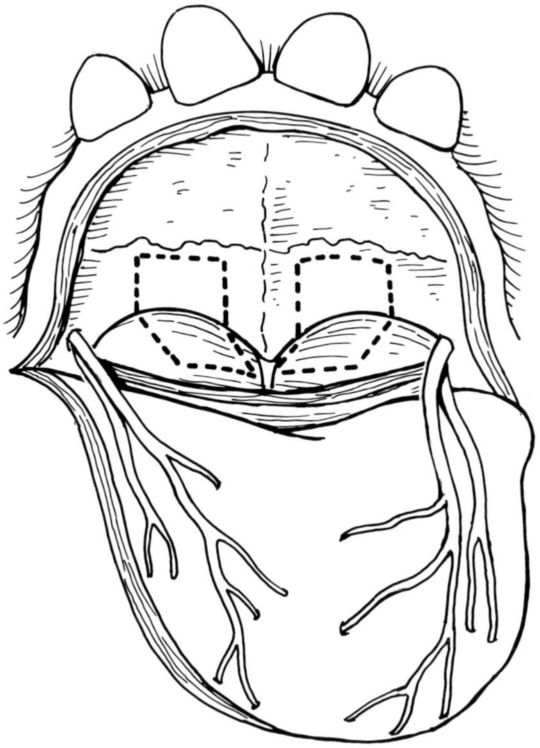

• **FIGURE 11–11.**

Dashed lines indicate areas of bone to be removed.

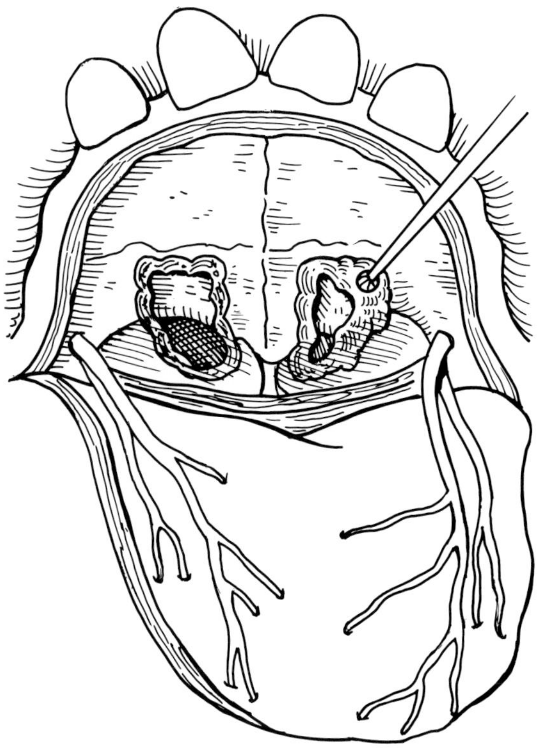

• **FIGURE 11–12.**

Cutting bur when removing the posterior edge of the hard palate.

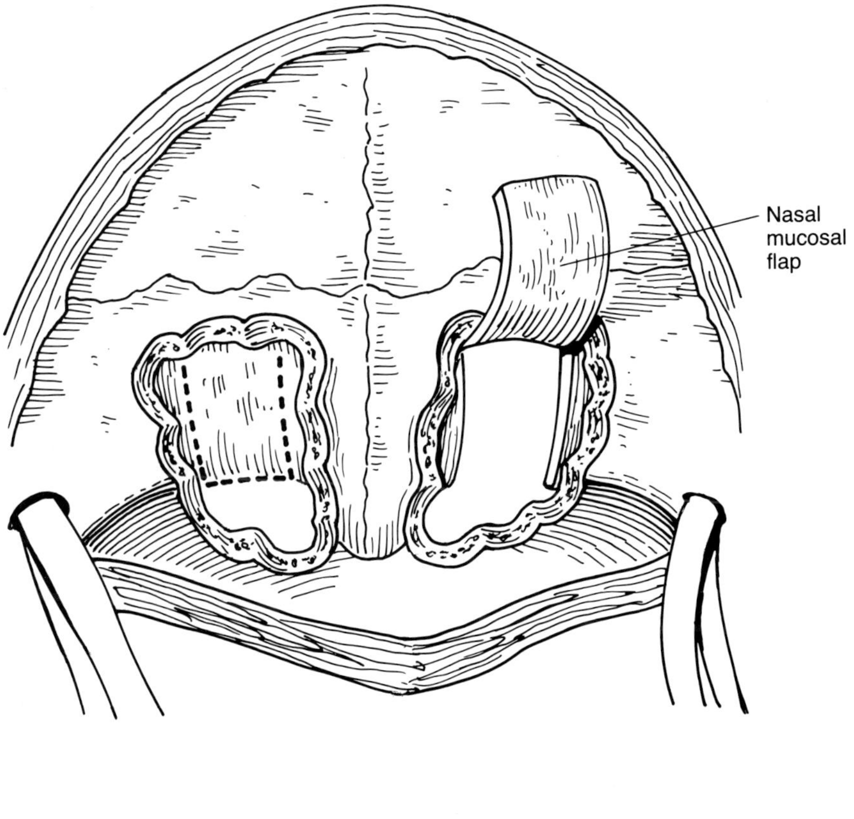

• **FIGURE 11–13.**

The technique for obtaining a mucoperiosteal flap from the membranous atresia.

Once atresia is removed, the new openings should be stented, both to maintain the opening(s) and to allow the child to breathe through the nose (Fig. 11–14 *A* to *C*). One continuous stent fastened anteriorly works well. The stent is made using an ET tube. The size depends on the size and age of the child, but a No. 3.5 or 4.0 is adequate for a full-term newborn. Suction catheters should pass easily through the stent into the nasopharynx. Design of the stent is shown in Figure 11–5. The stents should remain in place for several weeks, until re-epithelialization has taken place.

Postoperative care/complications

Postoperative care involves keeping the stents patent using saline and frequent suctioning. Even though the stents are sutured in place, they can become dislodged, and careful suctioning is always indicated.

Possible postoperative complications include palatal flap dehiscence, stent displacement or plugging, and restenosis once the stents are removed. The development of maxillary hypoplasia and an anterior crossbite have been documented following transpalatal repair and may result from removal of the midpalatal suture.[21]

LATERAL RHINOTOMY

Indications

This approach could be used for well-circumscribed unilateral intranasal lesions, such as dermoids and small encephaloceles, or lesions involving the inferior turbinate or anterior nasal floor.

Anesthetic considerations

The procedure should be performed under general anesthesia, with the airway secured by an ET or tracheotomy tube. Infiltration of the incision line with a local anesthetic agent with epinephrine facilitates hemostasis; an anesthesiologist should be consulted for the appropriate dosage. Vasoconstriction of the nasal mucosa can be achieved by the use of injected lidocaine with epinephrine, or the use of topical oxymetazoline or Neo-Synephrine.

Preparation

The entire face should be surgically prepared, and the eyelids should be closed using a stitch placed through the tarsal plate of the upper and lower eyelids. The entire nose and midface should be exposed.

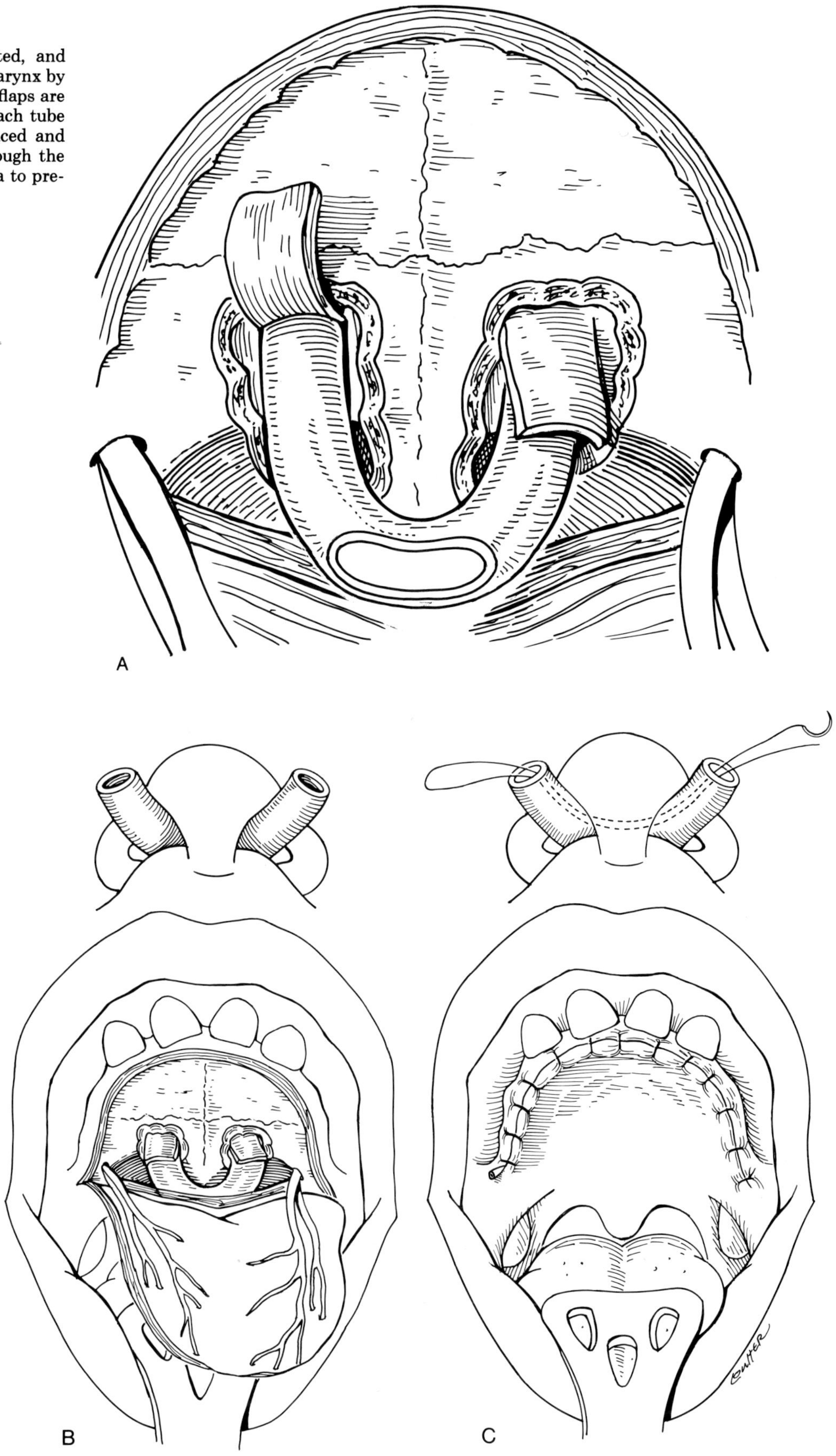

• FIGURE 11–14.

A, The mucosal flaps are elevated, and tubes are inserted into the nasopharynx by way of the nares. *B*, The mucosal flaps are placed on the inferior aspect of each tube before the palatal flaps are replaced and sutured. *C*, A suture is made through the nasal septum behind the columella to prevent displacement of the tubes.

Procedure

The incision begins just above the level of the inner canthus and is placed halfway between the inner canthus and the bony nasal dorsum (Fig. 11–15). It should be carried anteriorly to the nasomaxillary sulcus (for best cosmesis) and should then continue in the alar sulcus to the nasal vestibule. Each layer from skin to bone should be incised separately, which improves hemostasis by allowing the surgeon to ligate vessels as they are encountered.

The alar incision is carried through all layers of tissue until the bony edge of the maxillary process is reached (Fig. 11–16). A suture placed in the lateral alar region is helpful for retraction. If the periosteum of the nasal bone and ascending process of the maxilla is elevated, the underlying bone can be removed for better exposure.

Removal of lesions from the anterior nasal floor and the nasal septum is shown in Figure 11–17. Questionably malignant lesions should be removed with a good margin of normal mucous membrane. The floor of the nose lesion in this illustration has also had a small portion of palatal bone removed; however, in most children, this should be unnecessary, because most lesions are benign and are confined to the mucosa. This approach could be combined with a transpalatal approach for palatal lesions involving the posterior nasal floor.

Postoperative care/complications

If the incision is made posterior to the nasomaxillary suture, there may be some depression of the scar, which would be cosmetically more noticeable. Theoretically, bone removal could lead to asymmetric facial growth; if palatal bone is removed, growth of the palate could also be affected. Also, removal of the bony nasal floor could result in tooth bud injury.

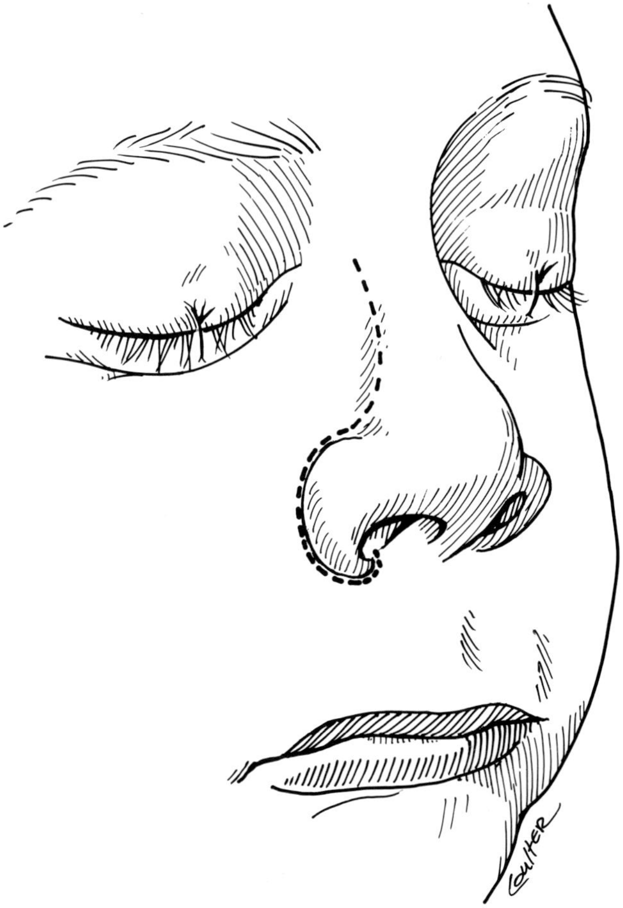

• FIGURE 11–15.

A nasal incision is shown.

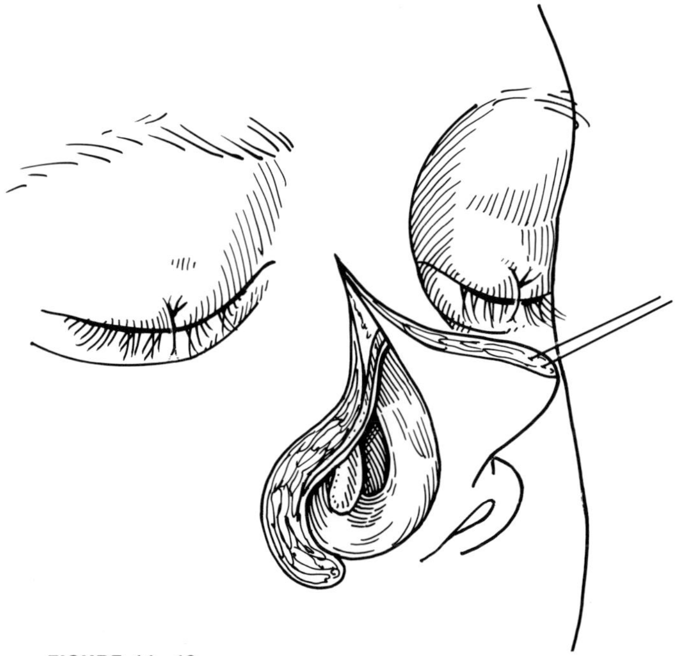

• FIGURE 11–16.

An alar incision is carried through all layers of tissue.

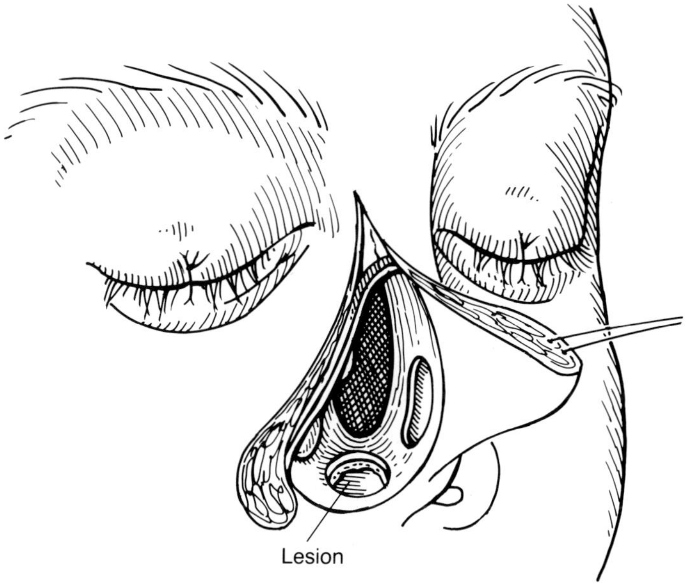

• FIGURE 11–17.

Demonstration of the removal of a lesion from the anterior nasal floor and nasal septum.

SUBLABIAL APPROACH TO PYRIFORM APERTURE STENOSIS

Indications

- The sublabial approach is appropriate for the repair of pyriform aperture stenosis. It could also be considered for removal of anterior nasal floor lesions.

Preparation

The operating microscope with the 300-mm lens should be used. Ear instruments and drills are precise and appropriate for use in the infant when performing this procedure.

Anesthetic considerations

A standard sublabial incision is used (Fig. 11–18 *A* and *B*). The mucosa and mucoperiosteum are elevated, and the pyriform aperture is exposed. Care should be taken with elevation of this flap to avoid injury to tooth buds.

Bone should be removed laterally but not along the nasal floor, because this could cause tooth bud injury (Fig. 11–19). If possible, the nasolacrimal ducts should be identified and preserved. The final nasal aperture should be wide enough to allow easy passage of a No. 3.5 ET tube stent. Because the stenosis in these children is anterior, the stents do not need to extend into the nasopharynx or posterior to the vomer.

Once sufficient bone has been removed and the stents are in place, the sublabial incision is closed using an absorbable suture (Fig. 11–20). The stents are left in place for 2 to 4 weeks.

Postoperative care/complications

Care of the nasal stents includes frequent suctioning and instillation of normal saline to prevent crusting and clogging. The stents should always be handled gently to avoid dislodging them.

Injury to tooth buds can occur if bone is removed in the area of the nasal floor, and nasolacrimal duct injury can occur if bone removal is carried posteriorly. Midfacial and nasal developmental hypoplasia can occur as a result of bone removal.

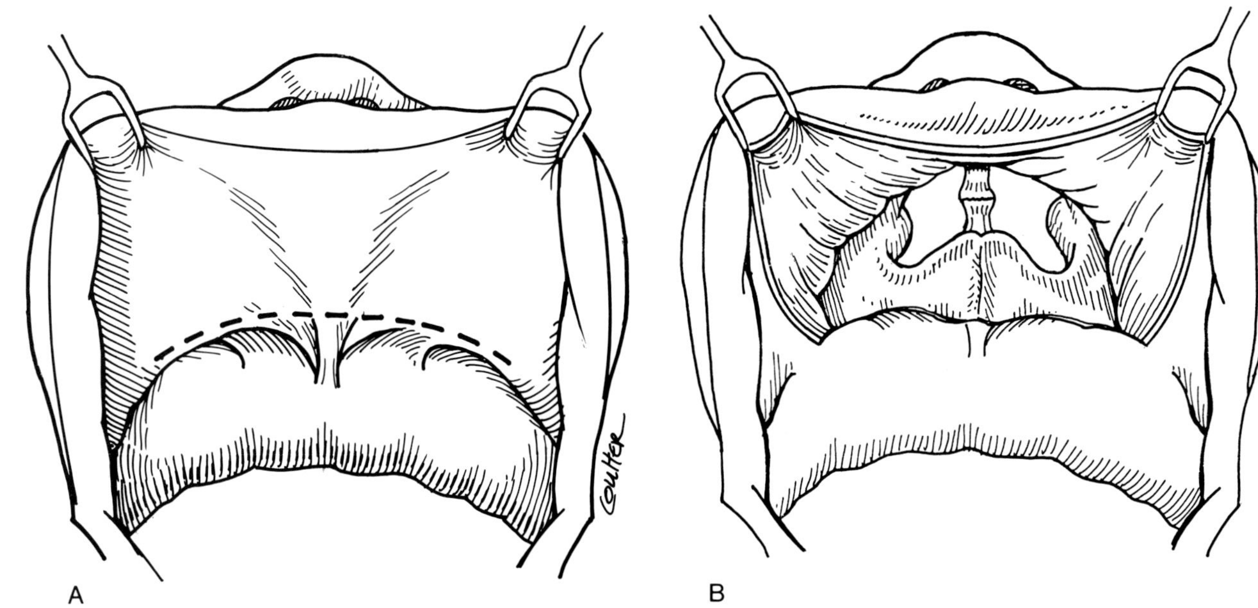

A B

• FIGURE 11-18.

A, A standard sublabial incision is used. *B*, The anterior spine is left attached to septal cartilage.

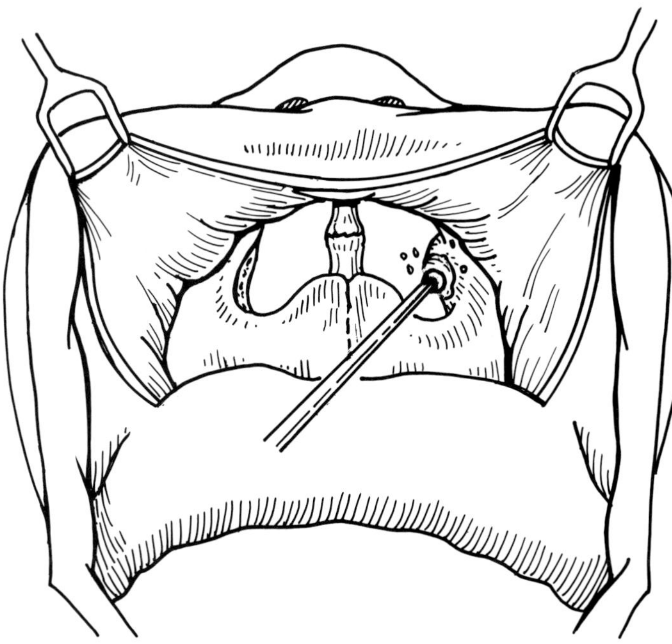

• FIGURE 11-19.

Removal of the bone of the pyriform aperture laterally and anteriorly.

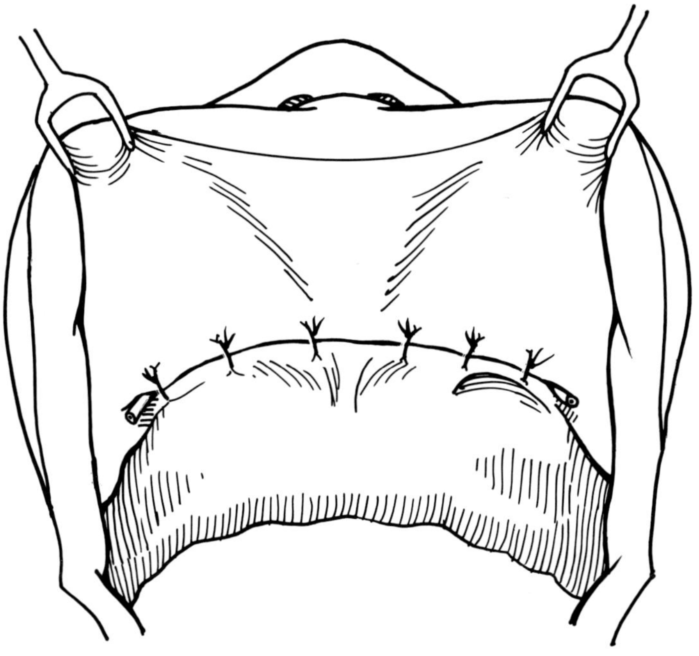

• FIGURE 11-20.

The sublabial incision is closed using an absorbable suture.

REFERENCES

1. Brown, OE, Myer CM, and Manning SC: Congenital nasal pyriform aperture stenosis. Laryngoscope 99:86–91, 1989.
2. Williams RG: An operation for relief of chronic nasal obstruction. J Laryngol Otol 89:527–530, 1975.
3. Hengerer AS and Newburg JA: Congenital malformations of the nose and paranasal sinuses. *In* Bluestone CD and Stool SE (eds): Pediatric Otolaryngology, 2nd ed. Philadelphia, WB Saunders, 1990, pp 718–728.
4. Hughes GB, Sharpino G, Hunt W, and Tucker HM: Management of the midline nasal mass: A review. Otolaryngol Head Neck Surg 2:222–233, 1980.
5. Pensler JM, Bauer BS, and Naidich TP: Craniofacial dermoids. Plast Reconstruct Surg 82:953–958, 1988.
6. Brown OE, Burns DK, Smith TH, and Rutledge JC: Bilateral posterior choanal atresia: A morphologic and histologic study, and computed tomographic correlation. Int J Pediatr Otorhinolaryngol 13:125–142, 1987.
7. Hengerer AS and Strome A: Choanal atresia: A new embryologic theory and its influence on surgical management. Laryngoscope 92:913–921, 1982.
8. Bergstrom L and Owens O: Posterior choanal atresia: A syndromal disorder. Laryngoscope 94:1273–1276, 1984.
9. Resouly A, Barnard JDW, and Purnell AN: Access by LeFort I osteotomy for correction of unilateral choanal atresia. Clin Otolaryngol 15:281–282, 1990.
10. Lang J: Clinical Anatomy of the Nose, Nasal and Paranasal Sinuses. New York, Thieme Medical Publishers, 1989.
11. Kenna MA: Transsphenoidal encephalocele. Ann Otol Rhinol Laryngol 94:520–522, 1985.
12. Krespi YP, Husain S, Levine TM, and Reede DL: Sublabial transseptal repair of choanal atresia or stenosis. Laryngoscope 97:1402–1406, 1987.
13. Stahl RS and Jurkiewicz MJ: Congenital posterior choanal atresia. Pediatrics 76:429–436, 1985.
14. Lantz HJ and Birck HG: Surgical correction of choanal atresia in the neonate. Laryngoscope 91:1629–1634, 1981.
15. Osguthorpe JD, Singleton GT, and Adkins WY: The surgical approach to bilateral choanal atresia. Arch Otolaryngol Head Neck Surg 108:366–369, 1982.
16. Healy GB, McGill T, Jako GJ et al: Management of choanal atresia with the carbon dioxide laser. Ann Otol Rhinol Laryngol 87:658–662, 1987.
17. Muntz H: Pitfalls to laser correction of choanal atresia. Ann Otol Rhinol Laryngol 96:43–46, 1987.
18. Stankiewicz JA: The endoscopic repair of choanal atresia. Otolaryngol Head Neck Surg 103:931–937, 1990.
19. Gleeson MJ and Hibbert J: A stent for the corrective management of bilateral choanal atresia. Laryngoscope 95:1409–1410, 1985.
20. Grundfast KM, Thomsen JR, and Barber CS: An improved stent method for choanal atresia repair. Laryngoscope 100:1132–1133, 1990.
21. Freng A: Growth in width of the dental arches after partial extirpation of the mid-palatal suture in man. Scand J Plast Reconstr Surg 12:267–272, 1978.

chapter

12

Cleft Lip and Palate

ROBERT W. SEIBERT, M.D.

ROTATION-ADVANCEMENT TECHNIQUE

Since first explained by Millard in the 1950s, the rotation-advancement (RA) technique has gained increasing acceptance as the method of choice for treatment of unilateral cleft lip. The basic principles of this technique have remained unchanged, although numerous, relatively minor refinements and modifications have been made. This is a flexible, "cut as you go" method that relies less on precise measurements and geometry than do other techniques, such as the triangular flap repair. Adjustments are relatively easy to make during the procedure, and precise positioning of the alar base and primary tip rhinoplasty are possible. Careful preoperative analysis of the individual patient's deformity, the specific challenges, and the best methods to meet these challenges accrue with experience and lead to optimal postoperative results.

Indications

- Any unilateral (and some milder bilateral) clefts (from minimal clefts to wide complete clefts, with or without a prior lip adhesion) are included. The "rule of ten" refers to deferment of the operation until the patient is at least 10 weeks of age, has 10 g/dl of hemoglobin, and weighs 10 lb. There has been a trend toward earlier lip closure, assuming that the child is otherwise healthy and that experienced pediatric anesthesia personnel are available.
- If a lip adhesion has been performed, the RA repair follows in 3 to 6 months. The RA repair may be done at 6 to 10 weeks of age if an adhesion is not required, assuming the aforementioned conditions.

Anesthetic considerations

General inhalation anesthesia by way of an endotracheal tube is usually used. A local anesthetic with a vasoconstrictor (Xylocaine 1% with epinephrine 1:100,000) may be infiltrated into the labial sulci and into areas of nasal incision for hemostasis, if desired.

Preparation

- An endotracheal tube is taped to the midline of the chin without distorting the lower lip.
- A roll is placed under the infant's shoulders to slightly extend the neck.
- The surgeon sits by the patient's head, and loupe magnification (2.5 to 3 ×) is usually used.
- A moist gauze pad (3 × 3″) is placed as an oropharyngeal pack.

Procedure

LANDMARKS (Fig. 12–1)

- The following points are determined and marked with gentian violet:

#1 — Nasal alar foot

#2 — Cupid's bow peak (lateral)

#3 — Cupid's bow midpoint

#4 — Cupid's bow peak (medial)

Distance #3 to #4 equals #2 to #3

NONCLEFT SIDE

#5 — The lateral limit of the *rotation incision* that raises the lip, curving laterally at the junction of the columella and the lip, does not extend into the normal philtral column but mirror-images it.

#6 — Limit of the *back-cut* of the rotation incision necessary in most cases to achieve enough downward rotation of the Cupid's bow.

#7 — Cupid's bow peak (lateral) corresponds to #4, usually located where the white roll above the vermillion cutaneous junction (VCJ) disappears.

CLEFT SIDE

#8 — The superior limit of the advancement flap is determined by the length from #4 to #6.

#9 — The distance along the alar crease (from #7 to #9) should equal that from #1 to #2 on the noncleft side for vertical lip lengths to be symmetric.

INCISIONS (Fig. 12–2)

- The labial sulci are injected with Xylocaine 1% with epinephrine 1:100,000.

- All incisions are made with a 6300 Beaver blade or a No. 15 Bard-Parker blade.

- The rotation incision (#4, #5, and #6) is made first until #4 lies at the same level as #2. Lip muscle is included in the back-cut, and lip is freed from the premaxilla as necessary. Skin that is left attached to the columella ("C" flap) may be used to lengthen the columella by advancing the flap on itself or to augment the medial nasal sill.

- A lateral cleft edge and circumalar incision are made (#7, #8, and #9) to create an advancement flap, which is freed from the maxilla in the supraperiosteal plane and is necessary in wider clefts, but dissection should be conservative.

- Incision in the nasal vestibule allows medial advancement of the alar base independent of the lip, which is unnecessary if the nasal deformity is mild.

- Mucosal flaps from the cleft edges or tissue of the lip adhesion may be used to close the alveolar cleft or may be discarded.

- The white roll flap just above the VCJ laterally is not cut until lip segments are approximated (see later). The white roll flap is a triangular flap of skin that measures the same height as the normal white roll and is usually $1\frac{1}{2}$ to $2\frac{1}{2}$ mm in length.

• FIGURE 12-1.

Rotation-advancement techniques. The landmarks and incisions described in the text are indicated. (Modified from Seibert RW and Bumstead RM: Cleft lip and palate. *In* Cummings CW, Fredrickson JM, Harker LA, et al [eds]: Otolaryngology—Head and Neck Surgery, 2nd ed., Vol II. St. Louis, Mosby-Year Book, 1991, p 1140.)

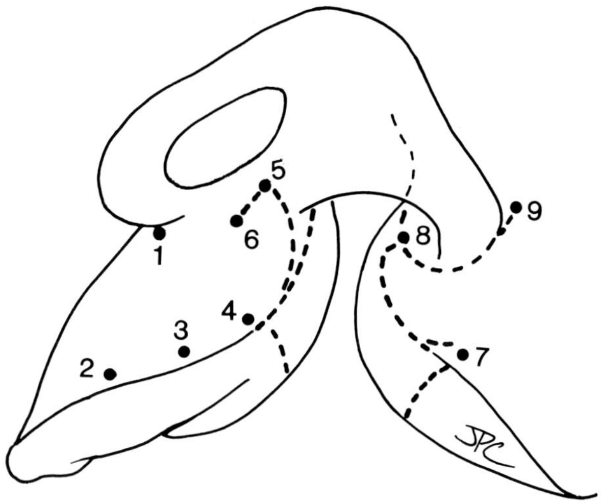

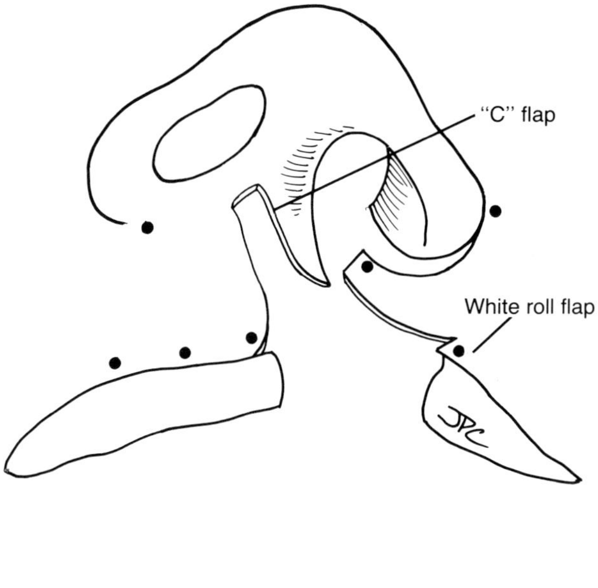

• FIGURE 12-2.

The flaps are incised and elevated. (Modified from Seibert RW and Bumstead RM: Cleft lip and palate. *In* Cummings CW, Fredrickson JM, Harker LA, et al [eds]: Otolaryngology—Head and Neck Surgery, 2nd ed., Vol II. St. Louis, Mosby-Year Book, 1991, p 1141.)

SUTURING (Figs. 12–3 and 12–4)

- A key suture (3-0 or 4-0 Vicryl) is placed deeply from the back-cut to the superior edge of the advancement flap at or lateral to #9. This advances the lateral lip better in wide clefts with deficient vertical height and produces more normal convexity to the lip.

- The alar base is sutured to the anterior nasal spine (using a 4-0 Vicryl suture) in symmetry with the noncleft side. Care is taken not to narrow the nostril too much. There should be minimal, if any, trimming of the alar foot to avoid excessive narrowing of the nostril, which is a difficult secondary deformity to correct later.

- Approximation of the orbicularis oris muscles with a 4-0 or 5-0 Vicryl suture is done, and care is taken not to shorten the lip.

- The skin edges are trimmed and slightly undermined as necessary.

- A white roll flap is cut, as described earlier. If rotation in a slightly more downward direction is required, an incision at the VCJ (#3) is made. If rotation is adequate, a triangular skin excision the same dimension as the flap is made. Subcutaneous 6-0 chromic or Vicryl suture approximates the flap medially.

- The "C" flap is advanced on itself to lengthen the columella or is trimmed for nasal sill reconstruction.

- Skin edges are sutured with a simple, everting 7-0 or 6-0 nylon suture.

- The vermillion is approximated snugly with 4-0 or 5-0 Vicryl in the muscle to avoid notching (whistle deformity).

- The mucosae are approximated with a 5-0 or 6-0 chromic suture. The incision may lend itself to broken line closure, or a Z-plasty may be done to help decrease any tendency to contracture with healing.

SUMMARY

- The goal is to create a perfectly symmetric lip/nose contour by matching the abnormal cleft to the normal noncleft side.

- The final appearance of the lip after healing and scar maturation will be what is achieved at the end of the operation. Scars will improve with time, but discrepancies in form will not. Constant assessment and adjustment during the procedure are required.

• FIGURE 12-3.

Placements of key suture advances on the lateral lip medially. (Modified from Seibert RW and Bumstead RM: Cleft lip and palate. *In* Cummings CW, Fredrickson JM, Harker LA, et al [eds]: Otolaryngology—Head and Neck Surgery, 2nd ed., Vol II. St. Louis, Mosby-Year Book, 1991, p 1141.)

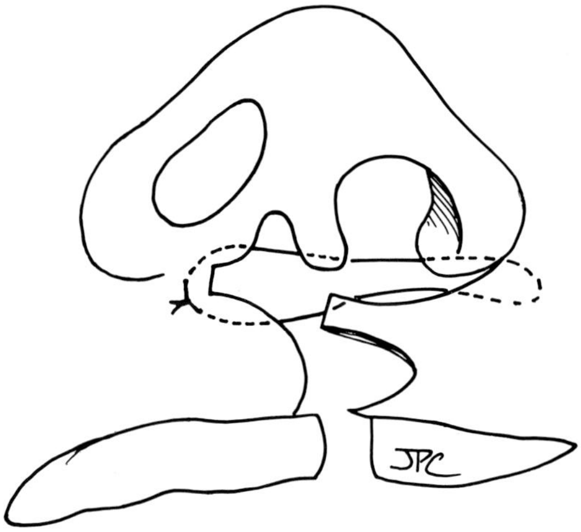

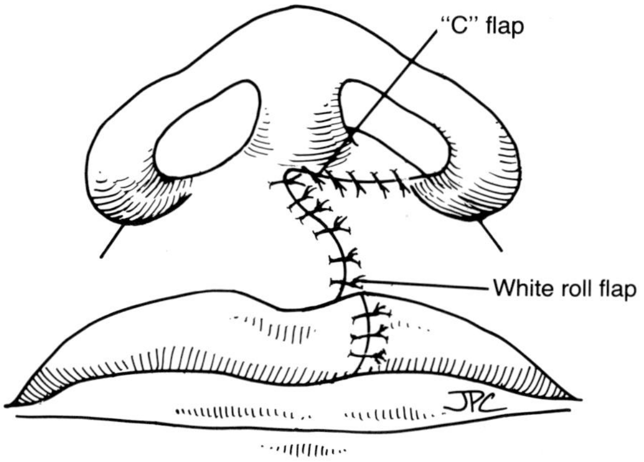

• FIGURE 12-4.

Final suturing. (Modified from Seibert RW and Bumstead RM: Cleft lip and palate. *In* Cummings CW, Fredrickson JM, Harker LA, et al [eds]: Otolaryngology—Head and Neck Surgery, 2nd ed., Vol II. St. Louis, Mosby-Year Book, 1991, p 1141.)

Postoperative care/complications

IMMEDIATE

- A tongue tip suture (3-0 silk) is placed to aid in airway management. The suture is usually removed in the recovery room.
- The pharyngeal pack is removed, and the throat and stomach are suctioned.
- Arm restraints are applied in the recovery room and are worn by the patient constantly for 10 days.

FEEDINGS

- Feedings begin on the morning after the procedure, using an Asepto syringe with rubber tubing, and are continued for 10 days.

SUTURE CARE

- A small amount of antibiotic ointment is applied to the sutures two to three times/day.
- Hydrogen peroxide cleaning of the sutures is not done unless there is a large amount of crusty, dried blood.
- The sutures are removed after 6 or 7 days with the patient under sedation (meperidine, 1 to 2 mg/kg intramuscularly [IM]).

COMPLICATIONS

- Wound infection is very rare. Stitch abscesses occur occasionally with the use of Vicryl.
- Hypertrophic scars with contraction and elevation of Cupid's bow peak occur occasionally but correct themselves as the scars mature.

LIP ADHESION

Lip adhesion operations are preliminary or first-stage procedures that are beneficial in the most severe and widest cleft lip deformities. Since described in the 1960s, they have been recognized as facilitating definitive lip closure (cheiloplasty) by decreasing tension, improving nasal symmetry, and narrowing alveolar clefts. The procedure may be performed either low in the lip (vermillion), which minimizes soft tissue undermining from the maxilla, or by a superior lip–nasal sill adhesion, which is the technique described below. Although often requiring some degree of dissection of the lip from the maxilla, this technique provides relief from excessive tension where the basic deficiency is greatest—high in the lip.

Indications

- A *very wide*, complete unilateral cleft lip in which a definitive procedure could be performed only under excessive tension
- The infant should be at least 3 to 4 weeks of age and should have gained weight and have no other significant, untreated medical problems.

Anesthetic considerations

- A general anesthetic is preferred, although a local anesthetic (Xylocaine 1% with epinephrine 1:100,000) may be used.

Preparation

- An endotracheal tube is taped to the midline of the chin without distorting the lower lip.
- A roll is placed under the infant's shoulders to slightly extend the neck.
- The surgeon sits by the patient's head, and loupe magnification (2.5 to 3 ×) is usually used.
- A moist gauze pad (3 × 3″) is placed as an oropharyngeal pack.

Procedure

LANDMARKS AND INCISIONS (Fig. 12–5)

- Landmarks for a definitive procedure are determined (see the RA method) and marked with gentian violet. Cleft edge mucosa/vermillion flaps are placed well away from definitive landmarks.

FLAP ELEVATION AND UNDERMINING (Fig. 12–6)

- A 6300 Beaver blade is used to incise and elevate the cleft edge mucosal flaps.
- Incisions along the pyramidal aperture of the nasal vestibule (*dotted line* in Fig. 12–6) free the alar sill for medial advancement.
- Undermining of the lip from the maxilla should be minimal, especially laterally and in the supraperiosteal plane.

SUTURING (Figs. 12–7 and 12–8)

- All deep sutures are placed before tying.
- A retention suture (3-0 nylon) is placed through the membranous septum, deep into the lateral lip/alar incision and back through the septum.
- Mucosal sutures, usually (three or four) of 4-0 or 5-0 chromic catgut are placed.
- Muscle/subcutaneous sutures (usually three or four) of 4-0 or 5-0 Vicryl are placed.
- All of the aforementioned sutures are tied in sequence.
- The skin/vermillion closure is completed with a 7-0 nylon suture.

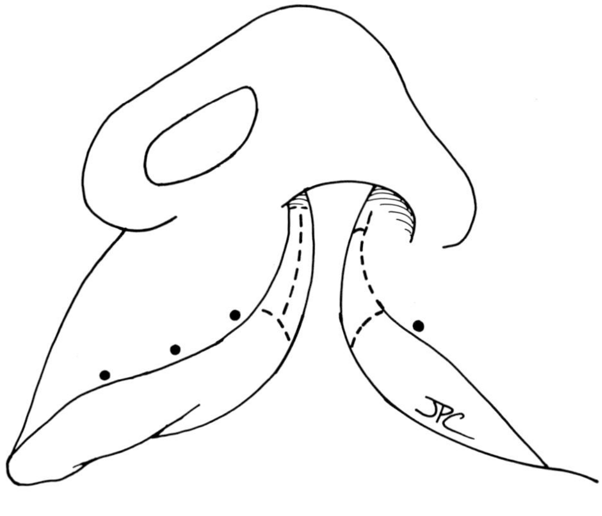

• FIGURE 12–5.

Unilateral lip adhesion: landmarks and incisions. (Modified from Seibert RW and Bumstead RM: Cleft lip and palate. *In* Cummings CW, Fredrickson JM, Harker LA, et al [eds]: Otolaryngology—Head and Neck Surgery, 2nd ed., Vol II. St. Louis, Mosby-Year Book, 1991, p 1137.)

• FIGURE 12-6.

The flaps are elevated and undermined (*stippled area*). (Modified from Seibert RW and Bumstead RM: Cleft lip and palate. *In* Cummings CW, Fredrickson JM, Harker LA, et al [eds]: Otolaryngology—Head and Neck Surgery, 2nd ed., Vol II. St. Louis, Mosby-Year Book, 1991, p 1137.)

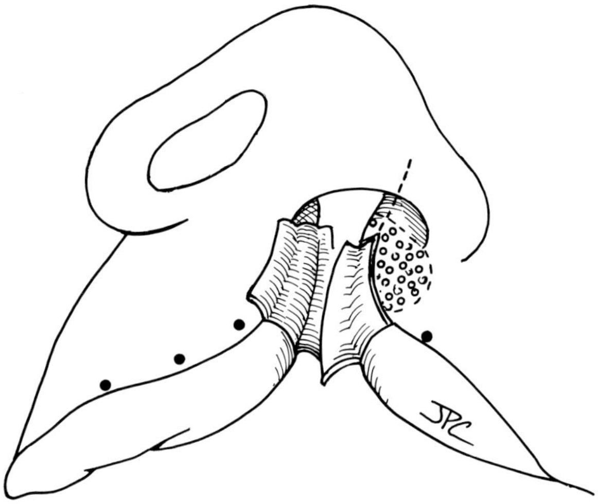

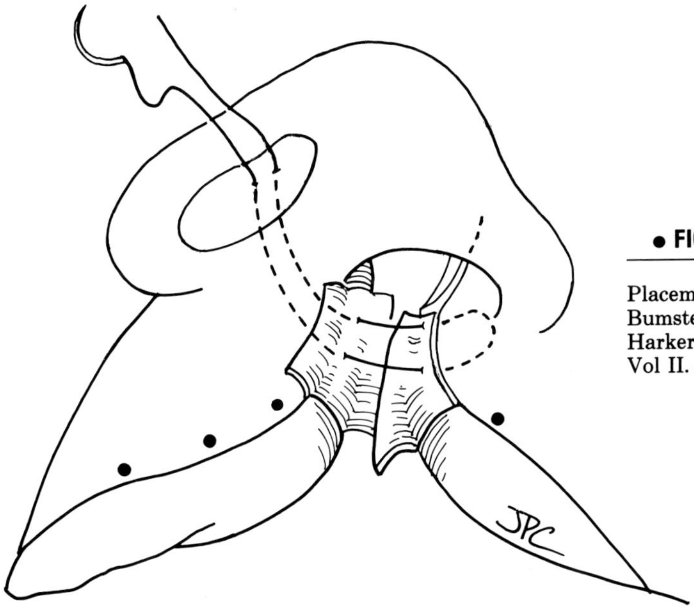

• FIGURE 12-7.

Placement of a 3-0 nylon retention suture. (Modified from Seibert RW and Bumstead RM: Cleft lip and palate. *In* Cummings CW, Fredrickson JM, Harker LA, et al [eds]: Otolaryngology—Head and Neck Surgery, 2nd ed., Vol II. St. Louis, Mosby-Year Book, 1991, p 1137.)

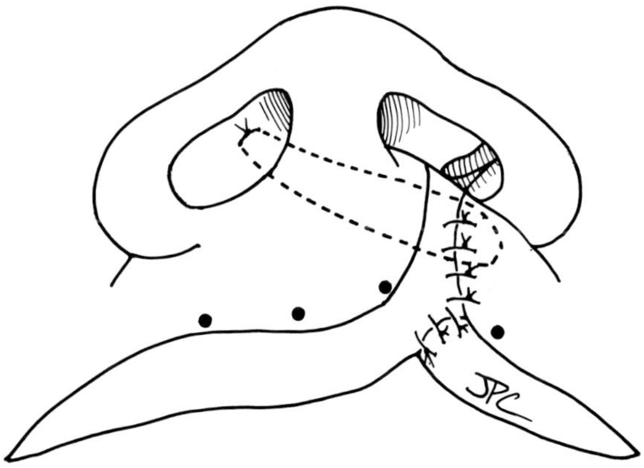

• FIGURE 12-8.

Final suturing. (Modified from Seibert RW and Bumstead RM: Cleft lip and palate. *In* Cummings CW, Fredrickson JM, Harker LA, et al [eds]: Otolaryngology—Head and Neck Surgery, 2nd ed., Vol II. St. Louis, Mosby-Year Book, 1991, p 1137.)

Postoperative care/complications

IMMEDIATE

- A tongue tip suture (3-0 silk) is placed to aid in airway management. The suture is usually removed in the recovery room.
- The pharyngeal pack is removed, and the throat and stomach are suctioned.
- Arm restraints are applied in the recovery room and are worn by the patient constantly for 10 days.

FEEDINGS

- Feedings begin on the morning after the procedure using an Asepto syringe with rubber tubing and are continued for 10 days.

SUTURE CARE

- A small amount of antibiotic ointment is applied to the sutures two to three times/day.
- Hydrogen peroxide cleaning of the sutures is not done unless there is a large amount of crusty, dried blood.
- The sutures are removed after 7 to 10 days with the patient under sedation (meperidine, 1 to 2 mg/kg intramuscularly [IM]).

COMPLICATIONS

- Breakdown of adhesion

  This is usually caused by excessive tension and not by infection.

  The incidence of complete separation is approximately 5%.

  Separation of the lower (vermillion) part of the adhesion is more common and does not affect the goals of the procedure.

- Scarring

  Interference with the definitive procedure is possible if landmarks are violated.

- Maxillary growth disturbance

  This is a controversial subject with no clear-cut (human) data; thus, it is best to avoid the maxillary periosteum.

CLEFT PALATE REPAIR—PALATOPLASTY

The purpose of palatoplasty is to construct an intact and physiologically adequate palatovelar mechanism for normal speech production. Its ultimate goals are normal naso-oral resonance, effortless production of non-nasal sounds in speech, and the absence of abnormal compensatory articulation patterns such as glottal stops and pharyngeal fricatives. Other goals include the anatomic separation of the nasal and oral cavities, elimination of nasal reflux of food and secretions, and possible improvement of eustachian tube function.

Indications

- Many methods of palatoplasty have been devised. Two single-stage procedures are described in this chapter: one for clefts of the secondary palate only (clefts that begin at or posterior to the incisive foramen)—the push-back palatoplasty or V-Y repair— and one for clefts of the secondary palate in which the alveolar ridge and the lip are involved as well—two-flap palatoplasty.
- The best age for palatoplasty is controversial. While delay of mucoperiosteal elevation from the hard palate may be optimal for maxillofacial growth, waiting for more than 18 months of age may result in more secondary operations (pharyngeal flaps) to achieve velopharyngeal competency for speech. Data suggest that the ideal age for speech production may be 9 to 12 months.
- Timing also depends on sufficient palatal shelf width for closure (it is *extremely* rare to have insufficient tissue) and adequate body size (at least 7 kg, which seems to minimize upper airway risks).

Anesthetic considerations

- A general anesthetic is always used.
- Xylocaine 1% with epinephrine 1:100,000 (0.5 ml/kg) is injected into the incision areas of the palate for hemostasis.

Preparation

- An endotracheal tube is taped in the midline to the lower lip and chin.
- The endotracheal tube is secured further by the slotted tongue blade of the Dingman oral retractor.
- The Dingman retractor is opened only widely enough to allow adequate exposure without undue pressure on the tongue or compression of the endotracheal tube.
- A folded towel may be placed beneath the retractor handle but is usually not suspended from the Mayo stand.
- A roll is placed under the patient's shoulders to slightly extend the neck.
- The surgeon sits or stands at the head of the table. Headlight illumination is desirable.

Procedure

PUSH-BACK (V-Y) PALATOPLASTY

Landmarks and Incisions (Figs. 12–9 and 12–10)

- Figure 12–9 shows a typical incomplete cleft of the secondary palate. Note the position of the neurovascular bundles (VB), the vomer (V), and the posterior edge of the hard palate (P). The shaded area represents the premaxilla, which, with the lip, comprises the primary palate.

- A medial (cleft edge) incision is made 2 to 3 mm lateral to the cleft margin.

- The lateral incision extends from slightly anterior to the cleft apex posteriorly to just behind the maxillary tuberosity over the hamular process of the medial pterygoid plate. The neurovascular bundle is just medial to the incision.

- Medial and lateral incisions are connected by an oblique incision. All incisions over the bone are made through the periosteum.

- An incision is made in the vomer midline if vomer flaps are used.

Flap Elevation and Undermining (Fig. 12–11)

- Mucoperiosteal flaps are elevated easily by blunt dissection with a Freer elevator.

- Blunt dissection posteriorly in a plane between the constrictor muscle and the pterygoid muscle allows medial mobility of the velar segments.

- Infracturing of the hamulus and stripping of the veli palatini tendon are necessary in wide clefts.

- The neurovascular bundle is preserved and may be lengthened by incising the periosteum on both sides of the bundle's attachment to the flap (see *inset* in Fig. 12–11). Bone medial to the bundle may be removed with a rongeur or drill to gain additional length in wide clefts.

- The mucoperiosteal flap is elevated from the vomer by dental-type (Woodson) elevators.

- All soft tissue is completely freed from the medial and posterior edges of the hard palate. Sharp dissection is necessary to elevate tissue from the suture just behind the neurovascular bundle.

- Care should be taken to avoid or minimize dissection at the vomeropremaxillary suture (growth center) in complete clefts.

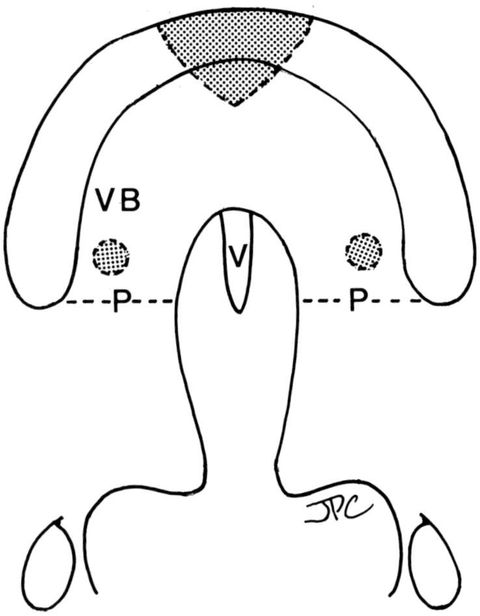

• FIGURE 12-9.

Landmarks in push-back palatoplasty.

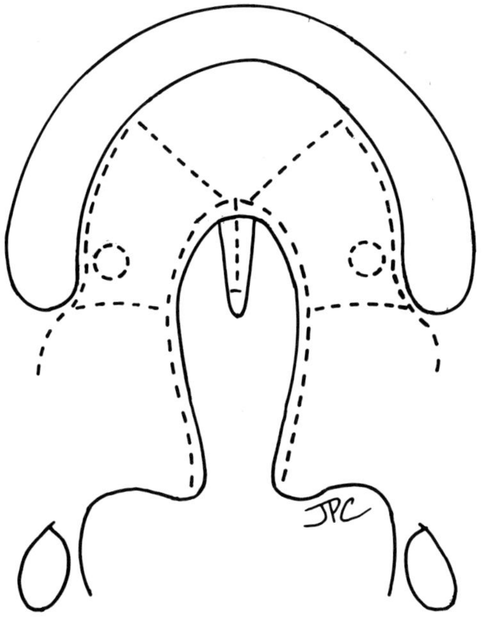

• FIGURE 12-10.

Incisions in push-back palatoplasty.

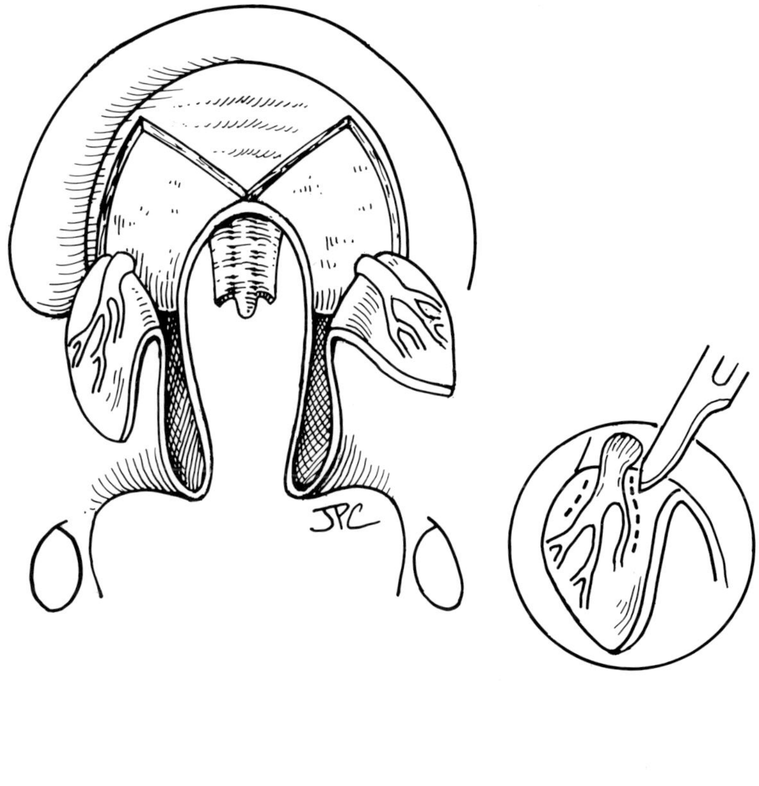

• FIGURE 12-11.

The flaps are elevated and undermined. The neurovascular bundle is preserved (*inset*).

Flap Suturing (Figs. 12–12 and 12–13)

- Closure begins by approximating the nasal mucoperiosteum side to side or to vomer flaps (using 4-0 or 5-0 chromic catgut or Vicryl) and by continuing posteriorly to the mucosa of the velum and the uvula, with knots placed on the nasal side.
- A levator muscle sling is reconstructed using several 4-0 or 3-0 Vicryl sutures, placed horizontally, to approximate the velar muscles.
- Closure is carried anteriorly along the periosteum of the oral layer.
- The oral and nasal layers are brought into contact with 4-0 Vicryl sutures.
- The oral mucosae are approximated with interrupted simple or running 4-0 or 5-0 chromic catgut sutures.
- Any gaping areas laterally are packed with microfibrillar collagen (Avitene) for hemostasis and for covering exposed bone.

TWO-FLAP PALATOPLASTY

Incisions (Fig. 12–14)

- The incision at the cleft edge extends to the vomeropremaxillary suture on the noncleft side, then laterally and just medial to the alveolar ridge, then posteriorly as described earlier for push-back palatoplasty.
- On the cleft side (lesser palatal) segment, a medial incision extends anteriorly to the alveolar ridge and curves laterally and then posteriorly.

• FIGURE 12-12.

The flaps are sutured.

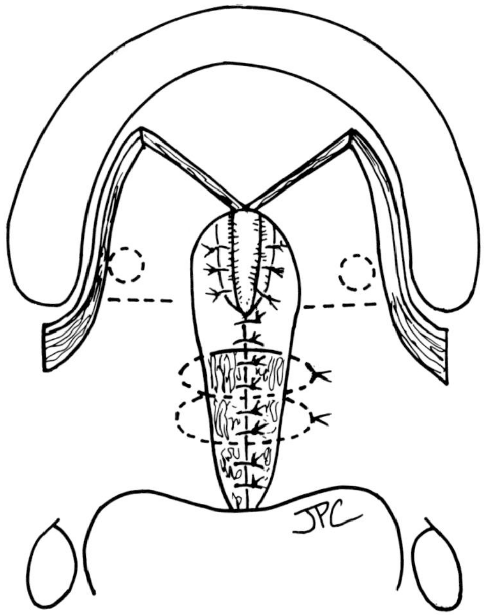

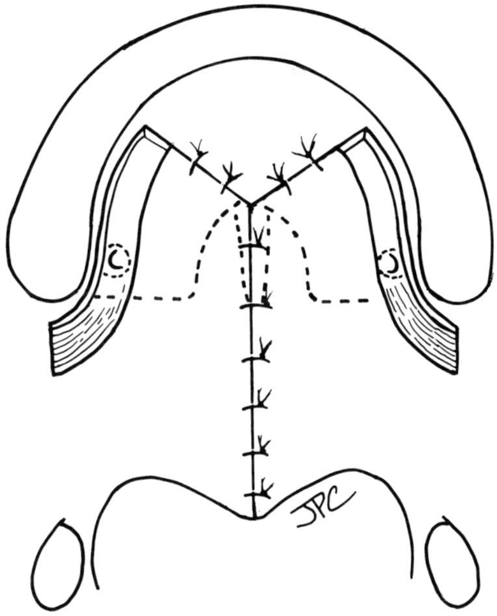

• FIGURE 12-13.

The closure is completed.

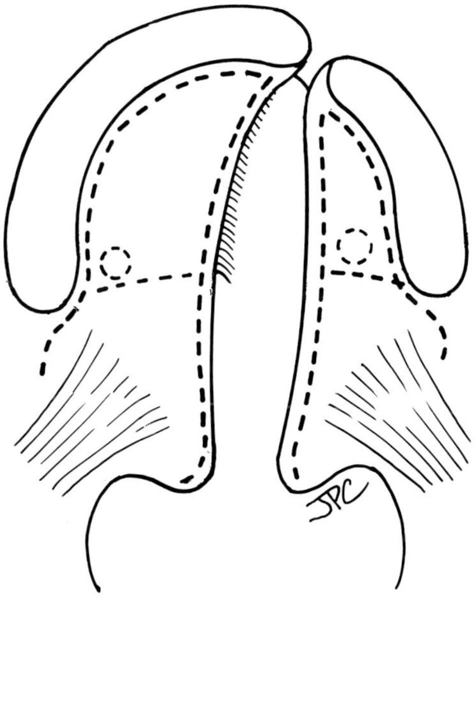

• FIGURE 12-14.

Incisions in a two-flap palatoplasty. (Modified from Seibert RW and Bumstead RM: Cleft lip and palate. *In* Cummings CW, Fredrickson JM, Harker LA, et al [eds]: Otolaryngology—Head and Neck Surgery, 2nd ed., Vol II. St. Louis, Mosby-Year Book, 1991, p 1150.)

Flap Elevation (Fig. 12–15)

- Mucoperiosteal flaps are elevated by a Woodson elevator from the vomer and the nasal layer of the hard palate (lesser segment).
- Large mucoperiosteal flaps are elevated from the hard palate by a Freer elevator.
- Dissection of the velum neurovascular bundles is the same as described earlier for push-back palatoplasty.

Suturing (Figs. 12–16 and 12–17)

- The vomer and nasal palatal mucoperiosteal flaps are approximated with 4-0 or 5-0 Vicryl or chromic catgut with the knots on the nasal side.
- The levator sling and oral closure are the same as for push-back palatoplasty.
- The anterior ends of the mucoperiosteal flaps are sutured to the alveolar mucoperiosteum to close the alveolar cleft, if possible.

Postoperative care/complications

- The main risk is airway obstruction and bleeding.
- Hemostasis is ensured by meticulous electrocautery; Avitene packing; and firm pressure held on the hard palate for 5 to 10 minutes, if necessary.
- If the tongue is severely compressed, to ensure airway patency the mouth gag is released for several minutes, every 15 minutes during the procedure.
- A suture is placed through the tip of the tongue to control the position of the tongue during recovery from anesthesia, and this suture is usually removed in the recovery room.
- The pharynx and nose are suctioned and the stomach is decompressed prior to extubation.

FEEDINGS

- The patient is given nothing by mouth (NPO) for 24 hours. Feedings are given using a cup or syringe, and the patient is discharged home when his or her oral intake is adequate.
- Bottle feeding is not allowed for 3 to 4 weeks.
- Arm restraints are worn for 3 to 4 weeks when the child is alone.
- The first postoperative recheck is in 3 to 4 weeks.

ANTIBIOTICS

- Parenteral penicillin, ampicillin, or cephalosporin is begun immediately preoperatively and is continued for 5 days orally.
- Analgesics such as acetaminophen are given, orally or by suppository (20 mg/kg), on discharge from the hospital.

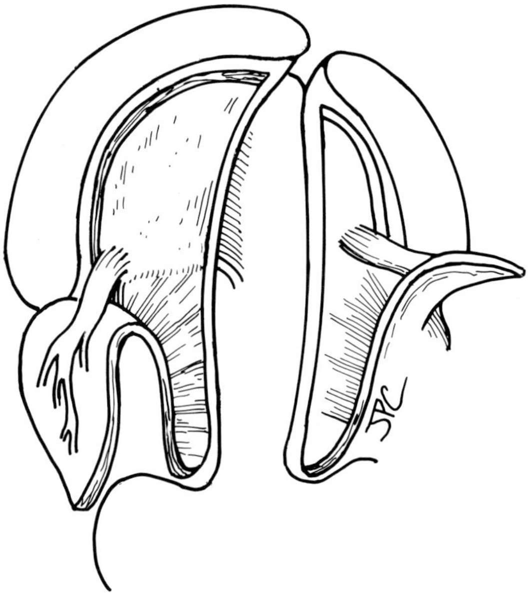

• FIGURE 12-15.

The flaps are incised and elevated. (Modified from Seibert RW and Bumstead RM: Cleft lip and palate. *In* Cummings CW, Fredrickson JM, Harker LA, et al [eds]: Otolaryngology—Head and Neck Surgery, 2nd ed., Vol II. St. Louis, Mosby-Year Book, 1991, p 1150.)

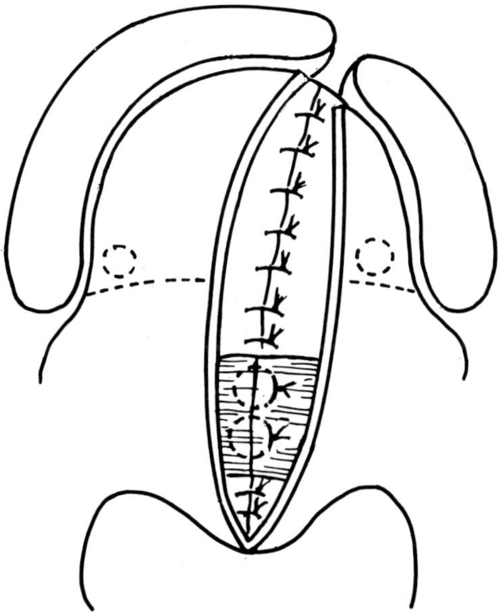

• FIGURE 12-16.

Nasal mucosa and mucoperiosteal closure and levator reconstruction. (Modified from Seibert RW and Bumstead RM: Cleft lip and palate. *In* Cummings CW, Fredrickson JM, Harker LA, et al [eds]: Otolaryngology—Head and Neck Surgery, 2nd ed., Vol II. St. Louis, Mosby-Year Book, 1991, p 1151.)

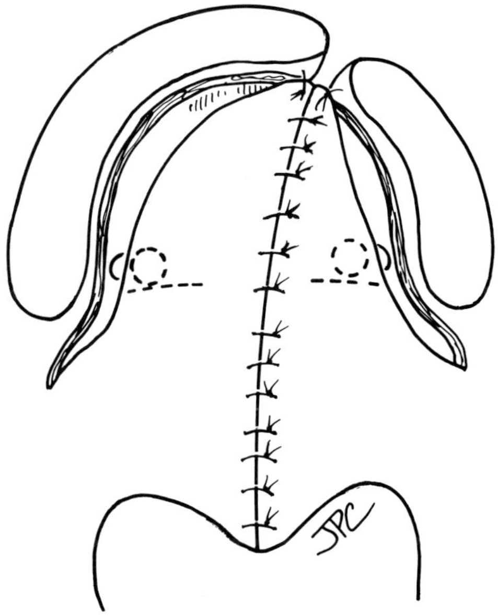

• FIGURE 12-17.

Oral layer closure. (Modified from Seibert RW and Bumstead RM: Cleft lip and palate. *In* Cummings CW, Fredrickson JM, Harker LA, et al [eds]: Otolaryngology—Head and Neck Surgery, 2nd ed., Vol II. St. Louis, Mosby-Year Book, 1991, p 1151.)

COMPLICATIONS

AIRWAY

- Severe or prolonged upper airway obstruction is uncommon unless an underlying anomaly (e.g., Robin's sequence, Treacher Collins syndrome) is present. Such patients may require prolonged observation in the intensive care unit. Airway management may range from maintaining tongue traction with a suture and positioning to prolonged intubation or tracheostomy in rare cases.

BLEEDING

- Late bleeding (5 to 7 days) from the raw edge of the flap is rare, especially if Avitene is used to pack relaxing incisions.

BREAKDOWN/FISTULA

- If the alveolar cleft is not closed at primary cheiloplasty, a fistula usually remains with a two-flap technique.
- A small (1- to 2-mm) fistula at the hard palate–soft palate junction, where the mucoperiosteum is thinnest, may occur with the push-back method.
- More extensive breakdown is rare unless the greater palatine artery is sacrificed by dividing the neurovascular bundle. Greater risk occurs with a two-flap technique, in which necrosis of the distal flap is possible. This occurs especially in older children and adults.

BIBLIOGRAPHY

Bardach J and Morris H: Multidisciplinary Management of Cleft Lip and Palate. Philadelphia, WB Saunders, 1990.

Millard DR Jr: Cleft Craft—The Evolution of Its Surgery. I: The Unilateral Deformity. Boston, Little, Brown, 1976.

Millard DR Jr: Cleft Craft—The Evolution of Its Surgery. III: Alveolar and Palatal Deformities. Boston, Little, Brown, 1980.

chapter

13

Pediatric Endoscopic Ethmoidectomy

RODNEY P. LUSK, M.D.

Considerable judgment needs to be used in deciding when to perform ethmoidectomy. There are no prospective studies to help guide this decision, and the indications for pediatric endoscopic sinus surgery are the subject of controversy. For example, questions remain about the role of adenoidectomy and nasal antral windows in the treatment of chronic sinusitis in children; these issues are discussed elsewhere.[1-7] As a matter of principle, all possible medical forms of management should be exhausted before proceeding to surgery.

Indications

- Chronic sinusitis that has failed to respond to aggressive medical management and evidence of disease on coronal computed tomography (CT) scan
- Recurrent acute sinusitis with anatomic abnormalities
- Persistent sinusitis after failed medical management of allergies
- Polyposis secondary to
  - Cystic fibrosis
  - Aspirin-sensitivity triad
  - Nonallergic NARES syndrome
- Mucocele of the sinuses
- Choanal antral polyps
- Complications of chronic sinusitis
  - Nasal obstruction
  - Headaches
  - Postnasal drip
- Symptomatic retention cysts
- Noninvasive mycoses

RELATIVE INDICATIONS

- Asthma in patients with chronic sinusitis
- Otitis media secondary to chronic sinusitis (proceed usually after failed adenoidectomy)
- Acute orbital complications such as subperiosteal abscess (requires superior surgical skill and judgment)
- Ethmoidectomy associated with intracranial complications
- Massive disease secondary to cystic fibrosis (requires extensive experience and skill)

RELATIVE CONTRAINDICATIONS

- Acute sinusitis
- Bleeding disorders that have not been corrected
- Recent history of aspirin ingestion (within 1 week)
- Any contraindication to a general anesthetic

CONDITIONS ASSOCIATED WITH ETHMOIDECTOMY

ADENOID HYPERTROPHY

Nasal obstruction secondary to an obstructive adenoid pad can mimic all the signs and symptoms of sinusitis. The keys to identifying nasal obstruction are hyponasal speech (best detected by saying the letter N or a series of n-sounds, like "*nine, nine, nine*"), lack of nasal airway, and bluish nasal mucosae noted on anterior rhinoscopy. If the child is old enough to blow the nose, clearing the secretions will improve visualization and help to ascertain nasal patency. Otherwise, the least invasive way to assess nasal patency is to place a large laryngeal mirror under each nostril. If the airway is patent, the mirror will fog; if there is no air movement, there will be no fogging. (The fogging is not quantitative, however; that is, the degree of patency cannot be measured in this manner.)

The next step is to vasoconstrict the airway with oxymetazoline (0.05%) and lidocaine 4% in a 1:1 solution. After several minutes the nose is re-examined with an otoscope, mirror, or flexible nasopharyngoscope. With the flexible scope, the nasopharynx can be examined and the degree of obstruction from the adenoid pad can be assessed. Assessment of significant obstruction is a judgment call. If there is doubt about the degree of obstruction, it is best to re-examine the patient after empiric treatment with a course of antibiotics.

SYSTEMIC DISEASES

Several systemic diseases predispose the patient to chronic sinusitis. In our experience, it is most cost-effective to evaluate the patient by taking a careful history and to select patients for a more extensive evaluation. It is important to diagnose systemic problems preoperatively so that the underlying problem can be treated and the parents can be given a realistic prediction of the surgical outcome. It is particularly important to rule out recurrent upper respiratory tract infections as a cause of chronic sinusitis-like symptoms.[8] Specific diseases to inquire about follow.

Cystic Fibrosis

Polyps in the nose of a child are relatively rare and may indicate an underlying systemic disease. The most likely systemic disease is cystic fibrosis, which has a very high incidence of polyposis. Although this condition is normally known prior to evaluation, we have had patients in whom the earliest manifestation of cystic fibrosis is sinusitis, with pulmonary infections or gastrointestinal symptoms yet to appear.

It is my impression that sinusitis has a variable expression in cystic fibrosis. Most patients with cystic fibrosis were suspected of having this disease when polyps were noted in the nose, and the diagnosis was confirmed by a sweat test. This test, which is relatively inexpensive and painless, should be considered in most pediatric patients. If polyps, recurrent bronchitis, or gastrointestinal symptoms are noted, the sweat test must be obtained preoperatively. If the patient has cystic fibrosis, the chance of a recurrence of polyps and sinus disease is much higher.

Immune Deficiency

Children with immune deficiencies also have a much higher incidence of chronic sinusitis.[9] The types of immune deficiencies range from transient selective IgG subtype deficiency to common variable immune deficiency. Treatment with broad-spectrum antibiotics and gamma globulin has virtually eliminated the life-threatening infections. However, chronic sinusitis remains a persistent problem.

DIAGNOSIS OF SINUSITIS

SIGNS AND SYMPTOMS

Although no signs and symptoms are diagnostic of sinusitis, the signs and symptoms are the reason for medical or surgical intervention. The symptoms most consistent with sinusitis are purulent nasal discharge, nasal obstruction, and cough that is more common at night but more significant if present during the day. Purulent rhinorrhea is more common in younger children, whereas postnasal drip (rarely documented in the office) is a common complaint in older children. Pain is reported variably as irritability, headache, or facial pain. Low-grade fever is a frequent complaint but is rarely documented in the office.

PHYSICAL EXAMINATION

The physical examination is not diagnostic for chronic sinusitis. In cooperative children, anterior rhinoscopy is all that can be performed, regardless of the method used. If the child struggles and moves the head, the speculum will hit the septum and cause more discomfort. Then the alae of the nose contract, making it difficult to insert the speculum. Crying and tearing further obstruct visualization of the nose. The flexible scope, however, can be placed without fear of damaging the nose or causing excess pain to the child. The flexible scope is best for examining the nasopharynx and the adenoid pad. It cannot be rolled into the middle meatus as a rigid scope can in adults. A 2.7-mm rigid Hopkins rod lens telescope can be used in cooperative children after the nose is anesthetized with a 1:1 mixture of 0.05% oxymetazoline and 4% lidocaine (Fig. 13–1).

We have found that anterior rhinoscopy can be performed most easily with an otoscope. Children are familiar with this instrument, and there is a good chance that a child who allows otoscopy will allow rhinoscopy. The otoscope has several advantages: (1) a good light source, (2) a speculum that will displace the vibracea of the nose, (3) a lens for magnification, and (4) a lens that will not fog if the child breathes through the nose.

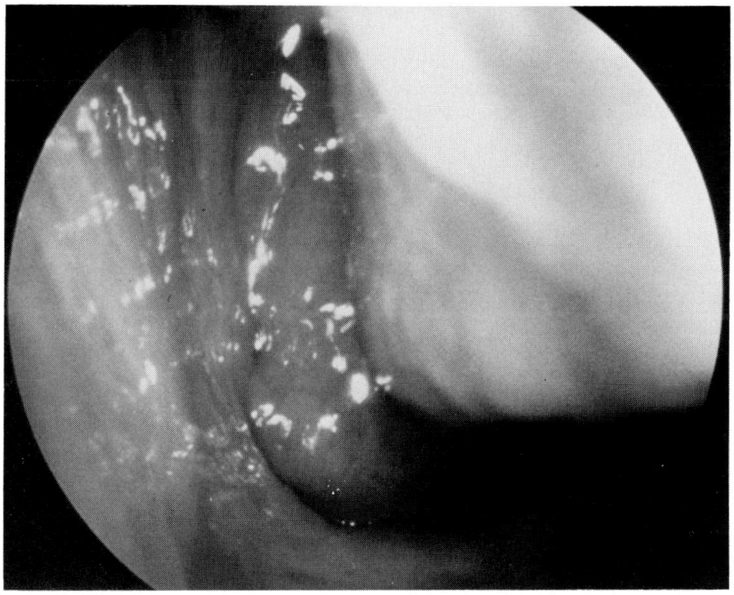

• FIGURE 13-1.

Adenoid hypertrophy causing symptoms of obstruction and sinusitis.

RADIOLOGY

Plain films have long been used to diagnose sinusitis, but it is now understood that they do not provide enough information to accurately assess the state of disease in the ethmoid sinuses. In a prospective study performed at St. Louis Children's Hospital,[10] a significant discrepancy was noted between plain films and coronal CT scans obtained within a few hours of one another. All patients had received aggressive medical management that failed and were being considered for ethmoidectomy. There was a lack of correlation between plain films and CT scans in 74% of the patients. Discrepancies between individual sinuses were 29% for the ethmoid sinuses and 23% for the maxillary sinuses. Mucosal thickening revealed by CT scans is usually seen as opacification on the plain films (Fig. 13–2*A* and *B*).

Because most acute sinusitis cases resolve spontaneously, and because CT scans cannot distinguish chronic from acute sinusitis, CT scans should be obtained only when sinus disease persists after full-dose antibiotic therapy for 3 to 4 weeks. Both the physician and the parents must ask themselves what they are going to do with the information from a scan. If the parents or the physician do not wish to proceed with surgery, there would appear to be little reason to do a scan, because the decision not to proceed with surgery has already been made.

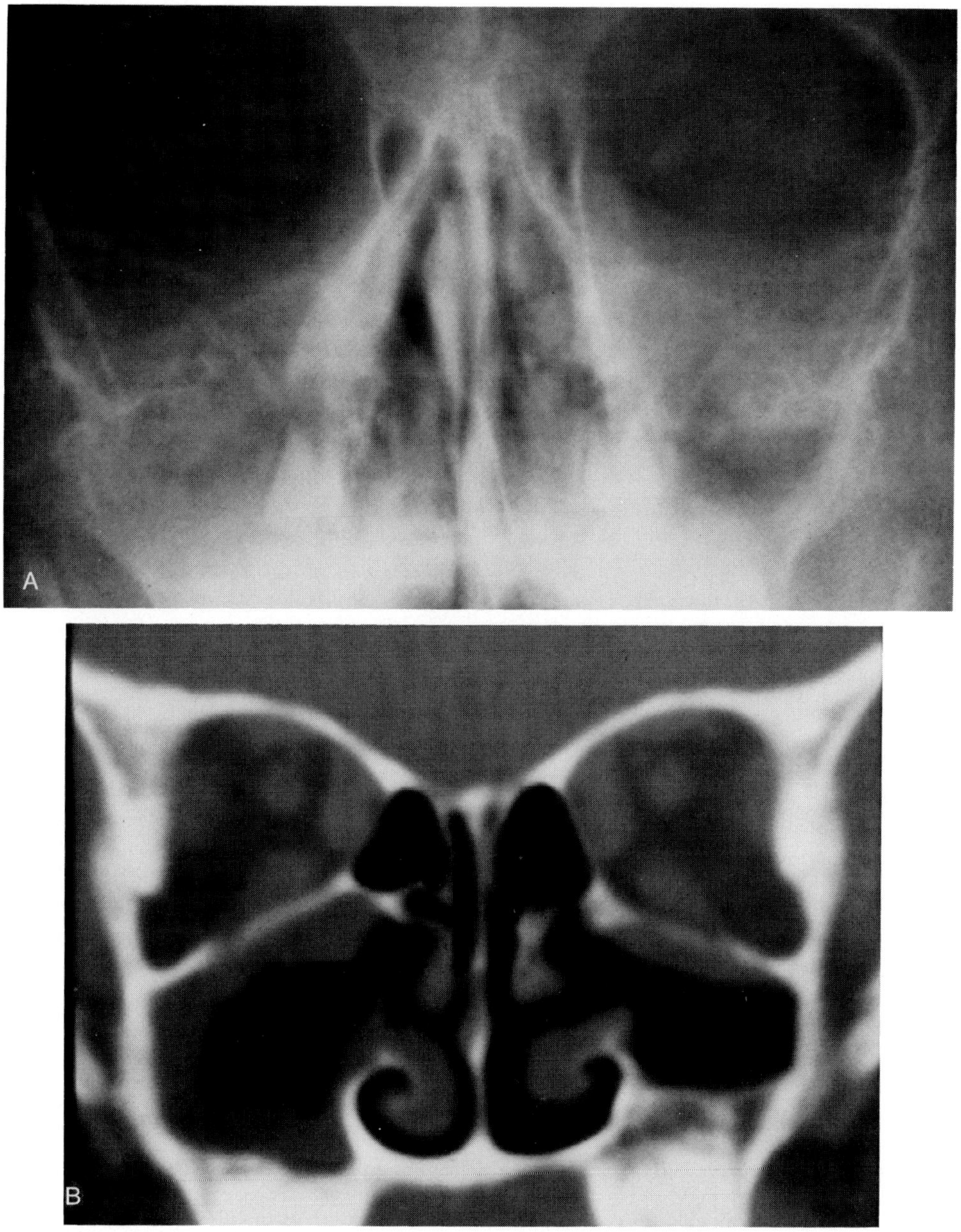

• FIGURE 13-2.

A, Plain film of a patient after an ethmoidectomy. Note the opacified right maxillary sinus and the mucosal thickening of the left maxillary sinus. *B*, CT of same patient taken within 2 hours of the plain film. Note the mucosal thickening of the right maxillary sinus and the small amount of thickening of the left maxillary sinus.

Anesthetic considerations

In children, ethmoidectomy must be performed under a general anesthetic. When the patient is intubated, an endotracheal tube large enough to prevent a leak of 15 to 20 cm H_2O should be used. As the case proceeds, the leak around the tube will increase, exposing the surgeon to anesthetic gases. In addition, blood from the nose is splashed onto the telescope as the gases pass through the nasal cavity. Packing the oropharynx or hypopharynx will not significantly decrease the leak for any length of time.

The vasoconstrictors used must be effective yet have minimal side effects when used with general anesthetic agents. In a double-blind study at my institution,[11] we found that the best vasoconstrictor was 0.05% oxymetazoline, because it caused no problems with arrhythmias and no excessive bleeding. We therefore recommend using topical 0.05% oxymetazoline with injections of 1% lidocaine and 1:100,000 epinephrine for vasoconstriction.

The topical vasoconstrictor is best applied on moistened, but not dripping, $\frac{1}{2}''$ neuropledgets. It is important to place the pledgets into the nose under direct visualization with a telescope to minimize the chance of traumatizing or abrading the mucosa. If the mucosa is traumatized, persistent bleeding will significantly compromise visualization throughout the remainder of the procedure.

Preparation

- The patient is best positioned with the head and shoulders inclined at 20 to 30 degrees and the neck extended approximately 15 degrees (Fig. 13–3*A* and *B*).

- The head is covered (but the eyes are not covered), and to allow intraoperative observation, the eyes are not taped. Lacrilube is placed into the eyes, and care is taken when passing instruments over the head. The surgical team members don gowns and gloves before the procedure for their own safety.

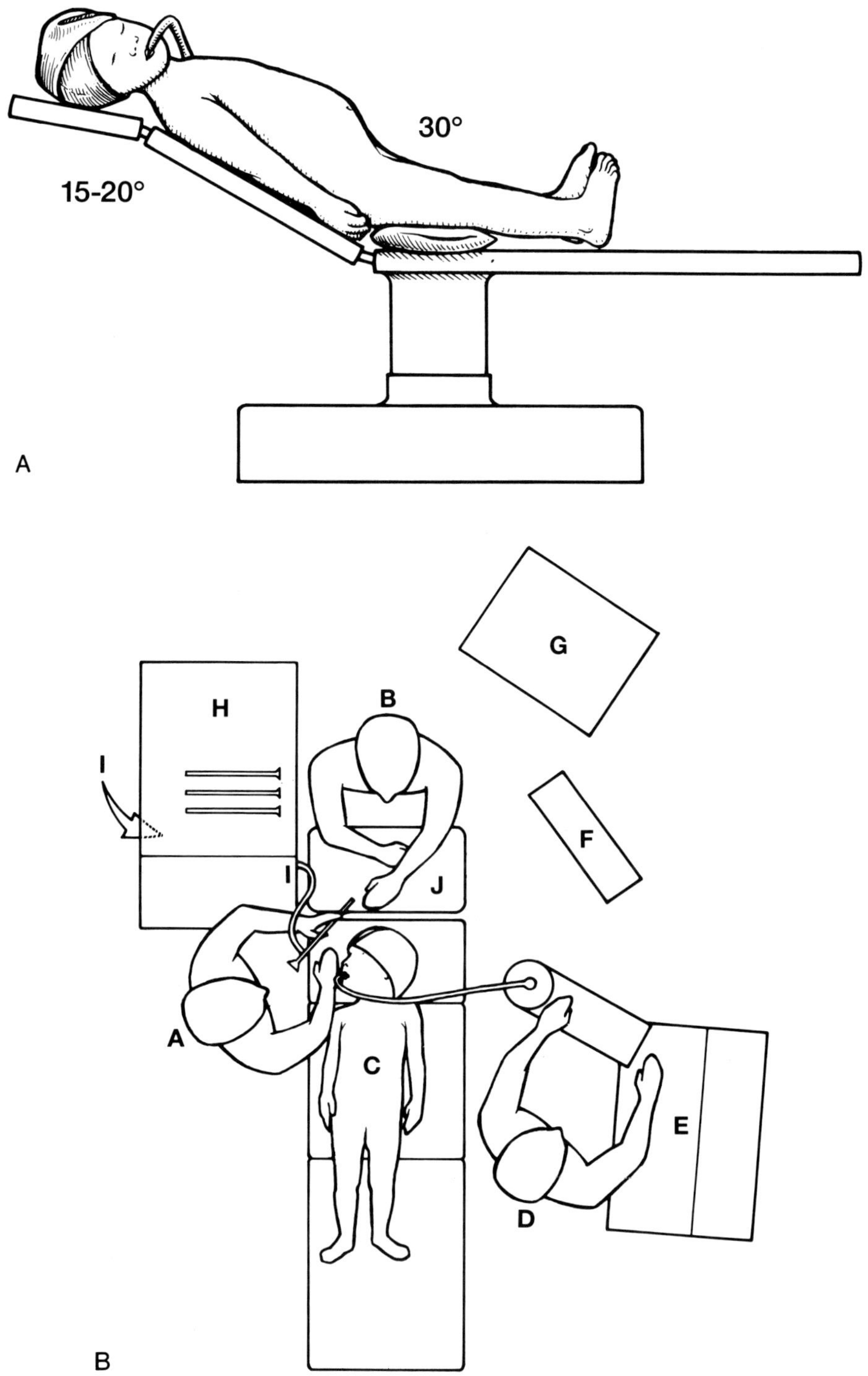

• FIGURE 13–3.

A, Position of the patient for ethmoidectomy. The head is elevated 30° and extended on the neck 15 to 20°. *B*, Position of operating room personnel. (A = Surgeon, B = scrub nurse; C = patient; D = anesthetist; E = anesthesia machine; F = x-ray view box; G = monitor and VHS recorder; H = back table for infrequently used instruments; I = light sources under table; J = Mayo stand for frequently used instruments.) (*A* and *B* from Lusk RP: Pediatric Sinusitis. New York, Raven Press, 1992.)

INSTRUMENTATION

Because adult instruments are much too large for a child's nose, special instrumentation must be used. In older children, a 4-mm telescope gives maximum light and visualization. In younger children, a 2.7-mm telescope is required, limiting the field of view and making the surgery more difficult to perform.

Smaller instruments are becoming available from several vendors. Cup forceps, in pediatric and adolescent sizes, allow for more precise removal of mucosa and bone (Fig. 13–4*A* and *B*). Suction forceps (Fig. 13–5*A* and *B*) are used when mucosal bleeding is increased. The seeker is used to identify the natural ostium of the maxillary sinus and to palpate the sinus lateralis and the frontal recess (Fig. 13–6). The J curette allows for precise opening of the ethmoid cells and intervening septa (Fig. 13–7). For small children only, narrow, short-jawed backbiters are appropriate (Fig. 13–8). The use of these instruments is described more fully in the discussion of the procedure.

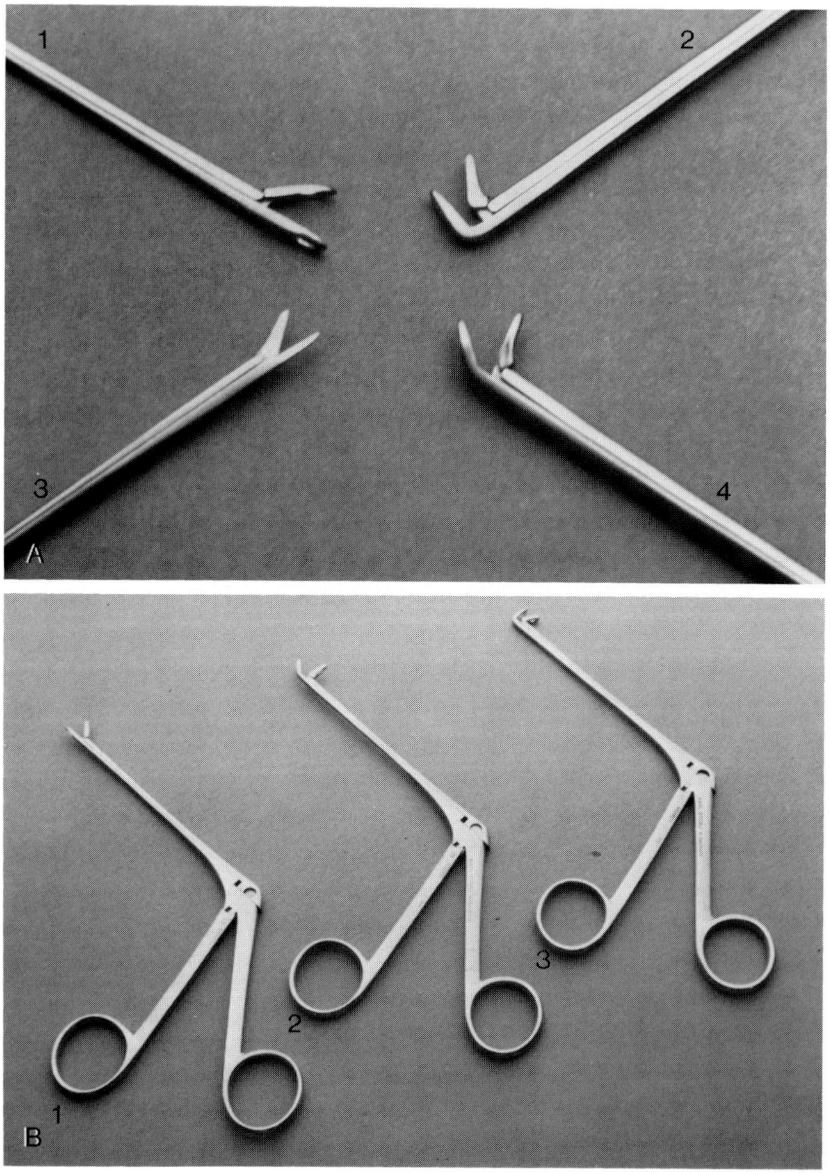

• FIGURE 13–4.

A, Pediatric cup forceps. (1) Straight forceps, (2) 90-degree forceps, (3) straight scissors, (4) 45-degree forceps. *B*, Adolescent cup forceps. (1) Straight forceps, (2) 45-degree forceps, (3) 90-degree forceps.

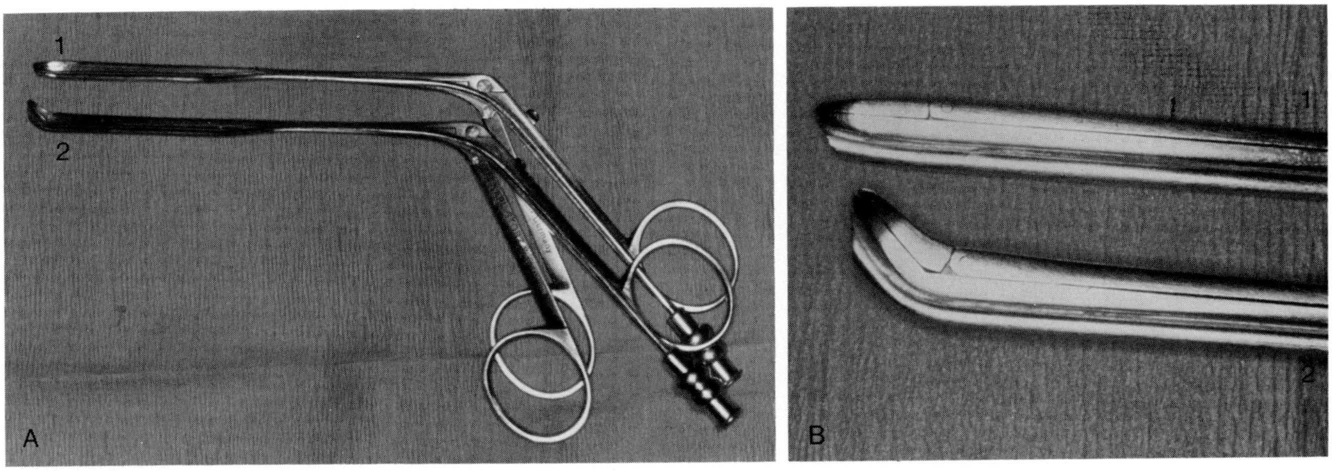

• **FIGURE 13-5.**

A, Pediatric suction forceps. (1) Straight forceps, (2) 45-degree forceps. *B*, Close-up of pediatric suction forceps. (1) Straight forceps, (2) 45-degree forceps.

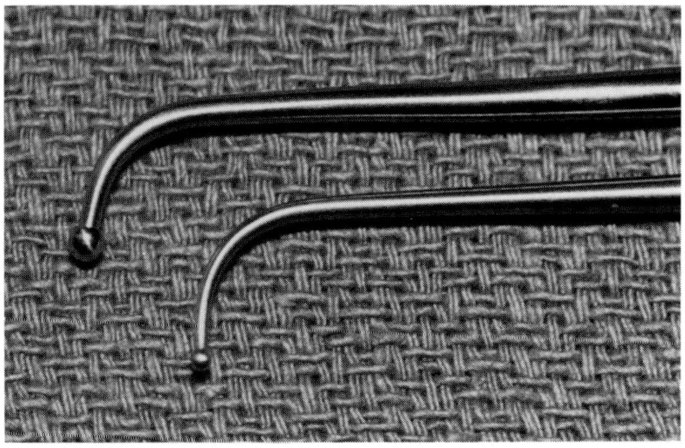

• **FIGURE 13-6.**

Seekers (large and small tips) used to palpate the natural ostium of the frontal and maxillary sinuses.

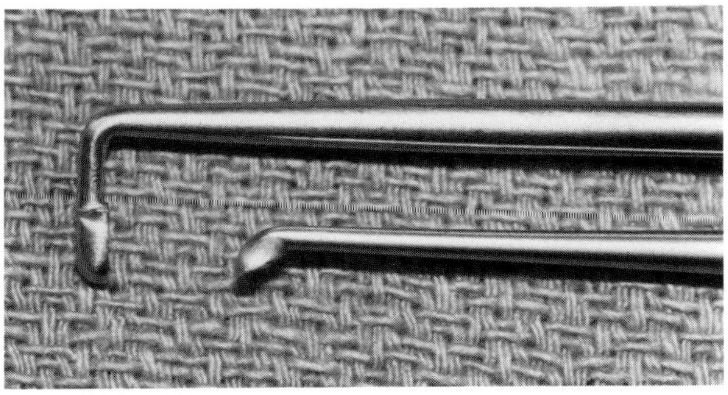

• **FIGURE 13-7.**

A J curette and a 90-degree J curette used for precise removal of bone.

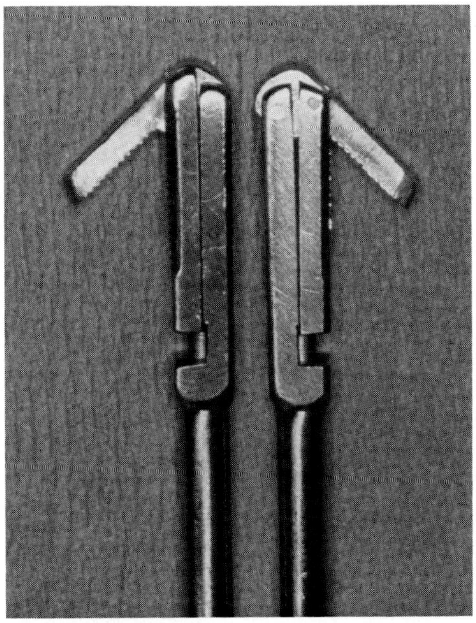

• **FIGURE 13-8.**

Narrow, short-jawed, right and left backbiters.

Procedure

EXAMINATION

Once the nose has been vasoconstricted, it is examined with a 2.7-mm 0-degree rigid scope. A 30-degree scope can also be used but is more likely to traumatize the mucosa. Vasoconstriction seems optimal when only one side is constricted at a time. When both sides are constricted, there appears to be a rebound phenomenon by the time the second side is operated on.

A first pass is made along the floor, and the nasopharynx is examined. The space medial to the middle turbinate is very narrow, and examination of the sphenoid recess is not easily accomplished at this time. An attempt to roll the telescope into the middle meatus is rarely successful, and the scope should not be forced because the mucosa is easily traumatized. An alternative method of examining the middle meatus is to retract the middle turbinate medially with a Freer elevator and to advance the telescope directly into the middle meatus. The lateral wall is inspected to identify the uncinate process, which may be palpated with the Freer elevator. The uncinate process is the only mobile structure in the lateral wall; careful observation will reveal a "break point" where it is attached, which can be used as a guide for the incision (Fig. 13–9*A* and *B*).

INJECTION

The base of the ground lamella, the uncinate process, and occasionally the area anterior to the uncinate process are injected with 1 to 2 ml of 1% lidocaine with 1:100,000 epinephrine (Fig. 13–10). The injection is best performed with a 25-gauge retrobulbar needle bent 10 degrees toward the bevel on a 3-ml syringe. A neuropledget of 0.05% oxymetazoline is then carefully placed into the middle meatus for an additional 5 to 7 minutes.

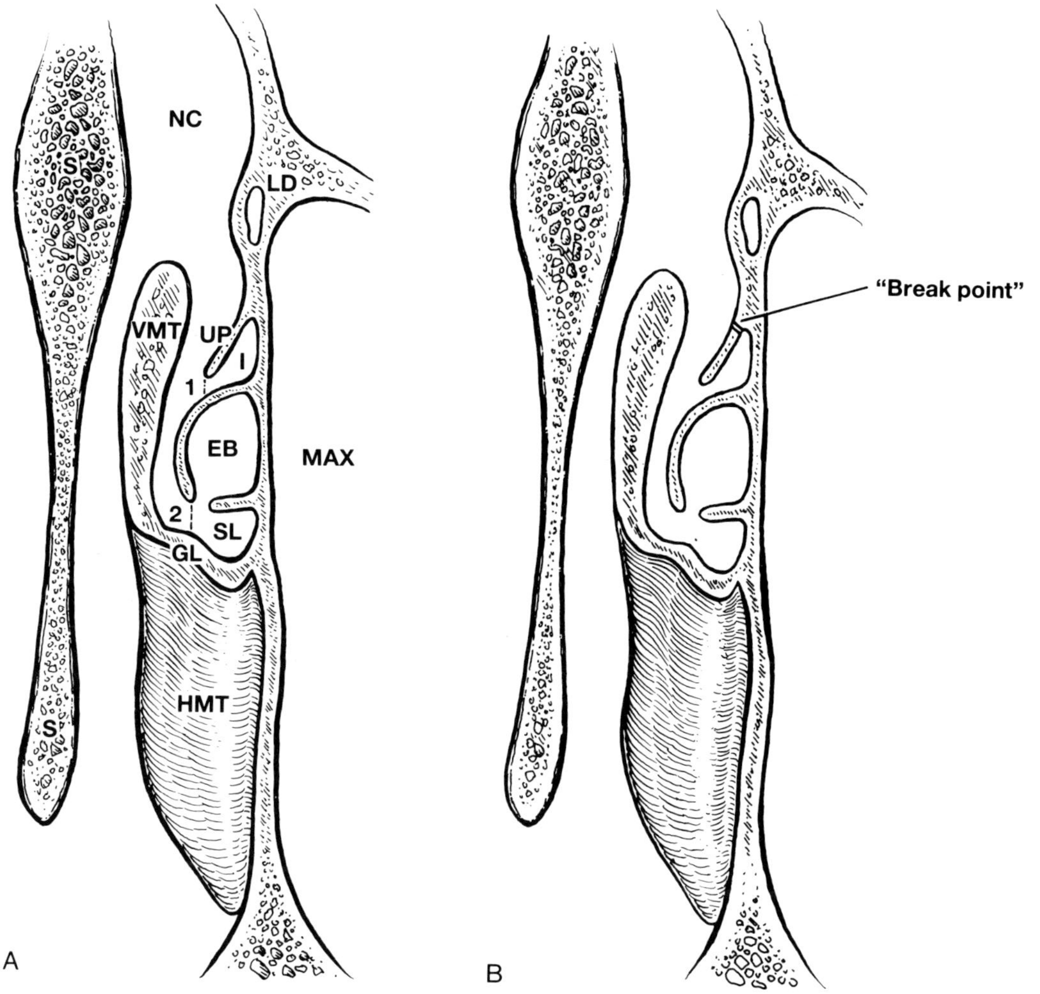

• **FIGURE 13-9.**

A, Axial diagram of anterior ethmoid cells. (NC = Nasal cavity; LD = lacrimal duct; VMT = vertical middle turbinate; UP = uncinate process; I = infundibulum; EB = ethmoid bulla; SL = sinus lateralis; GL = ground (basal or grand) lamella; HMT = horizontal lamella; S = septum; MAX = maxillary sinus; 1 = inferior hiatus semilunaris; 2 = superior hiatus semilunaris.) *B*, "Break point" of the uncinate process. (*A* and *B* from Lusk RP: Pediatric Sinusitis. New York, Raven Press, 1992.)

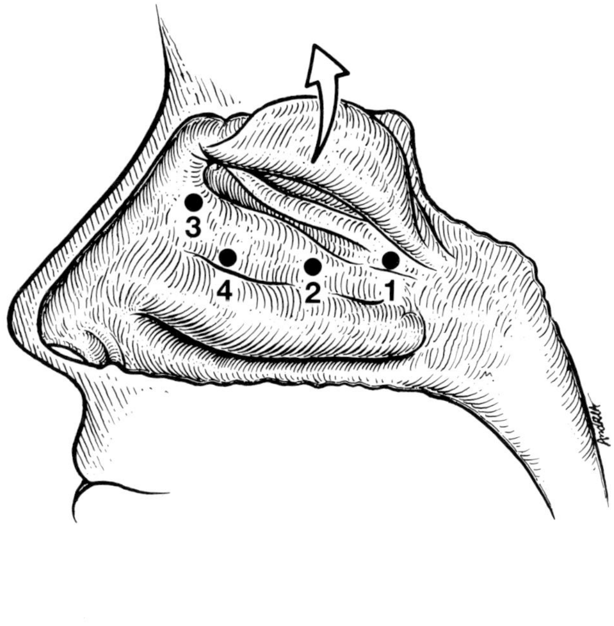

• **FIGURE 13-10.**

Injection sites for vasoconstriction (1% lidocaine with 1:100,000 epinephrine). Injections are placed in the order indicated. (From Lusk RP: Pediatric Sinusitis. New York, Raven Press, 1992.)

INCISION

The neuropledget is removed, the middle meatus is once again examined with a 0-degree telescope, and the uncinate is clearly identified. A sickle knife is used to make the incision through the first lamella or uncinate process and into the infundibulum. The incision may be started superiorly or inferiorly, but I have found that the inferior-to-superior approach is easiest. The incision must come through the mucosa inferior to the root of the middle turbinate to prevent tearing of the mucosa (Fig. 13–11). The uncinate process is then removed with a small cup forceps. If the mucosa starts to tear, it should be transected with a scissors. A J curette or seeker (see Fig. 13–6) is used to remove any residual uncinate process. This removal is important because it will maximize the opening into the middle meatus and minimize postoperative scarring. It is not unusual to be able to insert a 4-mm telescope after the meatus has been opened.

MAXILLARY OSTIUM

Most surgeons teaching adult surgery recommend performing the maxillary antrostomy at the end of the procedure. At the urging of Dr. Parsons at the University of Missouri, I now identify the ostium after removing the uncinate process. It is easiest to identify with a 30-degree telescope and a seeker, which is used to palpate posterior to the second mucosal incision in the posterior half of the infundibulum (Fig. 13–12). It is important not to force the seeker into what is believed to be the ostium, because the mucosa will tear from the roof of the maxillary sinus (Fig. 13–13). Once this occurs, it is very difficult to identify the natural ostium and prevent further separation of the mucosa from the bone. If the ostium is easily identified and does not appear to be diseased, then enlargement is not necessary; however, enlargement is frequently required.

• FIGURE 13-11.

Incision of the uncinate process does not extend into the root of the middle turbinate. (From Lusk RP: Pediatric Sinusitis. New York, Raven Press, 1992.)

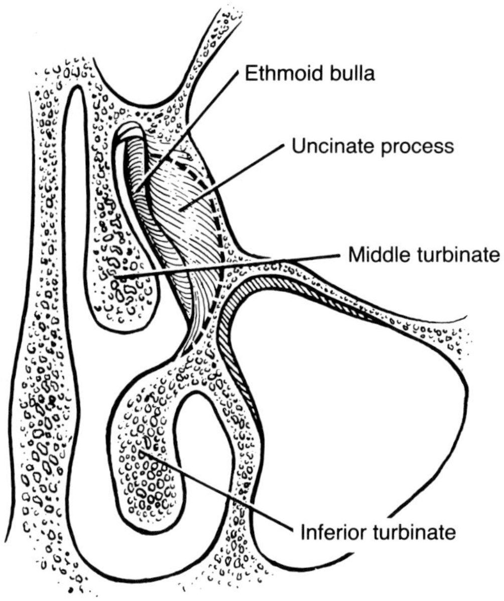

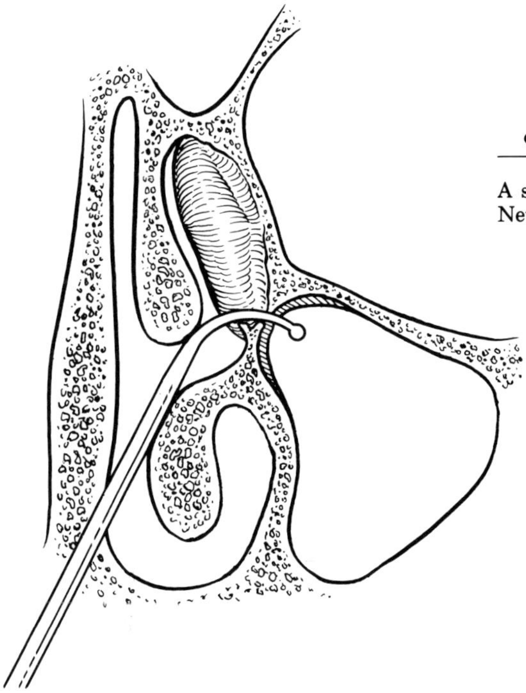

• FIGURE 13-12.

A seeker is used to palpate the maxillary ostium. (From Lusk RP: Pediatric Sinusitis. New York, Raven Press, 1992.)

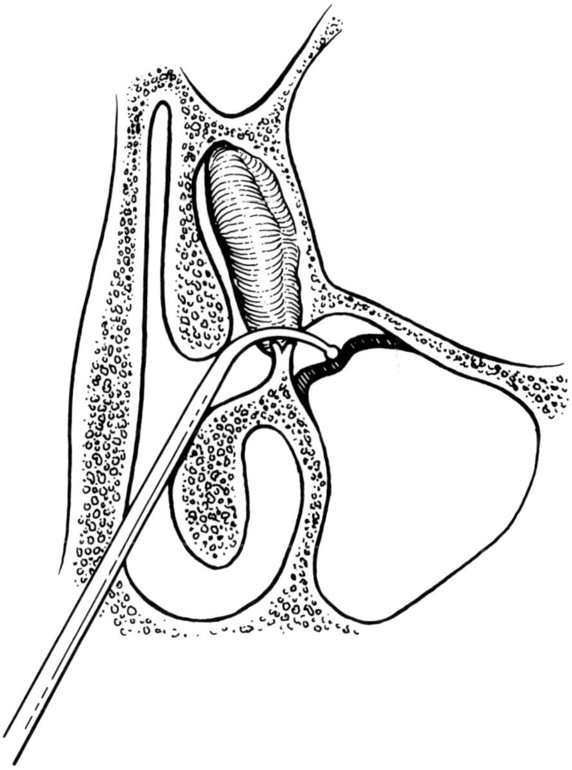

• FIGURE 13-13.

If a seeker is forced into the maxillary sinus, it will tear the mucosa from the medial and superior walls of the maxillary sinus. (From Lusk RP: Pediatric Sinusitis. New York, Raven Press, 1992.)

Once the seeker is in the ostium, it is rotated medially. The posterior fontanelle is incised with scissors, and the incision is curved inferiorly (Fig. 13–14). If necessary, the small backbiter is used to take a small bite of the anterior fontanelle (Fig. 13–15). Pediatric Blakesley forceps are used to remove the uncinate process while an attempt is made to avoid removing mucosa from the maxillary sinus. If this can be accomplished, the mucosa is rolled over the inferior edge, which will markedly reduce the amount of granulation tissue formed.

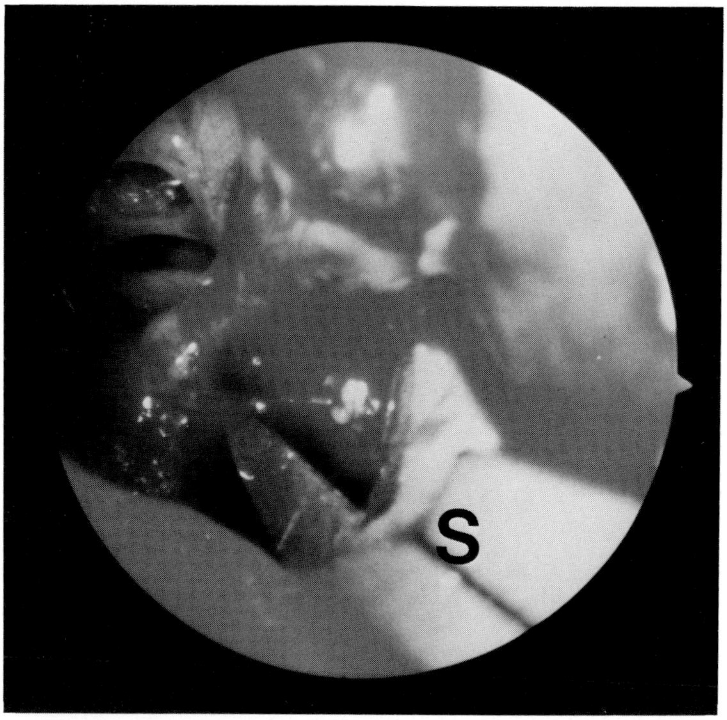

• FIGURE 13-14.

Scissors (S) incising the posterior fontanelle.

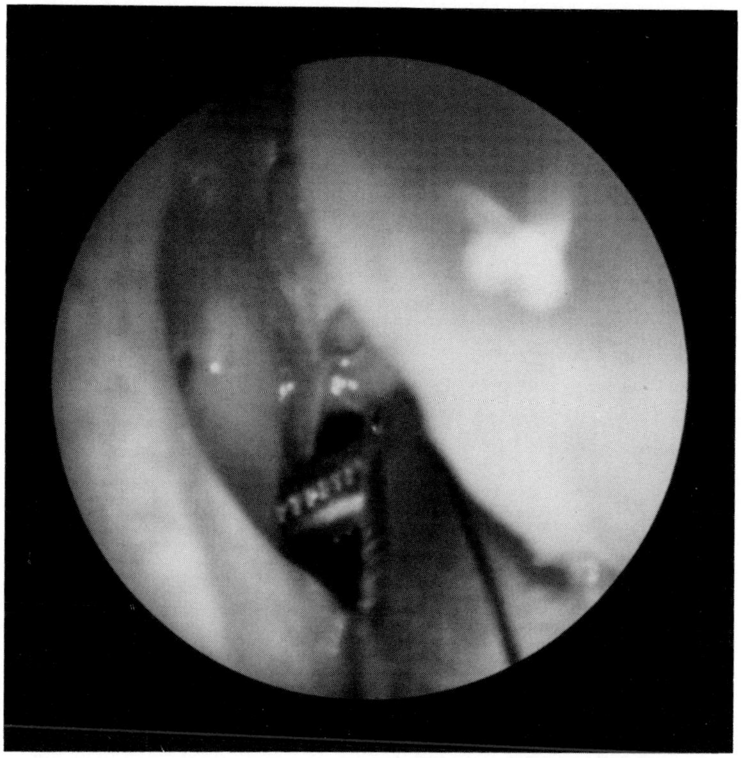

• FIGURE 13-15.

Backbiter removing a small portion of the anterior wall of the maxillary ostium.

ETHMOID BULLA

The second lamella or ethmoid bulla should now be readily identifiable. The bulla is entered in a controlled manner. This is accomplished by pushing a J curette into the bulla along the anterior, inferior, and medial borders (Fig. 13–16). The curette is then pushed upward and withdrawn. The contents of the bulla can then be observed. A 45-degree Blakesley forceps is used to remove the front wall of the bulla. The medial wall of the bulla is then removed with straight biting cup forceps while the sinus lateralis, if present, is carefully identified (Fig. 13–17). A 30-degree telescope is then used to remove the remainder of the ethmoid bulla and to identify the lamina papyracea. If there is a sinus lateralis, a space will be noted between the posterior ethmoid wall and the basal lamella. If there is no space, the juncture between the ethmoid bulla and the middle turbinate identifies the basal lamella (Fig. 13–18). These landmarks indicate the position of the basal lamella and the anteriormost posterior ethmoid cells. The most important factor in keeping oriented during an ethmoidectomy is to clearly understand what structures have been removed. The dissection can be carried superiorly to the frontal recess (see later), but if a posterior ethmoidectomy is to be performed, it is best to wait until the level of the roof of the ethmoid is identified in the posterior cells.

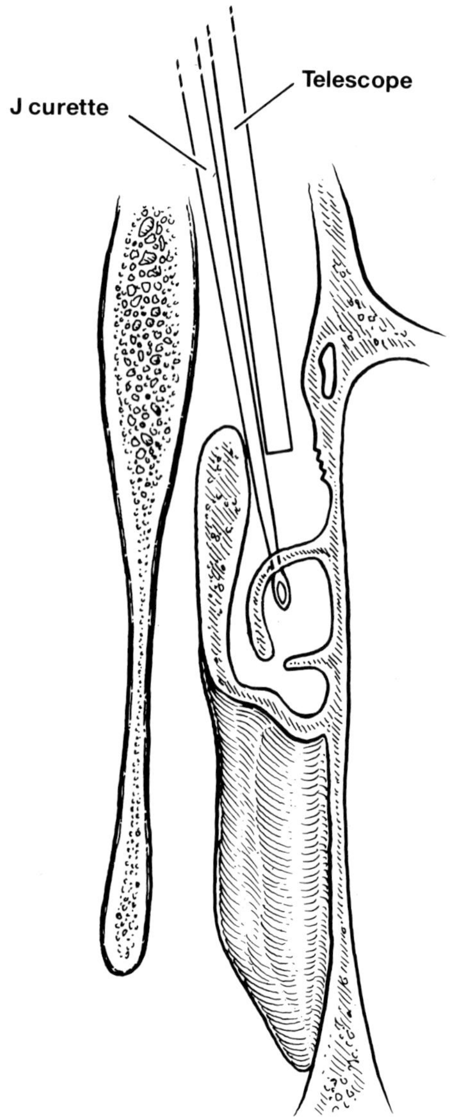

• FIGURE 13–16.

J curette opening the anterior wall of the ethmoid bulla. (From Lusk RP: Pediatric Sinusitis. New York, Raven Press, 1992.)

• FIGURE 13-17.

A 45-degree Blakesley forceps used to remove the anterior wall of the ethmoid bulla. (From Lusk RP: Pediatric Sinusitis. New York, Raven Press, 1992.)

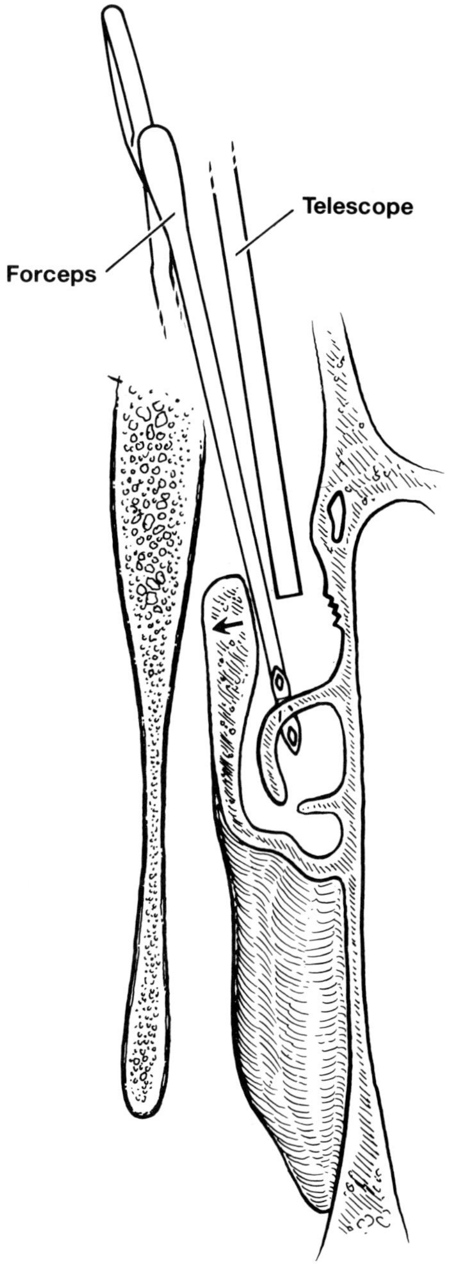

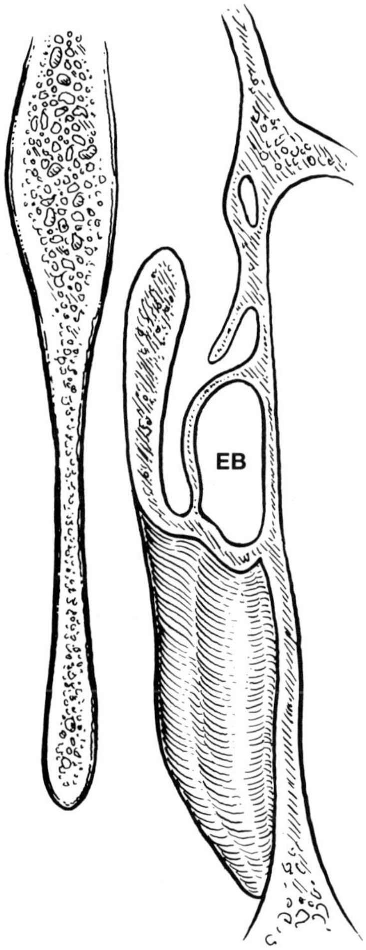

• FIGURE 13-18.

Diagram of the ethmoid bulla (EB) without any evidence of a sinus lateralis. (From Lusk RP: Pediatric Sinusitis. New York, Raven Press, 1992.)

POSTERIOR ETHMOID CELLS

The third lamella, or basal lamella, forms the anterior wall of the superior meatus. I prefer to enter the posterior ethmoid cells in the inferomedial region. It is best to enter the cells with a J curette, because if the meatus is normal the mucosa can be left intact and the cells unaltered. If the posterior cells are diseased, they are opened from an inferior to superior approach. The posterior cells are the largest, and from these cells it is easiest to identify the plane of the roof of the ethmoid cells. If at all possible, the mucosa should be left intact over the roof to promote faster healing with less granulation tissue. Even in children, the posteriormost ethmoid (Onodi) cell may be well developed and expose the optic nerve.

The sphenoid sinus is always located lower and more medial than would be expected. It is not often diseased in children and therefore not frequently opened. When a child's sphenoid sinus must be opened, it is almost always opened through the ethmoid sinus because of the narrow space medial to the middle and superior turbinates. If the sphenoid is not easily identified through the ethmoid, the position of the sphenoid ostium can be noted by following a line along the lower third of the middle and superior turbinates (Fig. 13–19). This can be accomplished best after the anterior and posterior ethmoidectomies have been performed, because the middle and superior turbinates can be very gently moved laterally to provide enough room to identify the sphenoid recess. Once the level of the sphenoid ostium is identified, the level of the roof of the sphenoid can be identified in the posterior ethmoids. The sphenoid sinus of some children is so small that it is difficult to use instruments within it.

FRONTAL RECESS AND AGGER NASI CELLS

If a posterior ethmoidectomy has been performed, the plane leading to the frontal recess is readily identified. If the posterior cells are not opened but disease is present in the frontal recess, the surgeon will have to decide if the frontal recess is best approached first through the anterior cells or through the posterior cells.

The frontal sinus recess is located medially in most children. The small end of the seeker can be used to gently probe this area under direct visualization with a 30-degree telescope. The seeker will rotate laterally if it is located in the frontal sinus. Diseased mucosa can be surgically stripped out of this region fairly easily. If a large area of mucosa has been surgically stripped from the region, the recess will need to be opened widely. When the frontal sinus is identified, every effort must be made to leave the mucosa intact around the opening. If the mucosa in the area of the frontal recess is normal, it should be left in place. The effects of surgery in the frontal recess of children are not known, so surgery in this area should be conservative.

• FIGURE 13-19.

Landmarks to the natural ostium of the sphenoid sinus. The telescope is placed along a line at the root of the inferior turbinate (1), at the lower $\frac{1}{3}$ of the middle turbinate (2), at the lower $\frac{1}{3}$ of the superior turbinate (3), and at the ostium of the sphenoid sinus (4). (From Lusk RP: Pediatric Sinusitis. New York, Raven Press, 1992.)

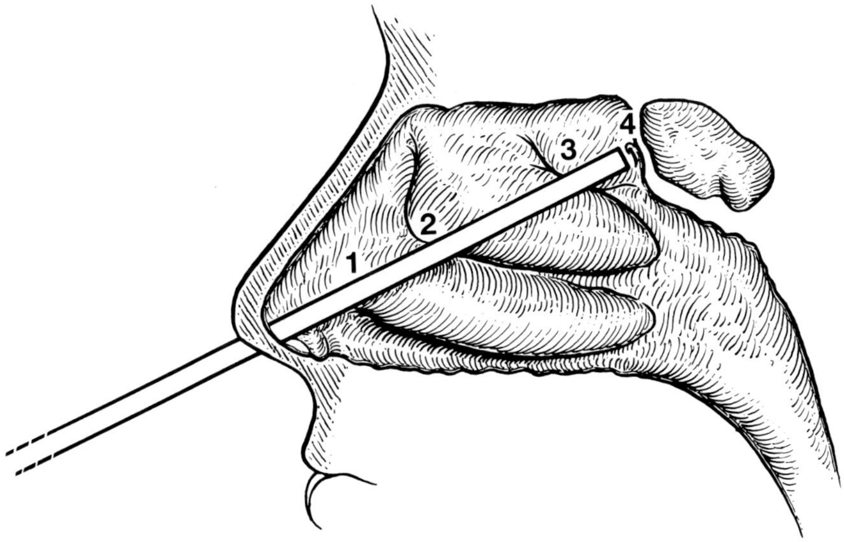

AVOIDANCE OF COMPLICATIONS

The best way to avoid complications is to have an appropriate preoperative evaluation with coronal CT scans, a thorough knowledge of the anatomy, good visualization of the operative field, and good judgment about when to discontinue the operation. My experience in the operating room and the laboratory indicates that the most likely cause of an orbital complication is penetration of the lamina papyracea at its junction with the roof of the maxillary sinus. This is more likely to occur on the left side. Obviously, care must be used in operating at this site. Great care must also be taken when operating medially in the ethmoid cavity. This is the area of the cribriform plate, and the site most likely to be penetrated is in the region of the anterior ethmoid artery.

Most complications occur when there is poor visualization secondary to bleeding. The bleeding is usually mucosal and not arterial. A patient, conservative approach is the key to successful surgery. If there is troublesome bleeding, a pledget with vasoconstrictor or Avitene (mixed with saline solution to form a slurry) should be placed into the cavity for several minutes. If problems persist, it is always better to stop and finish the operation at a later time.

Postoperative care

Most children will not allow postoperative cleaning of the ethmoid cavity in the office. Postoperative management, therefore, has to be altered from that used in the adults. We have found that a Gelfilm stent rolled in the middle meatus significantly decreases the amount of scarring (Fig. 13–20). Granulation tissue usually develops around the frontal recess and the antrostomy. We take the child back to the operating room to remove the stent under a second general anesthetic after 2 weeks. Granulation tissue at the frontal recess and maxillary ostium is also removed, but granulation tissue that has formed over the lamina papyracea and middle turbinate is not removed. A half pledget is rolled and placed back into the cavity and allowed to dissolve. The second stent remains in place for an additional 2 to 3 weeks and is allowed to be absorbed. The patient receives full-dose antibiotics as long as the stent is in place. Prophylactic antibiotics are used until the crusting is resolved. Although no prospective studies indicate the necessity for the second look or the postoperative use of antibiotics, this regimen has consistently given us our best results.

CONCLUSION

To date, more than 450 endoscopic sinus ethmoidectomy procedures have been performed at our institution without orbital complications. Small amounts of orbital fat have been noted, once at the time of cleaning granulation tissue and twice during the primary procedure. The exposed fat was recognized at an early stage, and the procedure was continued without problems. During our prospective study on vasoconstriction, two procedures were terminated because of excessive bleeding. Both patients were being treated with phenylephrine, which proved *not* to be an effective vasoconstrictor.

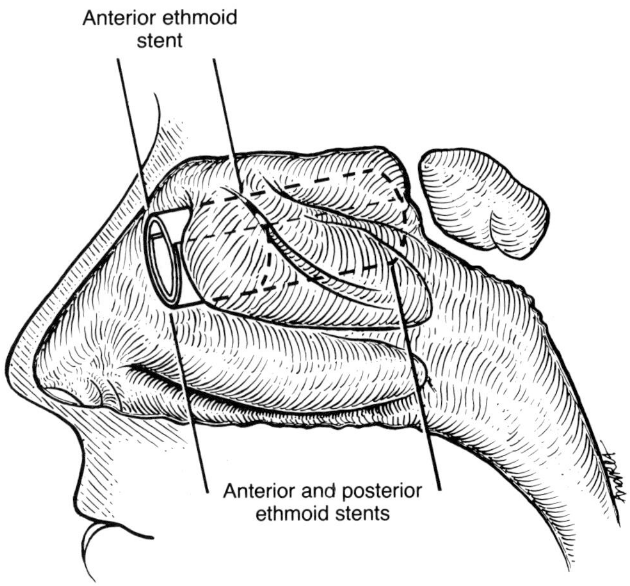

• FIGURE 13-20.

Diagram of absorbable gelatin film placed into the middle meatus from the lateral view. If an anterior ethmoidectomy has been performed, the stent is placed posteriorly to the basal lamella, and if a posterior ethmoidectomy has been performed, the stent is placed all the way back in the cavity. It is important to make sure that the stent is positioned high in the middle meatus to prevent scarring at the root of the middle meatus. (From Lusk RP: Pediatric Sinusitis. New York, Raven Press, 1992.)

REFERENCES

1. Paul D: Sinus infection and adenotonsillitis in pediatric patients. Laryngoscope 91:997–1000, 1981.
2. Hibbert J: The current status of adenoidectomy: A survey among otolaryngologists. Clin Otolaryngol 2:239–247, 1977.
3. Huggill PH and Ballantyne JC: An investigation into the relationship between adenoids and sinusitis in children. J Otolaryngol 66:84–91, 1952.
4. Merck W: Relationship between adenoidal enlargement and maxillary sinusitis. HNO 6:198–199, 1974.
5. Walker FM: Tonsillectomy and adenoidectomy: Unsatisfactory results due to chronic maxillary sinusitis. BMJ 2:908–910, 1947.
6. Lund VJ: Inferior meatal antrostomy: Fundamental considerations of design and function. J Laryngol Otol Suppl 15:1–18, 1988.
7. Muntz HR and Lusk RP: Nasal antral windows in children: A retrospective study. Laryngoscope 100:643–646, 1990.
8. Wald ER, Guerra N, and Byers C: Upper respiratory tract infections in young children: Duration of and frequency of complications. Pediatrics 87:129–133, 1991.
9. Lusk RP, Polmar SH, and Muntz HR: Endoscopic ethmoidectomy and maxillary antrostomy in immunodeficient patients. Arch Otolaryngol Head Neck Surg 117:60–63, 1991.
10. McAlister WH, Lusk RP, and Muntz HR: Comparison of plain radiographs and coronal CT scans in infants and children with recurrent sinusitis. Am J Roentgenol 153:1259–1264, 1989.
11. Riegle EV, Gunter JB, Lusk RP, et al: Comparison of vasoconstrictors for functional endoscopic sinus surgery in children. Laryngoscope 102:820–823, 1992.

chapter

14

Inflammation of the Nose and Paranasal Sinuses

ANDREW J. HOTALING, M.D.

NASAL POLYPECTOMY

- Children can have a variety of inflammatory and other nasal disorders that require surgical intervention. Many of the inflammatory disorders are amenable to endoscopic management, which will not be discussed in this section. Depending on the surgeon's training and experience, there are older, time-tested techniques available to manage some of the pathologies. Some of the available techniques are reviewed here.

- Although local anesthesia may be suitable for some children, general anesthesia is generally preferable because it will limit operative time and increase safety.

- A topical decongestant such as 0.25 to 0.5% phenylephrine (Neo-Synephrine) on cotton pledgets or neurosurgical cottonoids is helpful for many of these procedures. If the procedure is to be performed under local anesthesia, the addition of 2% tetracaine hydrochloride will suffice.

- Postoperative care is enhanced with the addition of normal saline (0.9 NaCl) drops or spray. One to two sprays or two to four drops in each naris every 4 hours while the patient is awake will help to keep the nasal cavity lubricated and minimize crusting and scabbing.

Indications

- Indicated for nasal polyps that are symptomatic

- Children with polyps should have a sweat test to rule out cystic fibrosis using the quantitative pilocarpine iontophoresis method used by Gibson and Cooke.[1]

Anesthetic considerations

- The procedure is usually performed under general anesthesia.

- Topical intranasal decongestion will assist in visualization.

- Greater palatine blocks and local intranasal injections of lidocaine with Neo-Synephrine will minimize blood loss. A palatine block can be performed with a No. 27 gauge $1\frac{1}{2}''$ needle inserted 25 to 28 mm into the foramen. After aspiration to ensure that the needle is not intravascular, 2 ml of 1% lidocaine can be injected into the pterygomaxillary fossa.[2]

Procedure

- Polyps can be removed under direct vision using Takahashi forceps or wire snares (Fig. 14–1).

- Endoscopic sinus surgical techniques can be used to improve visualization.

- When lack of hemostasis limits visualization, packing with $\frac{1}{2}$ to 1% Neo-Synephrine while working on the contralateral nasal cavity minimizes blood loss, improves visualization, and shortens operative time.

- Neurosurgical cottonoids, soaked in $\frac{1}{2}$ to 1% Neo-Synephrine drops, are placed intranasally and bilaterally as a dressing before the patient leaves the operating room, and these cottonoids are removed later in the recovery room.

- If bleeding occurs in the patient in the recovery room, $\frac{1}{2}$ to 1% Neo-Synephrine drops can be placed intranasally and bilaterally.

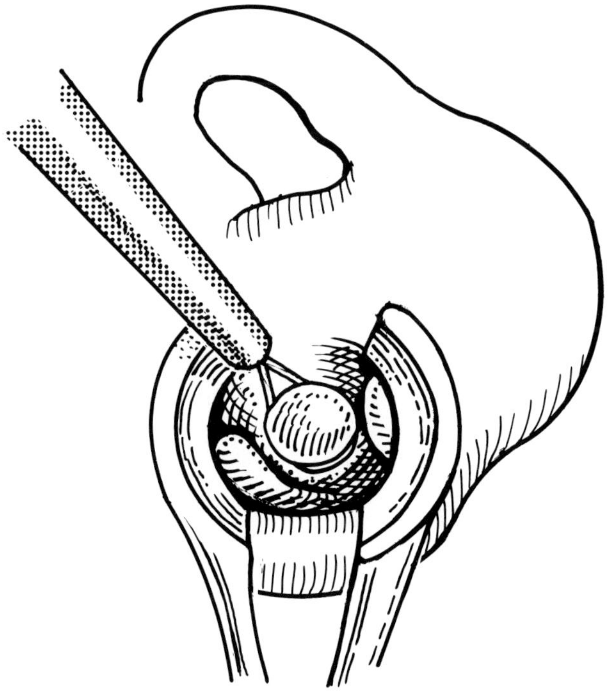

• FIGURE 14-1.

Removal of a polyp under direct vision using a wire snare.

Postoperative care

• As discussed earlier, saline spray or drops of one to two sprays or two to four drops in each nostril of 0.9 normal NaCl every 4 hours while the patient is awake will decrease crusting and improve humidification.

CLOSED REDUCTION OF NASAL FRACTURE

Indications

• The two primary indications for closed reduction are nasal dysfunction and unsatisfactory cosmesis.

• If there is significant edema, the procedure should be delayed until the edema resolves so that visualization and palpation are improved. The nasal bones can be manipulated for approximately 10 days post-trauma in most patients.

• X-rays are not usually necessary.

• An exact description of the mechanism of trauma is helpful when planning the closed reduction.

• Patients and parents are informed that if the closed reduction is unsatisfactory, an open reduction can be performed later.

Anesthetic considerations

The procedure is performed easily under general anesthesia with topical ($\frac{1}{4}$ to $\frac{1}{2}$%) Neo-Synephrine for decongestion.

Procedure

• After adequate decongestion, the nose is examined externally and intranasally (Fig. 14–2). The deformity can be corrected with a variety of elevators; a Sayre elevator works well in most situations.

Postoperative care

• The postoperative dressing is used to stabilize and protect the reduction as well as to remind the patient and playmates to avoid nasal trauma.

• For the dressing, a ready-made splint is the easiest to use. If these are not available, a plaster splint of six to eight layers can be used. Mastisol is first applied to the external nose, followed by paper Steri-Strips, then by another layer of mastisol. The splint is then applied and secured with two pieces of tape—vertically from the splint onto the forehead and bilaterally onto the cheeks.

• If bleeding occurs following reduction, neurosurgical cottonoids soaked in Neo-Synephrine may be applied in the operating room and may be removed in the recovery room.

• If bleeding occurs in the recovery room, Neo-Synephrine drops may be placed intranasally and bilaterally.

• The splint is removed in 5 to 7 days.

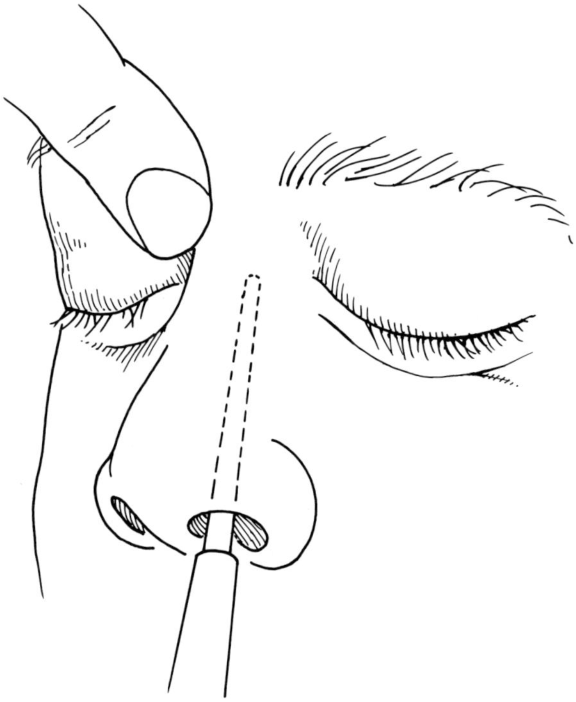

• FIGURE 14-2.

Closed reduction of a nasal fracture.

DRAINAGE OF SEPTAL ABSCESS OR HEMATOMA

Indications

- The primary cause is trauma, often secondary to nasal fracture. It is essential to perform a complete intranasal examination of the traumatized nose. If an abscess or hematoma is not diagnosed, there can be subsequent loss of cartilage that can lead to septal perforation.

Anesthetic considerations

- The procedure is usually performed under general anesthesia with intranasal decongestant ($\frac{1}{4}$ to $\frac{1}{2}$% Neo-Synephrine).

Procedure

- An incision is made over the abscess or hematoma, usually in the dependent portion to assist drainage. If pus is encountered, a culture may be taken (Fig. 14–3).
- After evacuation of the abscess or hematoma, a light nasal pack is placed against the traumatized site to prevent a recurrence. One-quarter-inch plain gauze with topical antibiotic ointment works well.

Postoperative care

- The pack is removed in 2 to 3 days. The site is reinspected in the office after 5 to 7 days to ensure that healing is satisfactory.

REMOVAL OF AN ANTROCHOANAL POLYP

Indications

- The antrochoanal polyp presents in two ways. The patient may have a nasal obstruction. Alternatively, there may be bulging of the soft palate or an irregular mass seen hanging below the palate from the nasopharynx into the oropharynx.
- The patient may be referred for a probable tumor of the nasopharynx. A complete head and neck examination and radiographic studies should be performed preoperatively.

Anesthetic considerations

- The procedure is usually performed under general anesthesia.
- Intranasal decongestion increases visualization during the procedure.

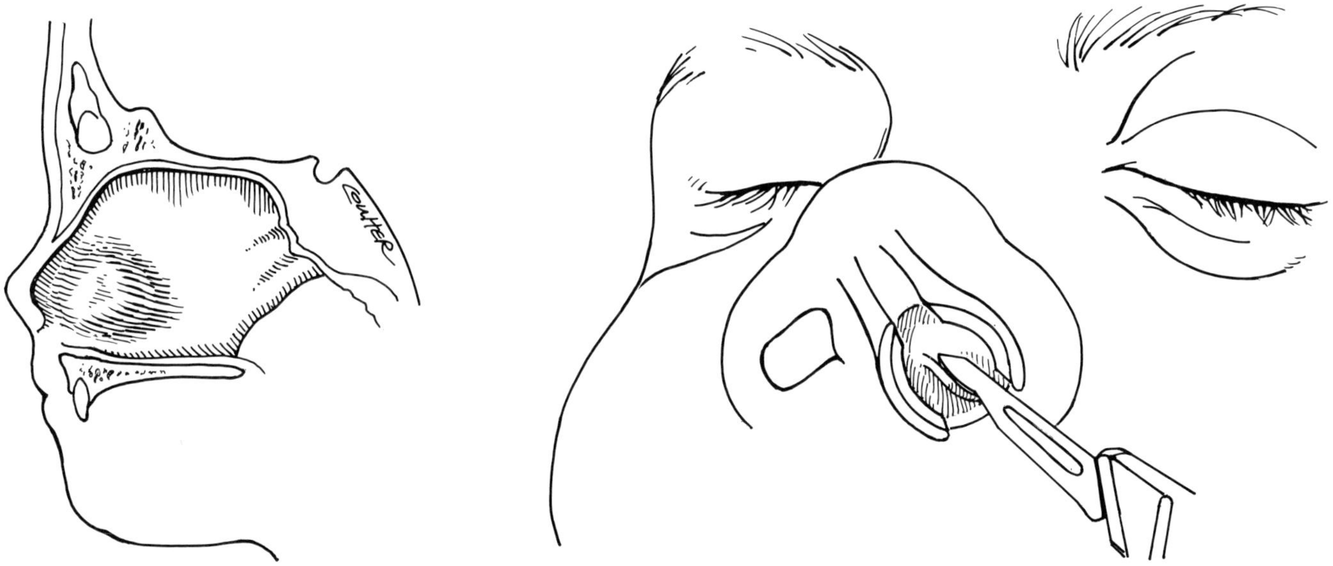

• FIGURE 14-3.

Drainage of a septal abscess.

Procedure

- The bilobed tumor can be removed transorally using a wire snare (Fig. 14–4). The heavier gauge wire on the tonsil snare is less likely to break than is the smaller gauge wire on the polyp snare. With the palate retracted, the snare is placed transorally around the choanal portion of the tumor and tightened. Steady inferior traction is then applied. Frequently, the entire tumor is removed using this technique. If the tumor breaks, the intranasal portion is removed transnasally using Takahashi forceps or endoscopic sinus surgical instruments.
- Intranasal inspection is performed with sinus endoscopy equipment to ensure that removal is complete.
- The maxillary antrostomy is usually adequate; if it is not, the os is enlarged as needed.
- If significant ethmoid sinusitis exists, this disease may also need to be treated concurrently with removal of the antrochoanal polyp.

Postoperative care

- A light intranasal packing of absorbable gelatin sponge, petroleum gauze, or synthetic surgical sponge may be required for 1 to 2 days postoperatively.

CILIARY BIOPSY

Indications

- To obtain a specimen suitable for electron microscopy to detect abnormal cilia

Anesthetic considerations

- The procedure can be performed easily under topical anesthesia. Some children will permit the biopsy to be done with no anesthesia.

Procedure

- Under direct vision, a small ear curette is used to gently scrape the mucosa over the inferior turbinate. The specimen is placed in a suitable medium for transport to the laboratory (Fig. 14–5).
- The procedure should not be performed during or just after an acute upper respiratory infection, because the cilia may be absent due to the infection.

Postoperative care

- No postoperative care is needed.

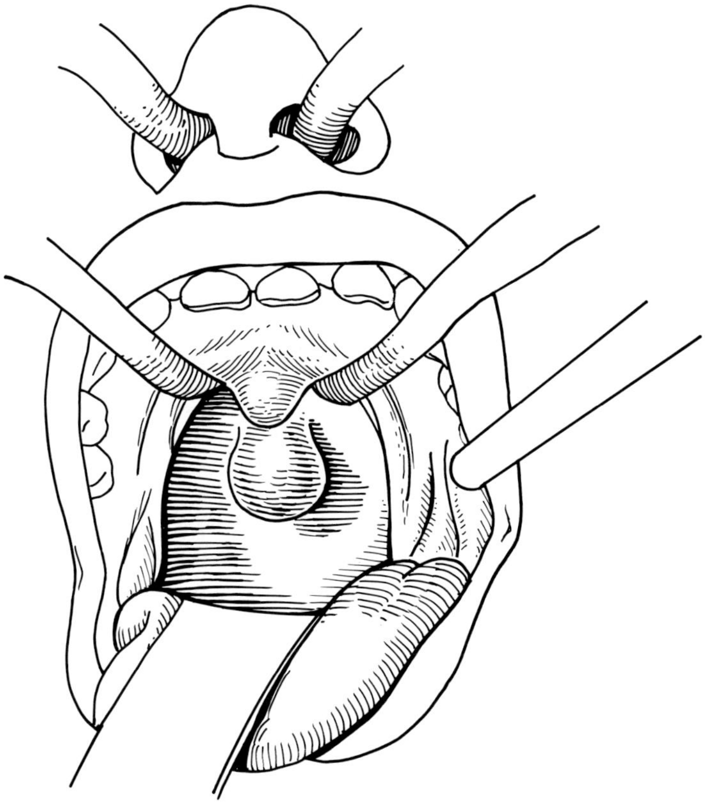

• FIGURE 14-4.

An antrochoanal polyp is removed.

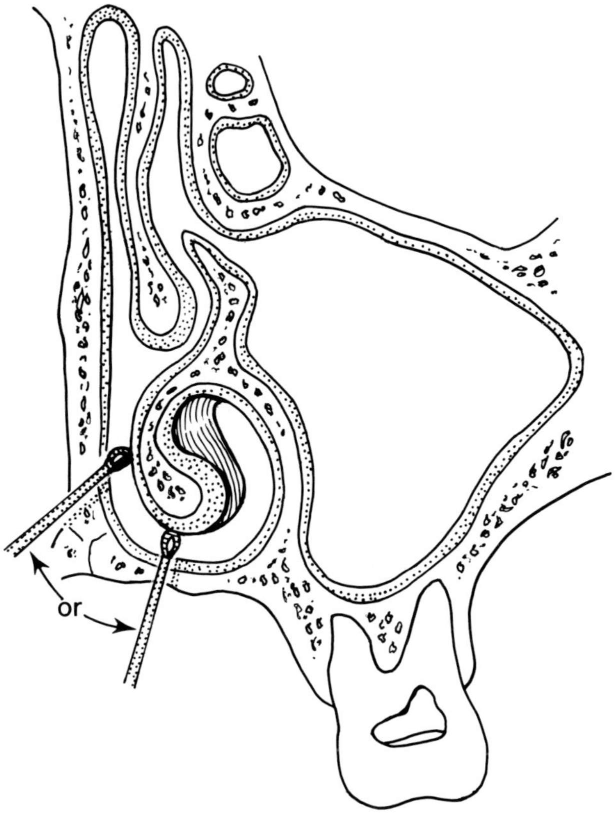

• FIGURE 14-5.

A cilia specimen is obtained by gently scraping the mucosa over the inferior turbinate with a small ear curette.

FRONTAL SINUS TREPHINATION

Indications

- Acute frontal sinusitis unresponsive to medical management
- Intracranial complication of frontal sinusitis

Anesthetic considerations

- The procedure is performed under general anesthesia.

Procedure

- A preoperative Caldwell film is used to determine the exact location of the incision made just posterior to the orbital rim in the superomedial aspect of the orbit under the medial eyebrow. The incision is marked and injected with local anesthetic with vasoconstrictor.
- A tarsorrhaphy will help to protect the globe (Fig. 14–6*A*).
- The periosteum is elevated inferiorly and superiorly.
- A cutting bur is used to make the trephination. Care is taken to open to only the anterior table (Fig. 14–6*B*).
- A culture is taken through the opening, after which a lacrimal probe is used to gently palpate all the walls of the sinus (Fig. 14–6*C*).
- The opening is made large enough to accept a small endotracheal tube, through which a smaller red rubber catheter is placed. The catheter extends beyond both ends of the endotracheal tube. The proximal end of the red rubber catheter is fitted with a blunt needle so that sinus irrigation can be performed through the red rubber catheter with outflow between the red rubber catheter and the endotracheal tube. The red rubber catheter is sewn to the endotracheal tube, which is sewn to the skin (Fig. 14–6*D*).
- The incision is closed, leaving an untied stitch at the drain site, which is tied when the drain is pulled.
- Irrigations are performed with sterile saline every 4 hours while the patient is awake until the patient has a consistent flow into the pharynx or nose.
- When the drain is pulled, the untied stitch is tied to complete wound closure.

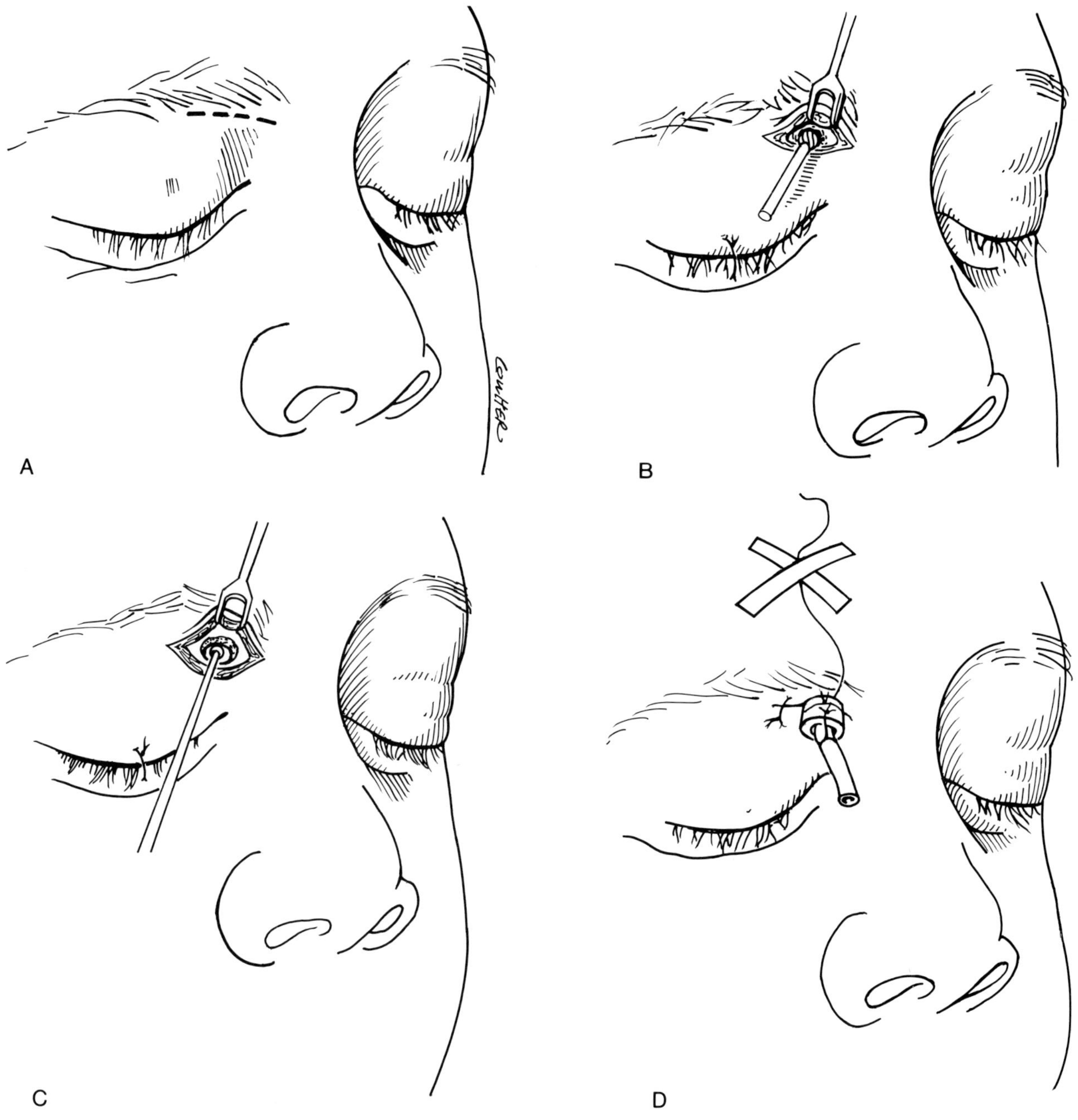

• **FIGURE 14-6.**

Frontal sinus trephination. *A*, The incision is marked. *B*, The anterior table is opened using a cutting bur. *C*, A culture is taken, and the sinus is probed with a lacrimal probe. *D*, A drain is sewn in place.

MAXILLARY SINUS ASPIRATION/NASOANTRAL WINDOW

Indications

- Acute maxillary sinusitis unresponsive to medical management
- Immunocompromised host with maxillary sinusitis with need for a culture specimen from the sinus

Anesthetic considerations

- The procedure is performed under general anesthesia or topical anesthesia with intravenous sedation.

Procedure

- After induction of anesthesia, the nose is decongested. This process can be performed easily with two small cottonoids soaked in Neo-Synephrine, which are placed along and under the inferior turbinate.
- A trocar is inserted into the posterior half of the inferior meatus, posterior to the nasolacrimal duct. The trocar is aimed toward the ipsilateral lateral canthus (Fig. 14–7).
- If the trocar does not enter the sinus with moderate pressure, the trocar can be moved posteriorly several millimeters; often, the bone is thinner more posteriorly.
- Once entered, the contents of the sinus can be aspirated with a syringe attached to the trocar. If the contents cannot be aspirated, instillation of nonbacteriostatic saline into the sinus with subsequent aspiration may be helpful. Palpation should be maintained over the ipsilateral orbit and cheek during irrigation to detect any displacement of the globe or cheek due to a misplaced trocar.
- After aspiration and washing, a small piece of absorbable gelatin sponge placed under the inferior turbinate will assist in hemostasis.
- If required, a nasoantral window can be constructed using a rat-tail rasp or a Cottle elevator.
- Alternatively, the maxillary sinus can be aspirated through the canine fossa, but care must be taken to avoid harming dentition.

Postoperative care

- One to two sprays or two to four drops of 0.9 NaCl every 4 hours will decrease crusting and improve humidification.

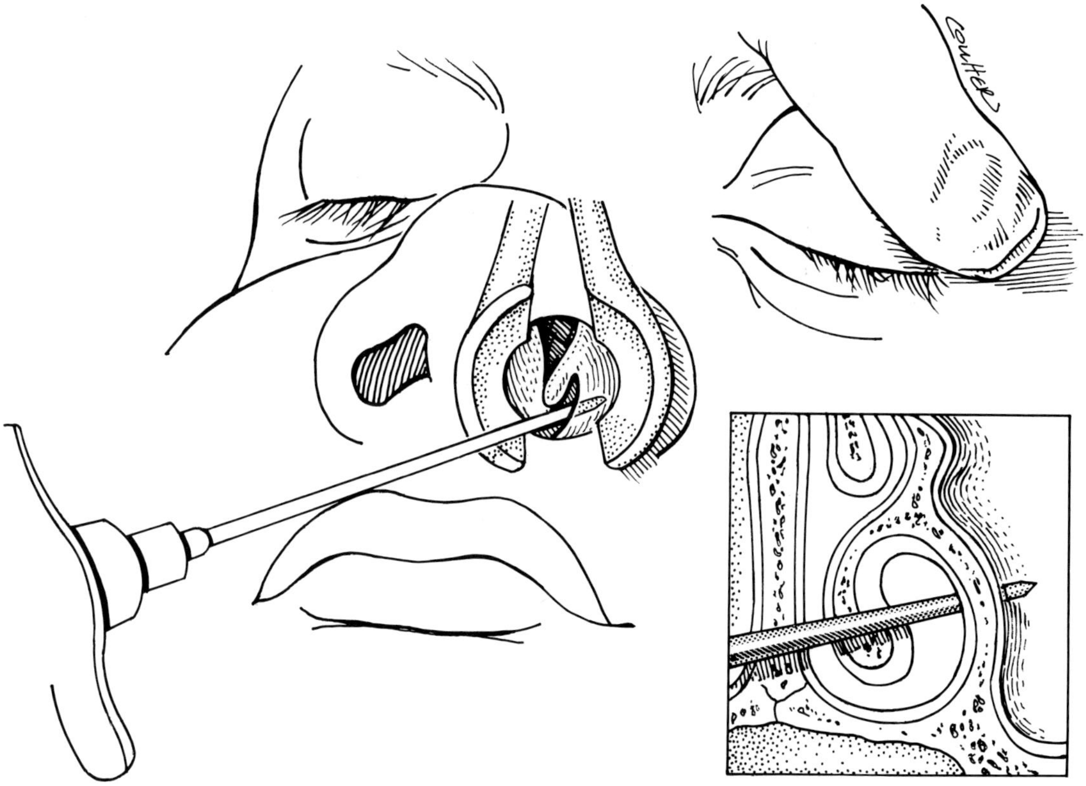

• FIGURE 14–7.

Aspiration of the maxillary sinus with a trocar.

CALDWELL-LUC PROCEDURE

Indications

- The primary indication is the presence of a mass within the sinus, such as a dentigerous cyst or a suspected neoplasm.
- The operation is not recommended for chronic sinusitis. The maxillary sinus usually improves when the ethmoid disease resolves following adequate medical or surgical treatment.

Anesthetic considerations

- The procedure is usually performed under general anesthesia.
- Local anesthesia with vasoconstriction is used in the gingivobuccal sulcus.
- Topical decongestion is used intranasally.

Procedure

- The incision is placed above the secondary dentition, whose location is determined with a plain radiograph.
- The mucosa is elevated until the intraorbital nerve is seen (Fig. 14–8*A*).
- An osteotome is used to outline a window over the antrum. After the bony cuts are made, the window can be elevated with a Freer elevator.
- A culture is taken.
- Once the limits of the sinus have been established by inspection and palpation, the window can be enlarged with Kerrison forceps, protecting the infraorbital nerve.
- The contents of the sinus are removed. The mucosal lining can be elevated for removal with ring curettes, if required.
- A nasoantral window is constructed, using a curved hemostat to enter the sinus from the nose through the inferior meatus. The window is enlarged as necessary to provide adequate aeration (Fig. 14–8*B*).
- The sinus is packed with a modified Foley catheter. The tip is cut just above the balloon. The catheter is inserted through the nares, through the nasoantral window, and into the sinus.
- The catheter is inflated with saline to fill the sinus, after which the mucosal incision is closed with an absorbable suture.
- The catheter is deflated on postoperative day 1 or 2.

Postoperative care

- Saline irrigations assist in postoperative healing and in removal of the catheter.

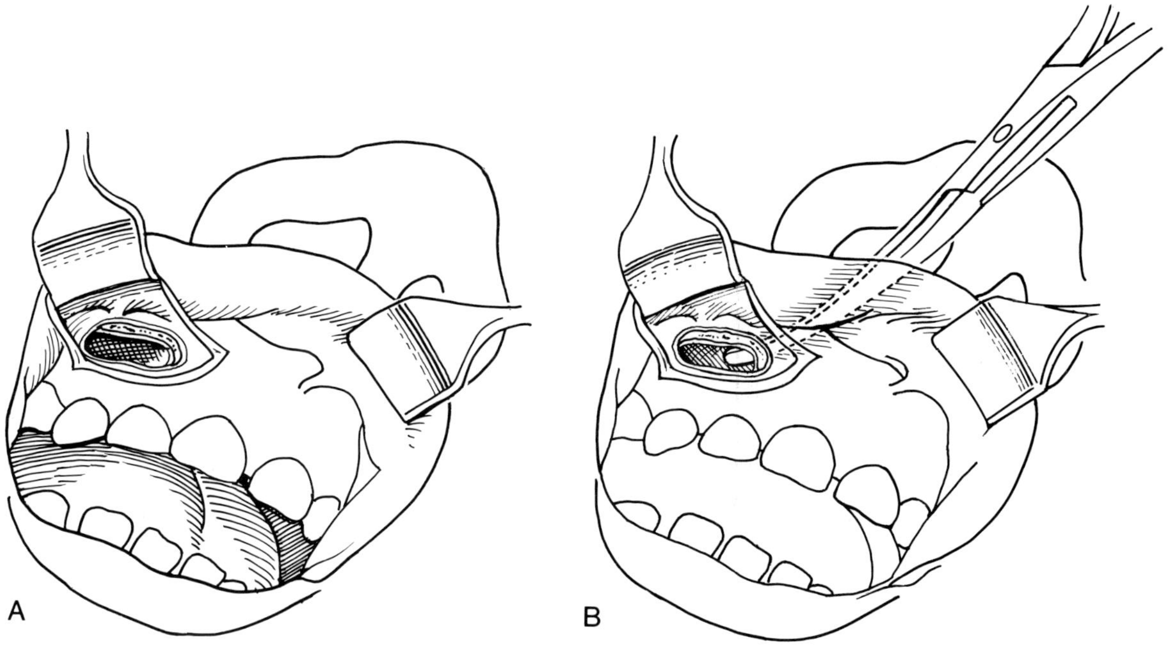

• FIGURE 14-8.

Caldwell-Luc procedure. *A*, An incision is made over the secondary dentition. The mucosa is elevated. *B*, A curved hemostat is inserted into the sinus through the inferior meatus.

EXTERNAL ETHMOIDECTOMY

Indications

- Acute or chronic ethmoid sinusitis unresponsive to medical management
- Orbital complication of sinusitis, such as subperiosteal abscess

Anesthetic considerations

The procedure is usually done under general anesthesia.

Procedure

- Endoscopic sinus surgical techniques can be used; however, unless the operator is skilled in this technique, an external approach is recommended for an orbital complication of ethmoid sinusitis.
- The nose is decongested topically.
- The curvilinear incision is outlined easily using the thumbnail to make an impression midway between the medial canthus and the midline of the nose. The resultant incision line is then marked and injected with local anesthetic with epinephrine (Fig. 14–9*A*).
- A tarsorrhaphy is performed on the ipsilateral eye for protection.
- The incision is made with a #15 scalpel blade.
- The periosteum is elevated medially to aid in closure. The lateral elevation will lift the lacrimal sac from its fossa along with its attachments superiorly and inferiorly (Fig. 14–9*B*).
- The orbital contents and lacrimal apparatus can be easily protected during further dissection by using a thin, malleable retractor for later retraction.
- If a subperiosteal infection is present, pus will be encountered during the dissection, which should be continued posteriorly to the anterior ethmoid artery or more posteriorly if required.
- Orbital contents can be inspected if required.
- Cultures are taken.
- The ethmoid complex is then entered through the lacrimal fossa or through the lamina papyracea, if it is not already dehiscent. The ethmoid complex can be easily drained into the nose using a mosquito hemostat through the incision into the ethmoid. The nose is viewed with a nasal speculum, and the hemostat is delivered into the middle meatus. A 4 × 4″ unfolded surgical sponge can then be pulled from the nose into the external wound and used as a rasp to open the ethmoid cells. The sponge is removed.
- The incision is closed in two layers and is drained externally with a rubber band (Fig 14–9*C*), leaving an untied stitch at the drain site to be tied when the drain is removed.
- An eye pad makes an excellent dressing.

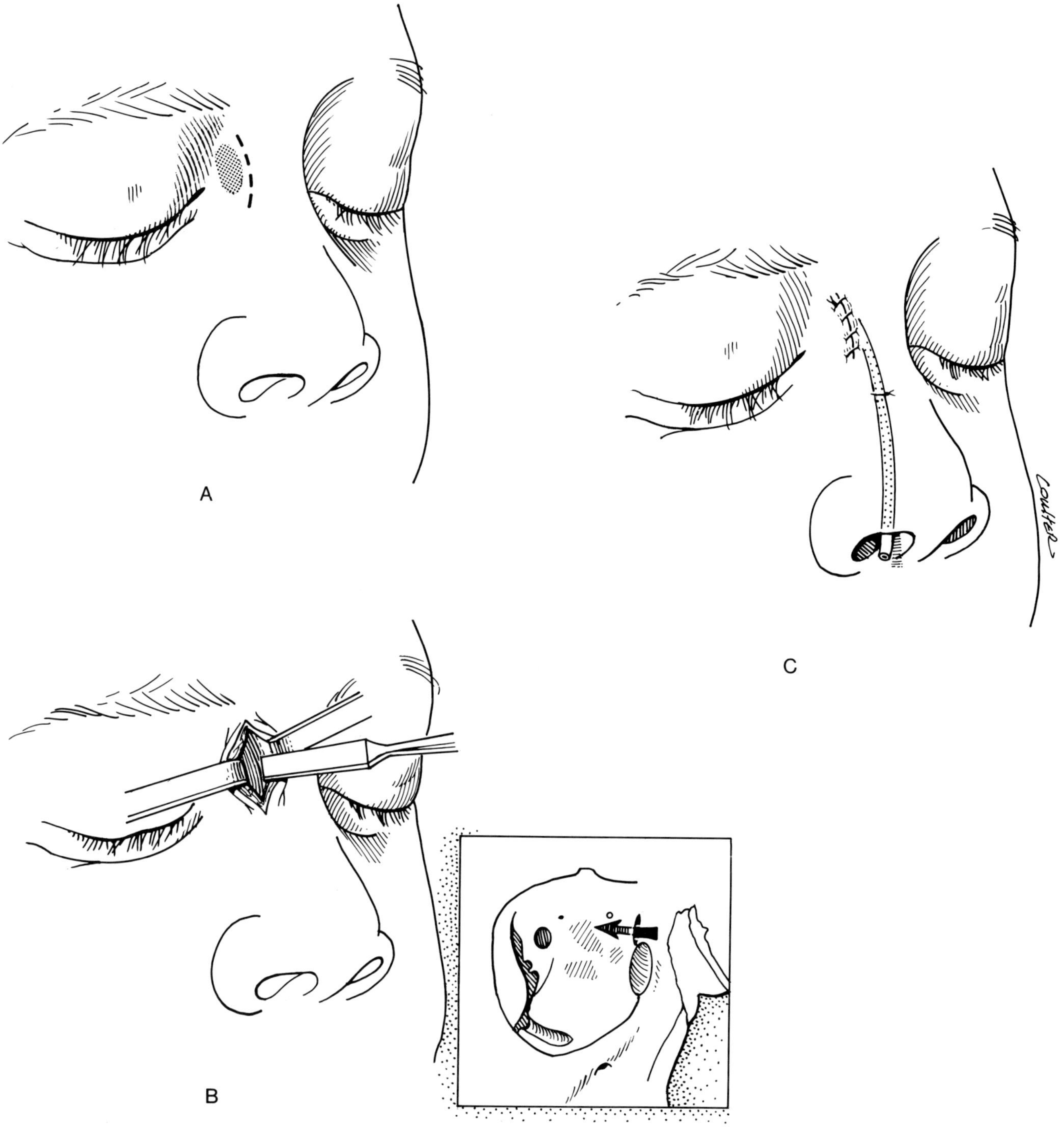

• **FIGURE 14–9.**

External ethmoidectomy. *A*, The incision site is marked with a thumbnail. *B*, A small osteotome is used to open the ethmoid sinus. *Inset*, Orbital cavity showing the lacrimal sac. *C*, The ethmoid complex is drained into the nose using a rubber band.

REFERENCES

1. Gibson LE and Cook RE: A test for concentration of electrolytes in sweat in cystic fibrosis of the pancreas utilizing pilocarpine by iontophoresis. Pediatrics 23:545–549, 1959.
2. Stankiewicz JA: Greater palatine foramen injection made easy. Laryngoscope 98:580, 1988.

chapter

15

Tonsillectomy and Adenoidectomy

LINDA BRODSKY, M.D.

Diseases of the tonsils and adenoids are among the most frequently encountered diseases in the pediatric population. Although the incidence of tonsillectomy and adenoidectomy has decreased greatly in the last 40 years, they are still the most common major surgical procedures performed on children in the United States today.[1] A better understanding of the natural history of tonsillar and adenoid diseases along with an expanded role for medical management has resulted in stricter indications for surgery.

Although the tonsils and adenoids are removed simultaneously, the indications for their removal should be considered separately. Furthermore, the efficacy of the surgical treatment depends on a precise clinical evaluation.[2] The otolaryngologist must be able to work with referring primary care physicians to establish which patients will benefit most from surgery.

Of all the surgeries that the otolaryngologist performs, tonsillectomy and adenoidectomy have the most variations in technique as well as recommendations for preoperative and postoperative management. My preferred method, with comments on the variations to this method, follows.

Indications

The indications for tonsillectomy and adenoidectomy can be divided into three basic categories: infection, obstruction, and neoplasia (Tables 15–1 and 15–2). The role of medical therapy has not yet been precisely defined. However, based on the acknowledged role of β-lactamase–producing microorganisms, multiple organisms, bacterial antigenic concentration, and encapsulated anaerobes in both chronic infection and hyperplasia,[3–5] it is necessary for each practitioner to assess the need for therapy and offer antibiotic therapy prior to surgery when appropriate.

Anesthetic considerations

- Careful planning of airway control in severely obstructed patients, patients with a craniofacial anomaly, and neurologically impaired patients
- Sharing of established airway by surgeon and anesthesiologist after intubation for handling the endotracheal tube and protecting the larynx
- Awareness by the anesthesiologist of possible complications of pulmonary edema after relief of airway obstruction, the status of the cervical spine in Down's syndrome, and family or patient history of malignant hyperthermia
- Avoidance of narcotics (which cause central respiratory depression) in patients with obstructive sleep apnea or neurologic impairment

• TABLE 15-1.

SURGICAL INDICATIONS FOR ADENOIDECTOMY

Infection	
Chronic purulent adenoiditis lasting for longer than 3 months despite medical therapy	
Recurrent acute adenoiditis (more than three attacks in 6 months) despite medical therapy	
Recurrent acute otitis media or chronic otitis media with effusion	
Chronic otitis media with perforation and otorrhea unresponsive to medical therapy	
Obstruction	
Obstructive adenoid hyperplasia resulting in:	
Sleep apnea or sleep disturbances	Not solely attributable to other causes
Obligate mouthbreathing	
Speech abnormalities	
Eating or swallowing disorders	
Failure to thrive	
Cor pulmonale	
Orofacial and dental abnormalities resulting in a narrow upper airway with adenoid hyperplasia	
Cardiac or pulmonary disease exacerbated by upper airway obstruction	
Neoplasia	
Suspected either benign or malignant neoplasia	

• TABLE 15-2.

SURGICAL INDICATIONS FOR TONSILLECTOMY

Infection	
Recurrent tonsillitis with more than 4 episodes in 1 year despite medical therapy	
Recurrent tonsillitis when complicated by:	
Peritonsillar abscess	
Febrile seizures	
Immune deficiency	
Abscessed cervical nodes	
Acute airway obstruction	
Recurrent tonsillitis associated with:	
Cardiac valve disease	
Recurrent or chronic otitis media	
Streptococcal carrier state unresponsive to medical therapy	
Chronic tonsillitis with one of the following (not attributable to other causes and unresponsive to medical therapy):	
Persistent sore throat	
Halitosis	
Tender cervical adenitis	
Tonsillolithiasis	
Obstruction	
Obstructive tonsillar hyperplasia resulting in:	
Sleep apnea or sleep disturbances	
Sleep abnormalities	Not solely attributable to other causes
Eating or swallowing disorders	
Cor pulmonale	
Failure to thrive	
Orofacial or dental anatomic abnormalities associated with a narrow upper airway	
Cardiac or pulmonary disease associated with upper airway obstruction	
Neoplasia	
Suspected either benign or malignant neoplasia	

Preparation

- Prepare the family and the patient for the procedure and postoperative course. Child life programs are helpful in this regard in children 4 years of age and older.
- Evaluate the integrity of the palate in children undergoing adenoidectomy.
- Establish a coagulation profile if there is a positive family history or easy bruisability.
- Evaluation of patients with Down's syndrome includes an evaluation for C1-C2 subluxation and cardiac abnormalities.
- Reserve a bed in the intensive care unit for the patient and possible overnight intubation in children with severe obstructive sleep apnea, neurologic abnormalities, craniofacial anomalies, or severe medical problems.

Procedure

POSITIONING AND DRAPING

- General endotracheal anesthesia is established.
- Anesthesia equipment is positioned at the side of the patient.
- A shoulder roll is placed to extend the neck.
- A head drape and down sheet are placed.

PLACEMENT OF THE RETRACTOR (Fig. 15–1)

- The endotracheal tube is centered on the tongue.
- A mouth gag with a ring tongue depressor is used to anchor the tube against the tongue.
- The mouth is retracted open, and care is taken not to pinch the tongue or lips on the teeth or dislodge the tube.
- The mouth gag is suspended from a Mayo stand on which the surgical instruments have been placed.

ADENOIDECTOMY

- A red rubber catheter is passed through one naris.
- Tension is held on the red rubber catheter with a clamp for palatal retraction.
- The nasopharynx is visualized using a defogged laryngeal mirror.
- A sharp curette is passed, using a mirror for guidance, to the caudal end of the septum. After pressing down until the posterior pharyngeal wall is met, the curette is brought forward with a seesaw motion to remove the adenoid pad intact (Fig. 15–2).
- Packing is placed in the nasopharynx and is left there while the tonsillectomy is performed. If only an adenoidectomy is being performed, the packing is removed, the nasopharynx is irrigated with saline, and hemostasis is obtained using a suction cautery under direct visualization using a mirror.

• FIGURE 15-1.

Placement of a mouth gag and suspension.

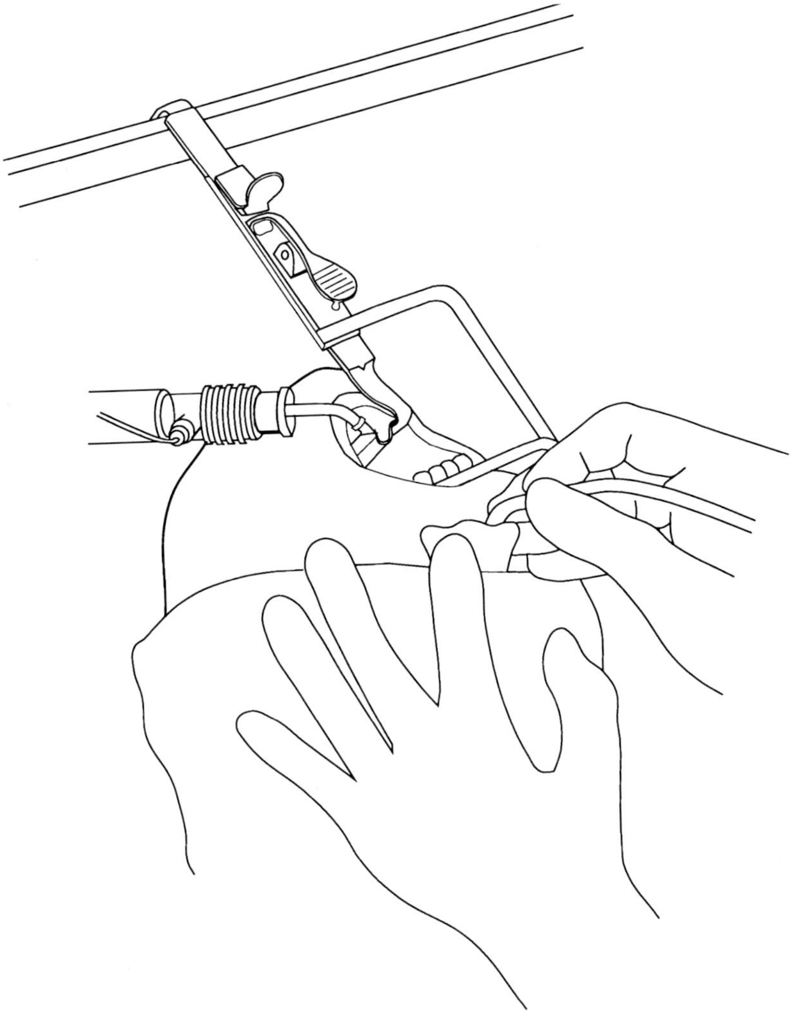

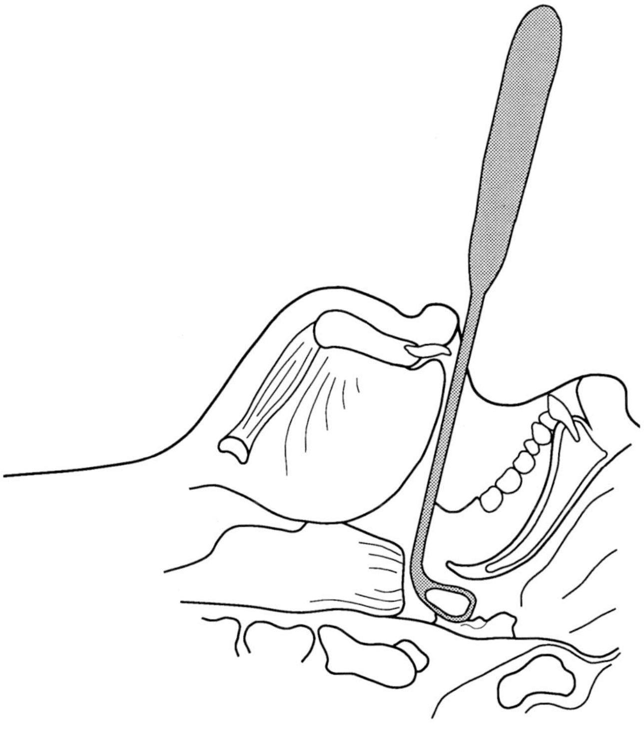

• FIGURE 15-2.

Removal of the adenoids with a curette.

TONSILLECTOMY

- An Allis clamp is applied to the superior pole of the tonsil, which is then retracted medially to identify the lateral extent of the tonsil submucosally.

- The anterior tonsillar pillar is incised through the mucosa. The incision is extended down to the base of the tonsil, both anteriorly and posteriorly (Fig. 15–3).

- Using blunt-tipped Metzenbaum scissors, a subcapsular plane of dissection is developed, with care taken to stay on the tonsil capsule (Fig. 15–4).

- Electrocautery of bleeders is accomplished when they are encountered. While the surgeon retracts the tonsil, the nurse simultaneously suctions and provides countertraction with a Yankauer suction in the tonsillar fossa.

- Taking care not to incise the lingual tonsils, the base of the tonsil is cut (Fig. 15–5).

- Packing is placed in the tonsillar fossae.

- Suction electrocautery is used to control residual bleeding after several minutes have elapsed. Visualization of the superior pole may be accomplished by use of a mirror. (Other methods of hemostasis include the use of suture ligatures, ties, bismuth subgallate, laser [KTP] tonsillectomy, and bipolar microdissection tonsillectomy.)

- The mouth gag is released, and the red rubber catheter is removed. If no further bleeding is noted after re-examination of the tonsillar fossae, the mouth gag is removed.

Postoperative care/complications

GENERAL CONSIDERATIONS

HOSPITAL DISCHARGE

- Same-day tonsillectomy is considered safe by some surgeons.

- I would *not* recommend it in the following instances: surgery for obstructive sleep apnea for children younger than 3 years of age; the presence of medical problems, craniofacial anomalies, or neurologic impairment; when the patient lives farther than 45 minutes from the hospital; when questionable caretaker or home environment is involved.

ACTIVITY

- Recommendations vary widely.

- Light activities can be undertaken for several days, with cautious return to full activities (including school) in 1 to 2 weeks.

DIET

- Recommendations vary widely from intake of liquids and soft foods for 7 to 10 days to an unlimited diet.

- Medication

    Antibiotics (usually ampicillin) are recommended for 10 days.

    Tylenol may be used, sometimes with codeine, for pain.
    NO ASPIRIN OR ASPIRIN-CONTAINING PRODUCTS
    IBUPROFEN SHOULD ALSO BE AVOIDED

    Perioperative steroids are used by some people.

• FIGURE 15-3.

Application of an Allis clamp onto the tonsil and incision of the anterior pillar.

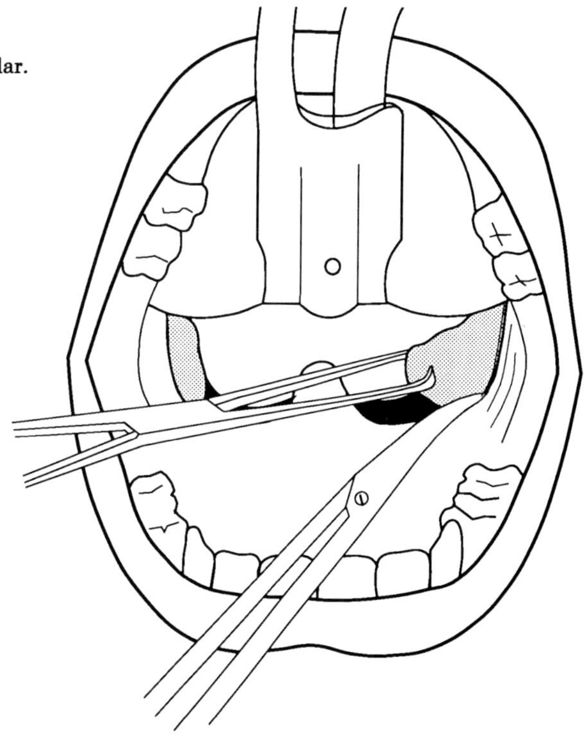

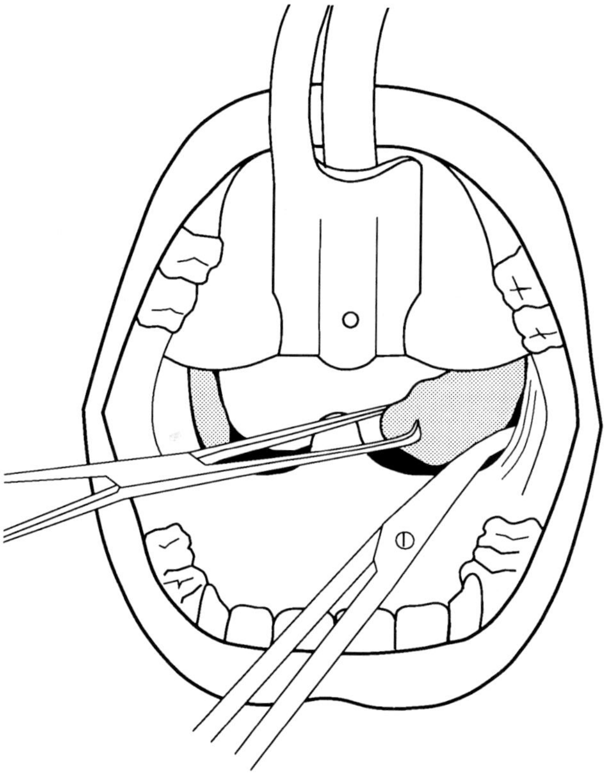

• FIGURE 15-4.

Scissor dissection of the tonsil.

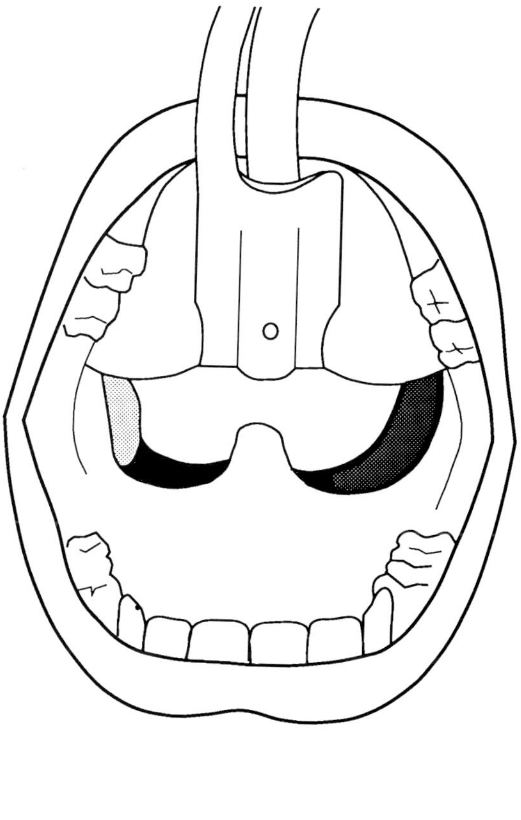

• FIGURE 15-5.

Tonsil dissection on one side is complete.

COMPLICATIONS

- Obstruction

  Planned overnight intubation and intensive care unit monitoring for a severely obstructed or medically unstable patient. In most severe cases, a tracheostomy tray should be kept at the bed.

  Consider placement of a nasopharyngeal tube.

  Steroids may be used to reduce palatal swelling.

- Bleeding

  Can be immediate or delayed (7 to 10 days)

  Most stop spontaneously but should be evaluated by a physician

  Local control in the emergency room with removal of a clot and vasoconstriction or cautery

  Return the patient to the operating room when bleeding is difficult to control. Rapid sequence induction—or, less favored, intubation while the patient is awake—is usually used by the anesthesiologist.

- Pulmonary edema after relief of upper airway obstruction

  Rare occurrence

  Should be suspected intraoperatively or postoperatively when difficulty occurs with oxygenation encountered after intubation for severe chronic upper airway obstruction

  Treated with diuretics, morphine sulfate, and positive-pressure ventilation

- Velopharyngeal insufficiency

  Frequently seen temporarily after a tonsillectomy and adenoidectomy from palatal splinting

  Persistent form seen occasionally after an adenoidectomy due to palatal insufficiency, often from an occult submucous cleft palate unrecognized preoperatively.

- Miscellaneous

  Torticollis is frequently seen for 1 to 2 weeks after an adenoidectomy. If torticollis is not resolved, one must suspect C1-C2 subluxation.

  Otitis media with effusion is seen occasionally after an adenoidectomy in a previously healthy ear. Expectant treatment or antibiotic therapy is used.

REFERENCES

1. Rutkow IM: Ear, nose and throat operations in the United States, 1979 to 1984. Arch Otolaryngol Head Neck Surg 112:873–876, 1986.
2. Brodsky L: Modern assessment of the tonsils and adenoids. Pediatr Clin North Am 36(6):1551–1569, 1989.
3. Brook I: The clinical microbiology of Waldmeyer's ring. Otolaryngol Clin North Am 20:259–272, 1987.
4. Brodsky L, Moore L, and Stanievich JF: The role of *Haemophilus influenzae* in the pathogenesis of tonsillar hypertrophy in children. Laryngoscope 98:1055–1060, 1988.
5. Brodsky L, Moore L, Stanievich JF, and Ogra PL: The immunology of tonsils in children: The effect of bacterial load on the presence of B and T-cell subsets. Laryngoscope 98:93–98, 1988.

chapter
16

Uvulopalato-pharyngoplasty

LINDA BRODSKY, M.D.

Upper airway obstruction, secondary to tonsil and adenoid hyperplasia, is the most common cause for obstructive sleep apnea in children.[1] Although in most of these children the problem resolves with tonsillectomy and adenoidectomy (see Chapter 15), some continue to have symptoms and require further treatment. Craniofacial anomalies, neuromuscular hypotonia, cerebral palsy, or severe mental insufficiency may often be contributing factors to obstructive sleep apnea.

Uvulopalatopharyngoplasty (UPPP) was first described in 1981 by Fujita and coworkers for the treatment of severe obstructive sleep apnea in adults as an alternative to permanent tracheostomy.[2] The application of this technique to children who have nasopharyngeal or oropharyngeal collapse as a cause of the obstruction has been advanced by several investigators.[1,3] As an alternative to tracheostomy, UPPP can be a valuable procedure for a select group of children with obstructive sleep apnea.

Indications

- Persistent obstructive sleep apnea not relieved by tonsillectomy and adenoidectomy
- Obstructive sleep apnea in the absence of tonsil or adenoid hyperplasia, which is due, at least in part, to nasopharyngeal or hypopharyngeal hypotonia and collapse.

This procedure seems to have its greatest applicability in children with cerebral palsy, neuromuscular hypotonia, craniofacial anomalies, or developmental deficiency.

PREOPERATIVE EVALUATION

- Multichannel sleep recording (polysomnogram) to identify the presence and degree of severity of the obstruction and the presence of arrhythmias and hypercapnia
- Direct visualization of the location(s) of the obstruction using a flexible fiberoptic nasopharyngoscope during sleep or with sleep videofluoroscopy

The best results are obtained when the obstruction is in the nasopharyngeal (palatal) or oropharyngeal area. An obstruction at the level of the base of the tongue or lower than that may require alternative forms of treatment. In the presence of mandibular retrognathia, a mandibular advancement procedure should be considered. Finally, tracheostomy may be needed for those who fail to respond to these alternatives. Parents should be well informed of the variability of the results and the possible need for additional surgery.

Anesthetic considerations

- Preoperative evaluation is similar to that for tonsillectomy and adenoidectomy; however, because these children tend to have severe and more complex medical problems, greater vigilance is necessary in the preoperative preparations.
- Careful planning of airway management is needed (see Chapter 15 for other anesthetic considerations).

  The following evaluations may be necessary: cardiac (to look for early right-sided heart enlargement), neurologic for seizure control, C-spine radiographs in patients with Down's syndrome, and a computed tomography (CT) evaluation of the foramen magnum in achondroplastic dwarfism or craniofacial anomalies.
- A bed in the intensive care unit should be reserved for the patient.
- Preparations for a tracheotomy should always be made for severely obstructed individuals.
- Perioperative sedation should be avoided, because acute airway obstruction may be precipitated or a central sleep apnea component may be enhanced.

Preparation

PREOPERATIVE

- Prepare the patient and the family for a potentially difficult postoperative course and the possible need for further surgical intervention.

POSITIONING AND DRAPING

- The procedure is performed in the same position as tonsillectomy and adenoidectomy.

  General orotracheal anesthesia is established.

  Anesthesia is positioned at the side of the patient.

  A shoulder roll is placed to extend the neck.

  A head drape and down sheet are placed.

Procedure

PLACEMENT OF THE RETRACTOR

- The endotracheal tube is centered on the tongue.
- A mouth gag with a ring tongue depressor is used to anchor the tube against the tongue.
- The mouth is retracted open, and care is taken not to pinch the tongue or lips on the teeth or dislodge the tube.
- The mouth gag is suspended from a Mayo stand on which the surgical instruments have been placed.

TONSILLECTOMY AND ADENOIDECTOMY

- If tonsillectomy and adenoidectomy has not yet been performed, this is done first. Some surgeons excise the tonsils in continuity with the soft palate and tonsillar pillars; however, this may reduce the precision of mucosal excision.

UPPP PROCEDURE

- If tonsillectomy has been done previously

  An anterior incision is made to include the mucosa of the tonsillar pillars and soft palate (Fig. 16–1).

  An incision is made on the posterior surface of the palate to include the uvula (Fig. 16–2).

- Determining the amount of mucosa to remove from the palate may be difficult; caution must be exercised to avoid excision of muscle, which could cause velopharyngeal insufficiency.
- Incise the mucosa at the corners of the vertical and horizontal limbs in a superolateral direction (Fig. 16–3).[4]

• FIGURE 16–1.

Incise the anterior palate to include the mucosa of the anterior tonsillar pillars and the free edge of the soft palate.

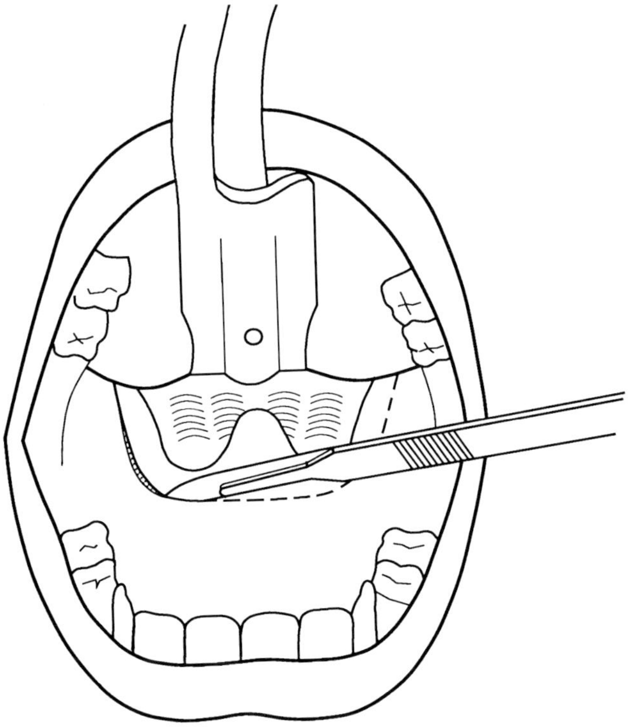

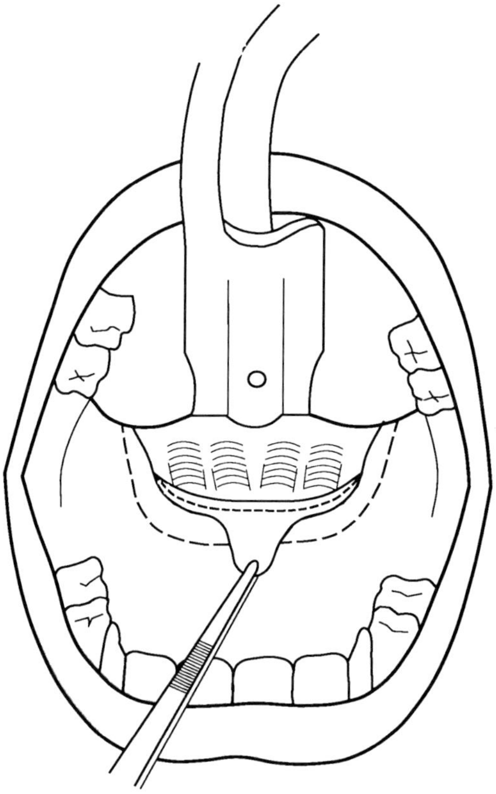

• FIGURE 16–2.

While holding the uvula with a forceps, make an incision on the posterior (nasal) side of the palate. Remove the incised mucosa without removing the underlying muscles.

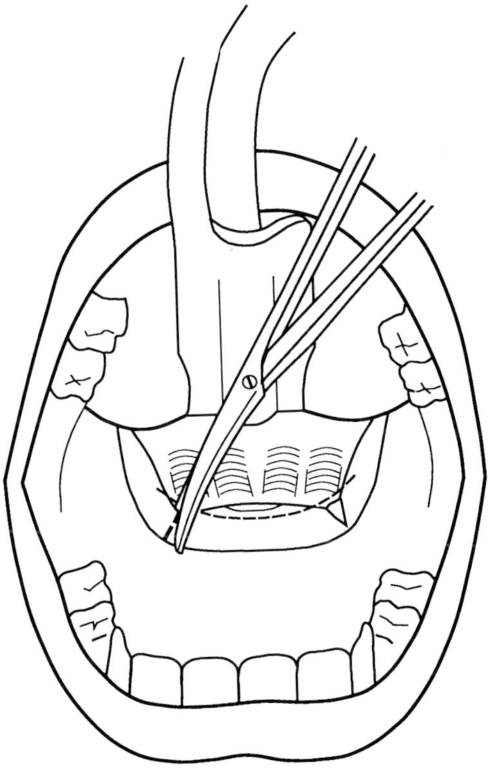

• FIGURE 16–3.

Incise the corners of the palate at the junction of the horizontal and vertical limbs.

- Suture the corners first using 4-0 Dexon or Vicryl.
- Excise and then close the mucosa of the palatoglossal and palatopharyngeal folds (anterior and posterior tonsillar pillars) (Fig. 16–4).
- Advance the palatal mucosa, and close the horizontal incision (Fig. 16–5). Use interrupted sutures for both closures.
- Place a nasopharyngeal tube under direct visualization and firmly secure it to the face with benzoin and tape.
- The mouth gag is released and removed.

Postoperative care/complications

GENERAL CONSIDERATIONS

- Admit the patient to the intensive care unit.
- Restraints may be necessary during the patient's recovery to prevent dislodgement of the nasopharyngeal tube.
- Prolonged orotracheal intubation may be necessary. The length of the procedure, the amount of swelling, the severity of the obstruction, and the underlying medical problems are considered.
- Activity

  Once the patient is discharged from the intensive care unit, activity may be resumed as tolerated.
- Diet

  Nothing should be taken by mouth for the first 24 hours; then give liquids and advance to a regular diet as tolerated.
- Medication

  Antibiotics are given for 10 days (usually ampicillin).

  Perioperative steroids may reduce palatal edema.

  Tylenol with codeine may be used if necessary.

COMPLICATIONS

- Airway obstruction from perioperative sedatives, failure to intubate, palatal or tongue swelling, or hemorrhage
- Wound dehiscence from tension of closure, infection, or intraoral trauma postoperatively (fingers or foreign bodies)
- Hemorrhage
- Palatal incompetence with velopharyngeal insufficiency or nasal regurgitation of liquids
- Nasopharyngeal stenosis

• FIGURE 16-4.

Suture the corner incisions first using 4-0 Dexon or Vicryl.

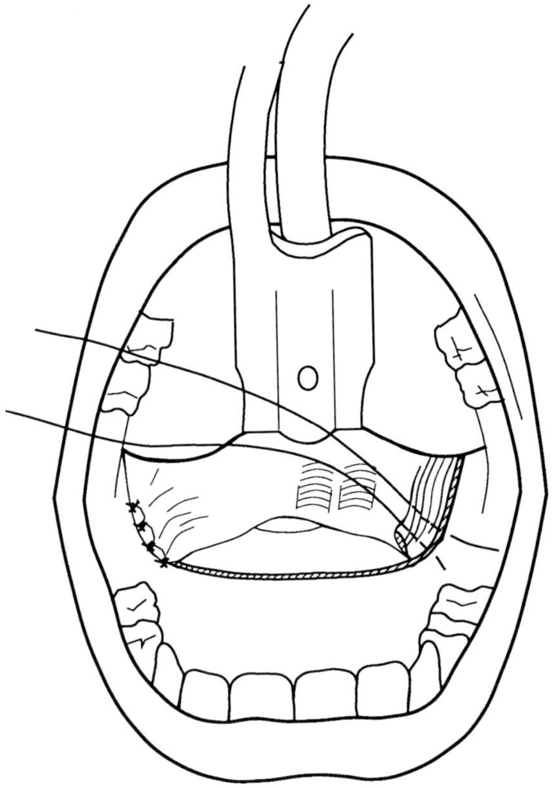

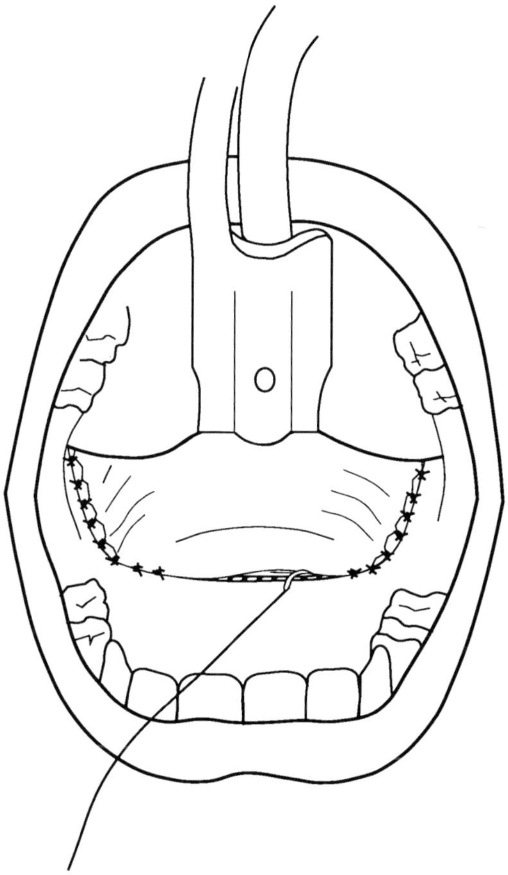

• FIGURE 16-5.

Excise redundant mucosa, and suture the anterior to the posterior tonsillar pillar. Advance the palatal mucosa, and close the horizontal incision with interrupted sutures.

REFERENCES

1. Seid AB, Martin PJ, Pransky SB, and Kearns CB: Surgical therapy of obstructive sleep apnea in children with severe mental insufficiency. Laryngoscope 100:507–510, 1990.
2. Fujita S, Conway W, Zorick F, and Roth T: Surgical correction of anatomic abnormalities of obstructive sleep apnea syndrome: Uvulopalatopharyngoplasty. Otolaryngol Head Neck Surg 89:923–927, 1981.
3. Koopmann CF and Moran WB: Surgical management of obstructive sleep apnea. Otolaryngol Clin North Am 23(4):787–808, 1990.
4. Fairbanks DNF: Operative techniques of uvulopalatopharyngoplasty. Oper Tech Otolaryngol Head Neck Surg 2(2):104–106, 1991.

chapter

17

Deep Neck Infections

CHARLES F. KOOPMANN, JR., M.D.

FASCIA LAYERS OF THE NECK (Figs. 17–1 and 17–2)

SUPERFICIAL CERVICAL FASCIA

The superficial cervical fascia of the neck encloses the voluntary muscles in its deepest portion (the platysma muscle) and surrounds the neck, being continuous with the superficial fascia of the muscles of facial expression superiorly and the deltoid, back, and pectoral areas inferiorly. Superficial lymph nodes on the external jugular vein also lie within this region.

DEEP CERVICAL FASCIA

Superficial Layer

The superficial layer of the deep cervical fascia is connected to the vertebral spinous processes and ligamentum nuchae. It completely encircles the neck and divides to surround the trapezius muscle. As it goes anteriorly, it divides again to enclose the sternocleidomastoid muscle.

The fascia forms a single layer anterior to the sternocleidomastoid muscle and meets its counterpart from the opposite side. This layer is attached to the hyoid bone and is important because it divides the neck into the areas above (suprahyoid) and below (infrahyoid). A superior part of this fascia encloses the submandibular and parotid glands and forms the stylomandibular ligament, which runs from the styloid process to the hyoid bone. The infrahyoid portion of the superficial layer attaches to the anterior and posterior portions of the sternum and forms the suprasternal space (space of Burns), where the anterior jugular veins and lymph nodes are found.

Middle (Pretracheal) Layer

The superficial muscular layer encloses the strap muscles (omohyoid, thyrohyoid, sternohyoid, and sternothyroid). This layer also passes in front of the trachea, esophagus, and thyroid gland, and as it courses inferiorly along the infrahyoid muscles behind the sternum, it fuses with the fibrous pericardium.

The carotid sheath (surrounding the internal jugular vein, common carotid artery, and vagus nerve) is found between the superficial layer, the pretracheal layer, and the prevertebral layer. The lateral portion of the pretracheal fascia fuses with the outer superficial fascia layer.

The visceral layer of the pretracheal fascia surrounds the constrictor muscles and attaches to the base of the skull, where it forms the anterior portion of the retropharyngeal space. This part of the fascia is sometimes called the buccopharyngeal portion.

Deep (Prevertebral) Layer

The prevertebral or deep layer of the deep cervical fascia may be thought of as originating from the cervical spinous processes and ligamentum nuchae. Anteriorly, it encloses the prevertebral muscles, brachial plexus, and subclavian artery.

• FIGURE 17-1.

Cross-section of the neck illustrating visceral structures and fascial planes. (Modified from Barrett G, Koopmann CF, and Coulthard SW: Retropharyngeal abscess—a ten year experience. Laryngoscope J 94[4]:455-463, 1984.)

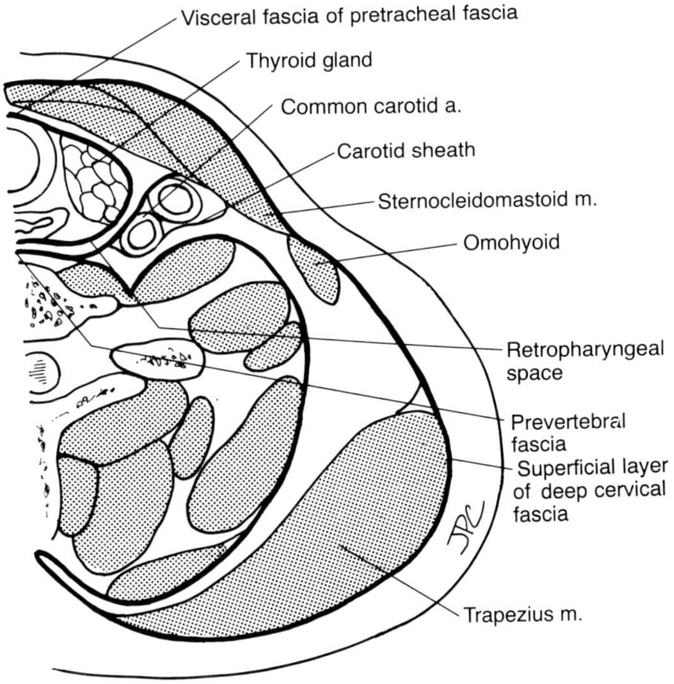

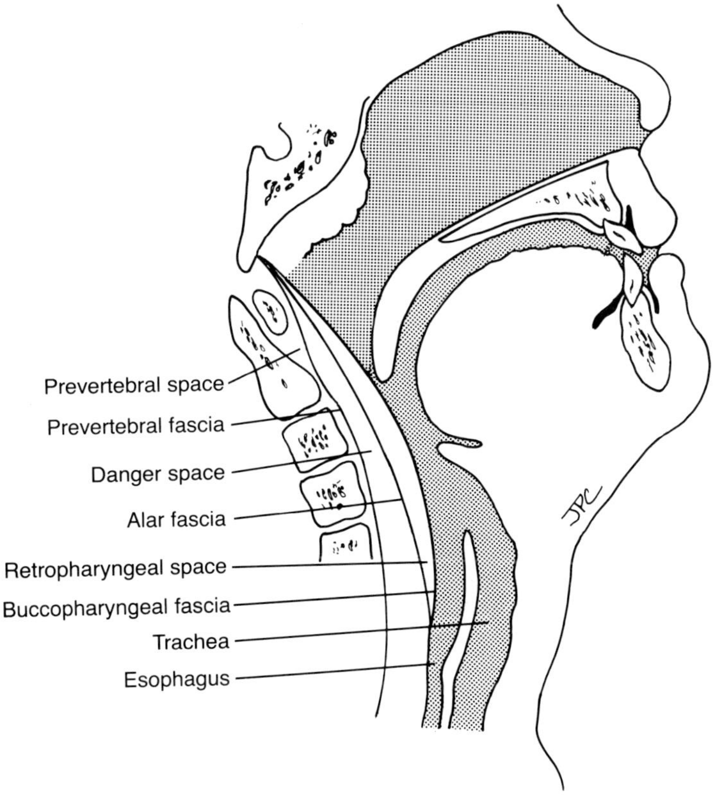

• FIGURE 17-2.

Lateral neck emphasizing retropharyngeal, prevertebral, and "danger" spaces. (Modified from Barrett G, Koopmann CF, and Coulthard SW: Retropharyngeal abscess—a ten year experience. Laryngoscope J 94[4]:455-463, 1984.)

A danger space exists near the posterior part of the trapezius muscle and the upper posterior triangle of the neck where the prevertebral layer splits into two definite layers anterior to the vertebral column. Both the anterior and posterior portions of this space originate at the base of the skull. The anterior layer blends with the fascia of the esophagus in the superior mediastinum and is considered the posterior wall of the retropharyngeal space. The posterior portion goes inferiorly to the coccyx.

CLASSIFICATION AND TREATMENT OF DEEP HEAD AND NECK SPACE INFECTIONS

SUPRAHYOID SPACES

Submandibular Space (Fig. 17–3)

The submandibular space is divided into the sublingual (supramylohyoid) space and the submandibular (inframylohyoid) space. The anterior belly of the digastric muscle forms a central component called the submental space, which is bounded by the mucosa of the floor of the mouth, the mandible, and the superficial layer of the deep cervical fascia. The sublingual and submaxillary spaces are frequently involved in odontogenic origin.

Indications

- Ludwig's angina

  The symptoms of infection in this specific entity include inflamed, swollen tissues of the floor of the mouth; displacement of the tongue upward and backward toward the soft palate; trismus; marked induration initially confined to the submandibular compartment but then spreading; and, if the angina is untreated, dyspnea.

- Poor response to antimicrobial therapy

  Surgical intervention is needed to avoid respiratory tract obstruction, aspiration pneumonia, progressive dehydration, or spread of infection from the lateral pharyngeal space to the carotid sheath, and then to the superior mediastinum.

Anesthetic considerations

The procedure must be performed under general anesthesia to control the airway and avoid aspiration. Nasotracheal or oral endotracheal anesthesia is preferred, but it may be difficult to obtain owing to trismus and superior and posterior displacement of the tissues of the floor of the mouth. A tracheostomy is then indicated under local anesthesia or under insufflation general anesthesia.

Preparation

- The skin is prepared with an antiseptic scrub of the surgeon's choice if an external approach is needed. The throat is packed with a gauze pack.

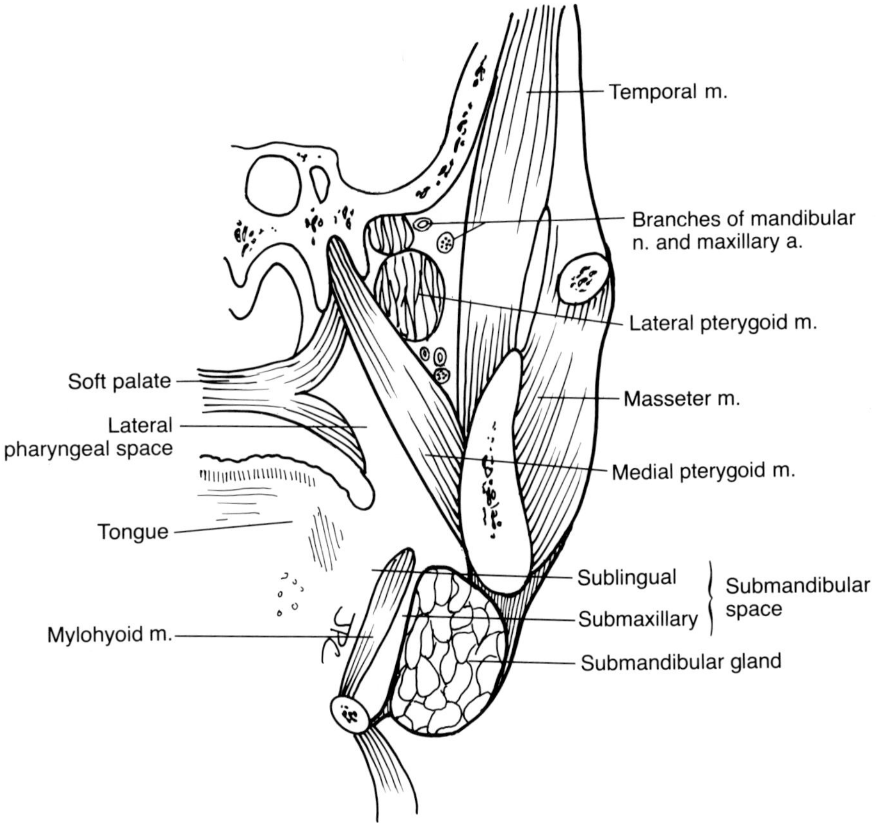

• FIGURE 17–3.

Submandibular and masticator space fascial planes. (Modified from Hollinshead WH: Anatomy for Surgeons Vol 1, 2nd ed. Hoeber, New York, 1968, pp 320–321. Used by permission of JB Lippincott.)

Procedure

The abscess in the sublingual space may respond adequately to intraoral drainage. In bilateral submandibular space infections, a submental incision is necessary (Fig. 17–4*A*). Especially in Ludwig's angina, a horizontal incision is placed approximately 1 cm above the hyoid bone (this may vary depending on the region of maximal induration) and extending laterally below the angle of the mandible in an attempt to avoid injury to the mandibular ramus branch of the facial nerve. The incision is carried through subcutaneous tissue and the platysma muscle to the deep cervical fascia, which is then incised. One can explore the neck bilaterally using a median raphe between the anterior bellies of the digastric and mylohyoid muscles. Blunt and sharp dissection are used, as necessary (Fig. 17–4*B*). The wound is irrigated copiously with either saline or an antibiotic and saline solution (bacitracin). Drains are placed (either Penrose or suction drains, such as Jackson-Pratt) (Fig. 17–4*C*). The suction drains may also be used for wound irrigation if necessary.

Postoperative care

Intravenous antibiotics are used for 4 to 5 days, followed by oral antibiotics for another 2 to 3 weeks. The drains are advanced slowly over several days.

Pharyngomaxillary (Lateral Pharyngeal) Space

This space is bounded by the petrous portion of the temporal bone superiorly; the superior constrictor muscle medially; the pterygoid muscles, mandible, and parotid gland laterally; the pterygomandibular raphe anteriorly; the buccopharyngeal and prevertebral fascia posteriorly; and the hyoid bone inferiorly.

The causes of infection in this space include odontogenic infections, penetrating wounds to the lateral pharyngeal wall, infections in the tonsil, a previous history of local infiltration such as dental injections or other oral local anesthetics, or peritonsillar cellulitis or abscess.

Indications

- The signs and symptoms include the general signs of toxicity (fever and chills), trismus, swelling of the lateral pharyngeal wall in the region posterior to the tonsil with occasional displacement of the tonsil medially or anteriorly, edema, and in some patients, generalized sepsis.
- The response to antibiotic therapy is unsatisfactory.
- Impending respiratory obstruction or extension of the abscess along the carotid sheath with rupture of the internal carotid artery is a possibility in this disorder.

Anesthetic considerations

The procedure should be performed under general anesthesia, preferably nasotracheal anesthesia in which a tube is placed in the contralateral naris. Oral endotracheal anesthesia is acceptable if the trismus is not too great; however, because of the swelling and trismus, a tracheostomy under local anesthesia or under general insufflation may be necessary.

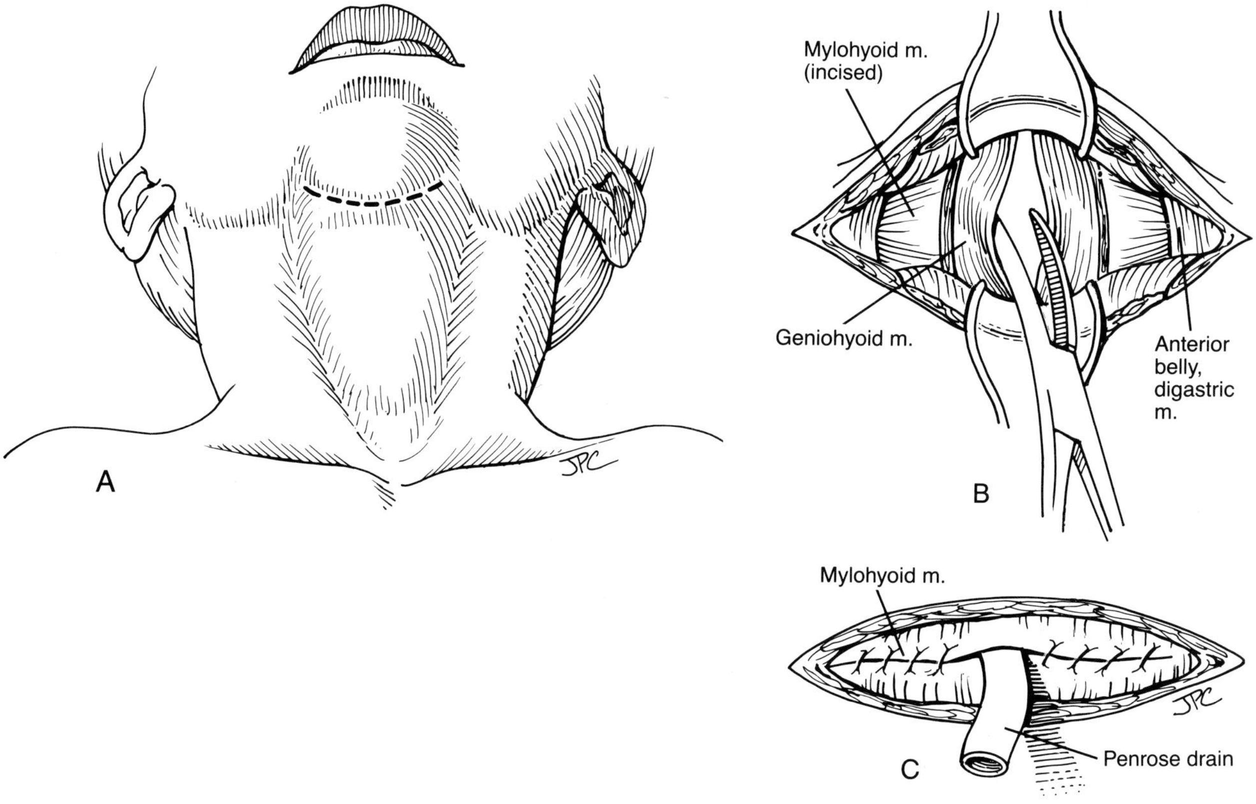

• FIGURE 17-4.

A, Incision for drainage of a submental space abscess or Ludwig's angina infection. *B*, Dissection between the geniohyoid muscles after the mylohyoid muscle has been incised. *C*, Drainage with a Penrose drain. (Modified from Lore J: An Atlas of Head Surgery, 3rd ed. Philadelphia, WB Saunders, 1988.)

Preparation

The skin is prepared with an antiseptic scrub of the surgeon's choice. The surgeon should have a nerve stimulator available.

Procedure

A horizontal incision or apron incision is made in the neck in the region of the infection. The dissection is carried through the skin and subcutaneous tissues.

Two subdivisions are made here. The posterior compartment contains the carotid sheath structures as well as cranial nerves IX to XII, and the anterior compartment contains fat, connective tissue, muscle, and lymph nodes. Normally, the dissection is carried anterior to the carotid sheath, and the carotid sheath structures are retracted laterally and posteriorly. The area of purulence is drained; cultures are taken for aerobic and anaerobic bacteria; the wound is copiously irrigated either with sterile saline or with sterile saline and antibiotic solution; and drainage is obtained through either a Penrose drain or a wall suction drain (Jackson-Pratt) (Fig. 17–5). The Jackson-Pratt system may be used if multiple drains are placed for concurrent irrigation and suction.

Postoperative care

Intravenous antibiotics are given for 5 to 7 days, followed by oral antibiotics for another 2 to 3 weeks. The drains are advanced slowly over 5 to 7 days.

Masticator Space (Fig. 17–6)

This space contains the masseter muscle, the pterygoid muscles, and the ramus of the mandible. It is formed by the deep cervical fascia as it covers the masseter muscle laterally and the pterygoid muscles medially.

The space becomes infected most commonly from odontogenic sources or from injections of oral anesthesia, especially attempts to block the inferior alveolar nerve. Also, infections from the zygoma, temporal bone, or mandible itself may occasionally spread to this region.

Indications

- Clinical signs and symptoms include general toxicity of acute onset, severe trismus, dysphagia, induration over the angle and ramus of the mandible externally, and oral swelling near the angle and ramus of the mandible, which may push the tonsil medially.
- The response to antibiotic therapy is unsatisfactory.
- Airway obstruction and asphyxia should be avoided.

Anesthetic considerations

General anesthesia is necessary. Nasotracheal or oral endotracheal anesthesia is preferred, although the trismus may preclude use of an oral tube. A tracheostomy is occasionally necessary.

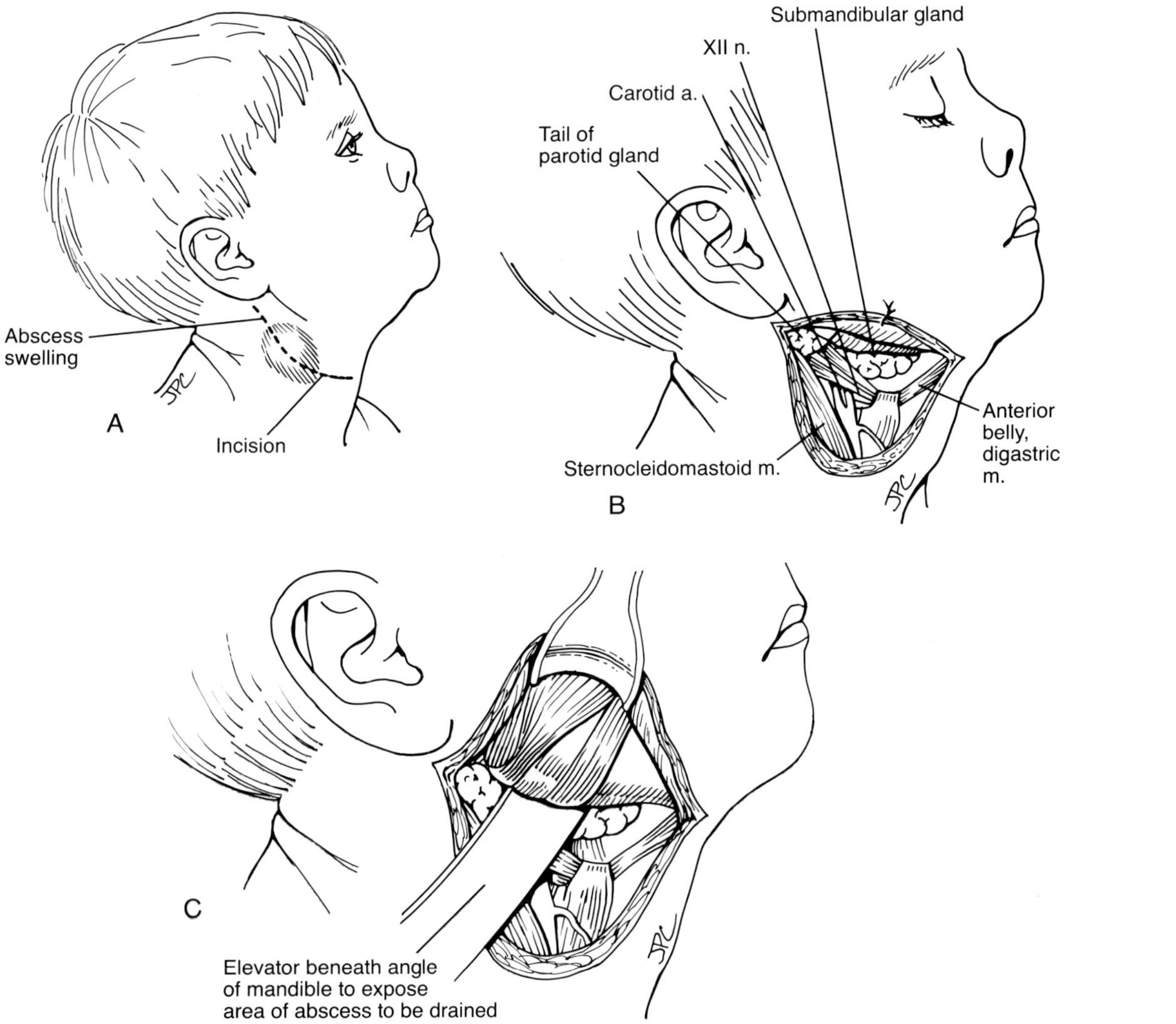

• FIGURE 17-5.

A to *C*, Drainage of the lateral pharyngeal space. (Modified from Lore J: An Atlas of Head and Neck Surgery, 3rd ed. Philadelphia, WB Saunders, 1988.)

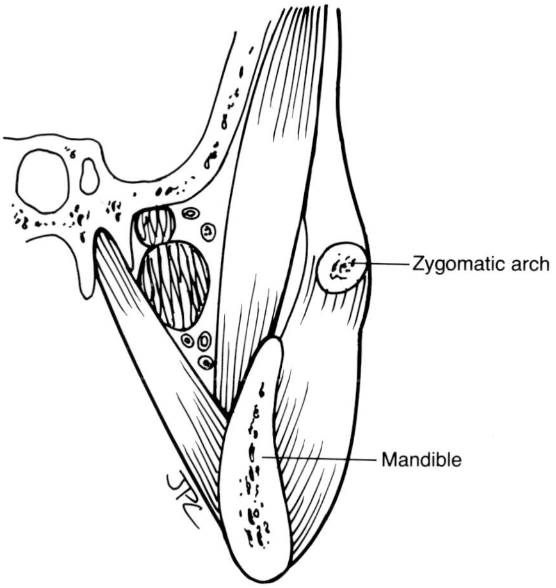

• FIGURE 17-6.

Masticator space. (Modified from Hollinshead WH: Anatomy for Surgeons Vol 1, 2nd ed. New York, Hoeber, 1968, pp 320–321. Used by permission of JB Lippincott.)

Preparation

If an external incision is necessary, the neck and facial skin is prepared with an antiseptic scrub of the surgeon's choice. If intraoral drainage is planned, the hypopharynx is packed with a gauze pack.

Procedure

External drainage is used if there is marked lateral swelling. The incision is made 2 to 3 cm below the angle of the mandible, and dissection is carried out in a plane beneath the mandibular ramus branch of the facial nerve. An incision is made through the periosteum of the mandible to enter the space and perform appropriate drainage. The wound is irrigated copiously with saline or a saline and antibiotic solution, and a Penrose drain or suction drain is inserted and advanced slowly.

If there is minimal or moderate external swelling, internal drainage may be performed in an attempt to avoid injury to the mandibular ramus branch of the facial nerve and also avoid an external incision. The incision must be made to avoid injury to the ductal system of the parotid gland. Blunt dissection is carried to the region of the abscess, and the abscess is drained intraorally. A drain may be sutured in the intraoral wound (Penrose type).

Postoperative care

Intravenous antibiotics are given for 5 to 7 days, followed by oral antibiotics for another 2 to 3 weeks. The drains are advanced over 4 to 7 days and, if the infection is extremely severe, the wound is packed with iodoform gauze soaked in Betadine solution. Additional Betadine solution is placed on the gauze as it is advanced over 3 to 4 days.

Parotid Space (Fig. 17–7)

The parotid space is formed by the superficial layer of the deep cervical fascia as it envelops the parotid gland, facial nerve, and parotid lymph nodes. The medial portion of the fascia is not complete and communicates with the pharyngomaxillary space. This allows the spread of parotid space abscesses into the pharyngomaxillary space and then to the prevertebral space.

Parotid space infections are most commonly caused by stasis of the parotid gland, dehydration after surgery or severe chronic or acute illness, salivary gland calculi, oral infections, or severe otitis externa. The causative bacterium is most commonly coagulase-positive *Staphylococcus aureus.*

Indications

- Generalized toxicity, dehydration (especially in postoperative or cachetic patients), painful swelling over the parotid gland, and, in the latter stages, pitting edema and erythema of the skin overlying the parotid gland are found.
- The response to antimicrobial therapy is unsatisfactory.

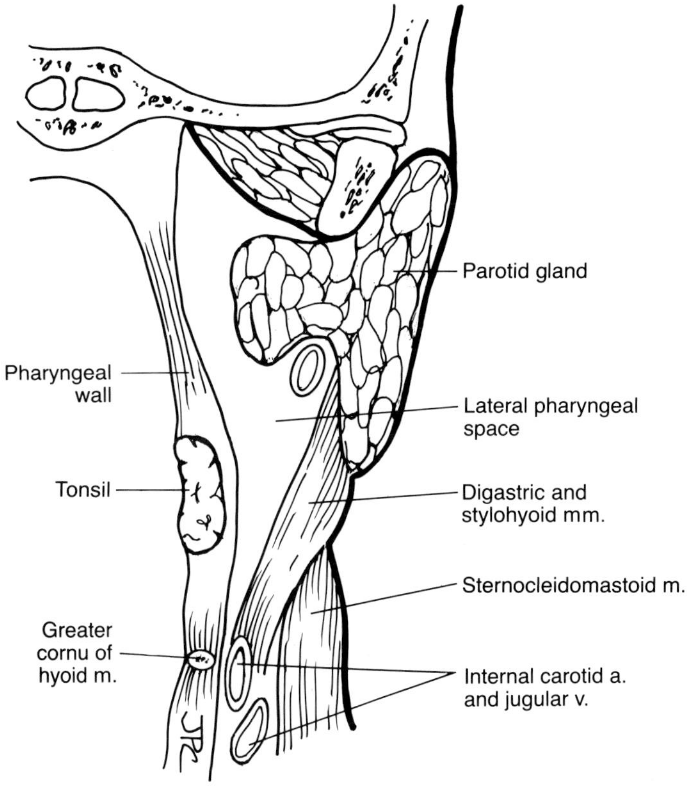

• FIGURE 17-7.

Parotid space. (Modified from Hollinshead WH: Anatomy for Surgeons, Vol 1, 2nd ed. New York, Hoeber, 1968. Used by permission of JB Lippincott.)

Anesthetic considerations

The procedure is usually performed under general oral endotracheal anesthesia.

Preparation

The skin is prepared with an antiseptic scrub of the surgeon's choice.

Procedure

An incision is made in the standard fashion used for a parotidectomy, with preauricular and retroauricular limbs curved in the standard fashion (Fig. 17–8). Skin and subcutaneous tissue are elevated over the parotid fascia. The parotid fascia is punctured in multiple areas with a curved, pointed mosquito hemostat, and the hemostat is opened in a direction parallel to the course of the facial nerve and its branches. Multiple openings are made in this fashion to allow drainage of the infected fluid. Because the infection involves multilocular abscesses, many areas of incision and opening of the mosquito hemostat are required.

An alternative method for drainage has been used most recently in the rare patient who also has bleeding diatheses. A small incision can be made in the usual parotidectomy outlined area, and a small liposuction cannula may be introduced through the incision to drain the multilocular areas. Care must be taken to perform this suction drainage parallel to the course of the facial nerve. This method allows the surgeon to avoid a long skin incision and flap elevation in the patient who has a bleeding disorder.

In either of the aforementioned methods, the wound is drained. In the first method, a Jackson-Pratt suction drain is used most commonly, although a Penrose drain could also be acceptable. In the second method, a Penrose drain is used most commonly.

In the patients with bleeding diatheses, a pressure dressing may be necessary.

Postoperative care

Intravenous antibiotics are given for 4 to 5 days, followed by oral antibiotics for 1 to 2 weeks. The drains are advanced over 4 to 5 days.

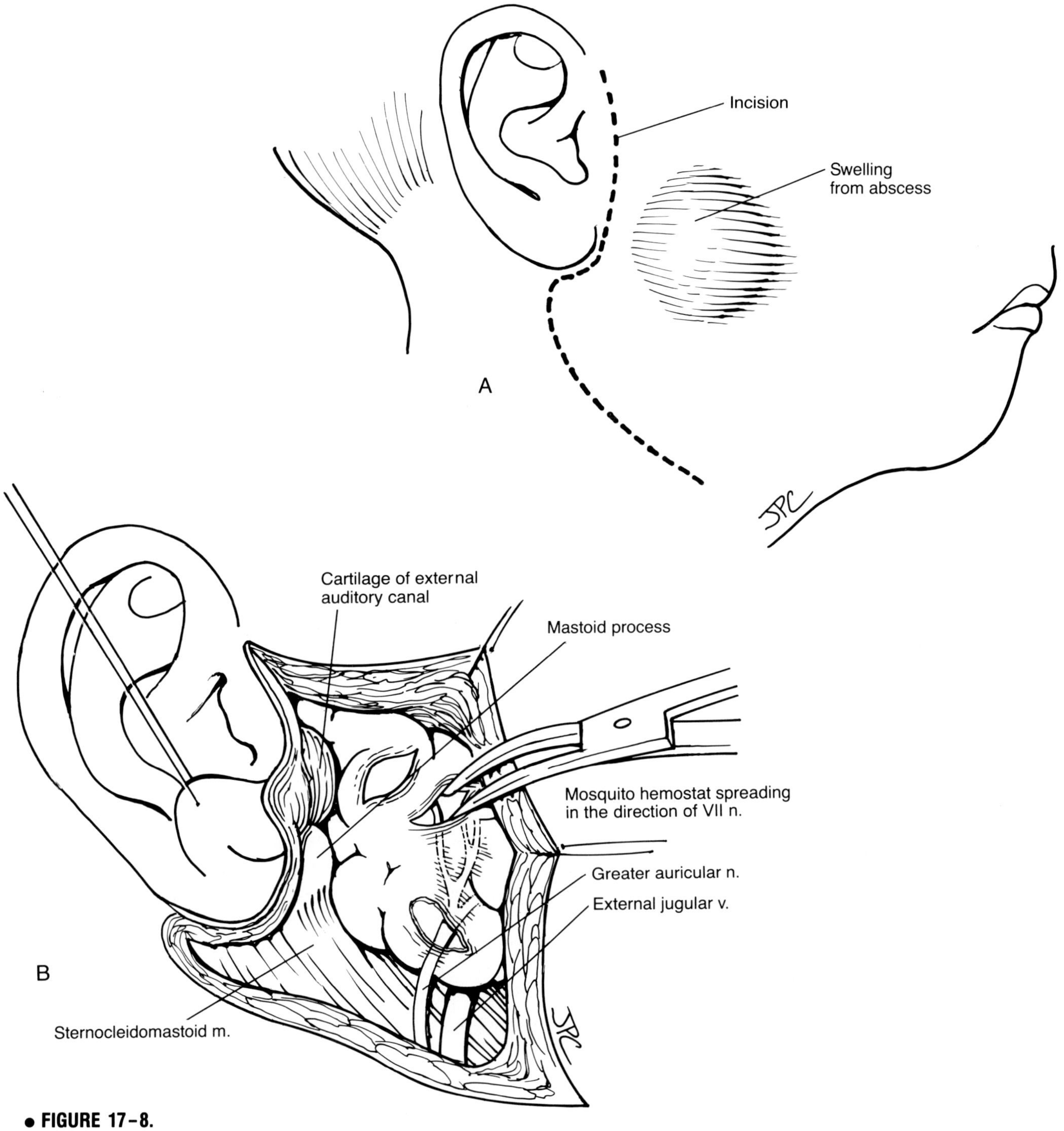

• FIGURE 17–8.

A and *B*, Incision for drainage of the parotid abscess. (Adapted from Lore J: An Atlas of Head and Neck Surgery, 3rd ed. Philadelphia, WB Saunders, 1988.)

Peritonsillar Space

The peritonsillar space is bounded by the capsule of the tonsil medially, the superior constrictor muscle laterally, and the tonsillar pillars anteriorly and posteriorly. Abscesses in the midportion may go through the superior constrictor into the lateral pharyngeal space.

Indications

- The signs and symptoms include dysphagia; trismus; swelling of the tonsillar pillars, the soft palate, and often the uvula, with displacement of the uvula to the contralateral side; displacement of the tonsil (also to the contralateral side); and a "hot potato" voice.
- The response to antimicrobial therapy, dehydration, and airway obstruction is unsatisfactory.

Anesthetic considerations

In younger children, a general anesthetic is necessary. In older children and teenagers, frequently topical and local anesthesia is adequate for needle aspiration. However, one must incise the area and place a hemostat for drainage; if an acute tonsillectomy is to be performed, general anesthesia is usually necessary.

Preparation

If the patient requires a general anesthetic, the throat should be packed with a gauze pack.

Procedure

The initial method of diagnosing and treating a peritonsillar abscess is with aspiration (Fig. 17–9). One uses a syringe with a 16- or 18-gauge needle and aspirates at the junction of the soft palate and superior tonsillar pillar (the area most likely to have purulence and also the area that is least dangerous for aspiration). If there is pointing in another area, or if the initial aspiration in this area fails, then one must go inferiorly and more medially.

If one is going to incise the tonsillar pillar, one would do this over the area that is most fluctuant and where the aspiration was positive for purulence. However, if the child must be placed on general anesthesia, a tonsillectomy is warranted. Most commonly, I use a coagulation cautery tonsillectomy to reduce the risk of bleeding. The contralateral tonsil is also removed at this stage, but only if the bleeding from the abscessed tonsil is not copious.

Postoperative care

If only aspiration has been used, the patient may be given intravenous antibiotics until oral intake is satisfactory to ensure compliance.

If a tonsillectomy or incision and drainage was performed, intravenous antibiotics are given until oral intake is satisfactory for discharge from the hospital.

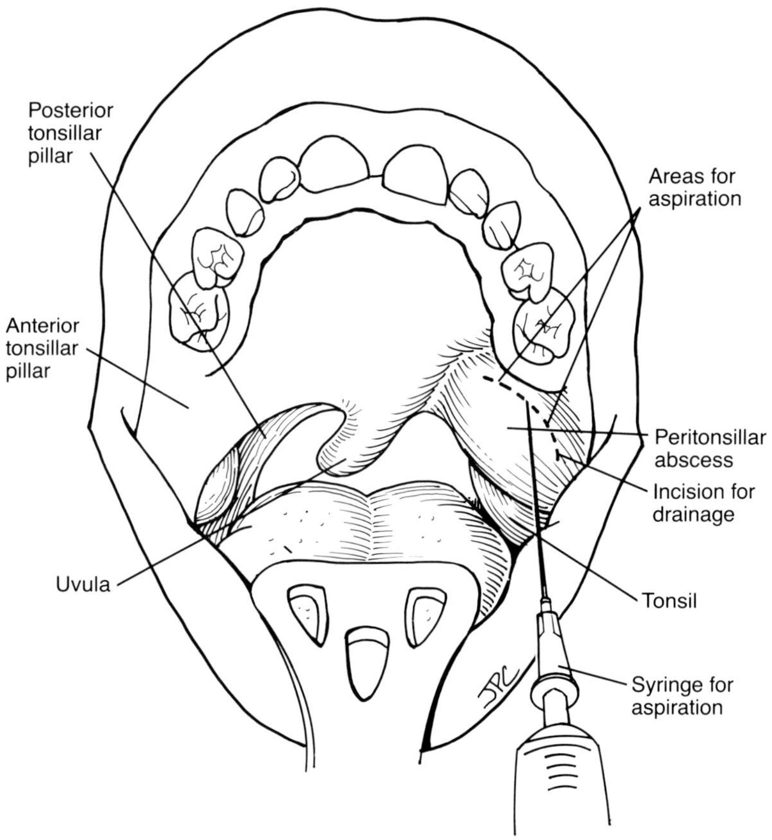

• FIGURE 17-9.

Peritonsillar abscess: aspiration and incision for drainage. (Adapted from Myer CM and Cotton RT: A Practical Approach to Pediatric Otolaryngology. Chicago, Year Book Medical Publishers, 1988.)

VISCERAL SPACE (SPACE INVOLVING INFRAHYOID)

The anatomic boundaries of this space are the visceral fascia (the superior border of which is the thyroid gland) and the inferior border, which is the mediastinum at the region of the aortic arch. Posteriorly, there is a communication with the posterior visceral space.

Causes of infections in this space include purulent thyroiditis, progression of pharyngitis, or perforation of or a foreign body in the cervical esophagus.

Indications

- Signs and symptoms include odynophagia, erythema and edema in the hypopharynx, dyspnea, and anterior neck swelling in the region of the thyroid glands and the midline cervical lymph nodes.
- The response to antibiotic therapy is unsatisfactory.

Anesthetic considerations

General anesthesia is usually used via the oral endotracheal route.

Preparation

The skin is prepared with an antiseptic scrub of the surgeon's choice.

Procedure

Surgical drainage uses an anterior horizontal skin incision similar to that of a tracheostomy. The skin and subcutaneous tissues are incised, and the dissection is carried through the midline fascia between the strap muscles. If the infection is lateral to the midline, dissection is carried to the involved side, and the abscess cavity is entered. Cultures are taken and the cavity is drained. The wound is irrigated with saline or a saline and antibiotic solution. A Penrose or wall suction drain is placed. The drains are advanced a small amount each day to allow the wound to close medially to laterally.

Postoperative care

Intravenous antibiotics are given for 4 to 5 days, followed by oral antibiotics for 2 to 3 weeks.

SPACES INVOLVING THE ENTIRE NECK

Retropharyngeal Space

The retropharyngeal space is bounded posteriorly by the alar fascia, anteriorly by the posterior pharyngeal wall, superiorly by the base of the skull, and inferiorly to the superior mediastinum at the level of T1, where the middle and deep cervical fascia layers fuse.

The sources of infections in this area are purulent diseases of the nasopharynx, the middle ear, the nose and paranasal sinuses, and the oral cavity as well as trauma (either from penetrating foreign body wounds or from iatrogenic endoscopy).

Indications

- A diagnosis is made by clinical findings of dysphagia, odynophagia, toxicity (fever, chills, malaise), nuchal rigidity, occasionally a hoarse or soft voice, and potentially progressive airway obstruction. Lateral neck x-rays may be positive, with a widening at the C2 level of more than 7 cm in both children and adults. At the C6 level, a widening of 14 mm occurs in children younger than 14 years of age, and a widening of 22 mm occurs in adults. Contrast computed tomography (CT) scans are recommended not only to evaluate potential extension into the mediastinum but also to rule out concomitant complications such as epidural abscesses, which are not unusual in severe cases of retropharyngeal space abscess.
- Neurologic findings are compatible with progressive spinal cord compression.
- Progressive airway obstruction is present.
- The response to antibiotic therapy is unsatisfactory.

Anesthetic considerations

This procedure must be performed under general anesthesia with protection of the airway by an endotracheal tube (cuffed in older children or teenagers, and hypopharyngeal packing in uncuffed tubes). If possible, an oral endotracheal tube is preferred; however, on rare occasions, a tracheostomy may be necessary. If an oral tube is used, it may be necessary to change to a nasotracheal tube after drainage if edema requires intubation in the postoperative period. The intubation should be performed by an experienced anesthesiologist, if possible.

Preparation

If an intraoral drainage is planned, the throat is packed with a gauze pack. If an external incision is planned, the skin is prepared with an antiseptic scrub of the surgeon's choice.

Procedure

If there is a question concerning the presence of purulence, aspiration with an 18-gauge needle into the upper retropharyngeal space is indicated.

If the abscess is limited to the upper retropharyngeal space, intraoral aspiration and drainage are recommended (Fig. 17–10*A* and *B*). The incision is carried through the posterior pharyngeal wall mucosa vertically through the edematous mucosa. I prefer to make this incision with the coagulation cautery to reduce blood loss. Dissection is then carried bluntly into the cavity. The cavity is drained completely, and an incision is made overlying the space. Cultures of the contents are taken. The drainage procedure is performed with the patient in the Rose position to prevent aspiration of the contents of the abscess. Intravenous antibiotics are administered.

An external approach (Fig. 17–10*C*) is used. When the abscess extends inferiorly to the hyoid bone, an external approach is preferred. The incision is made in an apron-like fashion, with a horizontal limb being made at the level of the midportion of the abscess cavity (judged on a lateral x-ray and on a CT scan) and the vertical portion carried along the anterior border of the sternocleidomastoid muscle superiorly. The dissection is carried down to the sternocleidomastoid muscle, which is retracted laterally. The carotid sheath is identified, and most commonly its contents are reflected laterally, with the dissection into the abscess cavity continued anterior to the carotid sheath. However, occasionally, when there is a large amount of induration and adhesions, it is technically more feasible to use a retrocarotid sheath dissection with the sheath being retracted anteriorly and the cavity drained posterior to the sheath. However, if the approach is anterior to the carotid sheath, the sheath contents are retracted laterally, and the larynx, trachea, and thyroid gland are retracted medially. The dissection is then carried down to the prevertebral muscles behind the inferior constrictors, and the cavity is opened bluntly. Using blunt dissection, the cavity is opened superiorly to inferiorly, and the contralateral extent is identified. The abscess cavity is irrigated with a saline and bacitracin solution, and wall suction (Jackson-Pratt) drains are inserted, both superiorly and inferiorly. I also like to use a third, and possibly a fourth, drain for irrigation, and all drains are marked according to their desired function (e.g., superior suction, inferior suction, superior irrigation, inferior irrigation). I use antibiotic ointment (Betadine ointment) and apply it to gauze packing (in the most severe cases) to pack the wound, in addition to the use of irrigation. The wound is dressed with a Montgomery dressing so that the abdominal gauze, which is used to soak up excess irrigation, can be changed easily.

Postoperative care

Betadine solution is added to the packing twice daily until all packing has been removed. The packing is advanced over 3 to 5 days. The irrigation drains are removed after 24 to 48 hours. The suction drains are advanced slowly beginning on the third to fourth postoperative day. Intravenous antibiotics are given for 7 to 10 days, followed by oral antibiotics for another 2 to 3 weeks.

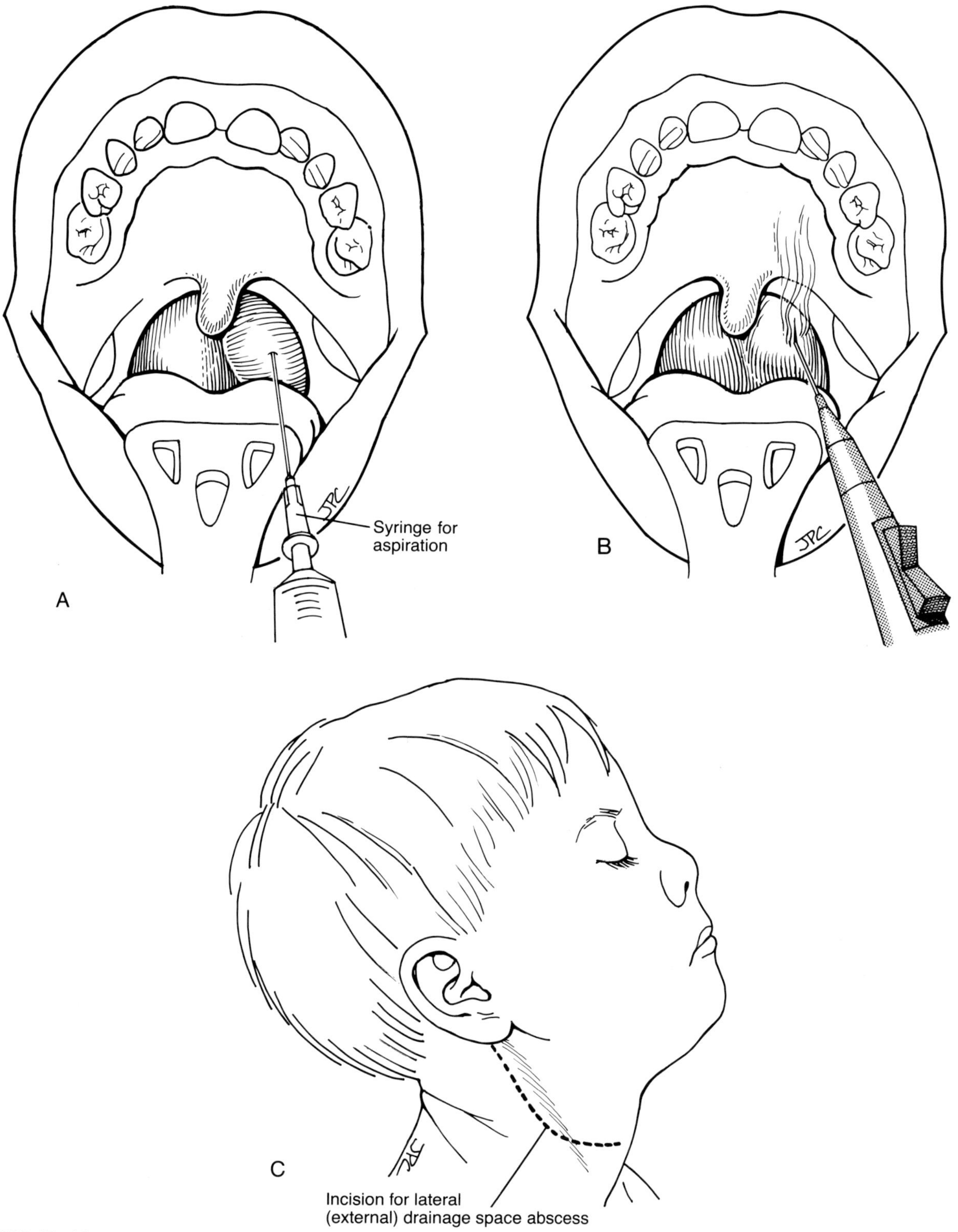

• FIGURE 17-10.

A, Retropharyngeal space: infection and aspiration. *B*, Intraoral incision for drainage of a retropharyngeal space abscess. (*A* and *B*, from Ballenger JJ: Diseases of the Nose, Throat, and Ear, 12th ed. Philadelphia, Lea & Febiger, 1977.) *C*, Incision for external (lateral) approach to a retropharyngeal space abscess. (Modified from Lore J: An Atlas of Head and Neck Surgery, 3rd ed. Philadelphia, WB Saunders, 1988.)

Prevertebral Space

The prevertebral space is found between the prevertebral layer of the deep cervical fascia and the osseous bodies of the cervical vertebrae extending from the base of skull to the coccyx.

Infections in this region are most commonly caused by distal disease, such as tuberculosis or cutaneous infections.

Indications

- The symptoms of infections in this space may be very subtle and include only localized or vague pain, torticollis of varying degrees, and malaise. If the cervical vertebrae are significantly infected, there may be neurologic symptoms. The diagnosis is confirmed by lateral radiographs of the neck and cervical spine, as well as by CT scans and magnetic resonance imaging (MRI).

Anesthetic considerations

The drainage of the prevertebral space abscess requires a general oral or nasal endotracheal anesthesia. If the edema is severe, the endotracheal tube should be maintained until the swelling has receded to allow a stable airway. Occasionally a tracheostomy is needed.

Preparation

The skin is prepared with an antiseptic scrub of the surgeon's choice.

Procedure

The treatment is directed at cervical drainage via a lateral approach in a fashion similar to that for the external method of treating retropharyngeal space abscesses. Concomitant medical management with appropriate antibiotics (e.g., antituberculosis drugs if tuberculosis is involved, or anti-staphylococcal drugs if *Staphylococcus aureus* is present). The wound should be drained with a Penrose drain or a Jackson-Pratt drain and packed in a fashion similar to that used for the retropharyngeal space abscess.

Postoperative care

The postsurgical care is similar to that of the retropharyngeal space abscess.

Vascular (Carotid) Space

The vascular space is a potential space within the carotid sheath, extending from the base of the skull to the superior mediastinum. The space is formed by all three layers of the deep cervical fascia. Consequently, infections in any of the other spaces (but especially the lateral pharyngeal space) may extend into the carotid sheath.

The source for infection in this space is either necrosis of a deep cervical lymph node or spread from other neck spatial planes, especially the lateral pharyngeal space.

Indications

- The signs and symptoms include more limitation of motion of the neck, profound swelling of the anterior or lateral neck, possibly pitting edema, and fever. A purplish discoloration may indicate hemorrhage. Spiking fevers and severe chills may indicate thrombosis of the internal jugular vein with septic emboli. Horner's syndrome is occasionally seen.
- There is a great danger of spontaneous carotid hemorrhage, cranial nerve deficits, Horner's syndrome, or thrombosis of the internal jugular vein, with septic emboli and potential spread to the brain by way of the lateral sinus.
- A poor response to antibiotic therapy also is a contributing factor.

Anesthetic considerations

The drainage of this space requires general oral endotracheal anesthesia. If the edema is severe, the tube must be left in place postoperatively to protect the airway. Occassionally a tracheostomy is needed.

Preparation

The skin is prepared with a surgical scrub of the surgeon's choice.

Procedure

An external approach is mandatory for the drainage of the vascular space abscess. The incision is placed along the anterior border of the sternocleidomatoid muscle in a fashion similar to the vertical limb of the apron incision. Dissection is carried down to the carotid sheath, and the abscess cavity is drained throughout its extent. If the internal jugular vein shows evidence of thrombosis, it may require ligation in an attempt to avoid spread to the lateral sinus and potentially to prevent distal abscesses or meningitis.

The wound is drained with a Jackson-Pratt drain or a Penrose drain. It is important to attempt to give good muscle coverage to the area because of the risk of vascular erosion and hemorrhage. This wound is usually not packed with gauze.

Postoperative care

The drains are advanced slowly over 5 to 10 days. Postoperative systemic antibiotic therapy is similar to that of the retropharyngeal space abscess.

"Danger" Space

The danger space lies between the two layers of deep prevertebral fascia, with the anterior wall being the alar layer and the posterior wall being the prevertebral layer of deep cervical fascia (Fig. 17–11).

Infections spreading to this space are usually found in the nose, paranasal sinus, nasopharynx, oropharynx, and hypopharynx.

Indications

- The signs and symptoms include odynophagia, dysphagia, spiking fevers, nuchal rigidity, a muffled voice, and swelling in the posterior pharyngeal wall.
- The response to antimicrobial therapy is unsatisfactory. Risks of infections in this space include airway obstruction, spread to the mediastinum or diaphragm, and involvement of the vertebrae or neural structures, including an epidural abscess.

Anesthetic considerations

The procedure is performed under general oral endotracheal anesthesia, if possible. If airway obstruction is impending, a tracheostomy must be performed.

Preparation

The skin is prepared with an antiseptic scrub of the surgeon's choice.

Procedure

If there is swelling in the upper neck region, aspiration via a transoral approach is appropriate prior to making an incision. If the area to be drained can be reached via a transoral approach, the posterior pharyngeal wall can be incised with the coagulation cautery and dissection can be carried through the prevertebral fascia. The space must be drained from the base of the skull to the most inferior aspect. The extent of the involvement is determined by CT scans (enhanced) and possibly by an MRI evaluation.

The external approach is taken for abscesses lower in the neck that are not accessible through a transoral approach or in infections that may extend from the base of the skull to the lower cervical vertebrae. The approach for this is similar to that taken for the retropharyngeal space.

The wound is cared for in a similar fashion to the retropharyngeal space abscess with drains in place, irrigation, packing, and Montgomery strap dressings.

Postoperative care

Postoperative systemic antibiotic therapy is similar to that of the retropharyngeal space abscess.

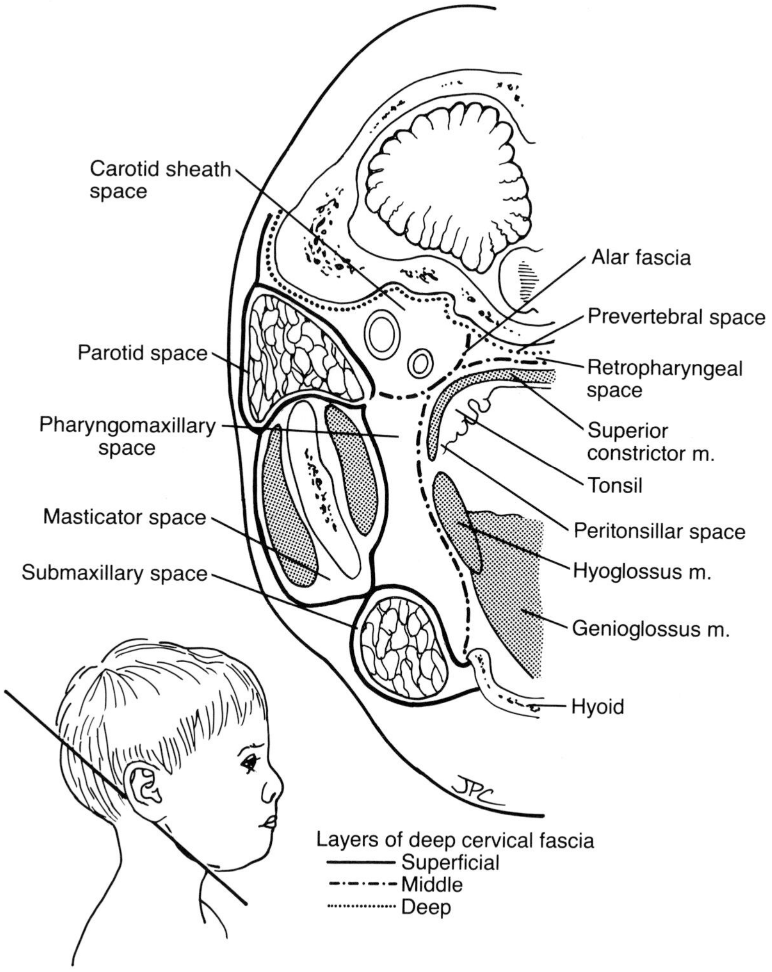

• FIGURE 17-11.

Vascular (carotid sheath) space. (Modified from Everts EC and Echevarria J: The pharynx and deep neck infections. *In* Paparella MM and Shumrick DA: Otolaryngology, Vol 3. Philadelphia, WB Saunders, 1973.)

BIBLIOGRAPHY

Ballenger JJ: Diseases of the Nose, Throat, and Ear, 12th ed. Philadelphia, Lea & Febiger, 1977.

Barrett G, Koopmann CF, and Coulthard SW: Retropharyngeal abscess—a ten year experience. Laryngoscope 94:455–463, 1984.

Everts EC and Echevarria J: The pharynx and deep neck infections. *In* Paparella MM and Shumrick DA: Otolaryngology, Vol 3, 2nd ed. Philadelphia, WB Saunders, 1980.

Gauthier M: Deep neck infections of the head and neck. *In* Katz A: Manual of Otolaryngology—Head and Neck Therapeutics. Philadelphia, Lea & Febiger, 1986.

Hollinshead WH: Anatomy for Surgeons, Vol 1, 2nd ed. New York, Hoeber, 1968.

Lore J: An Atlas of Head and Neck Surgery, 3rd ed. Philadelphia, WB Saunders, 1988.

Myer CM and Cotton RT: A Practical Approach to Pediatric Otolaryngology. Chicago, Year Book Medical Publishers, 1988.

Richardson M: The neck: Embryology and anatomy. *In* Bluestone CD and Stool SE: Pediatric Otolaryngology, Vol 2, 2nd ed. Philadelphia, WB Saunders, 1990.

chapter

18

Diseases of the Salivary Glands

WILLIAM S. CRYSDALE, M.D.
PAUL J. WALKER, M.B.B.S.

The operative procedures for excision of the submandibular gland and for superficial and deep parotidectomy are not unique to the pediatric age group and are well described in general surgical texts. Three procedures, however, are performed more commonly in children than in adults: (1) submandibular duct relocation; (2) sublingual gland excision; and (3) parotid duct ligation. The operative techniques of the senior author are presented here.

SUBMANDIBULAR DUCT RELOCATION

Indications

- Chronic significant drooling in the neurologically impaired patient that has not responded to nonsurgical measures—in particular, oral motor therapy intended to improve oral motor skills of the tongue, lips, and pharynx

CONTRAINDICATIONS

- Neurologic dysfunction that is not static (for which deterioration or improvement anticipated within 12 months)
- Chronic significant aspiration

ADVANTAGES

- The result obtained is usually maintained.
- The oral cavity remains moist and dentition remains healthy.

DISADVANTAGES

- Morbidity is significant and a hospital stay of 3 to 4 days is required.
- Ranula formation occurs usually within 6 months in approximately 8% of patients, unless the sublingual glands are removed simultaneously.
- Approximately 1% of the relocated ducts obstruct, resulting in the formation of a retention cyst that requires external excision of the ipsilateral submandibular gland.

Anesthetic considerations

- General anesthesia is maintained through a nasoendotracheal tube that is stabilized on the patient's forehead.
- A bolster is placed under the shoulders to extend the neck moderately. Draping around the head encompasses the endotracheal tube but leaves access to the mouth.
- The anesthetic machine is at the foot of the operating table to the left of the patient so that the surgical team has ample access to the patient's head.

Preparation

- The patient is placed in a slight reverse Trendelenburg position. A headlight facilitates visualization. The surgeon and the assistant sit at the head of the operating table.

- If a tonsillectomy has not been done previously, the tonsillar fossae are examined and the tonsils are removed if they are filling the fossae.

Procedure

- Exposure of the floor of the mouth is facilitated by inserting a two-pronged self-retaining retractor between the upper and lower dentitions and by suturing the tip of the tongue to the soft palate.

- The floor of the mouth anterior and posterior to the submandibular papillae is infiltrated with 5 ml of anesthetic agent containing 1:200,000 epinephrine.

- An island of mucosa 2 cm wide and 1 cm deep, encompassing the submandibular papillae, is created. The submandibular duct is found by grasping the posterior edge of the island and by elevating those tissues toward the lower dentition. It is then dissected with sharp scissors in a lateral direction from the midline just underneath the edge of the mucosal island (Fig. 18–1).

- Once both ducts have been found, they are freed of their attachments to the adjoining tissues down to the anterior aspect of the submandibular gland by blunt dissection along the axis of the duct, utilizing larger blunt scissors (Boyd). For this maneuver, appropriate retraction is crucial—the "anterior" retractor pulls laterally, holding the sublingual gland away from the duct, while the "posterior" retractor pushes the genioglossus muscle medially (Fig. 18–2*A*).

- A 4–0 chromic catgut suture is attached to both lateral corners of the mucosal island; the needle is left on. The island is then divided between the two papillae (Fig. 18–2*B*). The tip of the tongue suture is removed.

- With a towel clip in the lateral aspect of the tongue to provide countertraction, a mucosal tunnel from the anterior aspect of the submandibular gland to the tonsillar fossa is created by pushing a Kelly clamp through from the anterior incisional area.

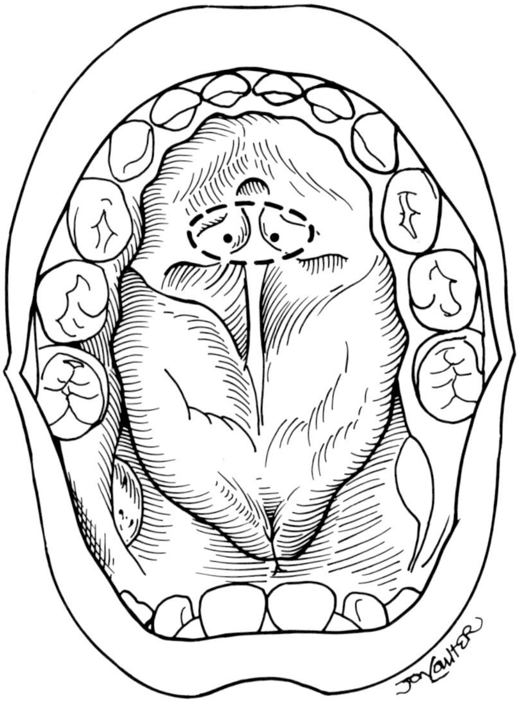

• FIGURE 18-1.

Creation of an island of mucosa.

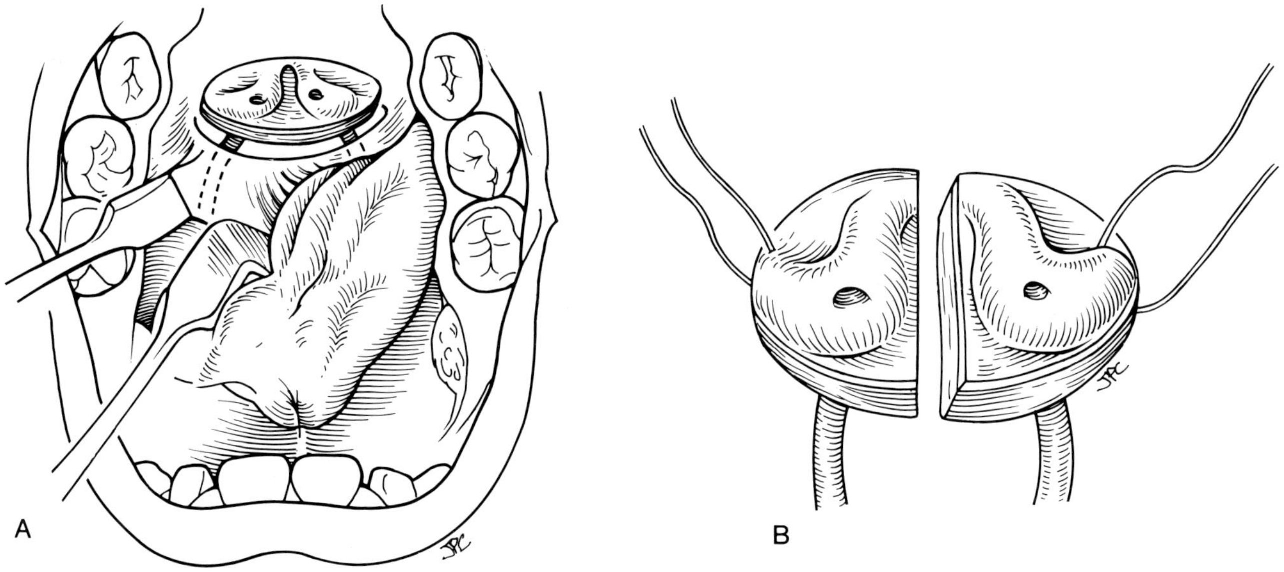

• FIGURE 18-2.

A, Freeing of the submandibular ducts using retractors. *B*, Division of the mucosal island between two papillae.

- The Kelly clamp is then used to pull a No. 10 suction catheter from the tonsillar fossa into the anterior incisional area (Fig. 18–3). The sutures attached to the mucosal islands are threaded through these catheters (Fig. 18–4) and then pulled through the submucosal tunnels into the tonsillar fossae. A single mattress suture attaches the mucosal island to the posterior aspect of the anterior tonsillar pillar close to the base of the tongue.
- Difficulty in relocating the duct posterior to the tonsillar fossa indicates that the anterior dissection of the submandibular duct off the adjacent tissues was not carried far enough posteriorly.
- If the sublingual glands are not removed, the anterior incision is closed with five or six simple sutures of 4–0 chromic catgut.

Postoperative care

- Airway obstruction requiring 24 to 48 hours of nasotracheal intubation may (rarely) occur if swelling of the tongue is excessive. This should be anticipated in patients with retrognathia who were difficult to intubate.
- Intravenous fluids are necessary for 24 to 48 hours postoperatively.
- Prophylactic antibiotics are recommended.
- Parental (or other caregiver) involvement in nursing care is encouraged because these patients frequently present as management problems during the first 48 hours.

SPECIAL CONSIDERATIONS

- The floor of mouth may take 4 to 6 weeks to close completely if closure of the anterior incision has been difficult.
- The result usually becomes apparent within 8 weeks.

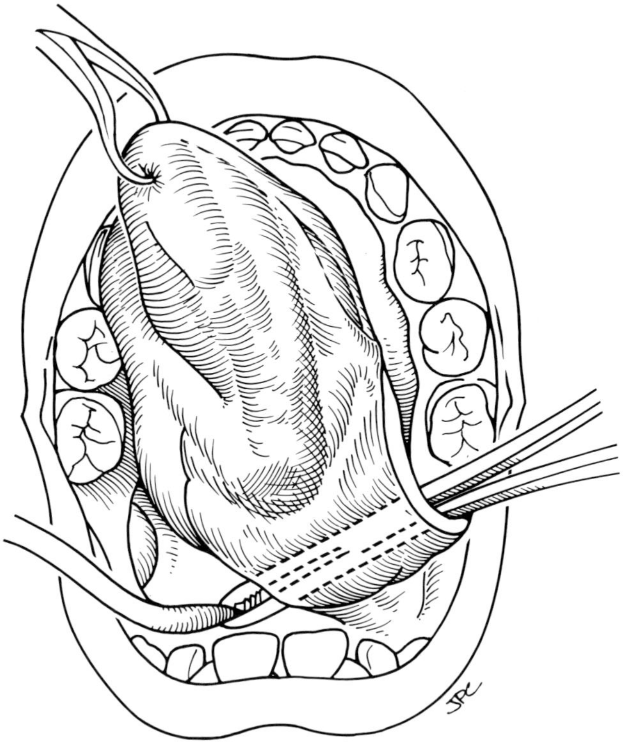

• **FIGURE 18-3.**

Pulling a catheter into the anterior incisional area.

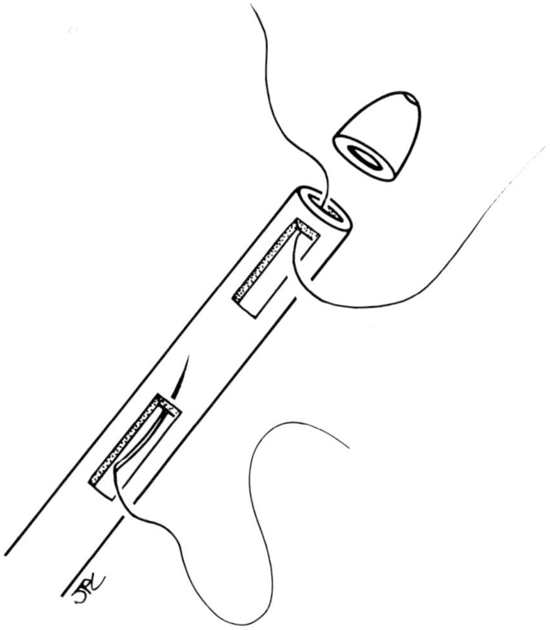

• **FIGURE 18-4.**

Threading of the sutures through the catheters.

SUBLINGUAL GLAND EXCISION

Indications

- Ranula (extravasation pseudocyst) unresponsive to simple incision and drainage or marsupialization
- Surgical procedures on the floor of mouth that are associated with a high probability of ranula formation (e.g., submandibular duct relocation, procedures on the proximal aspect of the submandibular duct [sialolithotomy], excision of benign tumors)

Anesthetic considerations

- General anesthesia is maintained through a nasoendotracheal tube that is stabilized on the patient's forehead.
- A bolster is placed under the patient's shoulders to extend the neck moderately. Draping around the head encompasses the endotracheal tube but leaves access to the mouth.
- The anesthetic machine is at the foot of the operating table to the left of the patient so that the surgical team has ample access to the patient's head.

Preparation

- The patient is placed in a slight reverse Trendelenburg position. A headlight facilitates dissection. The surgeon and the assistant sit at the head end of the operating table.

Procedure

- If sublingual gland excision is not to be combined with submandibular duct relocation, the incision on the floor of the mouth to access the sublingual gland must curve lateral to the papilla of the ipsilateral submandibular duct so that the duct may be identified and preserved. The attachment of the papilla in the midline is not disturbed. The incision in the floor of the mouth is placed medial to the alveolus and is extended posteriorly to facilitate primary closure (Fig. 18–5).
- The submandibular duct (if it is to remain in situ) is dissected off the sublingual gland posterior to the submandibular gland. The bulk of the sublingual gland is lateral to the submandibular duct.
- First, the anterior aspect of the sublingual gland is mobilized off the inner aspect of the mandible with blunt scissor dissection. The gland is then firmly grasped by a clamp and, via blunt dissection, is stripped posteriorly off the underlying muscles—the mylohyoid laterally and the genioglossus medially (Fig. 18–6).
- Next, the gland is freed of its attachment to the tongue. Scissors are used to create a tunnel between the gland and the tongue, avoiding large veins. The mucosa is then divided (Fig. 18–7).

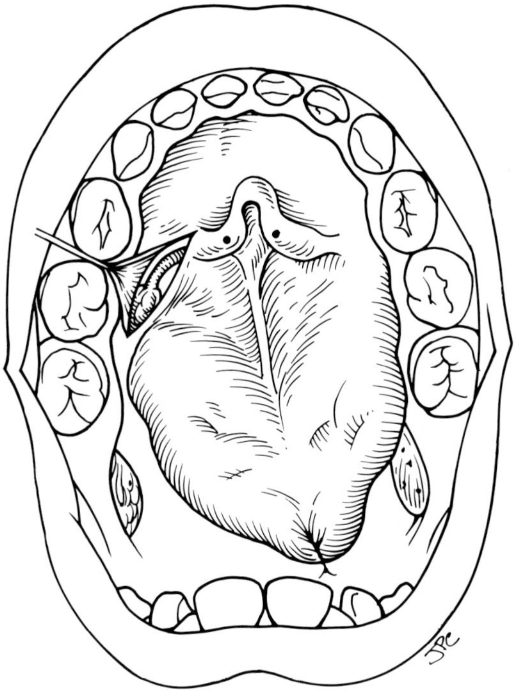

• FIGURE 18-5.

Placement of the incision on the floor of the mouth.

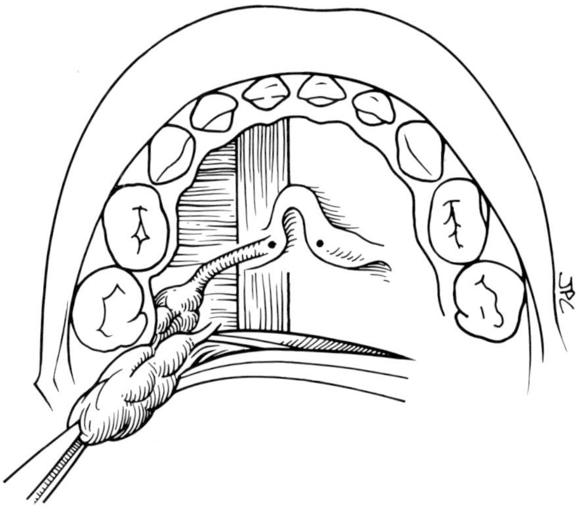

• FIGURE 18-6.

Dissection of the sublingual gland.

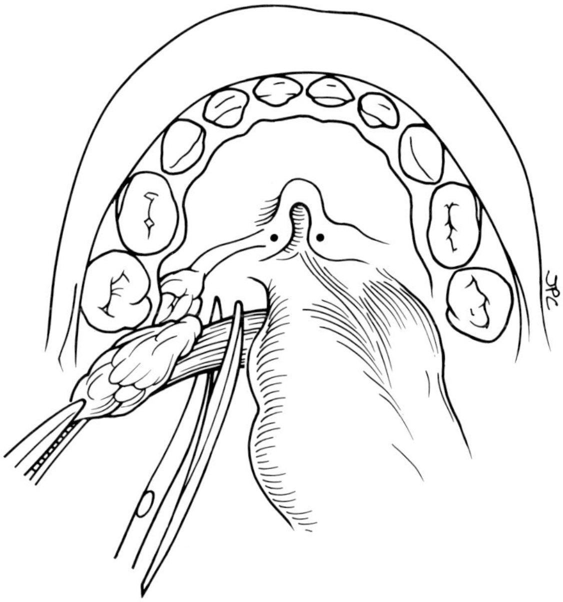

• FIGURE 18-7.

Freeing of the gland from the tongue.

• The lingual nerve is identified medially, and the sublingual gland is then dissected off the lingual nerve back to where the submandibular duct and the lingual nerve cross.

• If the submandibular duct has been relocated, one must watch that the duct is not still attached to the deep aspect of the sublingual gland, which is being retracted out of the oral cavity. The duct can be inadvertently divided as the gland is dissected off the nerve. A properly relocated duct that is totally dissected off the sublingual gland will be found resting posterior to the lingual nerve as the sublingual gland is being freed of its remaining attachments laterally.

• Hemostasis is crucial as one progresses through this dissection — electrocautery is essential. Particular care is required on the deep aspect of the gland laterally about midway back, because this is where the arterial supply from the lingual artery and branches of the submental artery to the gland enters.

PAROTID DUCT LIGATION

Indications

• Chronic sialorrhea of water-like saliva after submandibular duct relocation

• Recurrent parotitis

Anesthetic considerations

• An oral or nasal endotracheal tube should be used. If a nasal endotracheal tube is used, taping should be minimal to permit ready access to the buccal mucous membrane.

Preparation

• The patient's head is in a neutral position with a slight reverse Trendelenburg position.

Procedure

• The parotid duct is located and cannulated with a lacrimal probe. With the probe held in place, the soft tissues immediately anterior to the duct orifice are infiltrated with 2 to 3 ml of anesthetic agent containing 1:200,000 epinephrine.

• With the lacrimal probe held in place, an elliptical incision 1.5 cm in length is made 0.5 cm anterior to the duct orifice (Fig. 18–8). This incision should not be too far anterior to the duct orifice, or the duct will be difficult to locate.

• The duct quickly travels obliquely and posteriorly in a direction lateral to the gland; thus, dissection must be close to the duct orifice until the duct (with the probe inside) is identified.

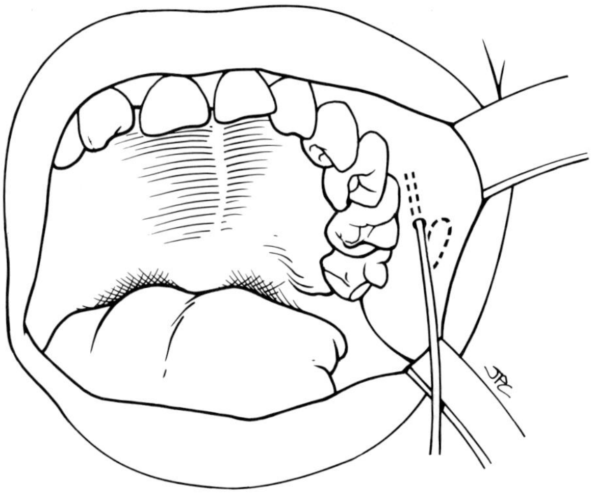

• FIGURE 18-8.

Location of the elliptical incision.

- When the duct is identified, it is cleared of excessive soft tissue for approximately 1 cm. Two tight ligatures of nonabsorbable suture (3–0 Mersilene) are placed around the duct.
- The duct is then cauterized (coagulating current) between the two ligatures. The duct is not divided.
- Buccal mucous membrane is closed with interrupted absorbable sutures.

Postoperative care

- Prophylactic antibiotics are recommended.
- Morbidity is minimal, and discharge is usually possible within 24 hours.

SPECIAL CONSIDERATIONS

- Fistulization of the duct with failure of the procedure may occur if cauterization is not done or if the duct is divided.

chapter

19

Tumors of the Mouth and Pharynx

CARLOS GONZALEZ, M.D.

Oral tumors constitute approximately 3% of all tumor-like growths in the oral cavity, jaws, and salivary glands in children in all age groups. The overwhelming majority of those tumors are benign.[1–5] However, a wide variety of congenital and acquired oral and pharyngeal neoplasms are encountered in the pediatric age group. The possibility of malignant lesions should always be considered. The head and neck area, excluding the central nervous system, is the site of 5 to 10% of all childhood malignancies. The majority of these lesions are either sarcomas (rhabdomyosarcoma being the most common) or epidermoid carcinomas.

TONGUE LESIONS

MOBILE TONGUE (ANTERIOR TWO THIRDS) TUMORS AND CYSTS

Tumors and cysts of the anterior two thirds of the tongue are usually benign and include hemangiomas, lymphangiomas, cystic lesions, fibrous tumors, epithelial tumors, and hamartomas.[1] Surgical intervention is usually limited to surgical excisional biopsy.

Indications

- Suspicion of malignancy
- Articulation disorder
- Bleeding

Anesthetic considerations

- For larger lesions or when the CO_2 laser is to be used, nasotracheal intubation can be considered. In most small lesions of the mobile tongue, oral intubation can be performed, and the tube is retracted out of the surgical field.
- Endotracheal tubes should be wrapped with a protective material (e.g., aluminum, Merocel tape), or special laser safety tubes should be used with CO_2 laser excision or vaporization.

Preparation

- The patient is supine with a shoulder roll in place or is in a semisitting position.
- When the CO_2 laser is used:

  All operating room personnel should wear appropriate eye protection.

  A separate suction line should be available to remove the laser plume.

  Moistened towels and sponges should be placed on all surrounding exposed skin and mucosal surfaces to avoid inadvertent laser burns.

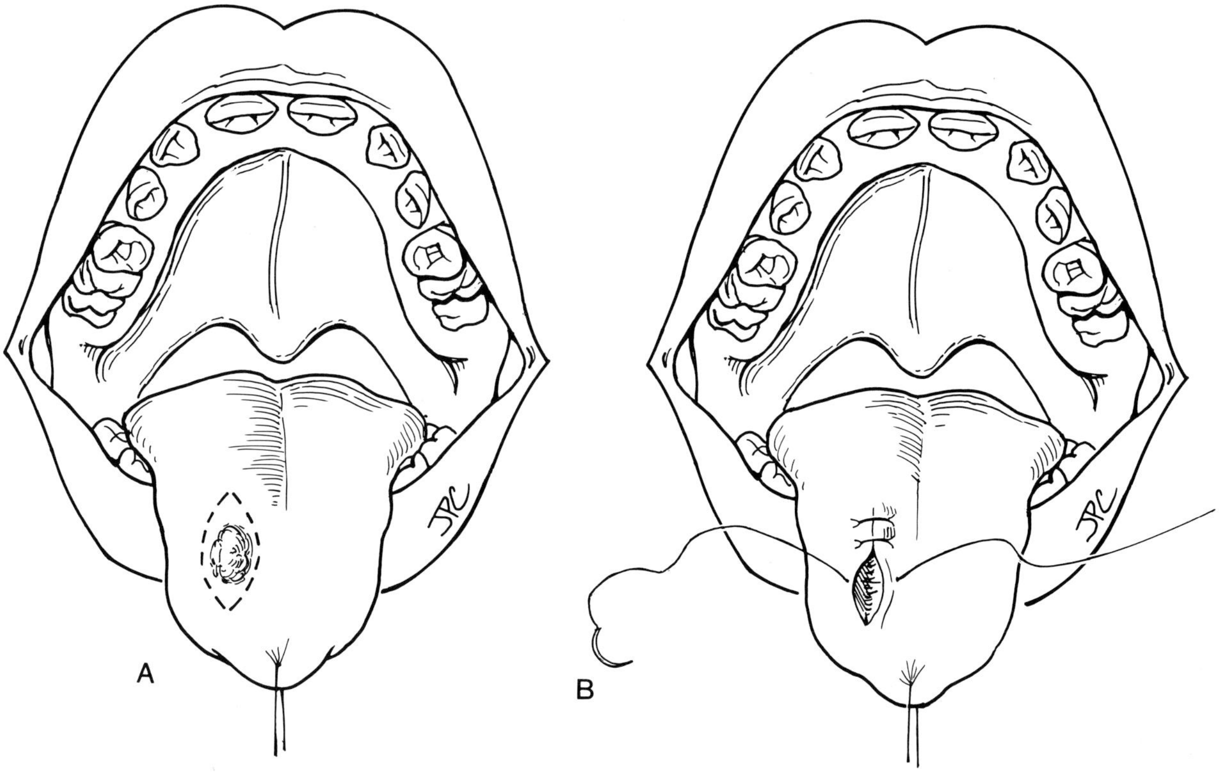

• FIGURE 19–1.

An excisional biopsy of a tongue lesion. *A*, Proposed elliptical incision allowing a cuff of normal tissue. *B*, Closure of the resulting defect. (Redrawn from Loré J. An Atlas of Head and Neck Surgery. Philadelphia, WB Saunders, 1988.)

Procedure

• A mouth retractor without tongue blade, such as the Jennings or bite block, is placed.

• A silk traction suture placed in the midline of the tongue will help in tongue retraction.

• When using the laser vaporization technique, laser energy can be applied using a handpiece or the operating microscope.

• For excisional biopsies, an elliptical incision is made around the lesion (Fig. 19–1*A*). Dissection is carried down through the tongue surface into the tongue musculature if necessary.

• The defect is closed in layers approximating the tongue musculature, followed by the mucosal edges, using absorbable suture material (Fig. 19–1*B*).

Postoperative care

• Feeding can resume shortly after surgery. Initially, a soft diet is better tolerated.

• Oral hygiene with normal saline solution increases the patient's comfort postoperatively.

MACROGLOSSIA

Abnormal enlargement of the tongue causing tongue protrusion at rest is known as macroglossia. Multiple causes for macroglossia have been described and include hypothyroidism, mucopolysaccharide and lipid storage diseases, lymphangioma, hemangioma, neurofibroma, and muscular macroglossia.[4] Persistent chronic macroglossia should be differentiated from acute parenchymatous glossitis due to various causes that often results in rapid tongue enlargement, causing airway distress.

Indications

- Chronic airway obstruction
- Maxillofacial deformity and malocclusion
- Recurrent hemorrhage from drying effects of chronic tongue protrusion
- Articulation disorder
- Cosmetic deformity

Anesthetic considerations

- Nasotracheal intubation or fiberoptic-guided intubation may be useful.
- Orotracheal or nasotracheal intubation may be difficult secondary to tongue size. A tracheostomy may be necessary prior to surgical treatment of the tongue.

Preparation

- The patient is supine with a shoulder roll in place or is in a semisitting position.
- When the CO_2 laser is used:

  All operating room personnel should wear appropriate eye protection.

  A separate suction line should be available to remove the laser plume.

  Moistened towels and sponges should be placed on all surrounding exposed skin and mucosal surfaces to avoid inadvertent laser burns.

Procedure

- A mouth retractor without a tongue blade, such as the Jennings or bite block, is placed (Fig. 19–2).
- A silk traction suture placed in the midline of the tongue will help in tongue retraction.

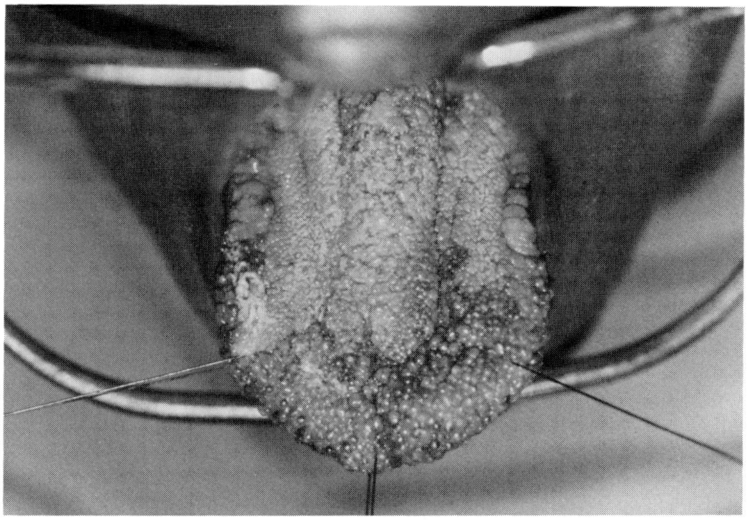

• FIGURE 19–2.

Macroglossia secondary to lymphangioma. A Jennings mouth gag and midline suture allow excellent exposure.

- Wedge resection of the tongue (Fig. 19–3) can be fashioned in several forms, depending on the amount of tongue that needs to be excised. One advantage of wedge resection is that more lateral tongue can be preserved, thus preserving taste and sensation.

  Simple wedge excision (see Fig. 19–3*A*)

  Extended wedge excision (see Fig. 19–3*B*)

  Keyhole wedge excision (see Fig. 19–3*C*)

- In certain cases wedge resection may result in a tongue that is too thin and pointed. In these cases, a tip reduction technique can be used (see Fig. 19–3*D*).

- Incision of the tongue surface and musculature is carried out using a surgical blade or an electrocautery, cutting toward deep musculature in order to have more mucosal surface to reapproximate and to decrease tension on the suture line.

- The tongue is closed in layers using an absorbable suture to reapproximate tongue musculature and mucosal surfaces (see Fig. 19–3*E* and *F*).

Postoperative care

- Postoperative edema of the tongue during the first 24 to 48 hours may cause significant airway distress. Overnight nasotracheal intubation versus tracheostomy must be considered.

- Patients and parents should be counseled for recurrent macroglossia, especially in cases of lymphangioma.

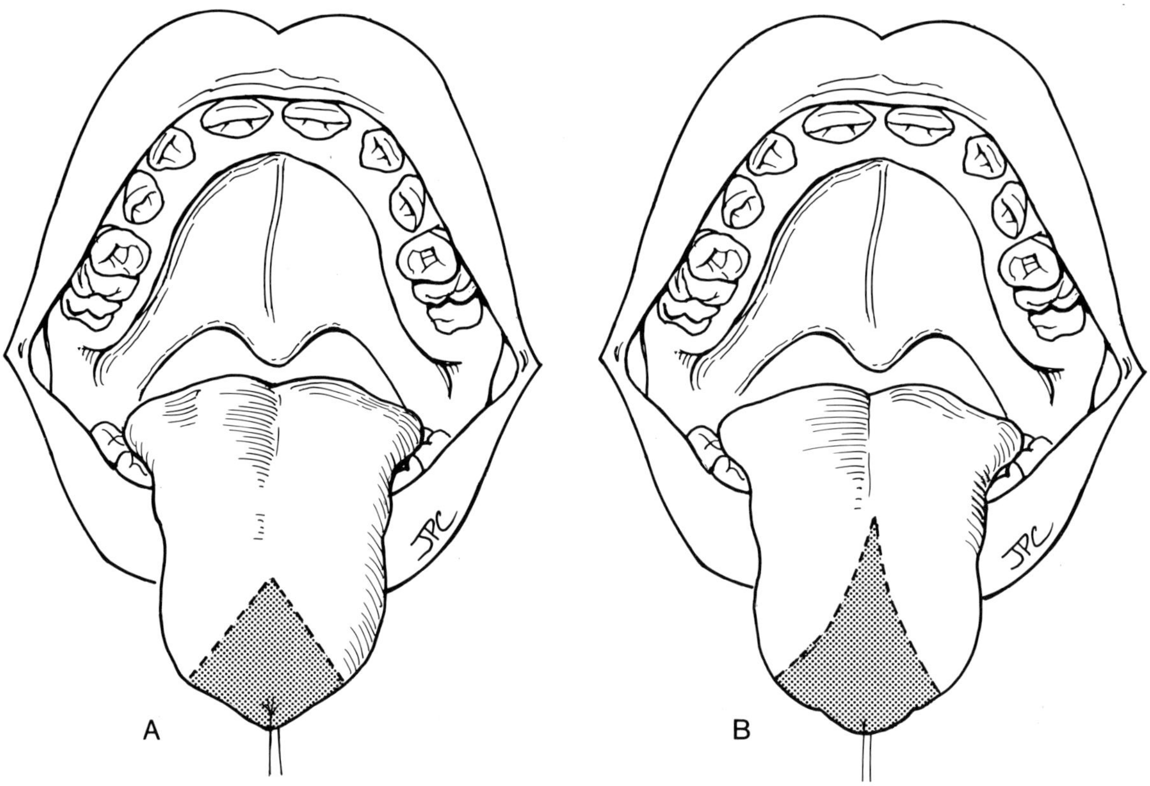

• FIGURE 19–3.

A, Simple wedge incision. *B*, Extended wedge incision.

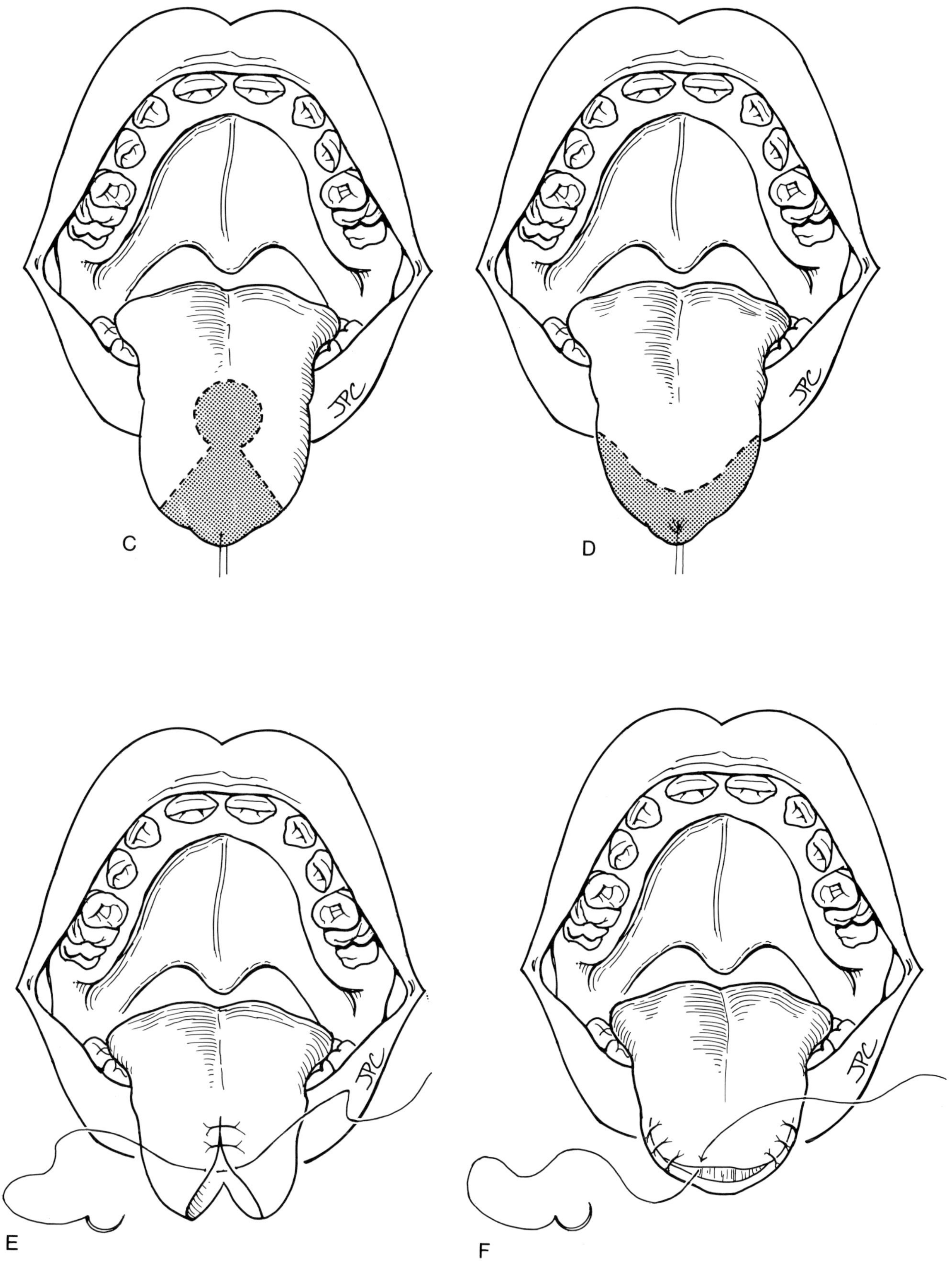

• **FIGURE 19–3.** *(continued)*

C, Keyhole wedge incision. *D*, Tip reduction. *E* and *F*, Closing technique. (Redrawn from Loré J. An Atlas of Head and Neck Surgery, Philadelphia, WB Saunders, 1988.)

BASE OF TONGUE CYSTS AND TUMORS INTRAORAL MARSUPIALIZATION OR EXCISIONAL BIOPSY

Mucoceles are commonly occurring lesions of the oral cavity. The lesions are usually painless, freely mobile, smooth, soft, fluctuant masses that vary in size from a few millimeters to several centimeters.[3–5] Larger lesions are usually located in the floor of the mouth or in the substance of the tongue. Mucoceles involving the base of the tongue region can enlarge enough to cause airway compromise. Histologically, the walls of most of the specimens consist of granulation tissue, and an epithelial lining is rarely identified.

Indications

- Upper airway obstruction
- Hemorrhage or risk of hemorrhage
- Dysphagia
- Speech impediment

Anesthetic considerations

- Nasotracheal intubation
- Orotracheal or nasotracheal intubation may be difficult secondary to the base of the tongue mass and size. A tracheostomy may be necessary prior to surgical treatment of the tongue.

Preparation

- The patient is supine with a shoulder roll in place or is in a semisitting position.

Procedure (marsupialization)

- A mouth retractor without tongue blade, such as the Jennings or bite block, is placed.
- A silk traction suture placed in the midline of the tongue will help in tongue retraction.
- The dome of the cyst is incised, and contents of the cyst are aspirated (Fig. 19–4*A*).
- The entire dome of the cyst is removed, leaving a granulation bed exposed to heal by second intention (Fig. 19–4*B*). Primary closure can also be performed in lesions that are completely excised.

Postoperative care

- Feeding can resume shortly after surgery. In cases of base of tongue lesions, feeding should start with liquids and can advance as tolerated.

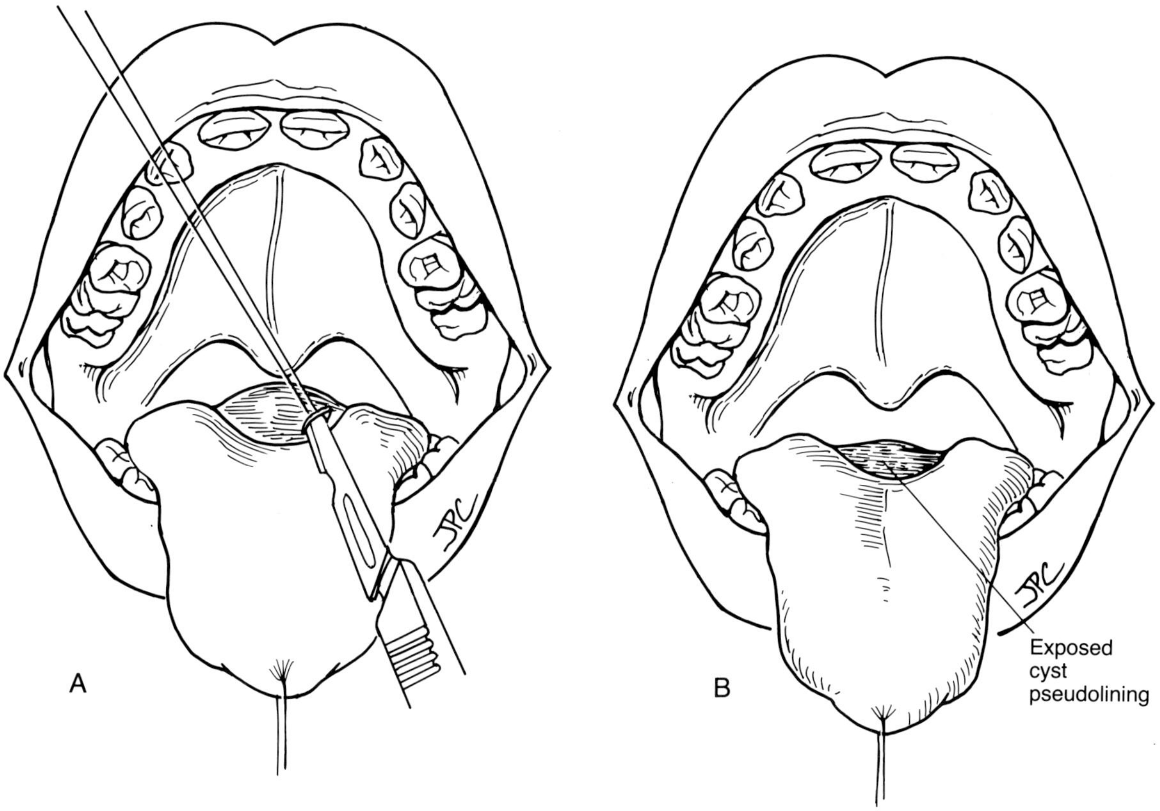

• FIGURE 19-4.

A and *B*, Intraoral marsupialization of a base of the tongue lesion.

EXTERNAL APPROACH

An external approach to a lesion of the base of the tongue is usually reserved for large cystic masses in which the inferior margin of dissection (vallecula) would be poorly visualized from an oral approach. Large thyroglossal duct cysts and mucoceles as well as lingual thyroids can be adequately excised using this approach.

Indications

- Upper airway obstruction
- Hemorrhage or risk of hemorrhage
- Dysphagia
- Speech impediment

Anesthetic considerations

- Nasotracheal intubation
- Orotracheal or nasotracheal intubation may be difficult secondary to the base of the tongue mass and size. A tracheostomy may be necessary before surgical treatment of the tongue.

Preparation

- The patient is supine with a shoulder roll in place to extend the neck fully.

Procedure

- Landmarks should be identified as follows: (1) suprasternal notch, (2) cricoid cartilage, (3) laryngeal cartilage, and (4) hyoid bone.
- A transverse incision is made in the neck fold over the hyoid bone (Fig. 19–5*A*). Subplatysmal superior and limited inferior flaps are developed.
- Suprasternal musculature is dissected and transected from the hyoid bone. Hyoid bone dissection should be carried out in the midline to avoid injury to lateral structures such as the hypoglossal nerve or superior laryngeal nerve. Dissection is carried down into pre-epiglottic fat pad (Fig. 19–5*B*). In cases of lingual thyroglossal duct cyst or lingual thyroid, the midportion of the hyoid bone can be freed of infrahyoid musculature and removed with the specimen, which is done with a Sistrunk procedure.[6]
- The pharyngeal mucosa is identified, and the pharynx is entered above the epiglottis (Fig. 19–5*C*). The lesion at the base of the tongue is identified and dissected free of the tongue musculature.
- The pharynx should be closed using a running Connell suture technique to invert the mucosal edges.
- Strap muscles are reapproximated, and the wound is closed in layers over a drain.

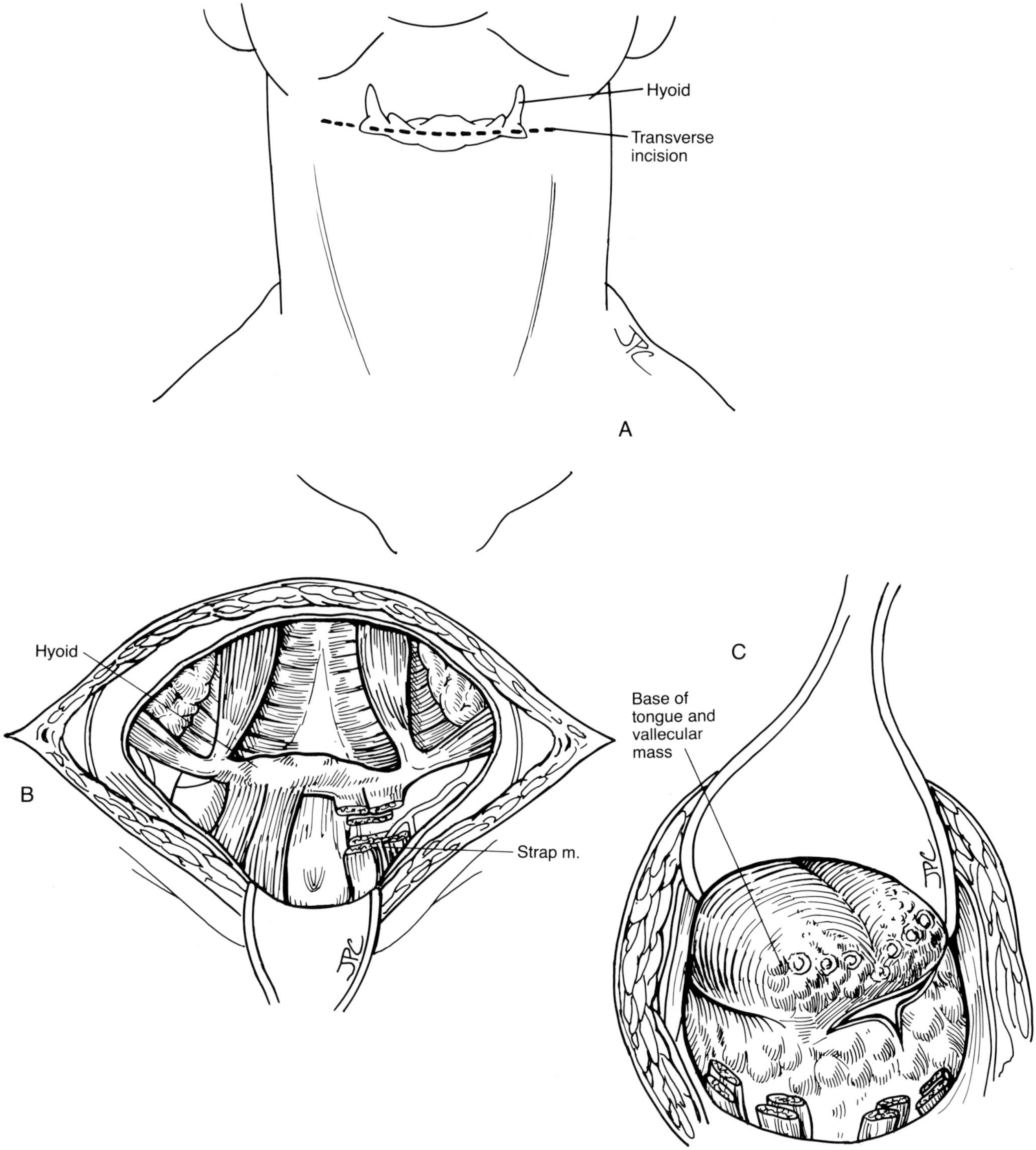

• FIGURE 19–5.

External approach to a base of the tongue lesion. *A*, Transverse incision over the hyoid bone. *B*, Surgical field identifying the supra and infrahyoid musculature, which is transected to gain access to the base of the tongue region. *C*, Visualization of the base of the tongue region through a midline neck approach.

Postoperative care

- Postoperative edema of the tongue during the first 24 to 28 hours may cause significant airway distress. Overnight nasotracheal intubation (versus tracheostomy) must be considered.
- Oral feeding can resume usually within 48 to 72 hours postoperatively, depending on the amount of dissection on the base of the tongue and on the reliability of the pharyngeal closure achieved.

FLOOR OF MOUTH LESIONS

MUCOCELE OR RANULA

Floor of the mouth lesions are usually bluish, transparent, and thin-walled cysts. Histologically, the walls of most specimens consist of granulation tissue, and rarely is an epithelial lining identified. Computed tomography may be beneficial to assess the true extent of a mass that appears in the oral cavity (Fig. 19–6). Treatment consists of surgical excision or marsupialization.

Surgical management of mucoceles depends on the size and extension of the lesion. Treatment options range from marsupialization to complete intraoral or cervical excision. When the intraoral mass is accompanied by a submaxillary, cervical, or parapharyngeal extension, the term plunging ranula is usually used. These lesions require external cervical approach excision as described for excision of the submandibular gland. Ranulas limited to the floor of the mouth can either be marsupialized (as described earlier for lesions of the base of the tongue) or be excised as follows.

Indications

- Dysphagia
- Speech impediment
- Recurrent infection
- Growth of lesion

Anesthetic considerations

- Nasotracheal intubation

Preparation

- The patient is supine with a shoulder roll in place or is in a semisitting position.

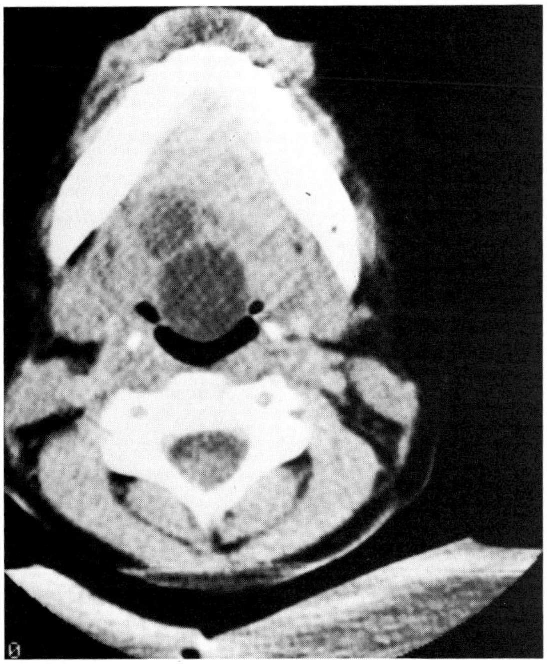

• **FIGURE 19-6.**

A computed tomography scan demonstrating vallecular mucocele with involvement of the deep musculature of the tongue. (From Gonzalez C: Tumors of the mouth and pharynx. *In* Bluestone CD and Stool CE: Pediatric Otolaryngology, 2nd ed. Philadelphia, WB Saunders, 1990.)

Procedure (marsupialization)

- A mouth retractor without a tongue blade, such as the Jennings or bite block, is placed.
- A silk traction suture placed in the midline of the tongue will help in tongue retraction.
- The orifice of the submandibular gland should be identified. Cannulation of the duct with a lacrimal duct probe may be useful in identifying the duct and in avoiding injury during dissection of the cyst.
- An elliptical incision is made over the dome of the cyst. Mucosa over the cyst is usually excised with the cyst and aids in retraction during dissection (Fig. 19–7*A*).
- Using blunt and sharp dissection, the cyst is separated of surrounding tissue. Care should be taken to identify and avoid injury to the lingual nerve and submandibular duct (Figs. 19–7*B* and *C*).
- The defect is closed using an absorbable suture to reapproximate the underlying soft tissues and mucosal edges (Fig. 19–7*D*). Meticulous hemostasis is imperative prior to mucosal closure.

Postoperative care/complications

- Postoperative edema of the floor of the mouth during the first 24 to 48 hours may cause significant airway distress. Overnight nasotracheal intubation versus tracheostomy should be considered.
- Oral feeding can usually resume within 24 to 48 hours postoperatively, depending on the degree of swelling on the floor of the mouth.

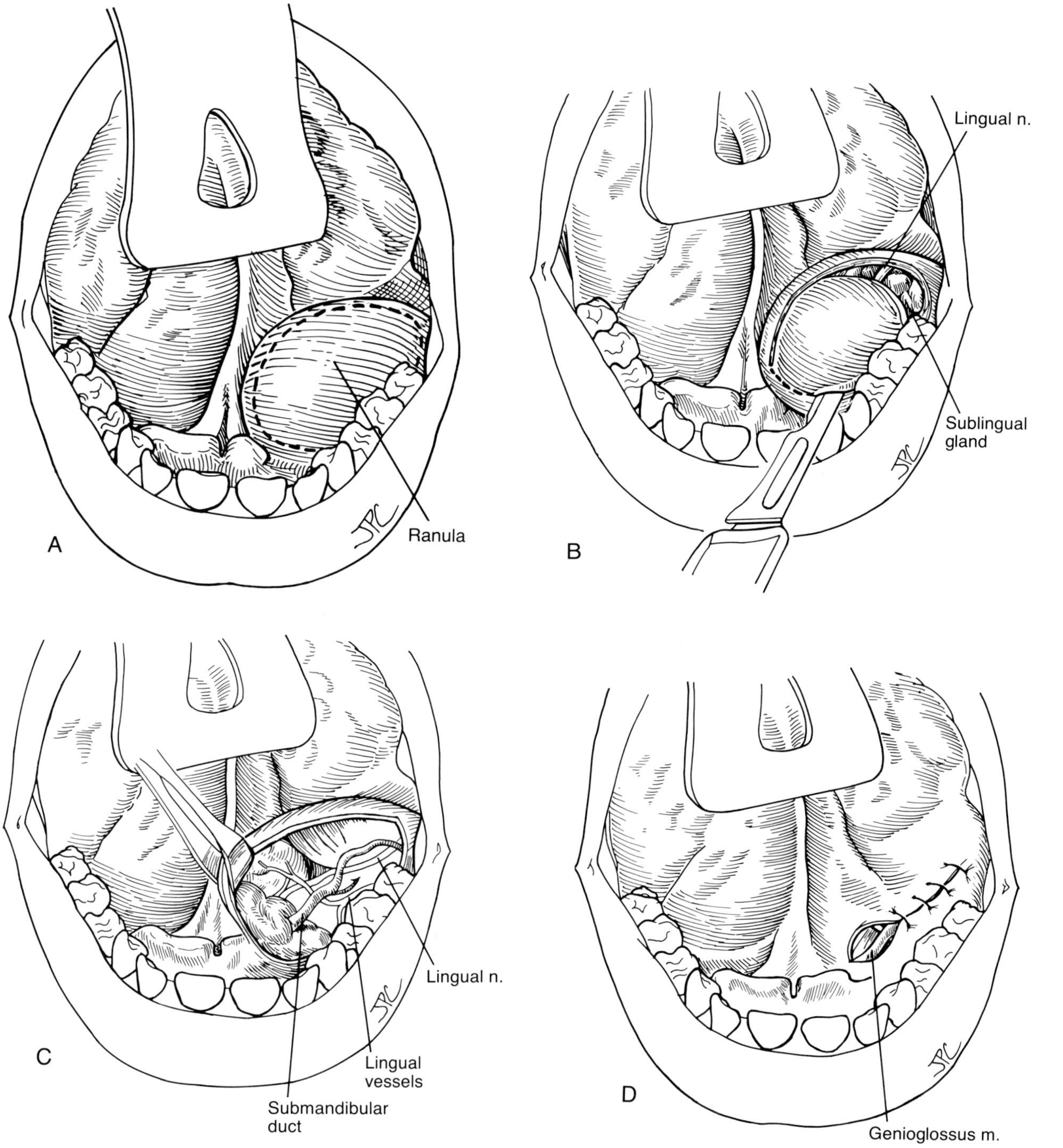

• FIGURE 19–7.

Marsupialization of a floor of the mouth lesion. *A*, Proposed incision over the dome of the ranula. *B* and *C*, Blunt and sharp dissection carried down to identify the submandibular duct and lingual nerve. *D*, Primary closure of the defect with absorbable suture.

REFERENCES

1. Balakrishnan A and Bailey CM: Lymphangioma of the tongue: A review of pathogenesis, treatment and use of surface laser photocoagulation. J Laryngol Otol 105:924–929, 1991.
2. Batsakis JG and McClatchey KD: Pathology consultation, cervical ranulas. Ann Otol Rhinol Laryngol 97(5, Pt 1):561–562, 1988.
3. Crysdale WS and Mendelsohn JD: Ranulas—mucoceles of the oral cavity: Experience in 26 children. Laryngoscope 98(3):296–298, 1988.
4. Gupta OP: Congenital macroglossia. Arch Otolaryngol Head Neck Surg 93:378–383, 1971.
5. Van Den Akker HP, Bays RA, and Becker AE: Plunging or cervical ranula: Review of the literature and report of 4 cases. J Maxillofac Surg 6:288–293, 1988.
6. Sistrunk WE: Technique of removal of cysts and sinuses of the thyroglossal duct. Surg Gynecol Obstet 46:109–112, 1928.

chapter

20

Endoscopic Surgery of the Upper Aerodigestive Tract

KENNY H. CHAN, M.D.
KEITH H. RIDING, M.D.
FRANCIS X. McGOWAN, M.D.
SYLVAN E. STOOL, M.D.

Endoscopy of the upper aerodigestive tract is an important component of the practice of a pediatric otolaryngologist. Historically, endoscopic procedures were limited by the instrumentation and anesthetics available to the pioneers in the early part of this century. However, technologic advances during the last 20 years have made endoscopic surgery useful and safe.

SELECTED AIRWAY PHYSIOLOGY

- Airflow is governed by the interplay of flow, pressure, and resistance. Under laminar flow conditions, resistance is proportional to the fourth power of the airway radius and is inversely related to airway length and viscosity. Under turbulent flow conditions, resistance is proportional to the fifth power of the radius, and thus decreased lumen size (from a pathologic process or a bronchoscope) is more critical.

- A greater flow rate is required to maintain the same driving pressure in the presence of turbulent flow. The smaller airways of infants require higher driving pressures to achieve gas flow, especially when flow is turbulent. Air in infants will desaturate more quickly because of the significantly higher metabolic rate and the modestly lower functional residual capacity.

- The incidence of abnormal control of breathing and apnea are increased in infants following general anesthesia. Older children with chronic upper airway obstruction (e.g., adenotonsillar hypertrophy, subglottic stenosis, Down's syndrome) also can have abnormal ventilatory drive and can be at increased risk of pulmonary hypertension, cor pulmonale, pulmonary edema, and postoperative respiratory obstruction.

PRINCIPLES OF ENDOSCOPIC SURGERY

The communication channel between the operative and anesthetic teams is maintained throughout the endoscopic procedure in order to accurately assess the depth and the duration of anesthesia. This coordinated effort is required to minimize potential complications.

The general principles of endoscopic surgery are as follows:

- Introduce instruments gently to avoid mucosal bleeding and edema.

- Advance the endoscope only when a lumen is present to prevent perforation of a viscus.

- The surgeon–anesthetist team approach is essential for a safe and successful outcome.

ENDOSCOPY OF THE ORAL CAVITY AND PHARYNX

Indications

- Adequate examination of the oral cavity and pharynx in uncooperative children sometimes requires anesthesia.
- The extent of trauma (blunt or sharp) or burns (caustic or electrical) can be assessed during pharyngoscopy.

Anesthetic considerations

INHALED ANESTHETICS

- Inhaled anesthetics can provide analgesia and amnesia and allow relatively accurate assessment and control of anesthetic depth. Dose-dependent respiratory depression is a feature common to almost all anesthetics. Anesthetic induction using inhalational anesthetics is usually faster in infants because of their higher minute ventilation, lower functional residual capacity, reduced blood gas solubility, and greater percentage of cardiac output delivered to the brain.
- Both halothane and isoflurane are bronchodilators. Halothane has the advantage of being less pungent and irritating to the airways. Halothane sensitizes the myocardium to the arrhythmogenic effects of catecholamines. Desflurane, a newer agent, may cause the least respiratory depression. This agent also promotes rapid induction; however, it can be irritating to the airways and cause laryngospasm on induction or emergence. Sevoflurane, another new agent under study, should provide rapid induction and emergence, minimal airway irritation, and minimal myocardial sensitization to catecholamines.

NARCOTICS

- Narcotics have been used as adjuncts to inhaled anesthetics to increase analgesia and as part of a nitrous oxide-narcotic-relaxant technique. All narcotics reduce respiratory rate (apnea occurs with sufficient doses). When used alone, narcotics do not control airway reflexes and do not provide reliable amnesia.
- Morphine may cause release of histamine and hypotension. Fentanyl and sufentanil are more potent than morphine, do not cause release of histamine, and (when used in judicious doses) can be relatively short-acting; short duration of action is particularly true of alfentanil.

ANTICHOLINERGICS

- Vagolysis is frequently employed prior to airway procedures to reduce secretions and to minimize bradycardia associated with airway instrumentation. All anticholinergics (with the possible exception of scopolamine) should be given immediately prior to the procedure for best effect.
- Atropine has been used most often, has a relatively short duration of action, and may cause delirium because it can cross the blood-brain barrier. Glycopyrrolate causes less tachycardia than does atropine. This drug may be more effective as an antisialagogue, lasts longer, and does not enter the central nervous system (CNS). Scopolamine is effective at reducing secretions, has long duration and minimal effect on heart rate, and has sedative properties that can be profound.

LIDOCAINE

- Topical lidocaine, applied as a 1 to 2% spray to the vocal cords or instilled into the trachea after induction of anesthesia, can be an important adjunct to diagnostic airway procedures by reducing the tendency toward laryngospasm or bronchospasm and by reducing inhaled anesthetic requirements. Intravenous lidocaine acts as a general anesthetic and can reduce airway reflex responses to laryngoscopy and intubation.

PROPOFOL

- The new intravenous hypnotic propofol has become the mainstay of our anesthetic approach to laryngeal laser surgery. This approach provides complete amnesia, good control of hemodynamic responses, the ability to use O_2/air for jet ventilation, and rapid emergence. Propofol may have antiemetic properties as well. Older children who have frequent procedures (e.g., laryngeal papillomatosis) now request this agent.

MUSCLE RELAXATION

- There are a number of muscle relaxants available to the anesthesiologist, so choice can now be tailored based on desired duration, mode of elimination, and side effects (e.g., tachycardia and histamine release).

- For the patient having airway endoscopy, a more fundamental consideration is whether to use relaxants at all and, if so, when? Possible advantages of spontaneous ventilation include (1) maintained gas exchange; (2) ability to assess vocal cord and airway motion; and (3) ability to obtain step-by-step control of the airway and avoid "bridge burning" (e.g., a muscle-relaxed patient who cannot be intubated or ventilated). On the other hand, prolonged spontaneous ventilation, especially with an unprotected airway, may increase the risk of aspiration.

Preparation

PREOPERATIVE MANAGEMENT

Complete historical and physical examination information must be known by all members of the surgical and anesthesia teams. Specific discussion about the severity, type, and presumed location of the airway abnormality should occur well in advance of beginning the anesthetic. The implications of significant coexisting diseases should also be taken into account. These measures allow for optimization of patient condition and ensure the availability of appropriate equipment, drugs, and personnel. It is useful for the anesthesiologist to view radiographs and computed tomography (CT) scans preoperatively to assess lesion location and airway caliber.

- All equipment that might possibly be necessary should be available, and its proper functioning should be ensured. Complications that require alternative techniques should be anticipated and discussed in advance.

- Our current practice requires continuous electrocardiography, automated blood pressure, pulse oximetry, precordial stethoscope, and temperature monitoring. A peripheral nerve stimulator (to assess muscle relaxation and its reversal) and the ability to measure end-tidal CO_2 are also necessary.

- The degree of airway obstruction should be assessed preoperatively, and the degree of difficulty to be anticipated should be assessed intraoperatively.

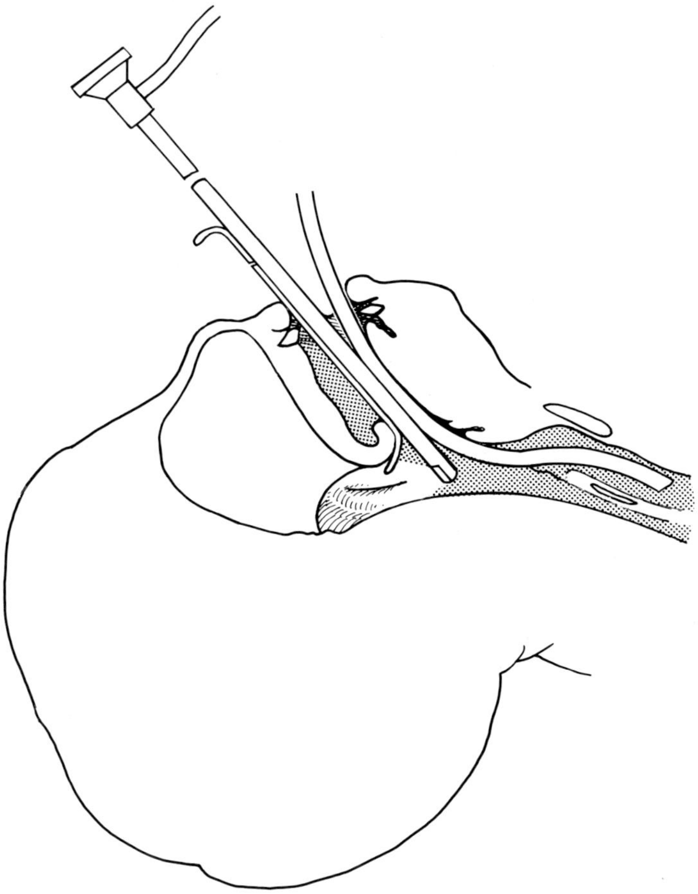

• **FIGURE 20–1.**

Examination of the nasopharynx using a 70-degree telescope.

INSTRUMENTATION

Various mouth gags are available for exposure. For endoscopic examination, a 70-degree telescope can be used (see Procedure).

Procedure

- Adequate illumination with a headlight is generally sufficient. For examination of the oral cavity and oropharynx, exposure is attained with either the Jennings or McIvor mouth gag. A Denhardt mouth gag is helpful for examination of the lateral tongue or alveolar ridge.
- Hypopharyngoscopy is part of the laryngeal examination (see Laryngoscopy).
- The nasopharynx can be examined alternatively with a 70-degree telescope from the oropharynx with the soft palate retracted (Fig. 20–1).

LARYNGOSCOPY

Indications

- Diagnostic laryngoscopy is used to
  - Assess alterations of anatomy
  - Determine physiology of the larynx
- Therapeutic laryngoscopy is used to
  - Ablate lesions
  - Remove foreign bodies
  - Dilatate stenoses

Anesthetic considerations

GENERAL CONSIDERATIONS

For general anesthetic considerations, refer to Endoscopy of the Oral Cavity and Pharynx.

LARYNGEAL AND VOCAL CORD ASSESSMENT

- Certain examinations of the larynx may be performed using flexible nasopharyngoscopy and are best facilitated by topical anesthesia using 2% lidocaine. Once the nasopharynx has been anesthetized, a nasal airway of appropriate size can be lubricated and passed into the nose to both dilate and lubricate. Gentle sedation (if not contraindicated by airway status) can be achieved with nitrous oxide (by oral or nasal cannula) or midazolam.

- Larynx and vocal cord mobility can be assessed in anesthetized, spontaneously breathing infants and children. One method is to perform a mask induction using inhalation agents. When sufficient depth is obtained, the vocal cords and larynx are sprayed with 3 to 4 mg/kg of 1 to 2% lidocaine. The mask is then reapplied to re-establish appropriate anesthetic depth with spontaneous ventilation; nitrous oxide is discontinued; and the table is turned to permit direct inspection of the larynx by the endoscopist. Close communication is required between the surgeon and the anesthesiologist, because anesthetic depth continually decreases during the period of inspection.

LASER SURGERY

- Possible techniques include spontaneous ventilation with and without an endotracheal tube, use of "laser-resistant" endotracheal tubes, or suspension laryngoscopy with Venturi ventilation. Regardless of the technique chosen, it is essential to confirm the ability to ventilate the patient using a mask before proceeding with muscle relaxation.

- No endotracheal tube (except metal), regardless of design or coating, is completely immune to ignition and combustion. Both oxygen and nitrous oxide will support combustion, and thus the inspired oxygen concentration should be diluted as close to 21% as can be tolerated with either air or nitrogen. The cuffs on cuffed endotracheal tubes are particularly vulnerable and should be filled with saline.

- We prefer to use suspension laryngoscopy with Venturi jet ventilation for the majority of laryngeal laser surgery procedures. Following successful induction and controlled mask ventilation, a muscle relaxant (usually atracurium or vecuronium) is given. Muscle relaxation is essential for this technique in order to maximize chest wall compliance and ensure vocal cord immobility. This technique is potentially dangerous in the small child with upper airway obstruction.

- Patients with significant obstruction in the region of the glottic opening may require debulking around an endotracheal tube to provide a sufficient opening for subsequent Venturi ventilation. As discussed previously, so-called total intravenous anesthesia using a propofol infusion and supplemental narcotic is an excellent choice for these patients.

- Once adequate ventilation and muscle relaxation are established, the table is turned and the suspension laryngoscope is placed. A catheter, connected via a length of flexible tubing to the high-pressure gas source/variable pressure–reducing valve, is aimed at the glottic opening. Both the surgeon and the anesthesiologist must confirm that this catheter is aimed appropriately, and its position must be constantly reassessed.

- Insufflation pressure is best titrated to chest excursion; in general, driving pressures between 6 and 8 psi for infants, 10 and 12 psi for children, and 12 and 16 psi for teenagers are adequate. Nonetheless, continuous clinical inspection of catheter position/aim, chest movement, and breath sounds is required. When performed correctly, gas exchange has been shown to be acceptable in infants and children ventilated in this manner.

- Complications of laser surgery include airway fires and extraneous tissue injury. Complications relating to the use of laser and jet ventilation are largely avoidable when a careful technique is employed.

- It is probably advisable to intubate most patients at the end of the procedure owing to the presence of secretions, blood, and edema. The patients are then extubated after emergence is completed with airway reflexes intact. Cool mist, intravenous dexamethasone, or nebulized racemic epinephrine may be useful to treat postprocedure stridor.

Preparation

PREOPERATIVE MANAGEMENT

For general considerations, refer to preoperative management in Endoscopy of the Oral Cavity and Pharynx.

INSTRUMENTATION

Pediatric laryngoscopes and forceps currently in use at our institutions are shown in Figures 20–2 and 20–3.

Procedure

GENERAL CONSIDERATIONS

- The use of anesthesia may be influenced by the age and overall medical condition of the parent. Awake diagnostic laryngoscopy is sometimes used in premature infants and infants younger than 3 months of age. The procedure is carried out by physically restraining the patient using a sheet.
- Because of potential synchronous lesions of the airway, laryngoscopy should generally be accompanied by bronchoscopy to completely assess the airway.
- Fiberoptic laryngoscopy using a fiberoptic nasopharyngoscope is an alternative to rigid laryngoscopy; however, because of the floppy epiglottis and the anteriorly placed larynx, this procedure is sometimes difficult in young infants. An evaluation of an infant with a compromised airway should be performed in the operating room.
- An excellent alternative to the use of standard rigid laryngoscopes is the use of a telescope with the aid of an anesthesia laryngoscope. The ability to attach a video camera to the telescope enhances resolution and facilitates teaching.

INTRODUCTION OF THE LARYNGOSCOPE

- The laryngoscope is held in the left hand, and the right index finger retracts the upper lip. In infants a tooth guard is usually not necessary; however, for older children it may be desirable to insert a tooth guard.
- The head (face forward) should be in the midline in a sniffing position.
- The laryngoscope is inserted on the right side of the tongue. The blade is rotated about 90 degrees in most infants and children; the tip is inserted into the vallecula, and the epiglottis is identified (Fig. 20–4).

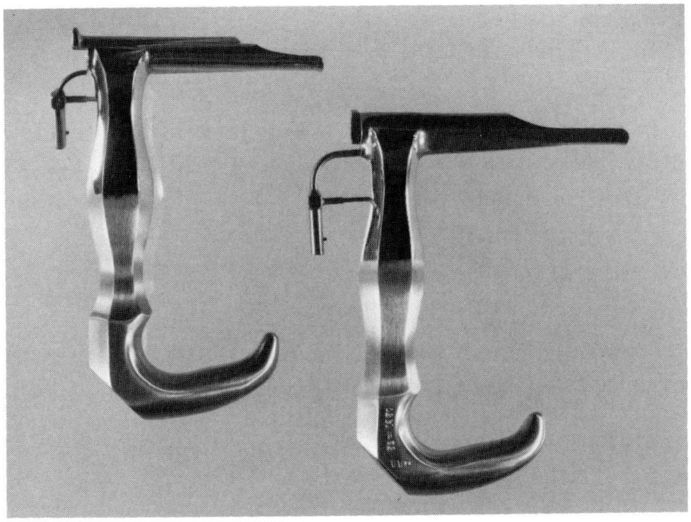

• FIGURE 20-2.

Sampling of pediatric laryngoscopes.

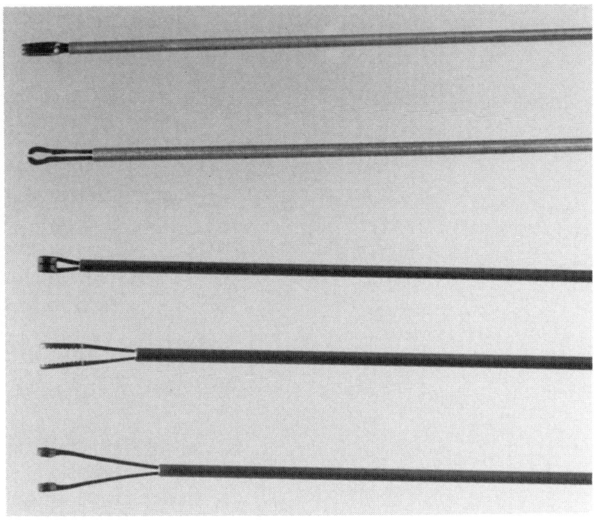

• FIGURE 20-3.

Sampling of the tips of forceps used in conjunction with laryngoscopy and bronchoscopy.

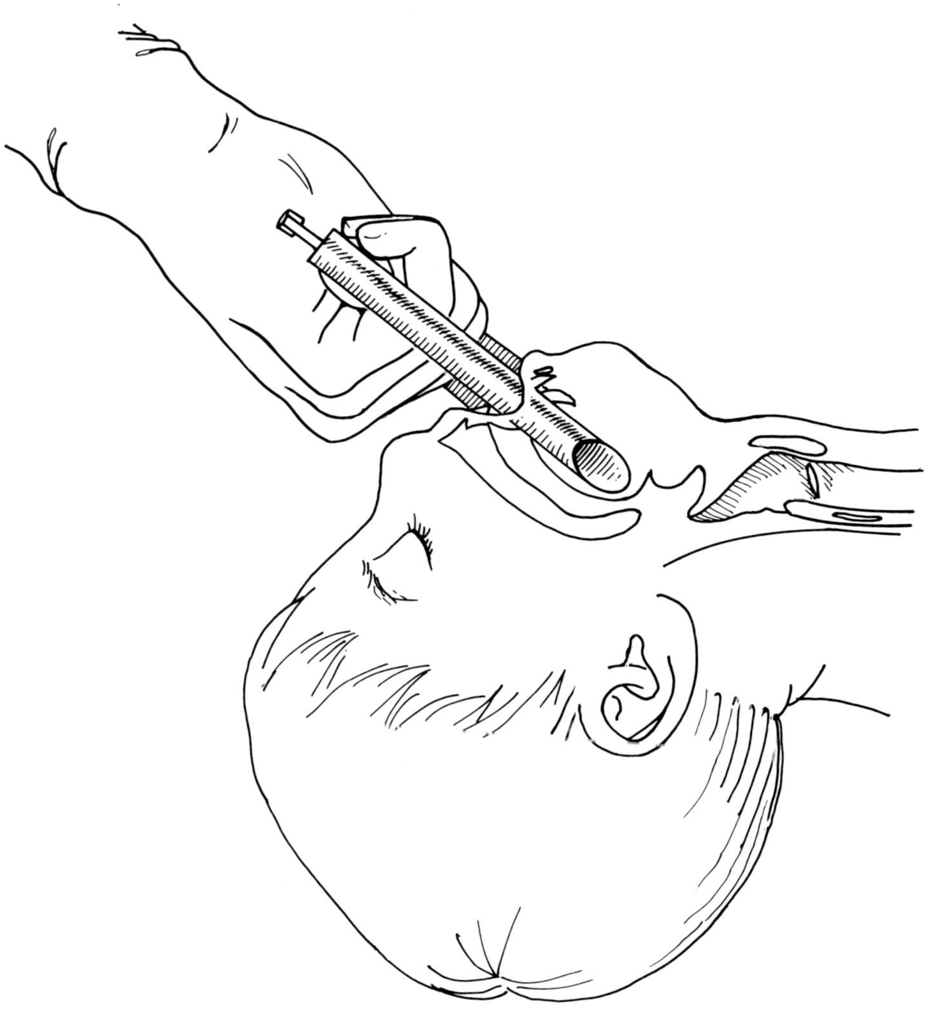

• FIGURE 20-4.

Laryngoscopy sequence I.

- Exposure of the larynx is accomplished by pulling the epiglottis forward, not by prying on the teeth (Fig. 20–5). The endoscopic view at this level is illustrated in Figure 20–6.

- The glottis can usually be visualized when the laryngoscope is advanced below the epiglottis. The endoscopic view at this level is shown in Figure 20–7. For an enhanced view, the rod-lens telescope can be used, and if a camera is attached, the vocal cord movement can be recorded (Fig. 20–8).

- If the glottis cannot be seen, it may be necessary to advance the tip of the laryngoscope down the laryngeal surface in the epiglottis.

- Caution should be used when inserting the instrument, because it is easy to advance it into the upper esophagus of a small child and cause airway obstruction.

SUSPENSION LARYNGOSCOPY

- Once the larynx is visualized, the cannula for jet ventilation is positioned to ensure adequate air exchange.

- Concurrently, the suspension device is attached to the laryngoscope.

- Refer to Chapter 23 for details on laser techniques.

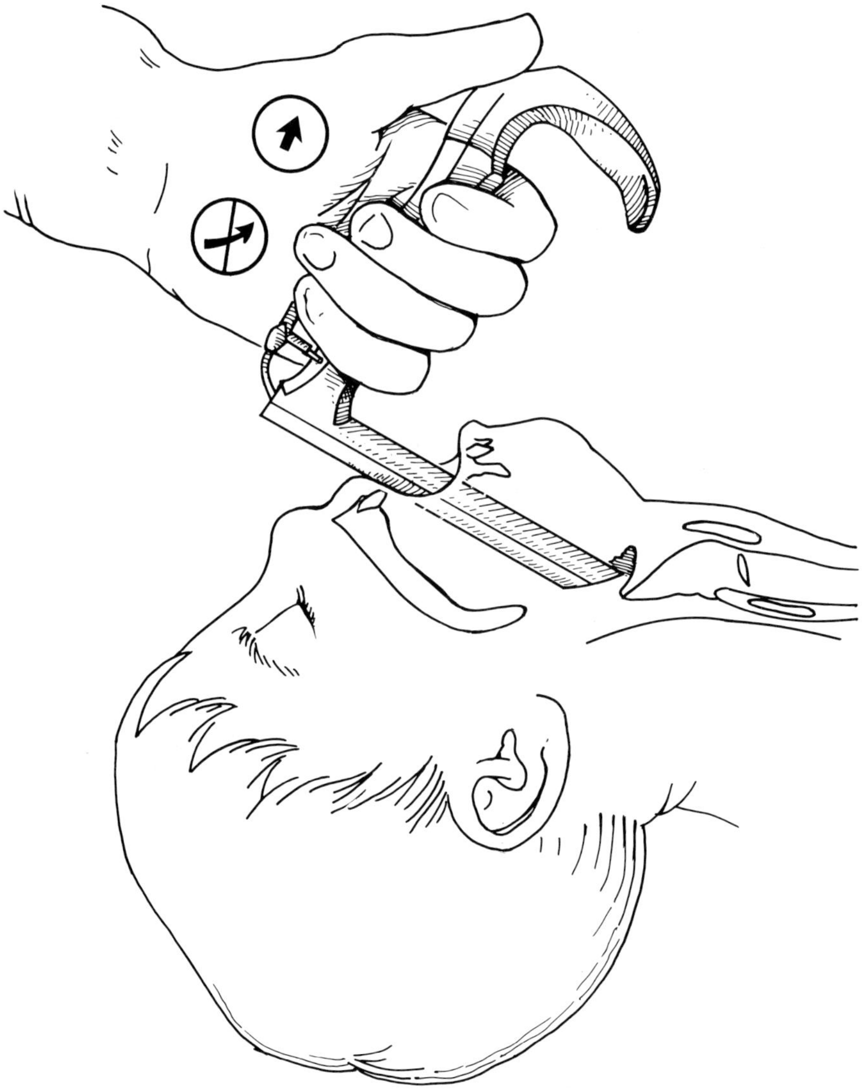

• FIGURE 20–5.

Laryngoscopy sequence II: correct and incorrect directions for lifting the laryngoscope.

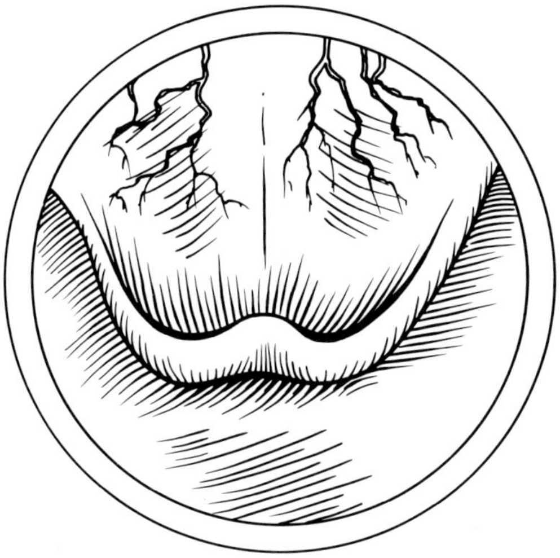

• **FIGURE 20–6.**

Endoscopic view during laryngoscopy sequence I.

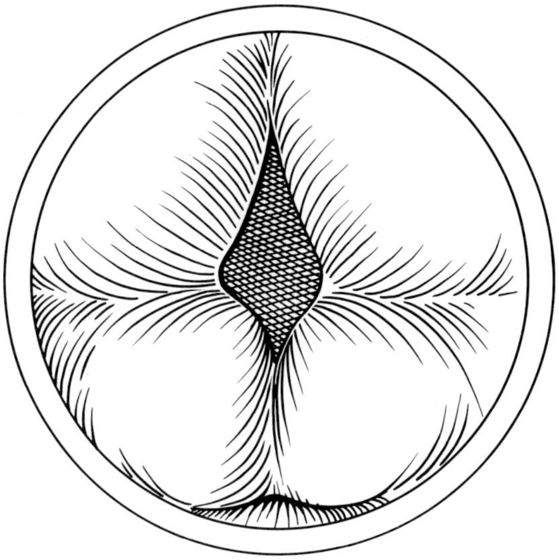

• **FIGURE 20–7.**

Endoscopic view during laryngoscopy sequence II.

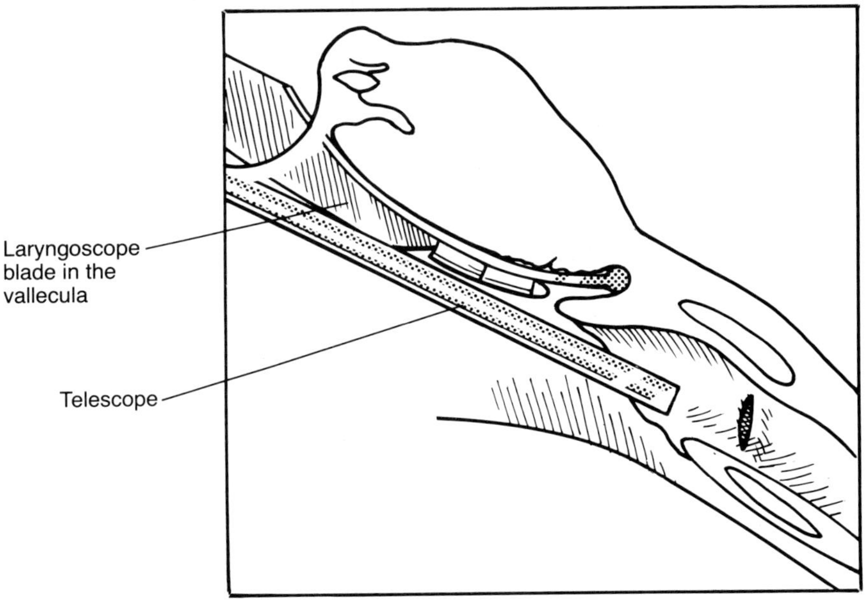

• **FIGURE 20–8.**

Alternative method to examine the larynx using a rod-lens telescope.

FOREIGN BODY REMOVAL

• Once the larynx is exposed, foreign bodies can be removed by choosing the appropriate grasping forceps (see Fig. 20–3).

LARYNGEAL DILATATION

• Laryngeal dilatation is generally performed in tracheostomized patients.

• Lubricated Jackson laryngeal dilators are inserted, conforming to the shape of the glottic opening in a serial fashion (Fig. 20–9).

BRONCHOSCOPY

Indications

• Diagnostic bronchoscopy is used to assess the tracheobronchial tree.

• Therapeutic bronchoscopy is used to remove tracheal and bronchial lesions and foreign bodies and to dilate stenoses.

Anesthetic considerations

GENERAL CONSIDERATIONS

For general anesthetic considerations, refer to Endoscopy of the Oral Cavity and Pharynx.

RIGID BRONCHOSCOPY

• Smaller bronchoscopes (especially < 4 mm) with the telescope in place may significantly increase airway resistance. Increased resistance may be tolerated for relatively brief periods by spontaneously breathing infants.

• Spontaneous ventilation may be optimal to diagnose dynamic lesions such as tracheomalacia or bronchomalacia. It may also be a crucial method to maintain adequate gas exchange in cases of severe obstruction (e.g., foreign body).

• In paralyzed subjects, the passive recoil properties of the lung and chest wall are the only forces producing expiratory gas flow. A slow, gentle pattern of manual ventilation is probably best, using larger-than-normal tidal volumes at reduced rates.

• Regardless of the mode of ventilation, frequent removal of the telescope (at least every 5 minutes; more frequently if the patient's condition so indicates) allows restoration of normocarbia and normoxia. Similarly, prolonged endobronchial intubation must be avoided.

• Suctioning can rapidly deplete lung oxygen content and accelerate the development of hypoxia. Suctioning should be brief and should be at reduced flow rates.

• Adequate ventilation may be impossible if the size of the patient (or that of the airway) requires the use of very small bronchoscopes (< 3 mm). A period of hyperventilation with 100% oxygen prior to telescope insertion, followed by apneic oxygenation during telescopic examination (pop-off and other valves open), may be best.

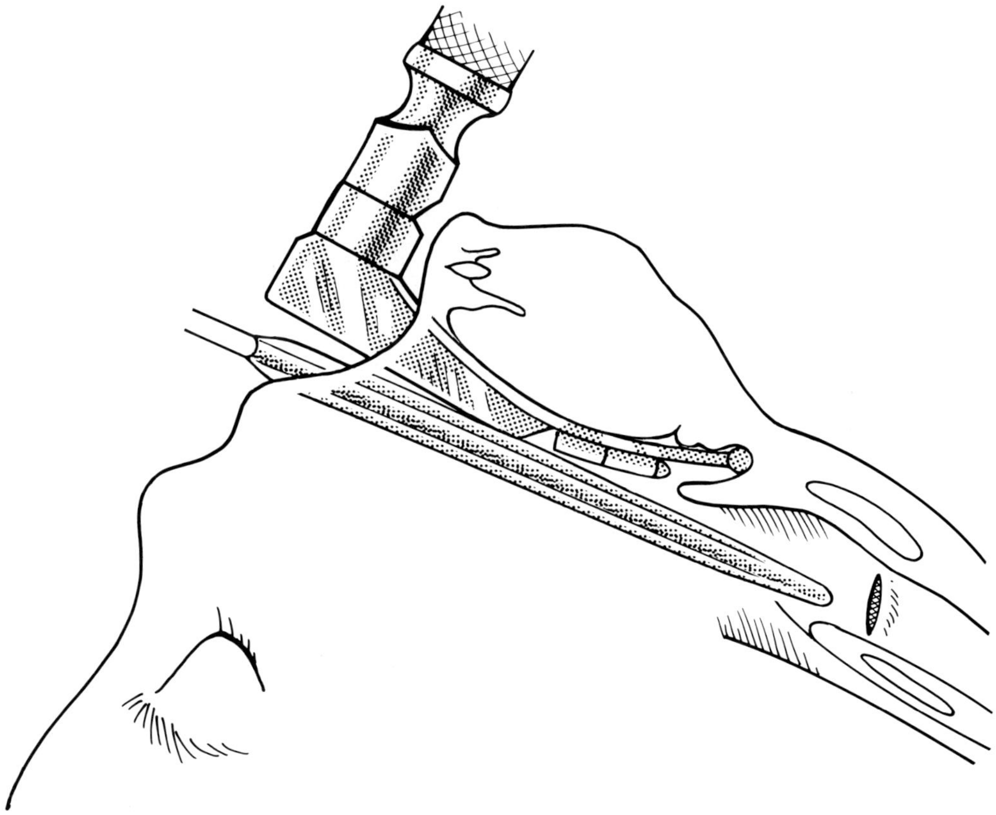

• **FIGURE 20-9.**

Laryngeal dilatation.

AIRWAY FOREIGN BODIES

- Anesthetic approaches for airway foreign bodies include rapid sequence induction with intubation, bronchoscopy and spontaneous ventilation, and bronchoscopy.

- We prefer to perform a careful, deep inhalational induction (the duration of which may be prolonged if obstruction is severe) and maintain spontaneous ventilation. Others prefer to use muscle relaxation during bronchoscopy and foreign body removal. Although this may simplify the technique, muscle relaxation should not be attempted until a careful sequence of assisted to controlled ventilation has demonstrated adequate gas exchange in the absence of spontaneous ventilation.

Preparation

PREOPERATIVE MANAGEMENT

For general considerations, refer to Endoscopy of the Oral Cavity and Pharynx.

INSTRUMENTATION

- Two main types of bronchoscopes are available: open bronchoscopes (Fig. 20–10) and rod-lens bronchoscopes (Fig. 20–11 *A* and *B*).

- Illumination during bronchoscopy is accomplished by three telescopes: proximal, distal, and rod-lens.

- Rod-lens telescopes offer the advantages of magnification, angled views (Fig. 20–12) if necessary, and video documentation.

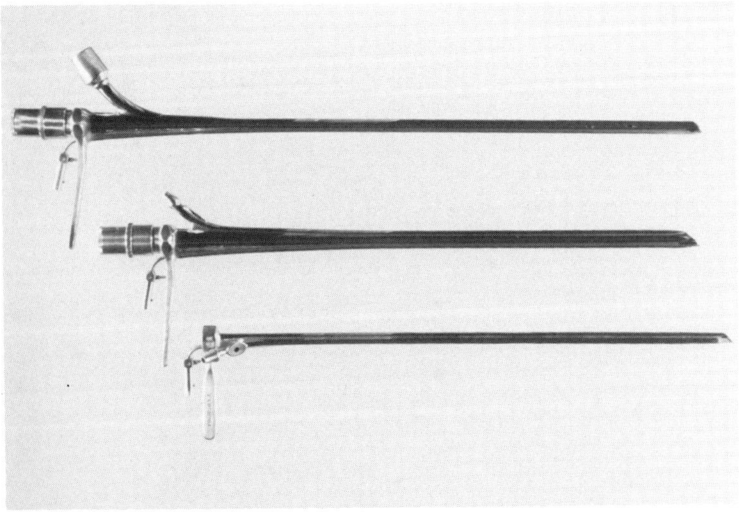

• FIGURE 20–10.

Open-type bronchoscopes.

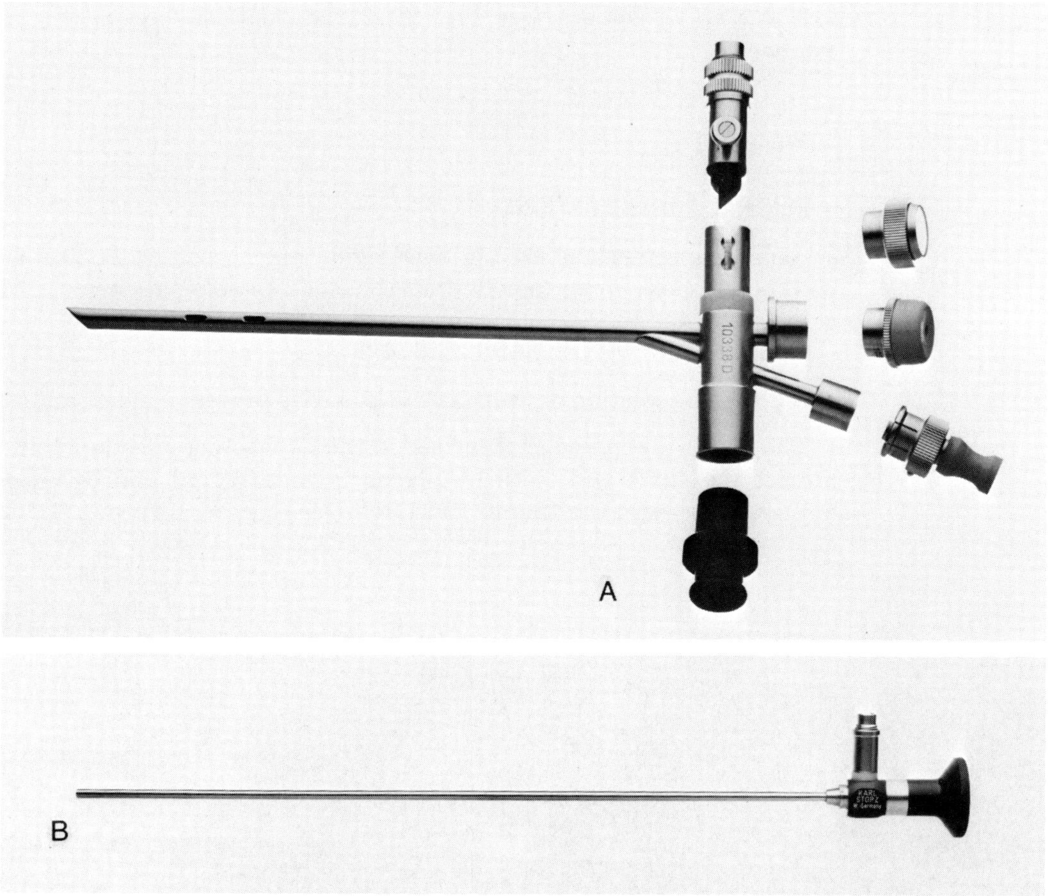

• FIGURE 20–11.

A, Parts of a rod-lens bronchoscope. *B*, A rod-lens telescope.

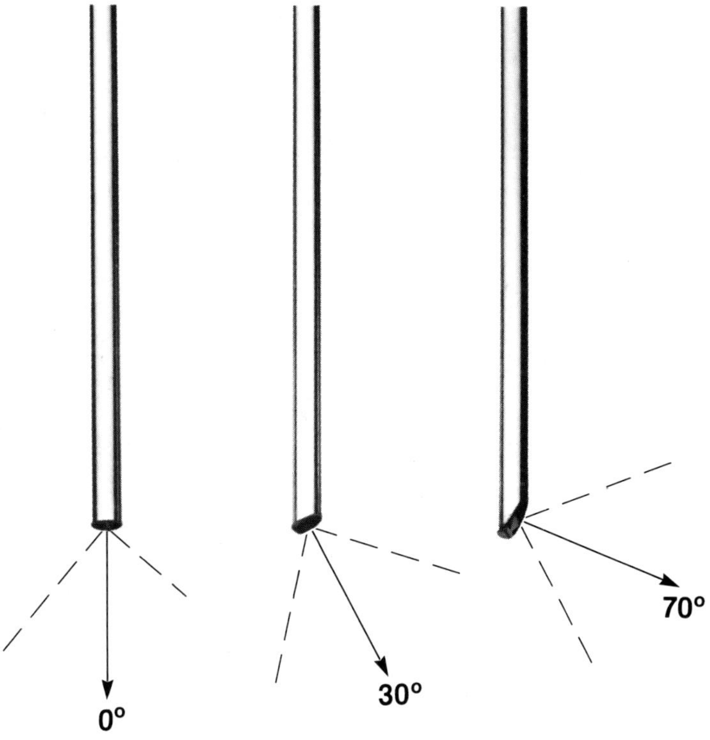

• FIGURE 20–12.

Angled views of rod-lens telescopes.

• A variety of forceps (see Fig. 20–3) and optical forceps (Fig. 20–13) are available.

Procedure

GENERAL CONSIDERATIONS

• General anesthesia is used in most rigid bronchoscopies. Topical anesthesia is used occasionally in extremely premature or unstable patients.

INTRODUCTION OF THE BRONCHOSCOPE

• A defogging solution or warm saline is used to prevent condensation on the lens.

• The larynx is exposed as described in the laryngoscopy section. Care is taken to protect the gums and teeth by placing a tooth guard and by suspending the bronchoscope with the thumb and forefinger (Fig. 20–14).

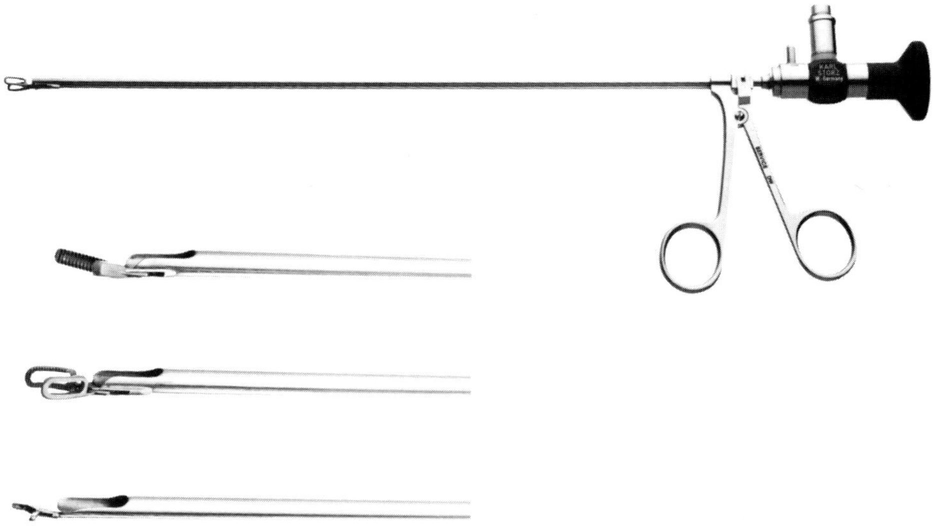

• FIGURE 20-13.

A variety of optical forceps for bronchoscopy and esophagoscopy.

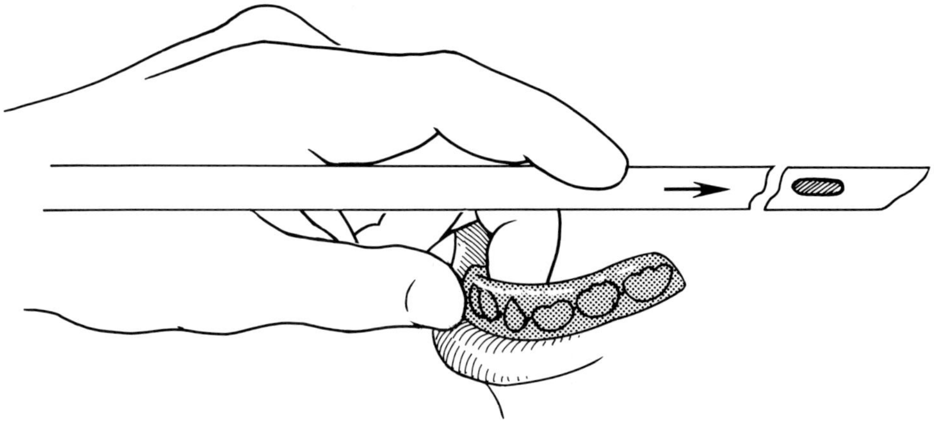

• FIGURE 20-14.

Gum and teeth protection using a tooth guard and suspension of the instrument.

- The bronchoscope is inserted alongside the laryngoscope (Fig. 20–15). The bronchoscope is turned 90 degrees to align the leading edge of the bronchoscope to the vocal cords (Fig. 20–16 *A* to *D*).

- In children, the larynx is usually exposed with a laryngoscope. This requires using an instrument with a slide that can be removed or an instrument with an open slot. In infants and young children, the cricoid is very prominent, and it is usually necessary to aim the instrument tip slightly posteriorly.

- The bronchoscope is introduced into the trachea, guided by the left hand; the laryngoscope is then removed. The index finger and thumb grasp the instrument, and the other fingers are inserted into the mouth to help stabilize the patient's head (see Fig. 20–14).

- The walls of the trachea appear somewhat white, and the posterior membranous party wall may be prominent.

- The carina is identified as a sharp vertical spur (Fig. 20–17). In the very young patient it may be blunt. To expose the right mainstem bronchus, the tip of the bronchoscope is turned to the right, slight lateral pressure is applied, and the child's face is rotated to the left. The endoscopic view is shown in Figure 20–18.

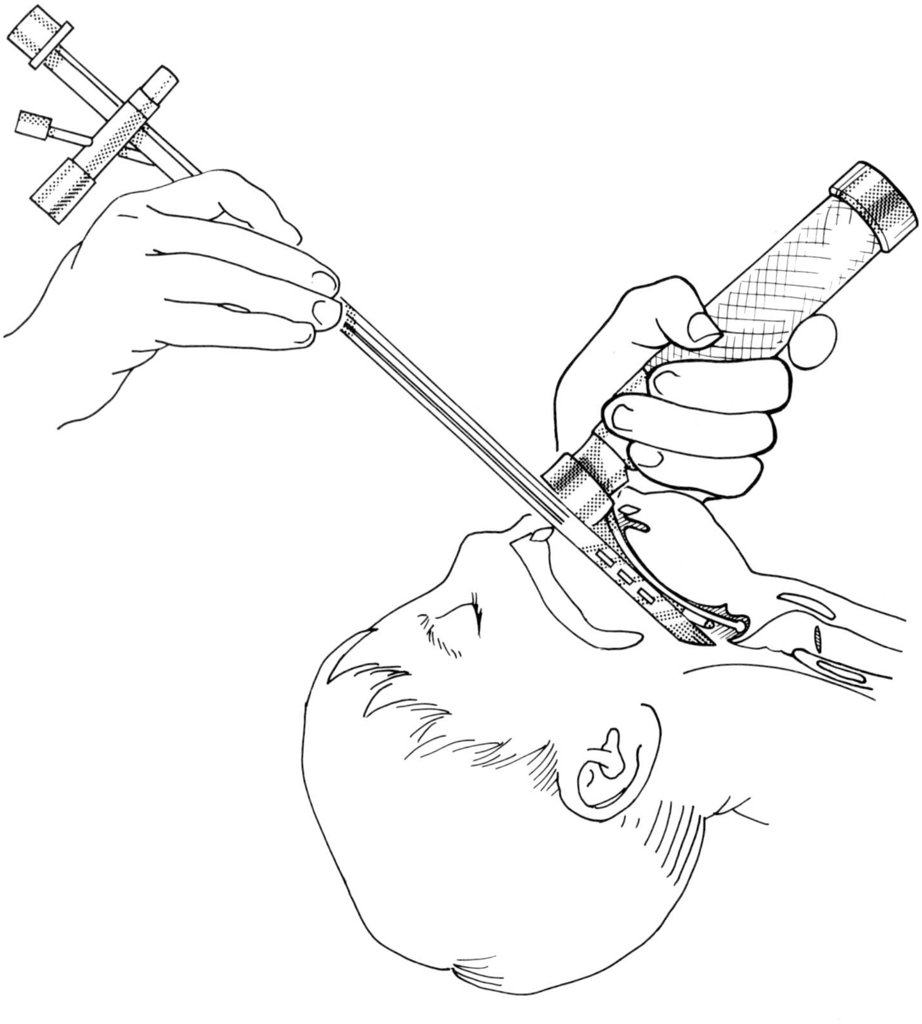

• FIGURE 20–15.

Insertion of a bronchoscope.

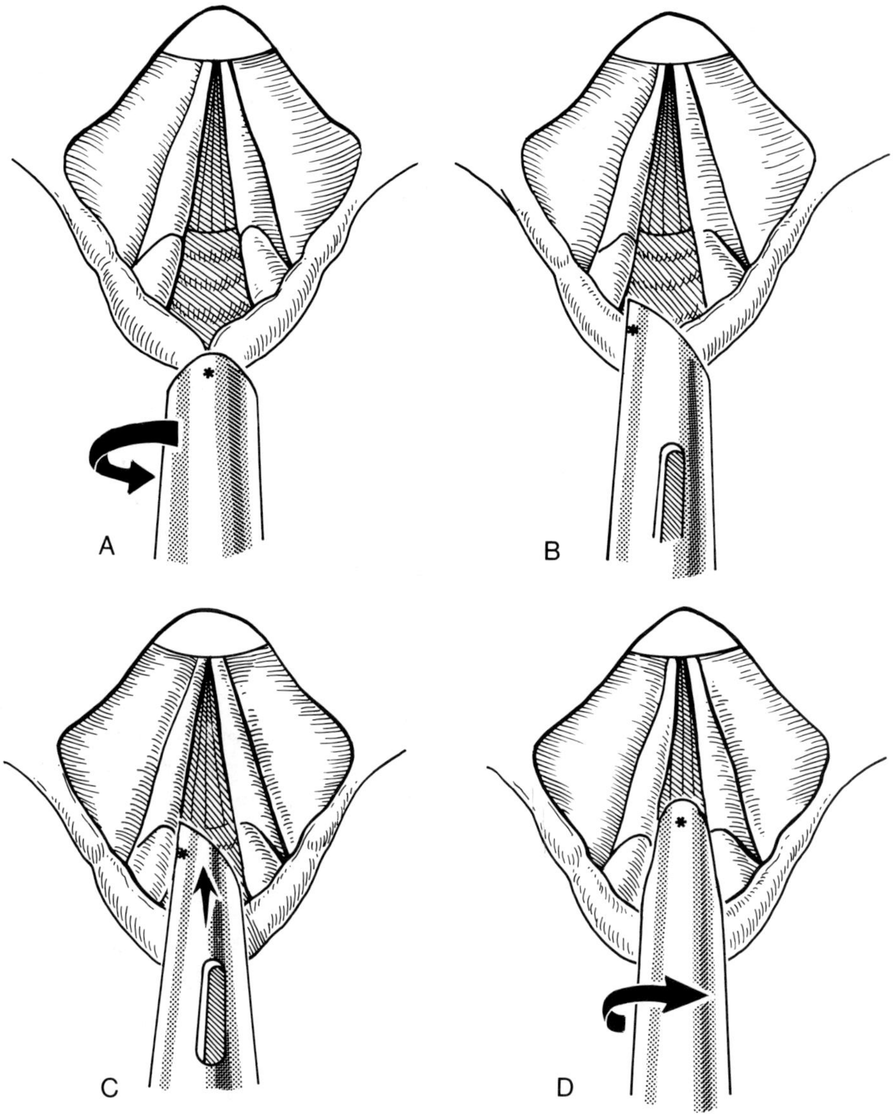

• FIGURE 20–16.

Sequence of passing the bronchoscope through the larynx. The asterisk indicates the orientation of the bronchoscope, and the arrows indicate the rotation and direction of the bronchoscope.

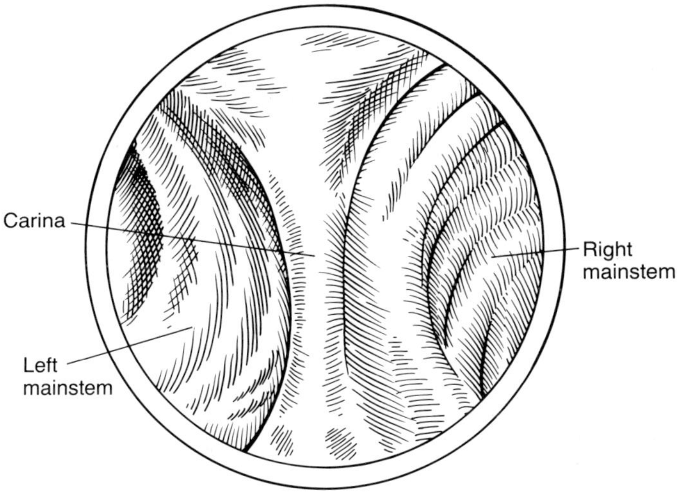

• FIGURE 20–17.

Endoscopic view of the carina.

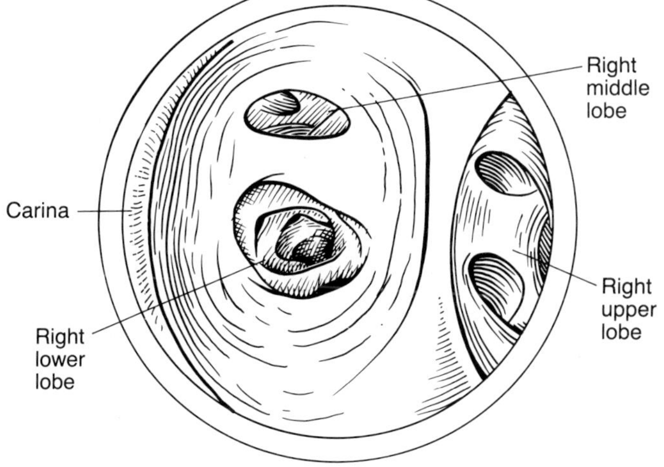

• FIGURE 20–18.

Endoscopic view of the right mainstem bronchus when the head is rotated to the left.

- To expose the left mainstem bronchus, the lip of the bronchoscope is rotated to the left, and the child's face is turned to the right.

- Most children are examined under general anesthesia, and cooperation between the anesthetist and the surgeon is important. The bronchoscopes have a male connector for the anesthesia adapters, and it is necessary for the anesthesiologist to support the tubing and adapters throughout the procedure.

- When using a small (3.0 mm) bronchoscope, it may become necessary to remove the telescope intermittently to improve ventilation.

REMOVAL OF SECRETIONS

- Secretions can be removed using a metal-tipped suction that is inserted proximally. A blunt-tipped suction is preferred to avoid mucosal trauma.

- Secretions can also be removed with polyethylene tubing (internal diameter 2 mm) that is inserted from the side channel. It is possible to direct the tubing into segmental bronchi for selective suctioning. Pneumothorax is a potential occurrence.

FOREIGN BODY REMOVAL

- The first objective of airway foreign body removal is the assessment of the airway itself. When the airway is reasonably secured, the feasibility of foreign body removal is entertained. More than one procedure is sometimes necessary to remove the entire foreign body. On a rare occasion, an open procedure by the thoracic surgeon may be necessary.

VEGETABLE MATTER

- The most frequently aspirated vegetable matter is a peanut. The most useful tool is an optical double-action peanut forceps. Cessation of ventilation at the time of removal is very important.

- The bronchoscope is positioned proximal to the foreign body, and the secretions are suctioned using the flexible catheter.

- The telescope is removed, and the optical forceps is inserted. The jaws of the forceps are opened once it is beyond the bronchoscope.

- The foreign body is engaged, and the forceps is withdrawn through the bronchoscope. Occasionally, a fragile foreign body is removed by sheathing it into the bronchoscope, and the bronchoscope and forceps are removed together.

- The airway distal to the foreign body should be examined to rule out additional foreign bodies and to remove secretions.

ROUND OBJECTS

- The forward-grasping forceps is introduced following placement. The remaining steps are identical as described earlier for vegetable matter. In some cases, distal lighting is advisable.

SHARP OBJECT

- The sharp point inside the bronchoscope is sheathed during retrieval. The grasping forceps and the bronchoscope are removed in unison, if necessary.

FOREIGN BODY WITH GRANULATION TISSUE

- Most foreign bodies incite surrounding inflammation and granulation tissue formation.

• **FIGURE 20-19.**

Angioplastic balloon and rigid bronchoscope instrumentation.

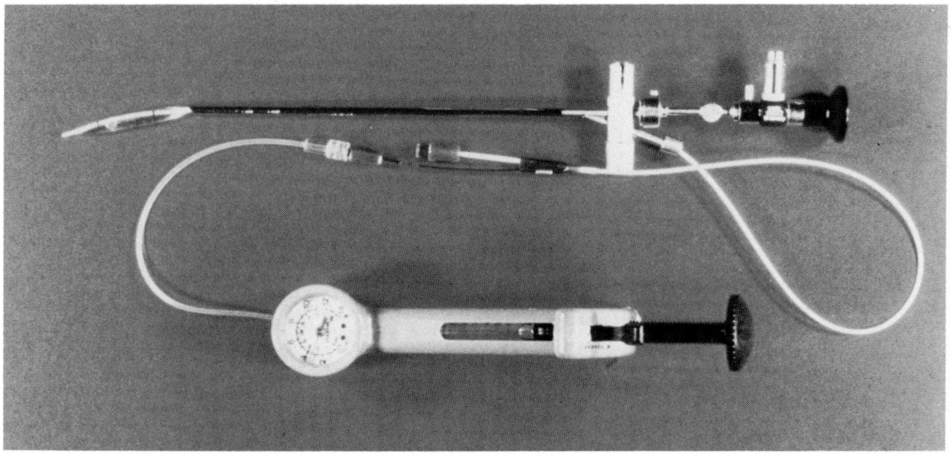

• The goal is to minimize bleeding during foreign body removal. Instillation of vasoconstrictive agents (e.g., Neo-Synephrine) via a flexible suction catheter is sometimes useful. The remaining granulation tissue following foreign body removal may be removed using a cup forceps.

LASER BRONCHOSCOPY

• Various laser bronchoscopy delivery systems are available. We have primarily used the CO_2 laser (Coherent) coupled with a laser bronchoscope system (Wolfe).

• Limitations exist in using the bronchoscope in infants and small children owing to their size relative to the instrument.

ELECTROCAUTERY

• The Bugby electrocautery unit (Karl Storz) can be used in conjunction with the rod-lens system.

• Lesions are cauterized by inserting the Bugby electrode down the side port until it extends beyond the bronchoscope.

• Controlled cauterization can be obtained by manipulating the bronchoscope.

TRACHEOBRONCHIAL DILATATION

• Tracheobronchial stenoses can sometimes be treated using successive dilatation with bronchoscopes, laser resection, and open surgical correction.

• Bronchial dilatation has been accomplished using an angioplastic balloon inserted through the side port (Fig. 20-19).

Postoperative care

• Postoperative observation is necessary if airway obstruction is anticipated. Postoperative monitoring devices, such as pulse oximetry, may be extremely useful. The nursing staff should be aware of the signs and symptoms of airway distress.

• A postoperative chest radiograph is often helpful when ruling out complications. One should be aware of postobstructive pulmonary edema and treat this entity aggressively.

ESOPHAGOSCOPY

Indications

- Diagnostic esophagoscopy in children is used to assess congenital and post-traumatic changes of the esophagus.
- Therapeutic esophagoscopy is used primarily to remove foreign bodies and to dilate stenoses.

Anesthetic considerations

GENERAL CONSIDERATIONS

Refer to the general anesthetic considerations under Endoscopy of the Oral Cavity and Pharynx as well as those for Airway Foreign Bodies.

Preparation

PREOPERATIVE MANAGEMENT

For general considerations, refer to preoperative management in Endoscopy of the Oral Cavity and Pharynx.

INSTRUMENTATION

- Similar to the bronchoscopes, esophagoscopes are classified as open (see Fig. 20–10) or telescopic (Fig. 20–20).

Procedure

GENERAL CONSIDERATIONS

- The rod-lens type of esophagoscope has advantages over the distal lighting esophagoscope in several areas: it provides better image resolution, it can be a teaching tool, and it can be adapted to a video camera.

INTRODUCTION OF THE ESOPHAGOSCOPE

- The use of a shoulder roll during esophagoscopy is optional.
- The esophagoscope is advanced using one of two methods. The esophagoscope can be advanced without guidance by identifying the cricopharyngeus (Fig. 20–21). The alternative technique is to place a nasogastric tube as a lumen finder.
- In children, this procedure is performed under general anesthesia (usually after endotracheal intubation).
- The hypopharynx is exposed using a laryngoscope in much the same manner as that described for direct laryngoscopy, except that the instrument is passed posteriorly so that the arytenoids can be identified.
- The cricopharyngeus is identified by its oval appearance and may be opened by forward traction on the larynx.
- If it is difficult to visualize the cricopharyngeus and there is no foreign body beneath it, it may be identified by passing a catheter through the nose into the hypopharynx and upper esophagus.

• **FIGURE 20-20.**

A rod-lens esophagoscope.

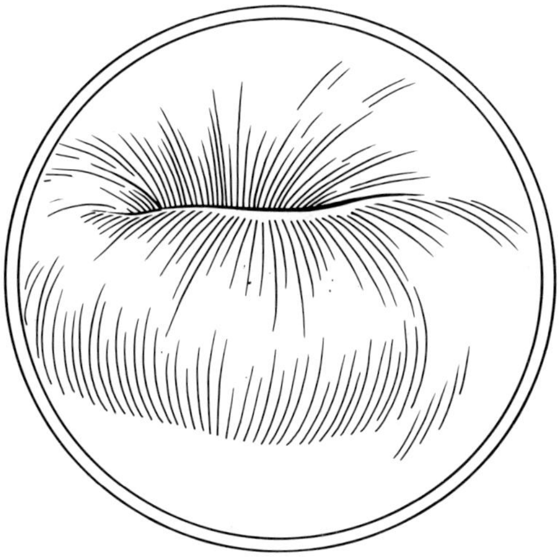

• **FIGURE 20-21.**

An endoscopic view of the cricopharyngeus muscle.

- When the cervical esophagus is entered, secretions may obscure visualization and thus are removed with suction. The rod-lens esophagoscope may be pulled back from the end of the esophagoscope so that it will not become clouded by secretions.

- The left hand guides the esophagoscope and protects the teeth with the thumb and index finger (identical with the insertion of the bronchoscope).

- As the instrument passes from the cervical to the thoracic esophagus, the patient's shoulders are elevated to visualize the thoracic esophagus. In the region of the heart, there is a prominent cardiac pulsation.

- The young child may be examined bimanually by placing the left hand behind the child's back and by manipulating the esophagoscope with the right hand.

- The esophagoscope is advanced slowly with the lumen under visualization. A small plastic tube can be passed down the instrument side port as a lumen finder.

FOREIGN BODY REMOVAL

- Similar instruments are used for esophageal foreign bodies as for airway foreign bodies.

- The timing for foreign body removal depends on the degree of distress. Removal in patients who are comfortable and who do not have potential airway compromise may be delayed for optimal timing.

- After foreign body removal, it is critical to examine the distal esophagus to rule out additional foreign bodies or other lesions. Not all esophageal foreign bodies are radiopaque.

- Because the endotracheal tube can easily be dislodged during passage of the foreign body and esophagoscope through the pharynx, the surgeon-anesthetist team approach is important.

COINS

- Coins can generally be safely removed by using an optical forceps through a rod-lens esophagoscope or a grasping forceps through an esophageal speculum.

ROUND OBJECTS

- Round objects are generally removed more easily by using the bead grasping forceps through a Jackson esophagoscope.

SHARP OBJECTS

- Sharp objects are sheathed into the esophagoscope using a grasping forceps through a rod-lens esophagoscope.

JACKSTONES

- Jackstones are difficult to remove because of their size and sharp points. Figure 20–22 illustrates how the sharp point is rotated into a Jackson esophagoscope and is removed using a grasping forceps. Mucosal tears are common and may result in periesophagitis.

SAFETY PINS

- Safety pins have rarely been seen at our institution during the past 2 decades. The original techniques described by Jackson are presented (Fig. 20–23).

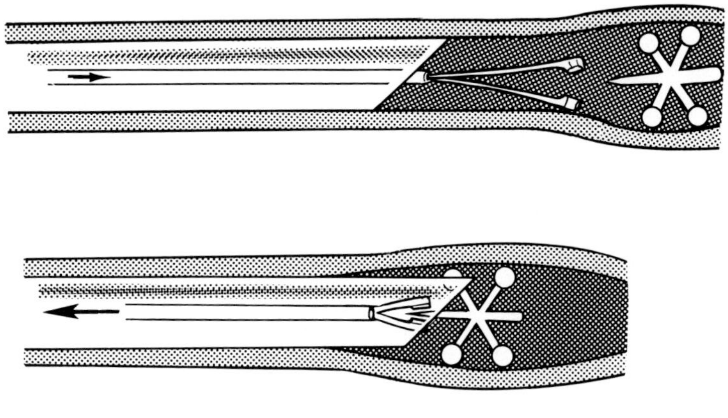

• FIGURE 20-22.

Removal of a jackstone.

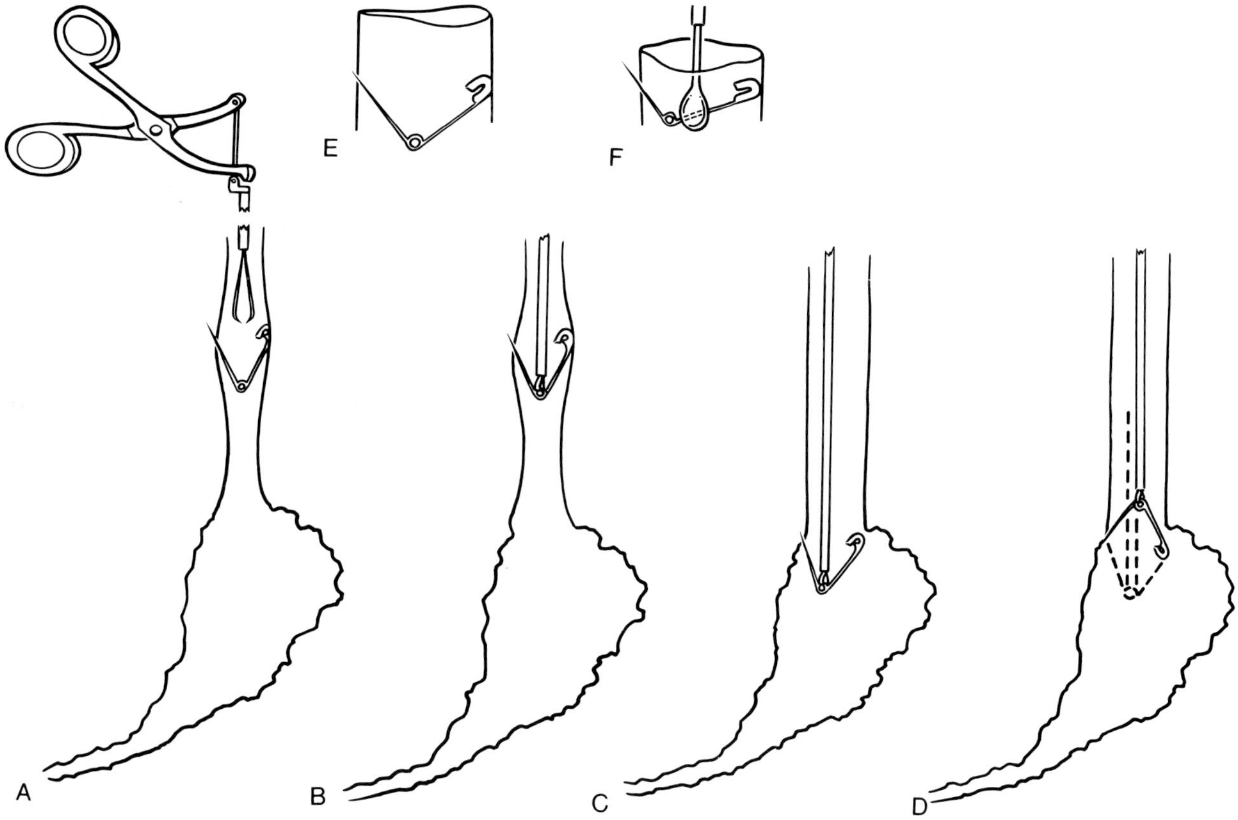

• FIGURE 20-23.

Safety pin removal sequence (Jackson's classic technique). *A*, The rotation forceps is shown before seizing the pin by the ring of the spring end. (Forcep jaws are shown opening in the wrong diameter.) *B*, The pin is seized in the ring by the points of the forceps. *C*, The pin is carried into the stomach and is about to be rotated by withdrawal. *D*, The withdrawal of the pin into the esophagoscope, which will thus close it. If the pin (*E*) is withdrawn by flat-jawed forceps (*F*), the esophageal wall would be fatally lacerated. (Modified from Jackson C: Bronchoscopy and Esophagoscopy. Philadelphia, WB Saunders, 1992, p. 104.)

INGESTION OF CAUSTIC MATERIALS

- Oral cavity and pharyngeal examination are not sufficient to determine the extent of esophageal injury.
- Life-threatening caustic burns may require immediate surgical intervention. Generally, caustic ingestion is evaluated within 24 hours after the event to assess the depth of the burn.
- The esophagus is examined, and the sites and depth of caustic burns are noted.
- When concentric third-degree burns are identified, the esophagoscope is not advanced. Our current management of a severe burn is to insert a small plastic tube through the side arm of the esophagoscope into the stomach. We perform a gastrotomy and retrieve the tube in the stomach. Either a string (monofilament suture) or a Silastic feeding tube can be pulled through the nose, esophagus, and gastrotomy to maintain a lumen. Hyperalimentation may be used. Feeding commences through the gastrotomy tube when satisfactory healing has occurred.

RETROGRADE DILATATION

- Retrograde dilatation is required when a repeat esophagoscopy shows the formation of stenosis. It can be started only following maturation of the gastrostomy.
- Before the dilatation procedure, Tucker bougies are attached to each other with sutures in the order of increasing calibers. The strength of each of the knots is tested individually.
- The loop of suture between the nostril and the gastrotomy stoma placed during the gastrotomy procedure is divided. The gastrotomy tube is then removed. Two sutures of the same length are pulled from the stoma through the nostril. One suture becomes the loop suture at the end of dilatation. The other suture is secured to the string of bougies.
- The suture that is attached to the bougies is pulled through the oral cavity. The Tucker bougies, coated with lubricant, are then pulled through the stoma individually (Fig. 20–24).
- Dilatation is completed when moderate resistance is encountered. The bougies are then separated by dividing the connecting suture and withdrawing it through the oral cavity. The remaining suture through the nostril is attached to the other end to form a loop. The gastrotomy is replaced.
- Erosion of the suture through the ala can be prevented by proper taping. Leakage of gastric content around the gastrotomy tube is commonly seen following dilatation.
- Although the above technique has been used for years, several institutions now use a Grüntzig balloon under radiographic control for this purpose.

PROGRADE DILATATION

- Prograde dilatation is used for isolated strictures or webs. It is also useful for strictures that have been adequately dilatated using the retrograde method.
- Esophagoscopes may be used as esophageal dilators through serial dilatations.
- Dilatation can be performed through an anesthesia laryngoscope for a high stricture or through an esophagoscope for a low stricture. Hurst and Maloney bougies are available for this type of dilatation.

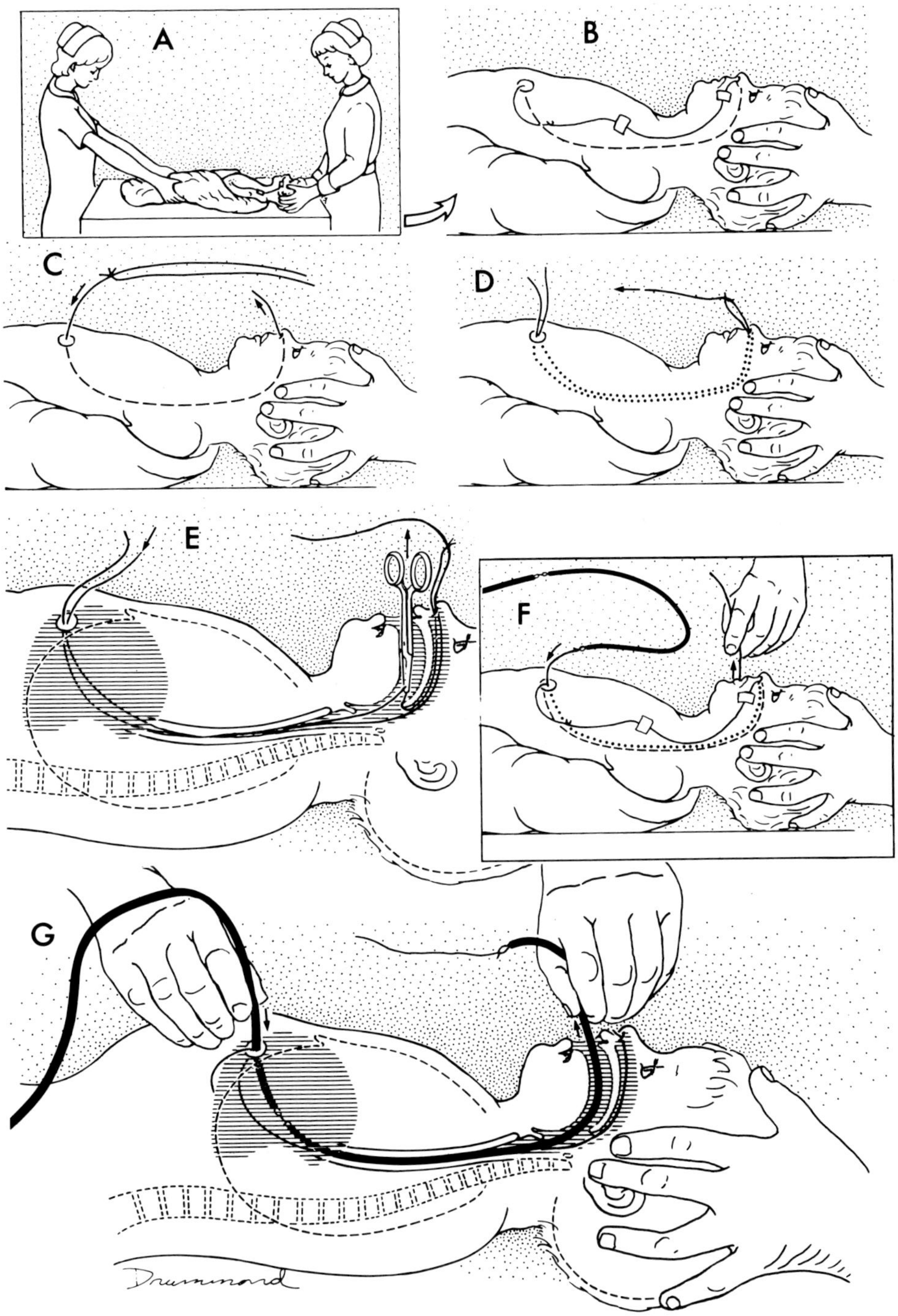

• **FIGURE 20–24.**

Retrograde esophageal dilatation. (From Riding KH and Bluestone CD: Burns and acquired strictures of the esophagus. *In* Bluestone CD and Stool SE [eds]; Pediatric Otolaryngology, 2nd ed. Philadelphia, WB Saunders, 1990, p 1004.)

chapter

21

Tracheostomy

MARGARETHA L. CASSELBRANT, M.D., PH.D.

Tracheostomy has a long history; however, very few cases have been reported in children prior to the late 19th century. The operation was considered dangerous for a child, and only after the introduction of tracheal intubation did it become relatively safe. The major impetus in the last 50 years has been the development of respiratory support devices that necessitate long-term intubation.

The name of the procedure has been a matter of controversy. The terms tracheotomy and tracheostomy are used almost interchangeably. Tracheostomy is the act of cutting a hole in the trachea and is also the name of the tube, whereas tracheotomy is the actual opening in the trachea.

Indications

- Respiratory obstruction
- Respiratory insufficiency
- Excessive secretions and prevention of aspiration

Anesthetic considerations

Use of general anesthesia is preferred, with an endotracheal tube or bronchoscope in place to establish a safe airway during the surgical procedure. If the airway cannot be secured owing to an anatomic abnormality or a cervical spine fracture, the tracheostomy can be carried out under local anesthesia.

Preparation

- To obtain maximal exposure of the trachea, a roll is placed under the shoulders to hyperextend the neck. The chin is held by the anesthesiologist and is kept in that position during the procedure to maintain hyperextension (Fig. 21–1). In a small infant, any esophageal tubings (e.g., nasogastric tube or esophageal stethoscope) should be removed to ensure correct identification of the trachea.

- The patient's neck is prepared and draped in such a way that the face is not covered. The neck is palpated, and the thyroid and cricoid cartilages are identified. The cartilages, suprasternal notch, and skin incision should be marked.

- Local anesthetic ($\frac{1}{2}$% lidocaine with 1:200,000 epinephrine) is injected intradermally and subcutaneously into the area of the planned skin incision for hemostasis.

Procedure

- The skin is generally incised one fingerbreadth above the suprasternal notch, either vertically or horizontally (Fig. 21–2), and the incision is carried through the subcutaneous tissue.

• FIGURE 21-1.

Positioning of the patient.

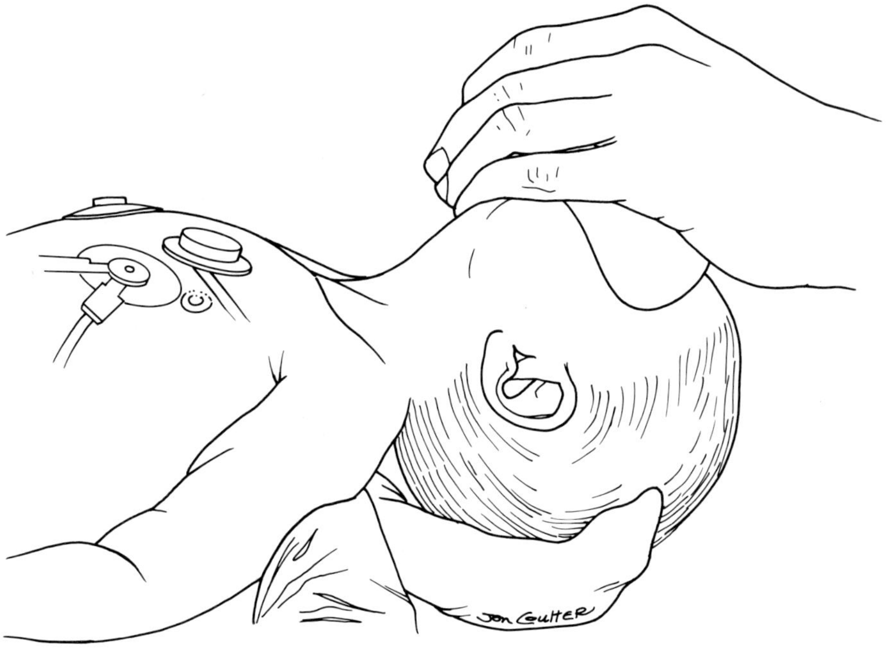

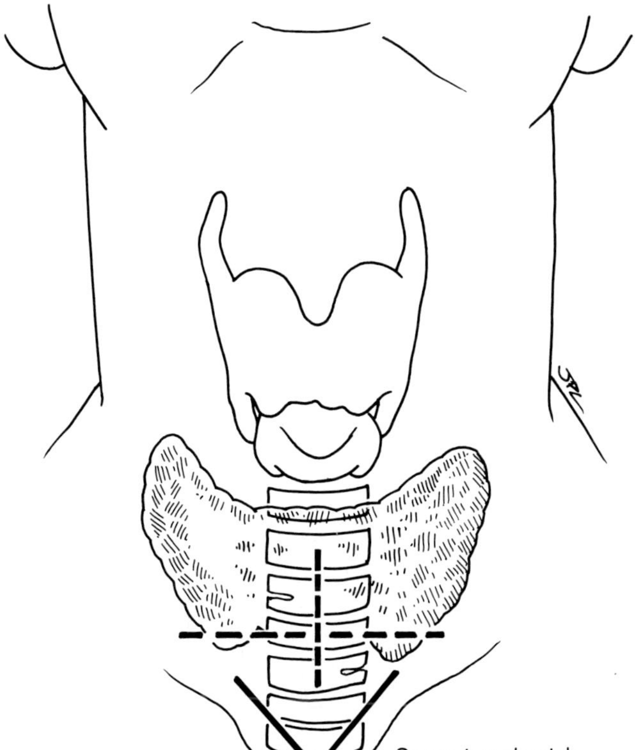

• FIGURE 21-2.

Anatomy of the neck and skin incisions.

- The trachea is palpated repeatedly during dissection to ensure an accurate approach to the trachea in the midline. The anterior jugular veins and the strap muscles should be identified (Fig. 21–3).

- The anterior jugular veins are retracted laterally. The strap muscles are separated in the midline in the following way: The fascia layer is grasped on each side of the midline with a hemostat and lifted; the fascia is opened between the two hemostats with scissors, and the edges are slightly undermined (Fig. 21–4). Senne retractors are used to retract the muscles laterally. Excessive lateral dissection should be avoided to prevent dissection of subcutaneous air, resulting in intrathoracic complications.

- The thyroid gland should be retracted if necessary. Rarely, the thyroid isthmus needs to be divided in children. When retraction is not possible, the isthmus is doubly clamped, divided, and suture-ligated.

- On completion of the dissection through the level of the pretracheal fascia, stay sutures (4-0 Neurolen) are placed bilaterally, approximatively 2 mm from the midline around at least two tracheal rings. After hemostasis has been obtained, a vertical incision is made in the midline of the second and third (or third and fourth) tracheal rings. No cartilage is removed in children (Fig. 21–5).

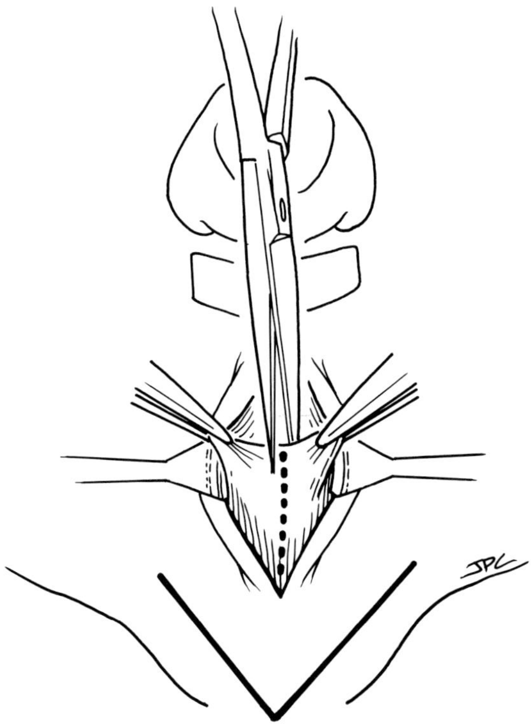

• FIGURE 21–3.

Identification of the strap muscles and the anterior jugular vein.

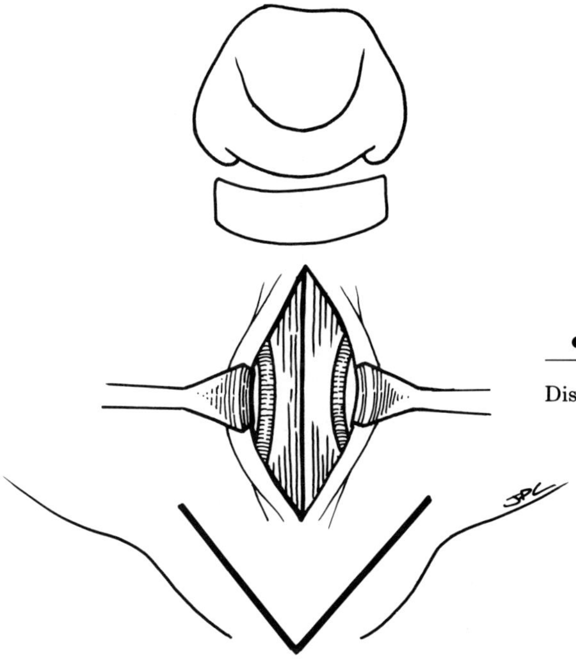

• FIGURE 21–4.

Dissection of the fascia in the midline.

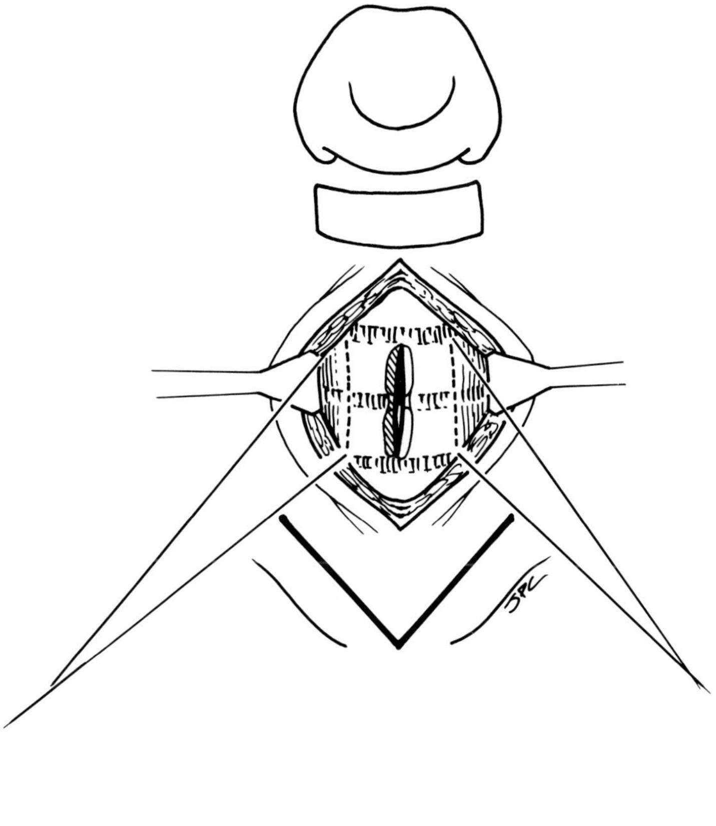

• FIGURE 21–5.

Placement of a stay suture and incision of the trachea.

• TABLE 21-1.

OPERATIVE COMPLICATIONS*

Hemorrhage: Coagulation defect, vascular anomalies
Air entry: Subcutaneous emphysema, mediastinal emphysema, pneumothorax, air embolus
Anatomic damage: Cricoid cartilage and laryngeal injury, esophageal puncture, recurrent laryngeal nerve injury
Tracheostomy tube problems: Incorrect choice of tube size, faulty placement (false passage into a bronchus)
Respiratory drive cessation: Cardiac and ventilatory arrest owing to a rapid change in carbon dioxide tension

*From Stool SE and Eavey RD: Tracheotomy. *In* Bluestone CD and Stool SE (eds): Pediatric Otolaryngology, 2nd ed. Philadelphia, WB Saunders, 1990.

• The tracheostomy tube is inserted after traction on the sutures opens the stoma. Prior to insertion of the tracheostomy tube, the endotracheal tube is pulled back above the stoma but *not* out of the trachea. It can be removed when satisfactory ventilation is established. Tapes are tied around the neck to secure the tube. One finger should be able to be passed under the tapes with the neck flexed. The stay sutures are taped to the chest without tension (Fig. 21-6).

• Tracheostomy tubes of different sizes and lengths are available. In infants and young children, the tracheostomy tube is "shaved" to avoid potential erosion of the skin below the tracheostomy tube (Figs. 21-7 and 21-8).

• Complications are summarized in Table 21-1.

Postoperative care/complications

• Intrathoracic complications are ruled out with a chest x-ray. The position of the tracheostomy tube is also assessed.

• The patient is observed in the intensive care unit or in a similar supervised setting during the first week. The patient should receive humidified air by way of a tracheotomy collar or ventilator. Suctioning is performed generally following instillation of normal saline.

• The first tracheostomy tube change is performed approximately 1 week after the procedure. A suction catheter inserted through the old tracheostomy tube is used as a guide over which the new tracheostomy tube is inserted.

• Complications are summarized in Table 21-2.

• TABLE 21-2.

POSTOPERATIVE COMPLICATIONS*

Hemorrhage: Wound ooze, tracheal erosion, paratracheal hematoma, tracheoarterial fistula
Air entry: Subcutaneous emphysema, mediastinal emphysema, pneumothorax, pneumopericardium
Anatomic (trachea) damage: Mucosal ulceration, stenosis, dilatation (caused by cuff), malacia, granuloma, crusting, fistulas (tracheocutaneous, tracheoesophageal, tracheopleural), skin-lined tube
Tracheostomy tube problems: Obstruction by crusts or mucous plug, displacement, cuff complications, malposition (false passage into a bronchus, excess tracheal wall pressure), difficult decannulation
Infection: Wound infection, neck cellulitis, perichondritis, tracheobronchitis, pneumonia, mediastinitis, lung abscess
Deglutition difficulty: Dysphagia, odynophagia, aspiration
Cosmesis: Tracheotomy scar, keloid, tracheocutaneous fistula
Laryngeal disuse
Delayed decannulation

*From Stool SE and Eavey RD: Tracheotomy. *In* Bluestone CD and Stool SE (eds): Pediatric Otolaryngology, 2nd ed. Philadelphia, WB Saunders, 1990.

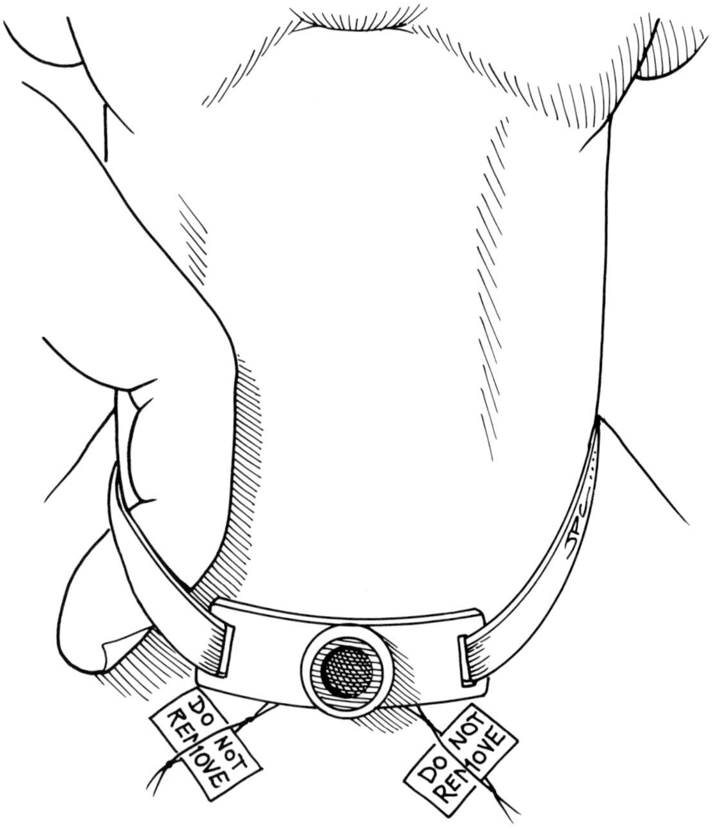

• **FIGURE 21-6.**

Position of the tracheal tube.

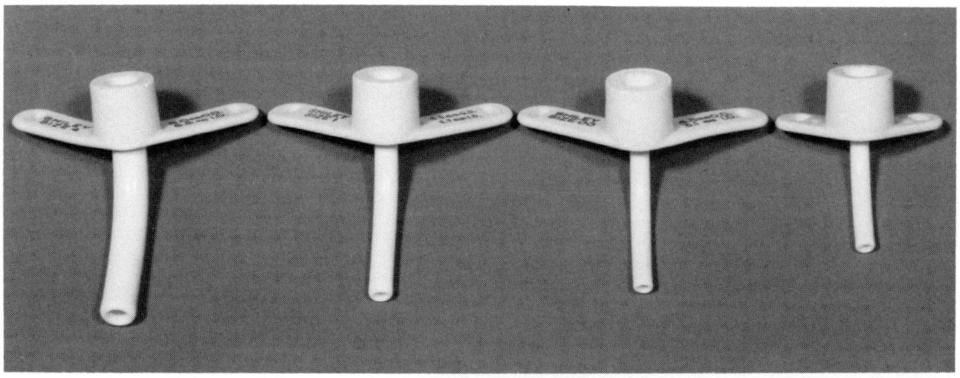

• **FIGURE 21-7.**

Different sizes of tracheostomy tubes are shown. The tubes from left to right are Shiley No. 4, No. 1, No. 00 pediatric, and No. 00 neonatal.

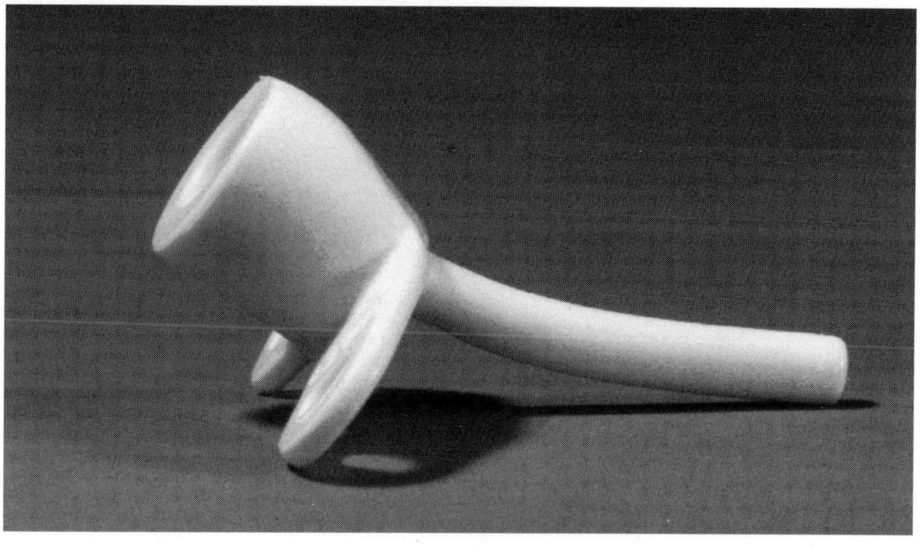

• **FIGURE 21-8.**

A "shaved" tracheostomy tube.

BIBLIOGRAPHY

Myers EN, Stool SE, and Johnson JT: Tracheotomy. New York, Churchill Livingstone, 1985.

Rothfield RE, Petruzzelli GJ, and Stool SE: Neonatal tracheotomy tube modification. Otolaryngol Head Neck Surg 103:133–134, 1990.

chapter

22

Surgery of the Larynx and Trachea

GERALD B. HEALY, M.D.

Disorders of the larynx and trachea that are encountered in childhood and are amenable to surgical intervention may be classified by region, such as supraglottic, glottic, subglottic, and tracheal regions. Although these disorders are encountered infrequently, surgical correction can be lifesaving or can improve the quality of life. The following four procedures represent those that are the most frequently performed in the pediatric population.

SUPRAGLOTTIC PROCEDURE

ARYTENOIDECTOMY

Bilateral vocal cord paralysis is a difficult and challenging problem (Fig. 22–1*A*). Arytenoidectomy offers an opportunity for decannulation in selected cases. Either an endoscopic or an open approach may be utilized.

Indications

- Bilateral vocal cord paralysis in patients in whom spontaneous resolution has not taken place within 18 months of onset
- Chronic arytenoid dislocation with obstruction of the glottis

Anesthetic considerations

- The procedure is performed under general anesthesia. If a tracheotomy is present, anesthesia is delivered through this port. If an endoscopic laser technique is employed, a noncombustible tracheostomy tube must be used.
- Maximal muscle relaxation facilitates the procedure.
- An intravenous line and oximeter are placed.

Preparation

- The patient is positioned with the shoulders elevated and the neck hyperextended.
- If an open procedure is used, the neck is prepared with Betadine solution and then draped. The incision area is infiltrated with 1:200,000 epinephrine (1 to 2 ml).
- The eyes and face are protected if the laser is used.
- 1:200,000 epinephrine solution (1 ml) is injected into the arytenoid area for hemostasis.

Procedure

ENDOSCOPIC

- Arytenoidectomy may be performed endoscopically using a suspension binocular laryngoscope and operating microscope. The CO_2 or KTP laser is extremely useful for the procedure.

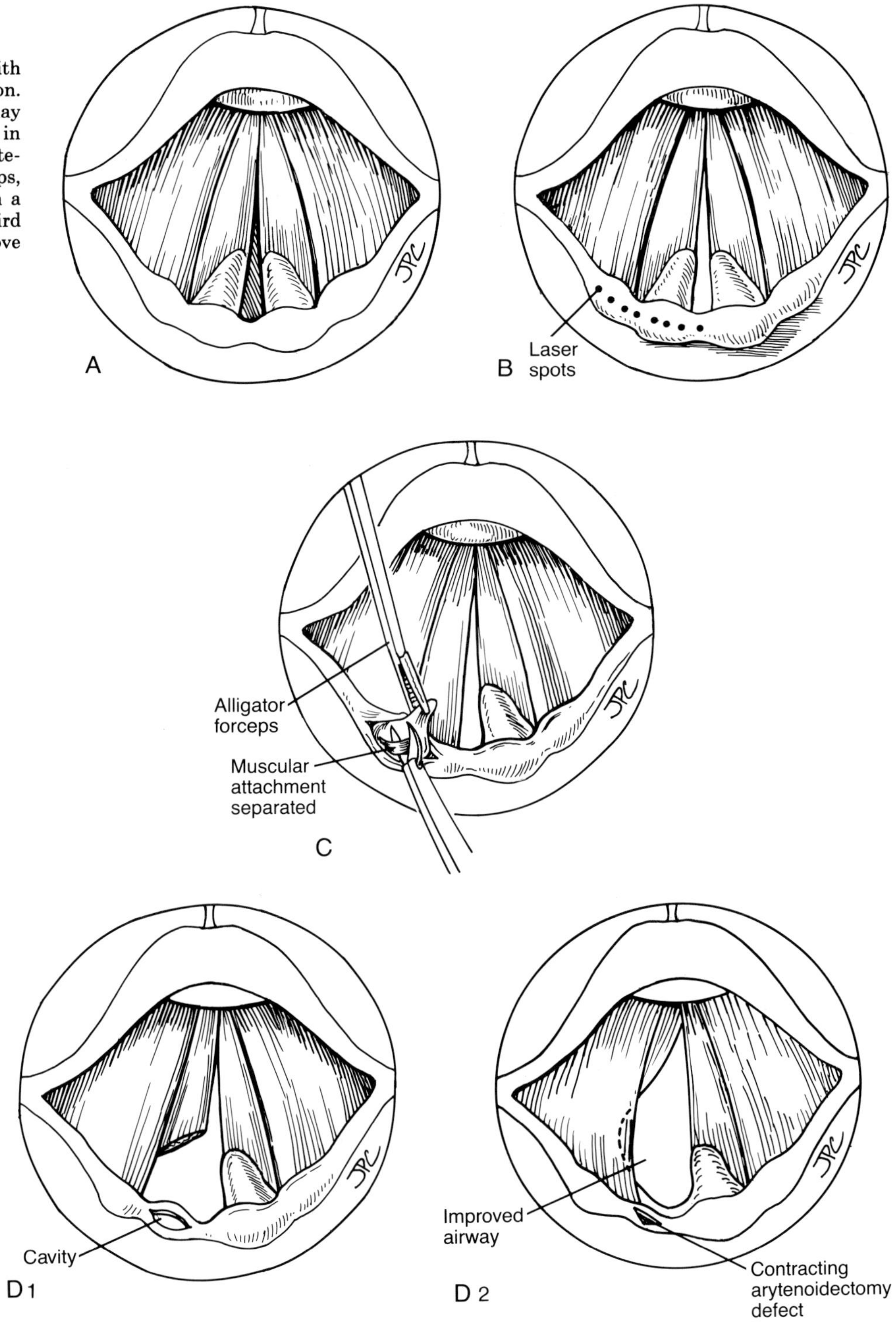

• FIGURE 22–1.

A, Bilateral abductor paralysis with vocal cords in the paramedian position. *B*, The incision over the arytenoid may be made with a laser or a sickle knife in the endoscopic approach. *C*, The arytenoid is grasped with alligator forceps, and attachments are separated with a laser or scissors. *D*, The posterior third of the true cord is resected to improve the glottic airway.

• A horizontal incision is made over the arytenoid cartilage, and the laser is used to resect the perichondrial attachments so that the cartilage may be removed (Fig. 22–1*B* and *C*).

• The posterior third of the true vocal cord is resected to improve the glottic aperture (Fig. 22–1*D*).

• The mucosal incision is closed with a 5-0 polyglactin 910 suture. A 2-0 polyglactin 910 suture is placed above and below the true vocal cord and tied externally over the thyroid lamina to improve lateralization.

• The wound is closed in layers over a drain.

OPEN TECHNIQUE

- If an open approach is employed, an external horizontal skin incision is made at the midlevel of the thyroid cartilage and is carried to the margins of the sternomastoid muscle (Fig. 22–2*A*).

- The dissection is carried subcutaneously through the platysma, exposing the external hyoid muscles. These muscles are separated in the midline to expose the thyrohyoid membrane, the anterior aspect of the thyroid cartilage, and the cricothyroid membrane.

- A vertical incision is made through the cricothyroid membrane and is carried up through the anterior thyroid cartilage in the midline (Fig. 22–2*B*). The thyroid laminae are retracted laterally.

- A vertical incision is made through the epithelium anterior to the vocal process of the arytenoid. The vocal process is dissected free, and then the posterior cricoarytenoid, the lateral cricoarytenoid, and the thyroarytenoid muscles are cut.

- The cricoarytenoid joint is transected, and the arytenoid is removed. The incision is closed with a 4-0 polyglactin 910 suture (Fig. 22–2*C*).

- A mattress suture is placed above and below the vocal cord with a 2-0 polyglactin 910 suture and then through the thyroid lamina and tied laterally. This lateralizes the vocal cord.

- The thyroid cartilage is closed with a 2-0 polyglactin 910 suture. The wound is closed in layers over a drain.

Postoperative care

- Wound care is accomplished twice a day.
- Systemic antibiotics are employed for 7 to 10 days.
- Meticulous tracheotomy care is encouraged.

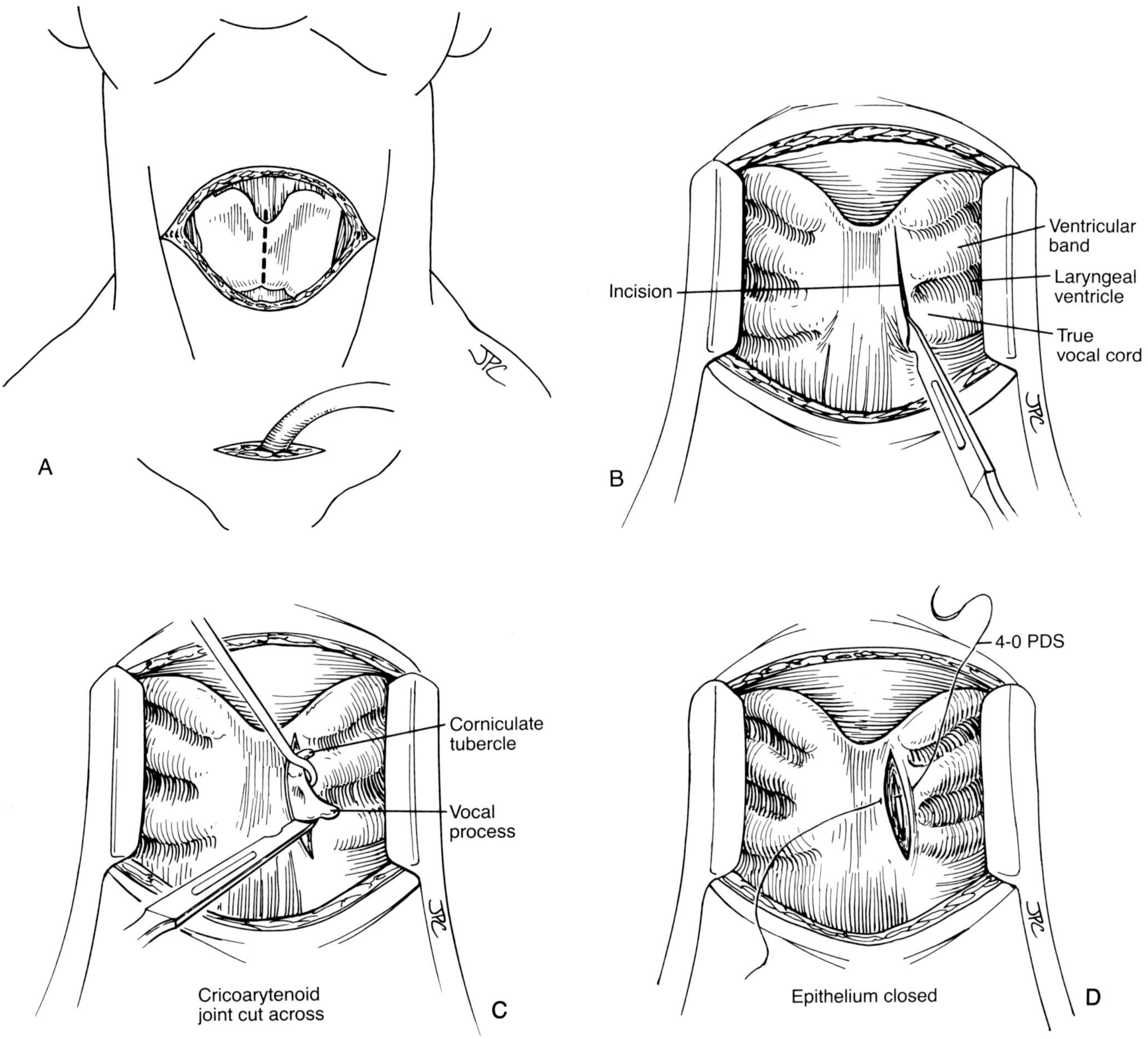

• FIGURE 22-2.

A, A horizontal skin incision is made at the midlevel of the thyroid cartilage, and the thyroid cartilage is visualized. A vertical incision is made in the thyroid cartilage in the midline. *B*, A vertical incision is made through the epithelium anterior to the vocal process. *C*, The incision is closed with a 4-0 polyglactin 910 suture.

SUPRAGLOTTOPLASTY

Congenital laryngeal stridor (laryngomalacia) is usually a self-limiting process that resolves with maturity. However, some patients afflicted with this disorder may demonstrate respiratory distress severe enough to require operative intervention to improve ventilatory function.

Indications

- Severe airway obstruction secondary to laryngomalacia (Fig. 22–3*A*)

Anesthetic considerations

- General anesthesia is employed in all cases. Combustion precautions are taken with the endotracheal tube if the laser is to be used.
- An intravenous line and an oximeter are placed.

Preparation

- The patient is positioned with the shoulders elevated and the neck hyperextended.
- The eyes and face are protected if the laser is used.
- Dexamethasone (1.5 mg/kg) up to 20 mg is given in a single intravenous dose.

Procedure

- Suspension microlaryngoscopy is employed in conjunction with the CO_2 or KTP laser.
- Vaporization of the cuneiform cartilages and excess mucosa over the arytenoids is accomplished (Fig. 22–3*B*)
- In severe obstruction, division of the aryepiglottic folds is completed with the laser to release the epiglottis.
- The mucosa may be trimmed from the lateral edges of the epiglottis, the aryepiglottic folds, and the arytenoid and corniculate cartilages (epiglottoplasty).

Postoperative care

- The patient is kept in a humidified atmosphere as much as possible.
- Systemic antibiotics are administered for 7 to 10 days.

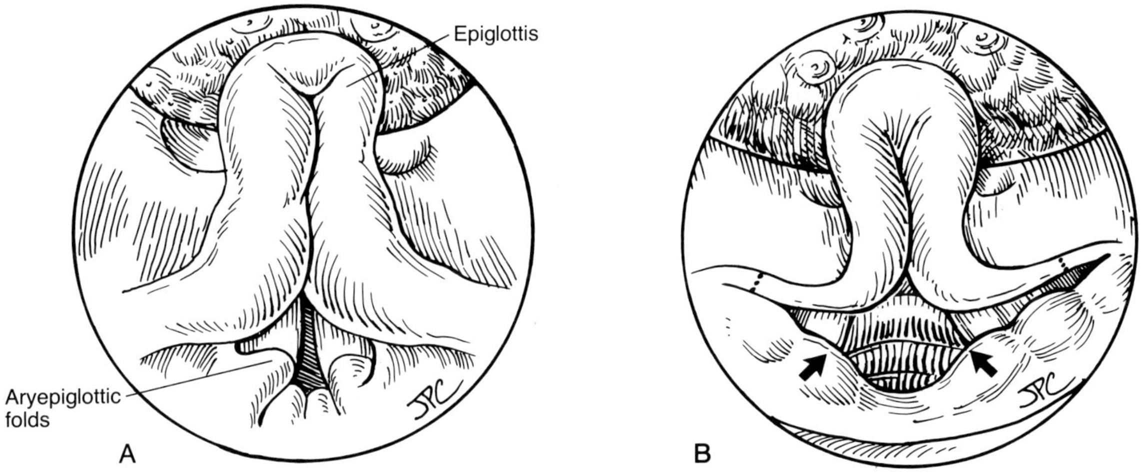

• **FIGURE 22-3.**

A, Supraglottic structures demonstrating significant obstruction. *B*, Cuneiform cartilages (*arrows*) are resected in conjunction with excess mucosa in this area.

GLOTTIC PROCEDURES

WEB

Congenital webs are commonly located in the anterior one half to two thirds of the glottis. These lesions may be thick or thin and may extend into the subglottic space. Patients usually present with aphonia and demonstrate varying degrees of respiratory distress, depending on the amount of obstruction present.

Webs occupying more than 50% of the glottis usually require treatment (Fig. 22–4*A*). Thin webs may be lysed, whereas thicker webs with subglottic extension may require a tracheostomy and more extensive treatment.

Indications

- Major indications for surgical intervention include webs occupying 50% or more of the glottic inlet and those causing respiratory distress or significant aphonia.

Anesthetic considerations

- General anesthesia is required in all cases.
- An intravenous line and an oximeter are placed.
- If possible, a small-bore fire-retardant endotracheal tube is inserted, and a short-acting paralytic agent is given to stop vocal cord activity.
- Dexamethasone (1.5 mg/kg) up to 20 mg is given in a single intravenous dose.
- If a tracheotomy is present, a fire-retardant tube should be inserted.

Preparation

- The patient is positioned with the shoulders elevated and the neck hyperextended.
- The eyes and face are protected if the laser is used.

Procedure

ENDOSCOPIC

- Microsurgical technique with or without laser is employed.
- Microscissors or a laser is used to divide the web along the free edge of one vocal cord (Fig. 22–4*B*). This can be easily accomplished if the web is thin.
- In thicker webs with subglottic extension, it may be necessary to keep the opposing raw surfaces apart. This may be accomplished with a keel, in which case a tracheostomy will be necessary. The alternative is to nasally intubate the patient for approximately 72 hours. In either case, prophylactic antibiotics are necessary while the keel or endotracheal tube is in place (Fig. 22–4*C*).

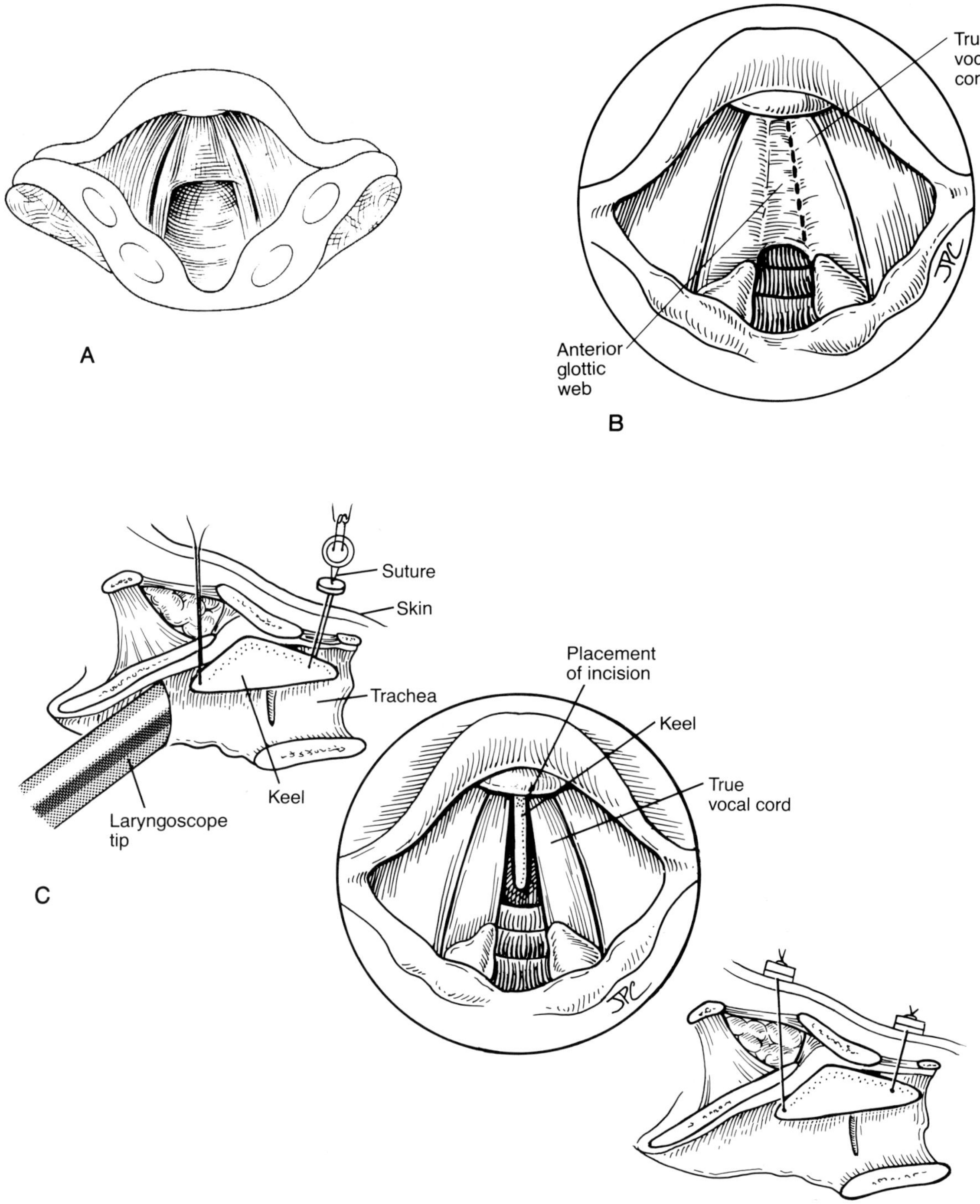

• FIGURE 22–4.

A, Congenital web occluding 75% of the glottic inlet. *B*, The web is divided with either a laser or scissors along the free edge of one cord. *C*, A keel is placed endoscopically and is left in place for 5 to 7 days. An endotracheal tube may also be inserted to prevent readhesion of the cords.

OPEN TECHNIQUE

- A horizontal incision is made at the upper level of the thyroid cartilage (Fig. 22–5*A*).

- The thyroid lamina is visualized and divided from the midportion inferiorly through the level of the cricoid (if subglottic extension is present). The mucosa is transected in the midline (Fig. 22–5*B*).

- A keel or endotracheal tube is placed for approximately 5 to 7 days (Fig. 22–5*C*).

- The wound is closed in layers over a drain.

Postoperative care

- Humidification is paramount. If an endotracheal tube is placed, the patient is sedated and is kept in a humidified atmosphere.

- Antibiotic ointment is applied to the wound for approximately 1 week. Systemic antibiotics are administered for 7 to 10 days.

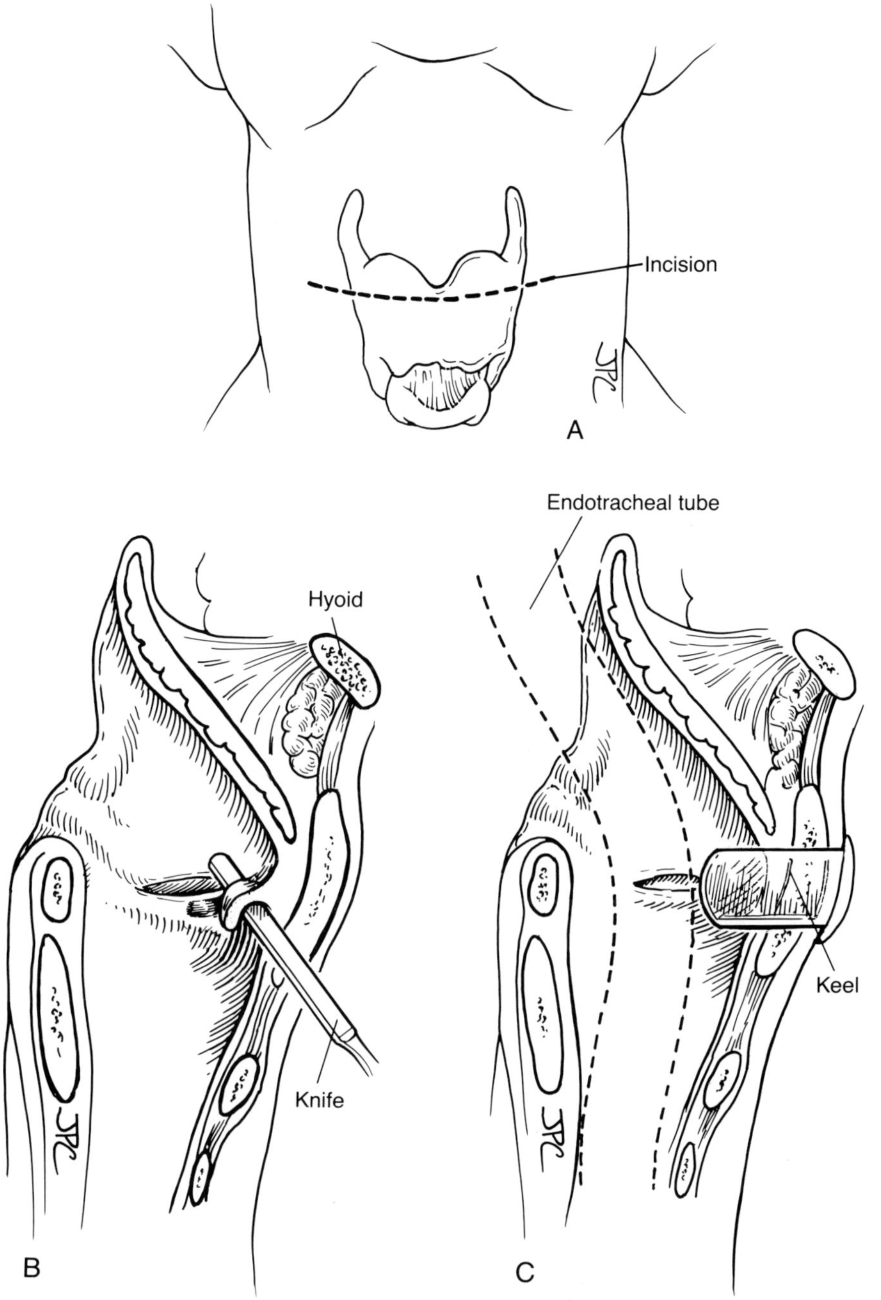

• FIGURE 22–5.

A, A horizontal skin incision at upper level of the thyroid cartilage. *B*, A cut (vertical) is made through the thyroid lamina, mucosa, and web. *C*, A keel (or endotracheal tube) is inserted for 5 to 7 days.

SUBGLOTTIC PROCEDURES

LARYNGEAL DECOMPRESSION (CRICOID SPLIT)

Prior to 1980, a tracheostomy was the only way to overcome complications secondary to endotracheal intubation. In 1980, the cricoid split procedure was introduced to decompress edematous mucosa in the subglottic space. More recently, however, it has been used to treat mild forms of congenital and acquired stenosis (Fig. 22–6*A*).

Indications

- Failure of extubation on at least two occasions
- Weight greater than 1500 g
- No assisted ventilation for 10 days prior to the procedure
- Oxygen requirement of less than 30%
- No congenital heart failure
- No evidence of upper or lower respiratory infection
- No antihypertensive medication requirement
- Mild forms of anterior acquired or congenital subglottic stenosis in infants or children

Anesthetic considerations

- General anesthesia is required and is administered through an indwelling endotracheal tube. A paralytic agent is used during the procedure.

Preparation

- The patient is positioned with the shoulders elevated and the neck hyperextended.
- Care must be taken to palpate and mark the landmarks, including the thyroid cartilage, cricoid cartilage, and sternal notch.
- 0.5% Xylocaine with 1:200,000 epinephrine is injected into the incision area for hemostasis.

Procedure

- A horizontal incision is made in the skin overlying the cricoid cartilage; the soft tissue is separated; and the cricoid, trachea, and lower border of the thyroid cartilage are identified (Fig. 22–6*B*).
- An incision is made through the cricoid cartilage and mucosa as well as through the first two tracheal rings and lower one third of the thyroid cartilage (Fig. 22–6*C*).
- Stay sutures are placed on both sides of the cricoid for emergency purposes.
- An endotracheal tube, 0.5 mm larger than might be expected for the age and weight of the patient, is inserted. This should be left in place for 7 days.
- The wound is closed loosely and drained.

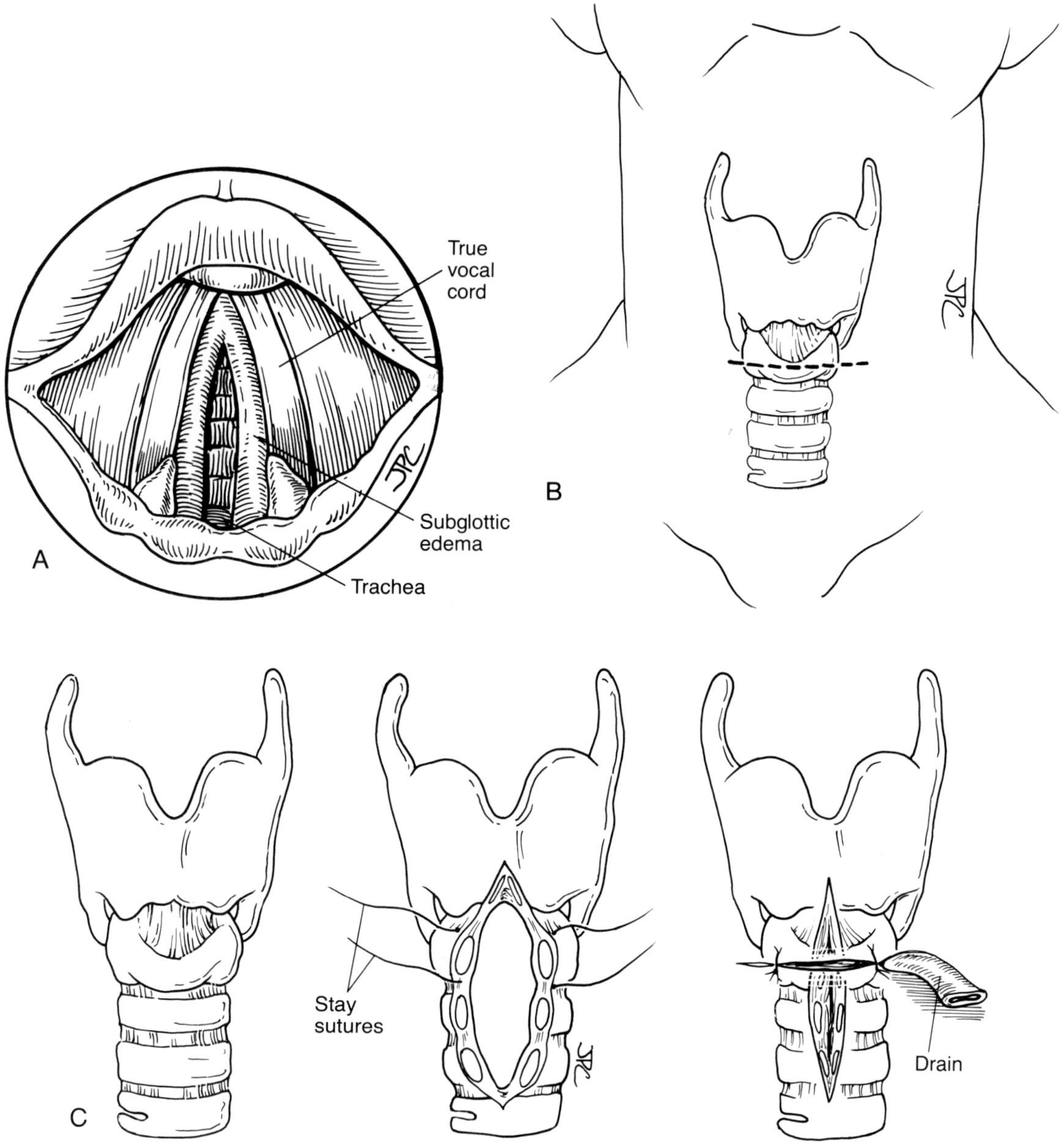

● **FIGURE 22–6.**

A, Subglottic edema preventing decannulation. *B*, The location of a skin incision for decompression. *C*, The location of a laryngotracheal incision for decompression of the subglottic space.

Postoperative care

- Sedation and humidity are necessary while the endotracheal tube is in place.
- Meticulous endotracheal tube care as well as wound care is given while awaiting extubation.
- Systemic antibiotics are administered for 7 to 10 days.
- Dexamethasone (1 mg/kg) is given approximately 6 hours before extubation.
- One or two treatments of racemic epinephrine may be useful after extubation.

SUBGLOTTIC STENOSIS

Subglottic stenosis is a rare and troublesome problem affecting the soft tissue and cartilaginous structures of the subglottic space. This condition may be congenital or acquired, but in either case, management presents a perplexing clinical challenge.

More than 90% of the cases in the pediatric population occur secondary to intubation injuries. In the milder cases, endoscopic management may be undertaken. In patients with more severe stenosis, one-stage laryngotracheoplasty is now recommended. However, in patients with significant stenosis — greater than 90% narrowing of the subglottic space — cartilaginous augmentation of the cricoid with stenting should be considered.

Augmentation Laryngoplasty With Cartilage Graft

Patients who fail laryngeal decompression or who have severe stenosis with either extreme congenital deformity of the cricoid or destruction of the cartilaginous framework owing to acquired chondritis usually require augmentation laryngoplasty or laryngotracheoplasty in order to achieve successful decannulation. The use of autologous costal cartilage to augment the cricoid seems to achieve the best results on a consistent basis.

Indications

- Severe (> 70%) congenital subglottic stenosis
- Anterior acquired subglottic stenosis with tracheotomy dependence
- Significant respiratory distress in congenital or acquired stenosis of less than 70%

Anesthetic considerations

- If a tracheotomy is in place, the patient is given general anesthesia via this route. Otherwise an endotracheal tube is utilized.
- An intravenous line and an oximeter are placed.
- The patient should be paralyzed for the duration of the procedure.

Preparation

- Endoscopy is undertaken first to update airway status and ascertain whether the operation is still necessary.
- The patient is positioned with the shoulders elevated and the neck hyperextended.
- 0.5% Xylocaine with 1:200,000 epinephrine is injected into the incision sites.
- The cartilage graft site is prepared on the anterior chest.

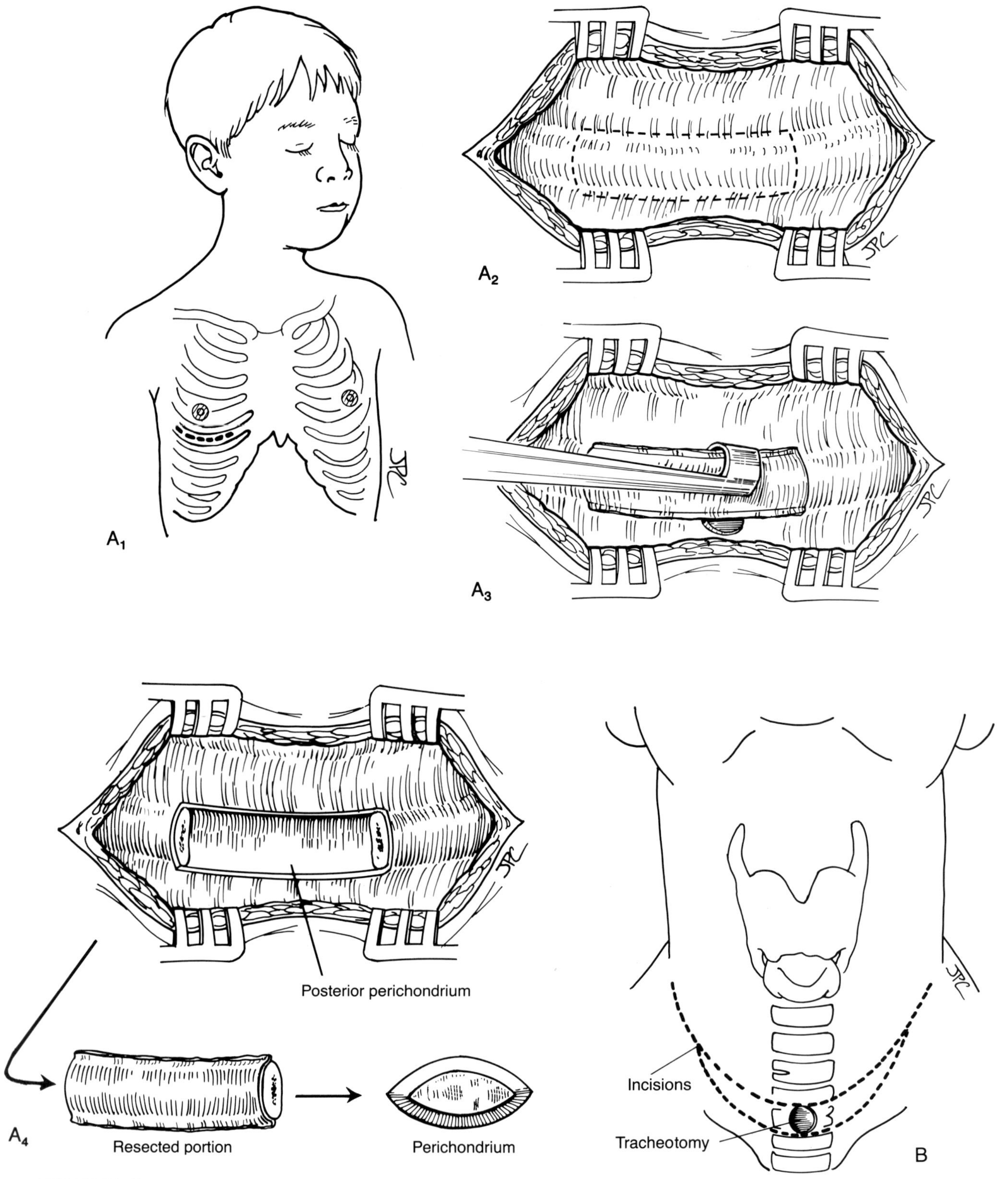

• FIGURE 22–7.

A, Rib graft donor showing resected cartilage graft with external perichondrium attached. *B*, Skin incision to include the tracheotomy site (if present).

• FIGURE 22–7. *(continued)*

C, A laryngotracheal incision with upper and lower extension, depending on the extent of stenosis. A cartilage graft is shown with the perichondrium internalized. A graft is sutured in position with a 4-0 polyglactin 910 suture.

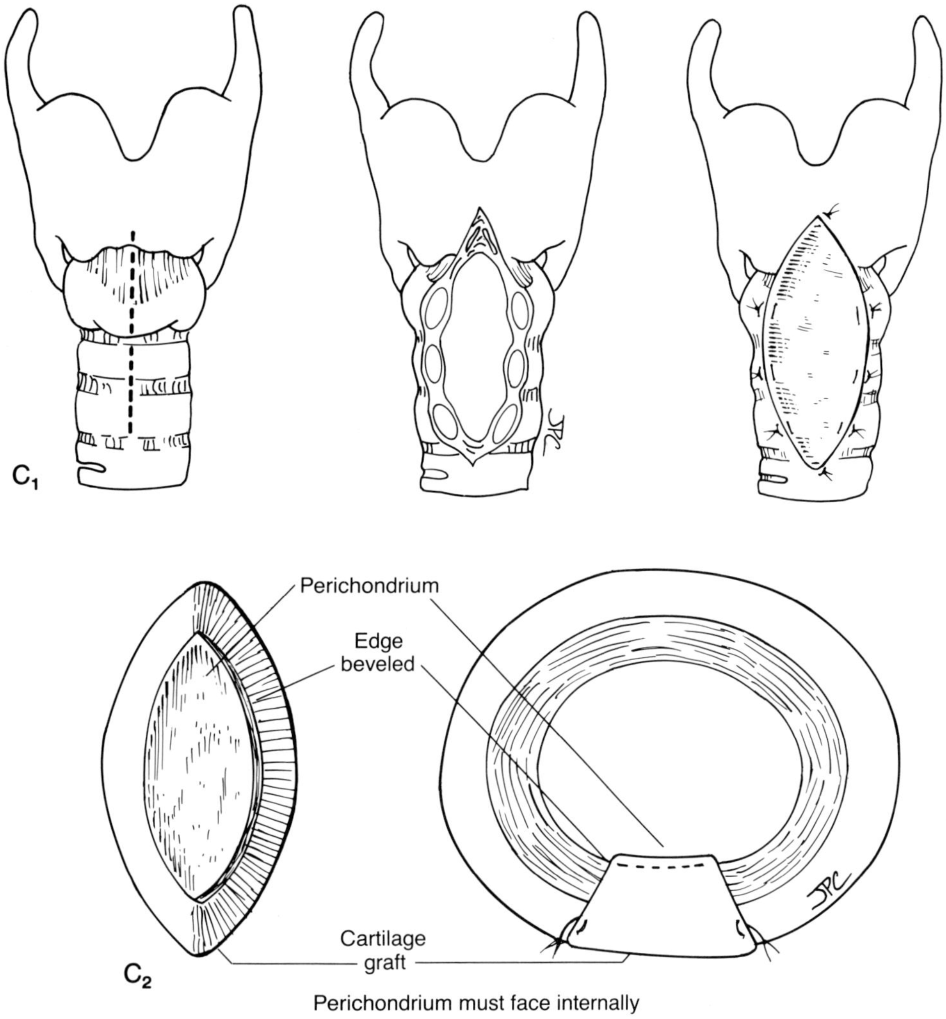

Procedure

- The autologous rib graft is removed with external perichondrium left attached (Fig. 22–7*A*). The chest wound is closed with a 4-0 polyglactin 910 suture.
- A horizontal neck incision is made and if a tracheotomy is in place, the stomal area should be included in this incision (Fig. 22–7*B*).
- The cricoid and thyroid cartilages are identified, as well as the upper trachea.
- A vertical incision is made through the cricoid, the lower end of the thyroid cartilage, and the upper two tracheal cartilages (Fig. 22–7*C*).
- The area of stenosis is then measured, and the cartilage graft is shaped appropriately.
- The costal cartilage with the perichondrium facing internally is fixed into position using a 4-0 polyglactin 910 suture.
- The wound is then closed in layers over a drain.

Postoperative care

- If the patient is left intubated, a nasotracheal tube is left in place for 7 to 10 days, with appropriate sedation being used.
- Meticulous endotracheal tube care is employed, and the patient is placed on broad-spectrum antibiotics for 7 days combined with twice-daily wound care.
- If an endotracheal tube is not placed, the patient's tracheostomy tube is replaced at the end of the operation, and approximately 6 weeks later the patient is re-endoscoped for a possible decannulation. Antibiotics are administered in prophylactic doses until endoscopy is done. Meticulous tracheotomy care is employed.

Augmentation Laryngoplasty With Cartilage Stent

Indications

- Significant subglottic stenosis with greater than 90% narrowing, either congenital or acquired (Fig. 22–8*A*)
- Significant tracheomalacia at the tracheotomy site
- Concomitant glottic and subglottic stenosis. In some cases, supraglottic stenosis may be present as well.

Anesthetic considerations

- Inhalational agents should be administered through the tracheostomy tube.
- An intravenous line and an oximeter are placed.
- A paralytic agent is used during the procedure.

Preparation

- Endoscopy is undertaken first to update airway status and ascertain whether the operation is still necessary.
- The patient is positioned with the shoulders elevated and the neck hyperextended.
- The costal cartilage graft site is prepared and the graft is obtained. The wound is closed with a 4-0 polyglactin 910 suture.
- A horizontal incision is made to include the old tracheotomy stoma. The incision is carried laterally to the level of the sternomastoid muscles (Fig. 22–8*B*).
- The thyroid and cricoid cartilages are visualized, as is the upper trachea. Care must be taken not to denude the perichondrium over these structures because this may disrupt the blood supply for the future cartilage graft.

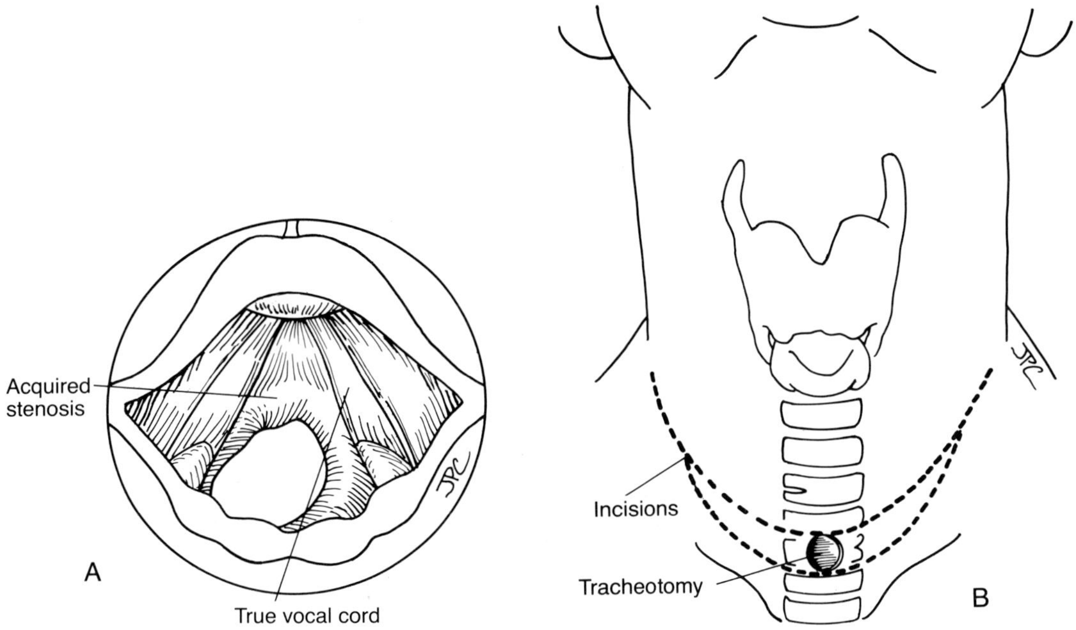

• FIGURE 22-8.

A, Severe congenital or acquired stenosis. *B*, Skin incision to include the tracheotomy site.

Illustration continued on following page

• A vertical incision is made through the cricoid and is carried as far superiorly and inferiorly as is necessary to expose the stenosis that may be present. This may include the supraglottic, glottic, and subglottic structures as well as the trachea (Fig. 22–8*C*). It may also be necessary to split the posterior cricoid lamina in severe cases (Fig. 22–8*D*). This is done carefully to avoid entering the esophagus.

• A Teflon stent is measured to the appropriate size and length. Superiorly, the stent should extend approximately to the level of the false cords if significant supraglottic stenosis is not present. Inferiorly, it should reside approximately 1.5 cm above the carina (Fig. 22–8*E*).

• The costal cartilage graft is shaped and measured to the appropriate length. The stent, with the attached tracheostomy tube, is inserted into the airway, and an endotracheal tube is inserted through the metal tracheostomy tube (the inner cannula is temporarily removed) as a temporary access for anesthesia.

• The costal cartilage graft, with the perichondrium facing the lumen, is inserted over the stent and sutured into position in the subglottic area (as well as to the thyroid cartilage and tracheal area, if necessary). A 4-0 polyglactin 910 suture is used (Fig. 22–8*F*).

• Before total closure is completed, an endoscopic view of the stent should be undertaken to be certain that it is appropriately positioned in the larynx.

• The tracheostomy tube is then wired to the stent, and the wound is closed in layers over a drain.

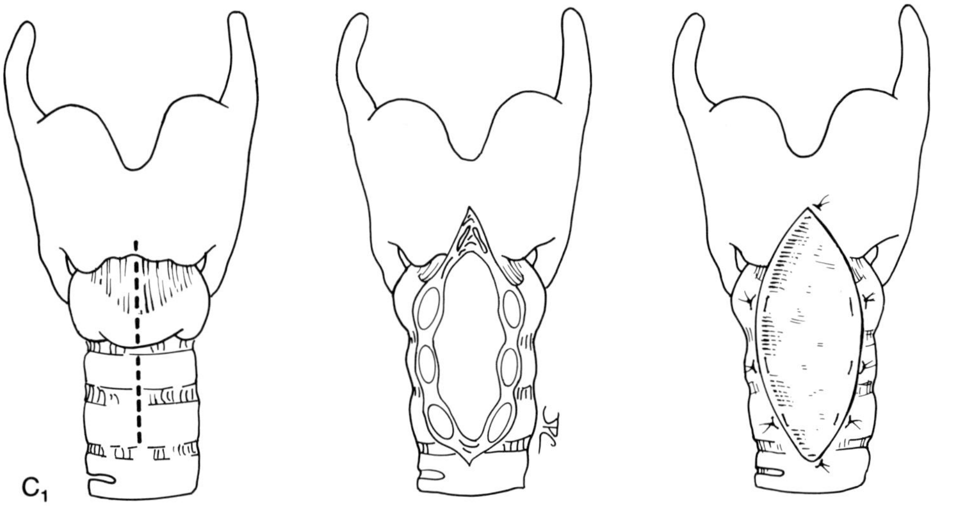

C_1

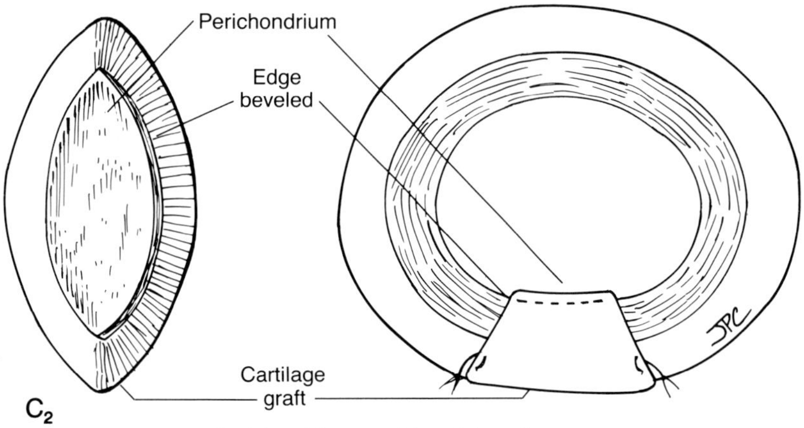

C_2

Perichondrium must face internally

• FIGURE 22–8. *(continued)*

C, A laryngotracheal incision extended superiorly and inferiorly as necessary.

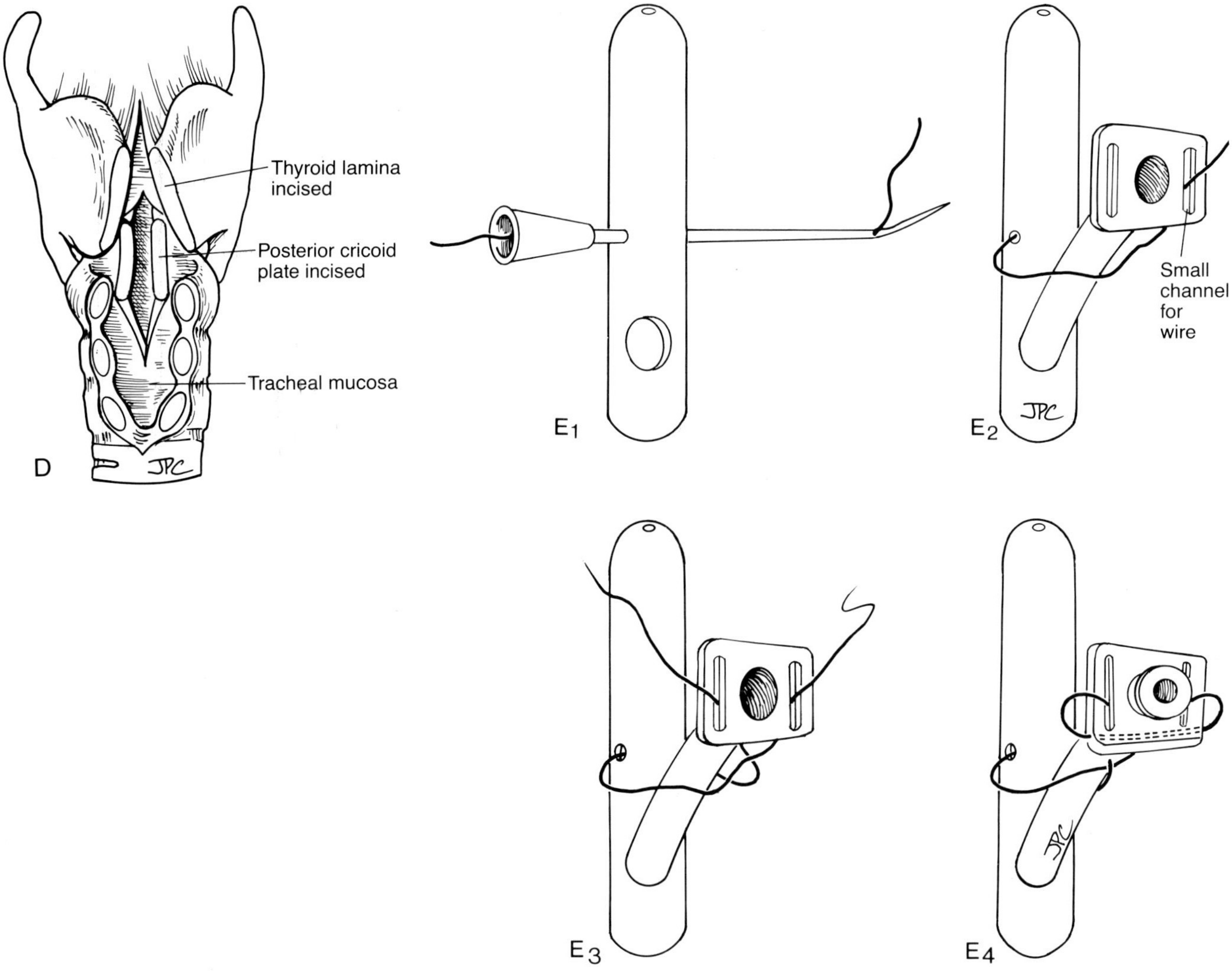

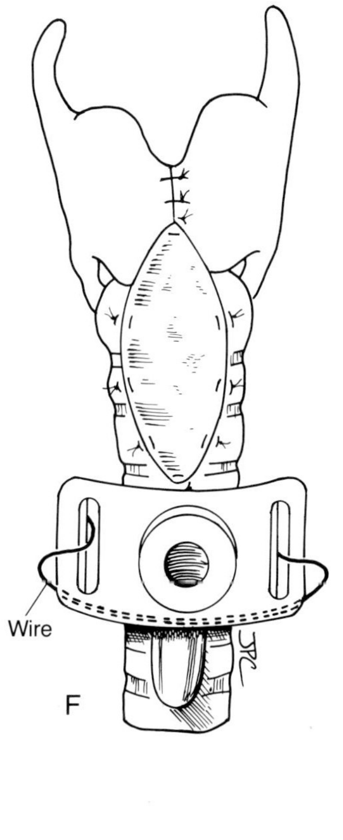

• FIGURE 22-8. *(continued)*

D, The posterior cricoid lamina is incised in severe cases. *E*, A method of preparation of a Teflon stent together with a Healy-Cotton modification of Holinger tracheostomy tube (Pilling). *F*, A stent is positioned in the laryngotracheal complex under the cartilage graft.

Postoperative care

- Humidification and meticulous tracheotomy care are essential, as is cleaning or change of the inner cannula.
- Wound care is conducted twice daily for 5 days, and the peristomal area is covered with antibiotic ointment. In addition, postoperative antibiotics are used in therapeutic doses for 7 days and then in prophylactic dosages until the stent is removed.

TRACHEAL PROCEDURES

SEGMENTAL TRACHEAL RESECTION

Tracheal stenosis may be congenital or acquired. In addition, the trachea may be affected by primary or secondary tracheomalacia. Complete assessment of the entire upper airway must be undertaken. Tracheal surgery on children may be performed either under cardiopulmonary bypass or using conventional endotracheal tube techniques for the delivery of anesthesia. Young infants seem to be better served by the use of cardiopulmonary bypass.

Indications

- Congenital or acquired segmental stenosis of the trachea, occluding more than 50% of the lumen of the airway
- Frequent episodes of respiratory distress or recurrent pneumonitis secondary to inability to clear secretions past a narrowed or stenotic area
- Segmental tracheomalacia of either a primary or a secondary nature

Anesthetic considerations

- Communication with the anesthesiologist is critical so that an appropriate technique may be devised.
- In patients with a complete ring, intubation is undertaken to place the endotracheal tube at a level just above the narrowing, and then induction of anesthesia is continued.
- If the patient is to undergo surgery using cardiopulmonary bypass, bypass is undertaken at this time.

Preparation

- The patient is positioned with the shoulders elevated and the neck hyperextended.
- The skin is prepared from the chin to the umbilicus.
- The incision area is infiltrated with 1:200,000 epinephrine (1 to 2 ml).

Procedure

- If cervical stenosis is present, a transverse incision is made just above the sternal notch to include the tracheotomy site (Fig. 22–9*A*).

- The trachea is mobilized, with care taken not to disrupt the recurrent laryngeal nerves. The thyroid is dissected free from the trachea.

- The area of narrowing or malacia is identified, and the trachea is opened to include this area. If a standard anesthetic technique is used, the endotracheal tube is advanced into the distal portion of the trachea (Fig. 22–9*B*).

- The diseased segment is resected, and the trachea is tested for adequate mobility of the remaining segments by simulating reapproximation (Fig. 21–9*B*). The shoulders are returned to the normal position, and the neck is flexed to facilitate anastomosis. If adequate length is not achieved, a suprahyoid laryngeal release is done.

- The trachea is anastomosed with a 3-0 or 4-0 polyglactin 910 suture, depending on the age of the patient (Fig. 22–9*C*).

- The wound is copiously irrigated and is closed in layers over a drain. Drainage should be kept in place for a minimum of 5 days because of potential for air leakage around the wound.

- A nasotracheal tube is left in place for 5 days, and the patient is sedated but is allowed to breathe spontaneously.

- The endotracheal tube is removed in the operating room, and direct bronchoscopic visualization of the anastomotic site is undertaken to confirm the integrity of the repair.

- For lower stenoses, it is advisable to undertake a median sternotomy, and with the assistance of the cardiothoracic surgeon, the patient is placed on bypass. Resection is undertaken in the method described earlier.

Postoperative care

- A posterior cervical collar is fitted to the patient for 1 week to prevent hyperextension of the neck.

- Antibiotics are administered in therapeutic doses for 7 days, and meticulous twice-daily wound care is employed.

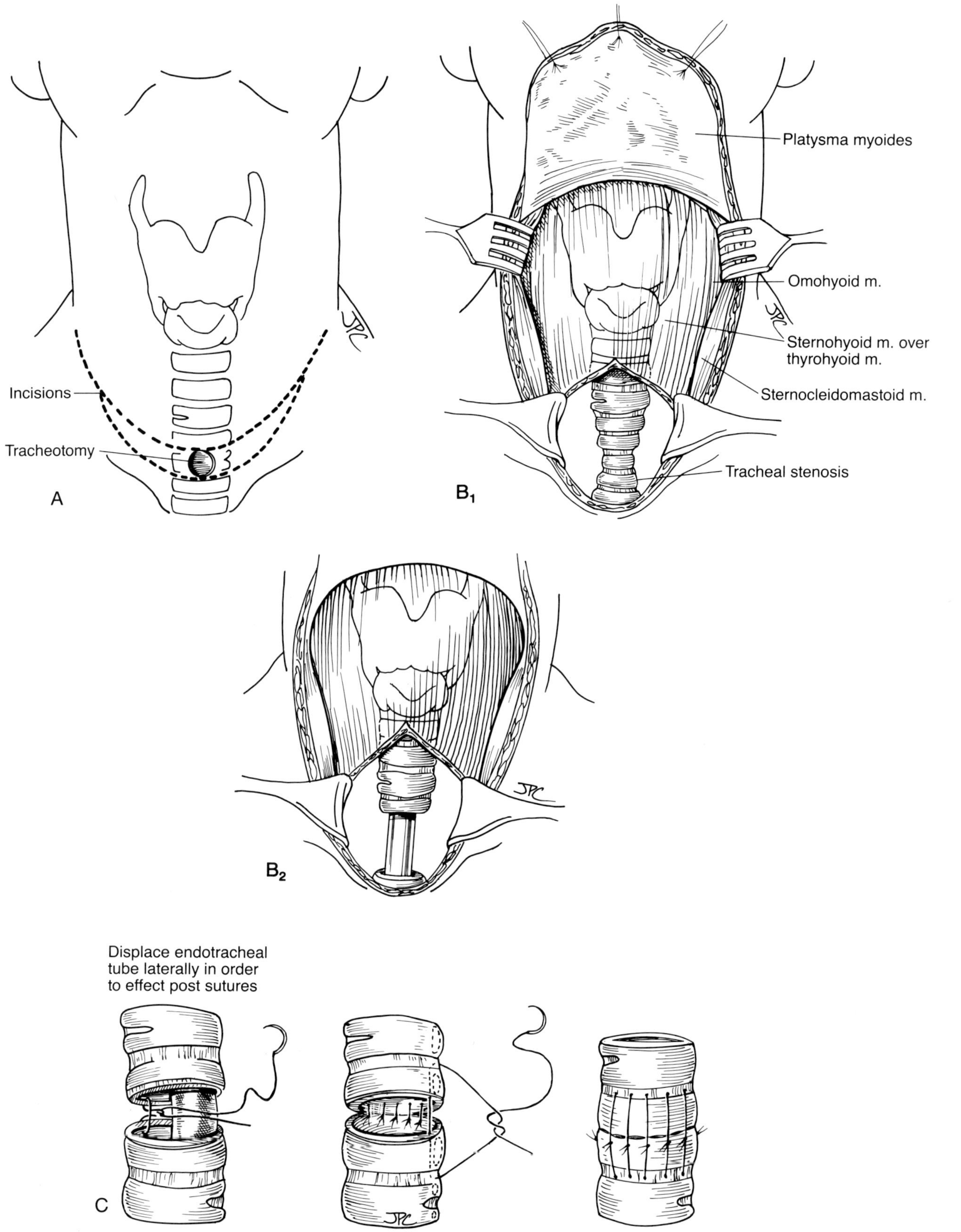

• FIGURE 22-9.

A, Cervical exposure to the trachea in cases of high tracheal stenosis. *B*, The area of stenosis is exposed and resected. *C*, Reanastomosis is accomplished with a 3-0 polyglactin 910 suture.

BIBLIOGRAPHY

Cotton RT: Management of subglottic stenosis in infancy and childhood: A review of consecutive series of cases managed by surgical reconstruction. Ann Otol Rhinol Laryngol 87:649, 1978.

Cotton RT and Seid AB: Management of the extubation problem in the premature child: Anterior cricoid split as an alternative to tracheotomy. Ann Otol Rhinol Laryngol 89:508, 1980.

Cotton RT, Myer CM, Bratcher GO et al: Anterior cricoid split. Arch Otolaryngol 114:1300, 1988.

Dedo H: Endoscopic Teflon keel for anterior glottic web. Ann Otol Rhinol Laryngol 88:467, 1979.

Healy GB, Schuster SR, Jonas RA, and McGill TJ: The correction of segmental tracheal stenosis in children. Ann Otol Rhinol Laryngol 97:444–447, 1988.

Holinger LD and Konior RJ: Surgical management of severe laryngomalacia. Laryngoscope 99:136, 1989.

Montgomery WH: Surgery of the Upper Respiratory System, Vol. 2. Philadelphia, Lea & Febiger, 1973.

Ossoff RH, Dunkavage JA, Shapshay SM et al: Endoscopic laser arytenoidectomy revisited. Ann Otol Rhinol Laryngol 99:764, 1990.

Seid AB, Park SM, Kearns MJ et al: Laser division of the aryepiglottic folds for severe laryngomalacia. Int J Pediatr Otorhinolaryngol 10:153, 1985.

Thornell WC: Intralaryngeal approach of arytenoidectomy in bilateral abductor vocal cord paralysis. Arch Otolaryngol 47:505, 1948

Woodman DG and Pennington CL: Bilateral abductor paralysis: Thirty years' experience with arytenoidectomy. Ann Otol Rhinol Laryngol 85:437, 1976.

Zalzal GH: Use of stents in laryngotracheal reconstruction in children: Indications, technical considerations and complications. Laryngoscope 98:849, 1988.

Zalzal GH, Anon JB, and Cotton RT: Epiglottoplasty for the treatment of laryngomalacia. Ann Otol Rhinol Laryngol 96:72, 1987.

chapter

23

Laryngotracheal Laser Surgery

JAY C. WERKHAVEN, M.D.

The use of lasers for pediatric laryngotracheal diseases is expanding as developing technology allows the delivery of the laser beam into smaller spaces. Experience gained with the use of lasers in the adult airway has naturally led to pediatric applications. However, the unique nature of some pediatric laryngotracheal diseases has necessitated the development of unique approaches to their treatment.

Although this chapter discusses the use of the laser for these pathologic processes, in many cases nonlaser techniques also work well. In certain instances the laser provides unique advantages, whereas in other cases (e.g., laryngeal papilloma and subglottic hemangioma) the laser is the most appropriate instrument.

LASERS, INSTRUMENTS, AND GENERAL TECHNIQUES

CARBON DIOXIDE LASER

The carbon dioxide (CO_2) laser is the most common laser used in otolaryngology–head and neck surgery. Since the first endolaryngeal application by Jako in 1972, the applications for this laser have grown significantly. Newer advances in technology and instrumentation have continued to keep the CO_2 laser the instrument of choice for many laryngeal and tracheal applications.

The CO_2 laser operates at a wavelength of 10,600 nm and is absorbed well by water. Because tissue is between 70 and 80% water, the CO_2 laser is very effective for tissue vaporization. The optical penetration depth of this laser is approximately 50 μm, and the thermal effect (coagulation lateral to the zone of vaporization) is usually between 120 and 240 μm. The implications of the thermal effect are that blood vessels up to slightly less than 0.5 mm may be coagulated with this laser, and vessels larger than this need to be dealt with by another modality. The thermal effect from the CO_2 laser depends on tissue water content or vascularity and the characteristics of the beam itself. Thermal coagulation decreases with increasing water content or vascularity, and coagulation also decreases with shorter pulse durations, if the tissue is allowed to cool between pulses. Another important caveat with use of the CO_2 laser is the removal of the carbonaceous char from the operative field. This char may function as a heat sink and allow production of local temperatures of approximately 2000° F. The laser parameters for normal use include 5 to 10 watts of power with pulse durations of 0.01 to 0.05 seconds.

The delivery of the CO_2 beam to the tissue is accomplished by way of an articulated arm from the laser to a delivery device. This delivery device may be a micromanipulator attached to the microscope or a bronchoscopic coupler for tracheobronchial applications. The standard for microscopic applications is now the "microspot micromanipulator." These newer micromanipulators yield spot sizes of 250 μm with a beam that is coincident with the optical path. Older micromanipulators often had a parallax error wherein the laser beam was offset below the optical path, such that the laser beam might contact the rim of the laryngoscope or the lip of the patient. The newer microspot micromanipulators eliminate this parallax problem and allow access to much smaller areas. For example, the CO_2 laser may now be used through the neonatal subglottiscope with the smallest 3-mm blade.

The bronchoscopic applications of the CO_2 laser require the attachment of the articulated arm assembly to a bronchoscopic coupler. Within this coupler is a vapor barrier window to prevent the deposition of secretions and saliva on the internal optical components. This vapor barrier window may form condensation due to the humidity within the system and may limit the visualization of the target. This is especially bothersome with the small bronchoscopes that are used in the pediatric and neonatal trachea. Two methods may be used to overcome this condensation. One method is to heat the vapor barrier window in very hot water immediately prior to use of the laser. The other technique is to coat the vapor barrier window with an antifog agent before use. The antifog agent must be allowed to evaporate and dry completely, because these agents often use an alcohol solvent base that is potentially flammable if not allowed to completely evaporate.

It has been found helpful to prefocus the bronchoscopic coupler for the appropriate length of bronchoscope. It is also helpful to center the CO_2 beam directly down the bore of the bronchoscope and to point the bronchoscope at the target rather than to move the joystick micromanipulator on the coupler.

Ventilation of the patient may be accomplished through the side arm of the bronchoscope, but the humidifier circuit in normal use on most anesthesia machines should be disconnected to minimize condensation on the vapor window.

KTP AND ARGON LASERS

The KTP and argon lasers operate in the green and blue/green wavelength range of the spectrum. They are well absorbed by pigmented tissue, especially hemoglobin. Hence, they have found widespread application for certain lesions, such as hemangiomas and granulation tissue. The optical penetration depth and thermal coagulation for these lasers is deeper than that of the CO_2 laser, with coagulation as deep as 1.5 mm. Because of this deep coagulation, care must be taken when using these lasers around sensitive structures, such as the vocalis muscle or the vocal process. Undesired scarring with permanent alteration of vocal vibratory function may result.

The KTP laser has a micromanipulator for laryngeal (and otologic) applications. Because of the absorption of this beam by hemoglobin, this laser is well absorbed by the vasculature but is not as readily absorbed by the white surface of the vocal cords until protein denaturization or charring occurs. At this point, laser beam absorption proceeds quickly, and the surgeon must be aware of this increase in absorption during laser application. The argon laser does not as yet have a micromanipulator.

Both of these lasers may be transmitted through fibers. This makes direct application down the side port of an operating bronchoscope feasible. The argon laser has fibers available as small as 200 μm, allowing application through the side port of even the smallest bronchoscope. These lasers may also be used through some of the smaller flexible pediatric bronchoscopes, but there are some limitations to this technique. These limitations include the lack of ventilation with the use of the flexible bronchoscope and the caution that the fiber must extend far enough from the bronchoscope to prevent reflected energy from melting the tip of the bronchoscope.

NEODYMIUM-YTTRIUM-ALUMINUM-GARNET LASER

The neodymium-yttrium-aluminum-garnet (Nd:YAG) laser operates at a wavelength of 1064 nm in the near-infrared. Its depth of optical penetration and thermal coagulation is deeper than the preceding lasers. Thermal coagulation may be as deep as 3 to 4 mm. The wavelength of the Nd:YAG laser is absorbed generally by tissue and does not have a specific chromophore.

The Nd:YAG laser does not have a micromanipulator but does have a wide range of contact tips and flexible fibers for delivery. These fibers may be directed down the laryngoscope or the side suction port on a ventilating bronchoscope.

Laryngeal applications of the Nd:YAG laser are limited due to the deep thermal effect, but tracheobronchial applications exist where this effect is a benefit. The ablation of granulation tissue, mixed capillary/cavernous hemangioma, or obstructing vascular tumors may be accomplished successfully with the Nd:YAG laser.

PREPARATION AND INTRAOPERATIVE PRECAUTIONS

The safety precautions for the use of each laser are unique for that particular wavelength. The surgeon should not attempt to use a new wavelength until he or she has obtained hands-on training and is familiar with all safety considerations as well as the expected tissue response from the laser.

Appropriate eye protection should be provided for both the patient and the operating room personnel. With the CO_2 laser, the patient's eyes should be taped closed and then protected with wet saline gauze pads taped over the eyes. It is recommended that the patient's eyes be taped before the eye pads are placed to prevent the accidental opening of the eyes if anesthesia becomes too light, with subsequent possible corneal abrasion. Operating room personnel who use the CO_2 laser should wear clear glasses with side shields. The surgeon is protected behind the eyepieces of the microscope and the bronchoscope coupler but should be aware of potential damage due to stray beams if the laser is accidentally left in the "on" position when not in use.

The visible wavelength laser beams (argon and KTP) can be transmitted through clear glass and water. The patient's eyes should be protected as with a CO_2 laser, with the addition of aluminum foil or other opaque, nonflammable material on top of the eye pads. Operating room personnel should wear appropriate laser-specific goggles for the wavelength in operation. In addition, because this wavelength may be transmitted through glass, the windows of the operating room must be covered with an opaque material to prevent a stray beam from causing damage outside the operating room itself.

The Nd:YAG laser operates in the near-infrared and is therefore an invisible beam. The patient's eyes should be protected as with the argon and KTP lasers, and all operating room personnel should wear appropriate wavelength-specific protective goggles. In addition, all operating room windows should be covered with opaque material.

In general, manipulation of structures within the airway should be kept to a minimum to avoid undue trauma. Intraoperative steroids are a useful adjunct in most procedures. Dexamethasone (Decadron), 0.5 kg, is usually given intravenously. Use of dexamethasone at an early stage allows tissue distribution and has been shown to decrease edema after the impact of the laser. Occasionally, epinephrine on a neurosurgical pledget may be applied topically to control any excessive bleeding. This technique is generally not used when the patient is under Venturi jet ventilation, which may obstruct the airway. The homeostatic properties of the laser generally obviate the need for topical epinephrine.

GENERAL PRINCIPLES OF POSTOPERATIVE CARE

The guidelines in this section are for general care of the patient undergoing an upper airway procedure, and specific recommendations will be made under each procedure.

Postoperatively, close attention is directed to evaluating the airway for any signs of edema and respiratory distress. Racemic epinephrine may be required in the recovery room. In addition, humidification and supplemental oxygen may be beneficial in selected cases. Postoperative edema is usually greatest within the first several hours, so postoperative evaluations should extend for several hours.

Pain following most of these procedures is usually minimal. Acetaminophen (Tylenol), or rarely acetaminophen with codeine, may be given as needed for relief of pain.

In procedures involving the true cords or the conus elasticus and subglottic region, postoperative voice rest is desirable. Realistically, however, it is difficult to achieve voice rest in the pediatric population.

APPLICATIONS

EPIGLOTTIC CYSTS

Indications

Epiglottic cysts may be found along the laryngeal surface of the epiglottis or occasionally along the aryepiglottic fold. These cysts vary in size (Fig. 23–1*A*).

Anesthetic considerations

Suspension microlaryngoscopy with endotracheal intubation using a laser-resistant tube is most often used. Because of the location of the cyst, it is difficult to employ Venturi jet or apneic ventilation.

Procedure

- Traction may be applied to the cyst with a grasping forceps or a cup forceps (Fig. 23–1*B*). Gentle dissection is performed using a low-power CO_2 laser (3 to 6 watts, 0.01 to 0.05 second, 250-μm spot size) to dissect the cyst from the underlying stroma (Fig. 23–1*C*).
- Large cysts may be marsupialized with the use of the CO_2 laser. The cyst is grasped with a cup forceps, and gentle traction is applied as the major portion of the cyst wall is resected with the CO_2 laser (Fig. 23–1*D*).
- Once the top of the cyst has been resected, the CO_2 laser may be used on slightly higher powers (8 to 12 watts) in a defocused mode to ablate the lining of the cyst.

Postoperative care

See General Principles of Postoperative Care.

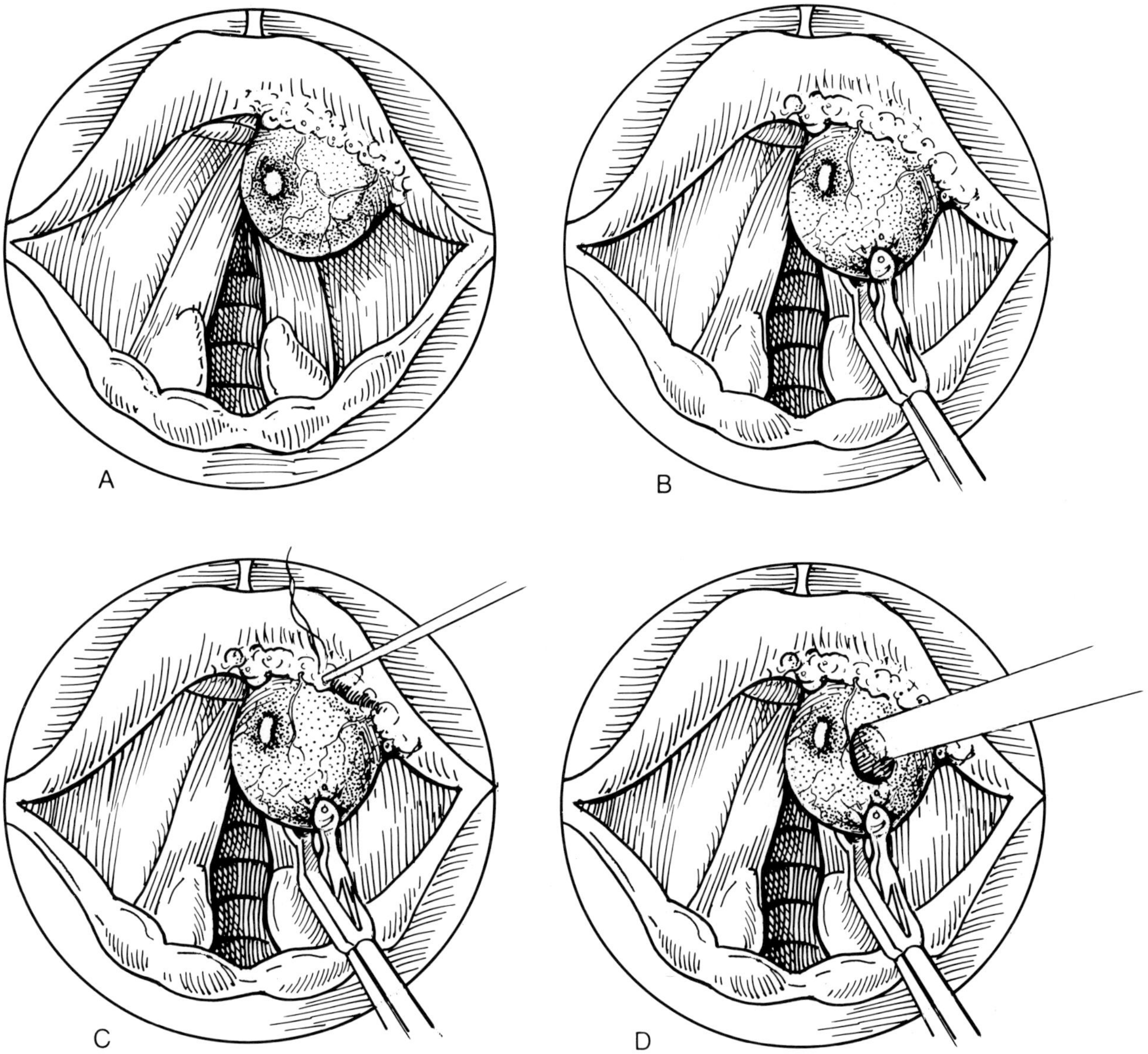

• FIGURE 23–1.

A, An epiglottic cyst. *B*, Traction is applied to the cyst with a cup forceps. *C*, A low-power CO_2 laser dissects the cyst from the underlying stroma. *D*, Resection of a large cyst with the CO_2 laser.

VENTRICULAR CYSTS

Indications

Ventricular cysts are often mucous cysts and may be seen protruding from the ventricle.

Anesthetic considerations

Suspension microlaryngoscopy with Venturi jet ventilation, apneic ventilation, or endotracheal intubation with a laser-resistant tube may be used.

Procedure

- The cyst is grasped with a cup forceps and is retracted medially, giving exposure to the base of the cyst and the ventricle (Fig. 23–2*A* and *B*).
- The CO_2 laser is used on low-power settings (3 to 6 watts of power, 0.01- to 0.05-second pulse duration, and 250-μm spot size) to cut across the base of the cyst. The CO_2 laser is very effective for this type of excision because it provides a bloodless field for dissection (Fig. 23–2*C*).

Postoperative care

See General Principles of Postoperative Care.

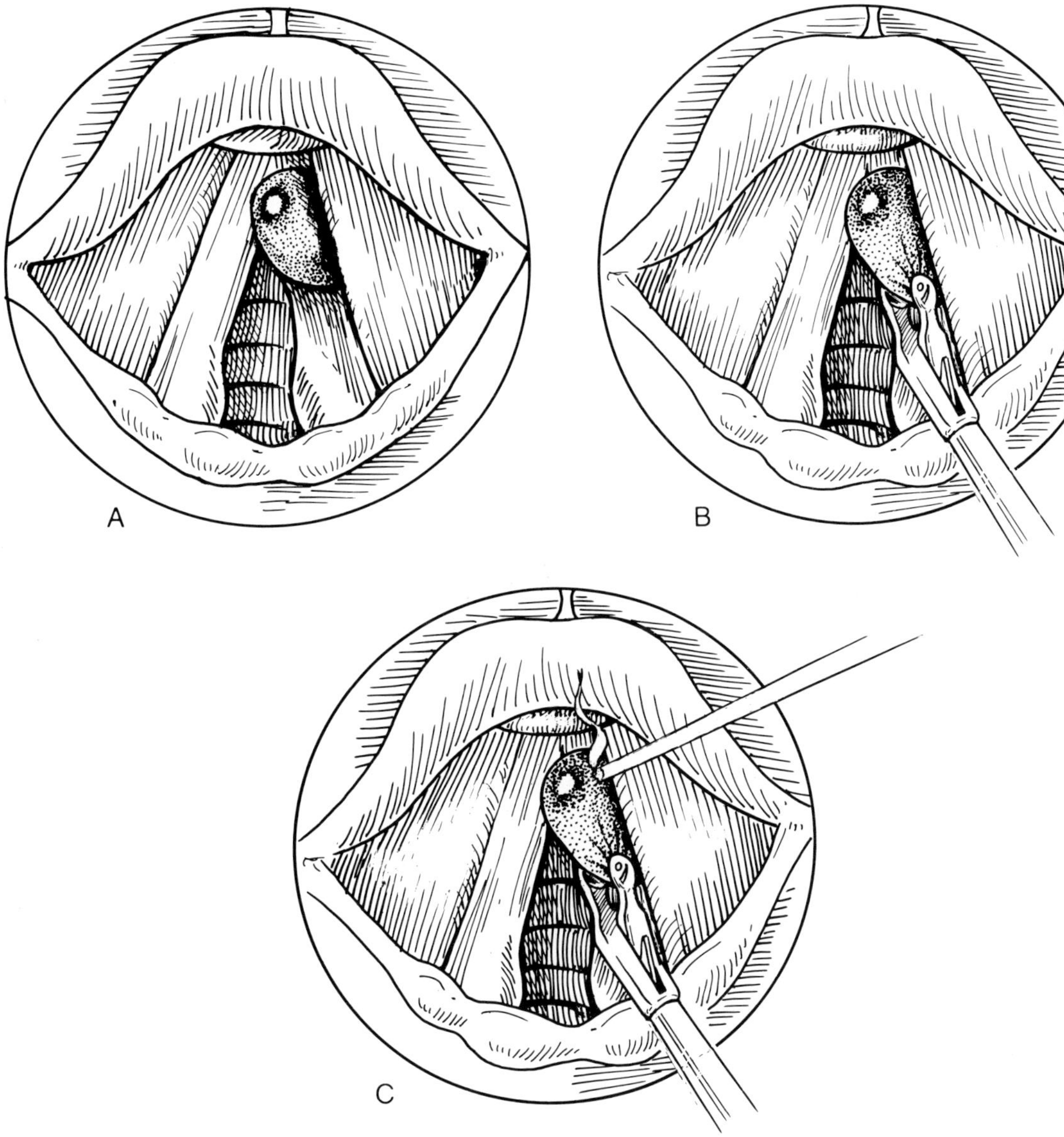

• **FIGURE 23-2.**

A, A ventricular cyst. *B*, The cyst is grasped and retracted medially. *C*, Excision using the CO_2 laser on low power.

INTRACORDAL CYSTS

Indications

Cysts of the true vocal fold are often mucous cysts, more rarely epidermoid cysts. They are most often located submucosally in the membranous portion of the vocal fold.

Anesthetic considerations

Suspension microlaryngoscopy under general anesthesia, using Venturi jet ventilation, apneic ventilation, or a laser-resistant endotracheal tube, may be used. If tracheal intubation is employed, a small-diameter endotracheal tube should be used.

Procedure

- An incision is made over the supralateral aspect of the vocal fold and is carried down through the mucosa. This incision may be made with the CO_2 laser to minimize hemorrhage and improve visualization but may also be made with a pair of scissors or a laryngeal knife (Fig. 23–3*A*).
- The mucosa is gently elevated using a blunt probe, with the medial mucosa carefully preserved. Gentle dissection with this probe may deliver the entire cyst.
- Sometimes, however, the cyst is bound down with tight scar tissue, and the enveloping fibrotic tissue must be ablated with the CO_2 laser. In this case, the cyst is grasped with a cup forceps, and traction is applied medially while the CO_2 laser is used on low power (3 to 6 watts, 0.01- to 0.05-second pulse duration, 250-μm spot size) to gently dissect the cyst (Fig. 23–3*B*).
- Once the cyst has been removed, the mucosa is then redraped over the superior aspect of the vocal fold, and any excess mucosa is trimmed with either the laser or a pair of scissors. The edges of the mucosa may be welded together using a milliwatt CO_2 laser.

Postoperative care

Postoperative care following removal of an intracordal cyst includes emphasis on avoidance of vocal strain. Quiet talking is generally acceptable, but strained whispering and loud talking, shouting, or screaming should generally be avoided.

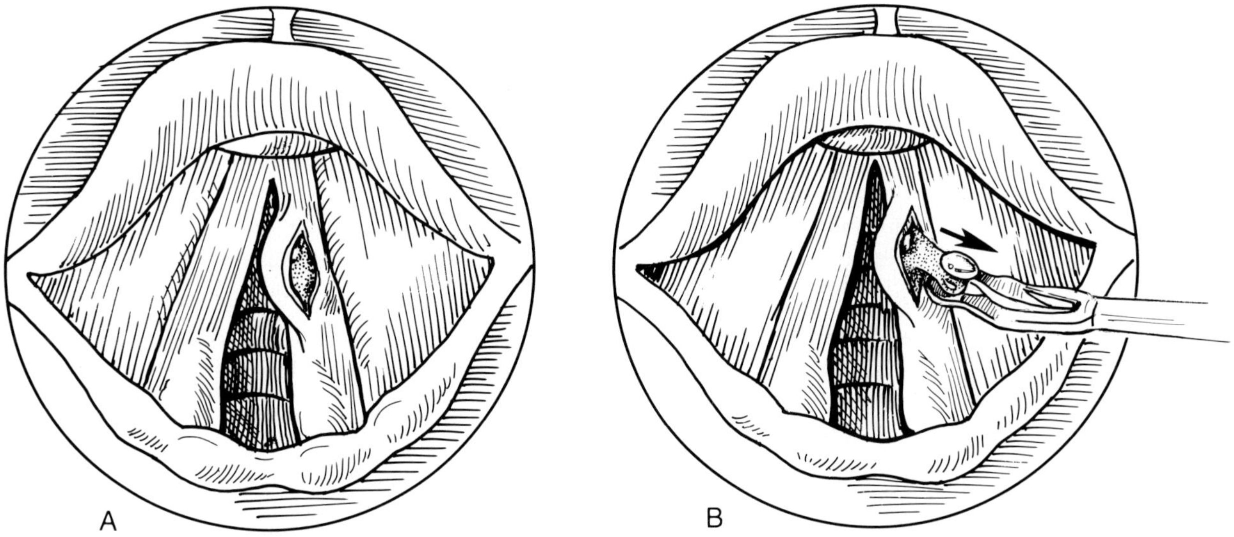

• **FIGURE 23-3.**

A, An intracordal cyst. *B*, The cyst is grasped with a cup forceps, and traction is applied medially while the CO_2 laser is used on low power to dissect the cyst.

VOCAL PROCESS GRANULOMAS

Indications

In pediatric patients, vocal process granulomas are usually a sequela of trauma or prolonged intubation. Very rarely, a granuloma may be the result of chronic gastroesophageal reflux.

Anesthetic considerations

Suspension microlaryngoscopy with Venturi jet ventilation, apneic ventilation, or endotracheal intubation is employed. If an endotracheal intubation anesthetic technique is to be used, a posterior commissure laryngoscope must be available in order to give adequate exposure.

Procedure

- Because granulomas often consist of small capillary vessels, the CO_2 laser is usually adequate for removal of these granulomas. The CO_2 laser is used in a coagulation/vaporization mode (5 to 8 watts, 0.05- to 0.2-second pulse duration, 250-μm spot size or slightly defocused). The granulation tissue is ablated to re-establish the contour of the vocal process, but care is taken to minimize the thermal damage to the cartilage. Great effort must be made not to expose the cartilage itself, because this may predispose to reformation of the granuloma (Fig. 23–4).

- Adjunctive measures in the treatment of vocal cord granulomas may include a triamcinolone (Kenalog) injection into the field of the granuloma.

Postoperative care

Postoperative care of resection of vocal process granuloma emphasizes minimizing postoperative cough. If cartilage is exposed accidentally during excision of the granuloma, postoperative antibiotics may be helpful in preventing the development of perichondritis or chondritis.

If the vocal process granuloma is a sequela of trauma, resolution is generally good. However, if the vocal process granuloma is a result of gastroesophageal reflux, appropriate therapy for gastroesophageal reflux should be instituted.

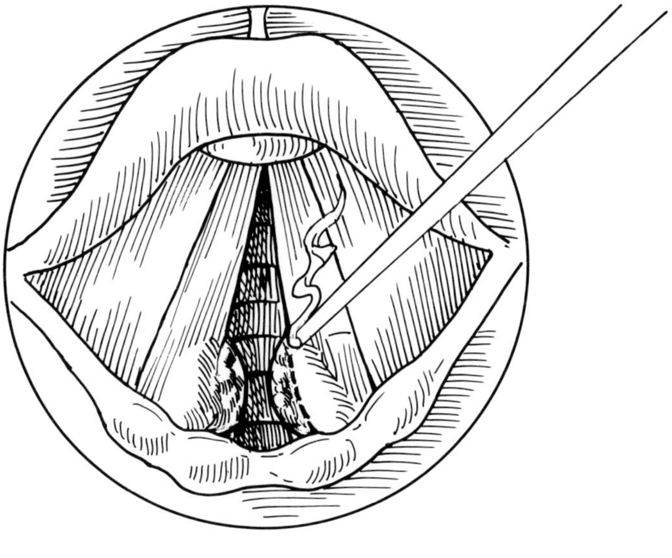

• FIGURE 23-4.

Removal of a vocal process granuloma using the CO_2 laser in a coagulation/vaporization mode. Care is taken not to expose the cartilage, which could lead to reformation of the granuloma.

LARYNGEAL PAPILLOMATOSIS

Indications

The CO_2 laser is the instrument of choice for palliation of laryngeal papillomatosis. The goal of papilloma surgery is control of the papilloma without deleterious scar formation within the glottis.

Anesthetic considerations

Suspension microlaryngoscopy under general anesthesia, using Venturi jet ventilation, apneic ventilation, or a laser-resistant endotracheal tube, is used. The Venturi and apneic techniques have the advantage of better exposure.

Procedure

- High magnification with the microscope is often required to accurately identify the borders of papilloma involvement.
- The papilloma is vaporized or ablated to the level of the mucosa or submucosa. Vaporization deeper than these layers may result in unwanted scarring (Fig. 23–5*A*).
- When operating in the anterior or posterior commissure, a commissure retractor should be used to protect the opposite side. At no time should both sides of the anterior and posterior commissures be vaporized at the same surgical setting, because this frequently results in the formation of a web (Fig. 23–5*B*).
- Laser power settings used initially are 5 to 8 watts of continuous power to debulk the majority of the papilloma. However, once the bulk of papilloma has been vaporized, the parameters should be returned to 0.01- to 0.05-second pulse duration to limit the thermal damage.

Postoperative care

See General Principles of Postoperative Care.

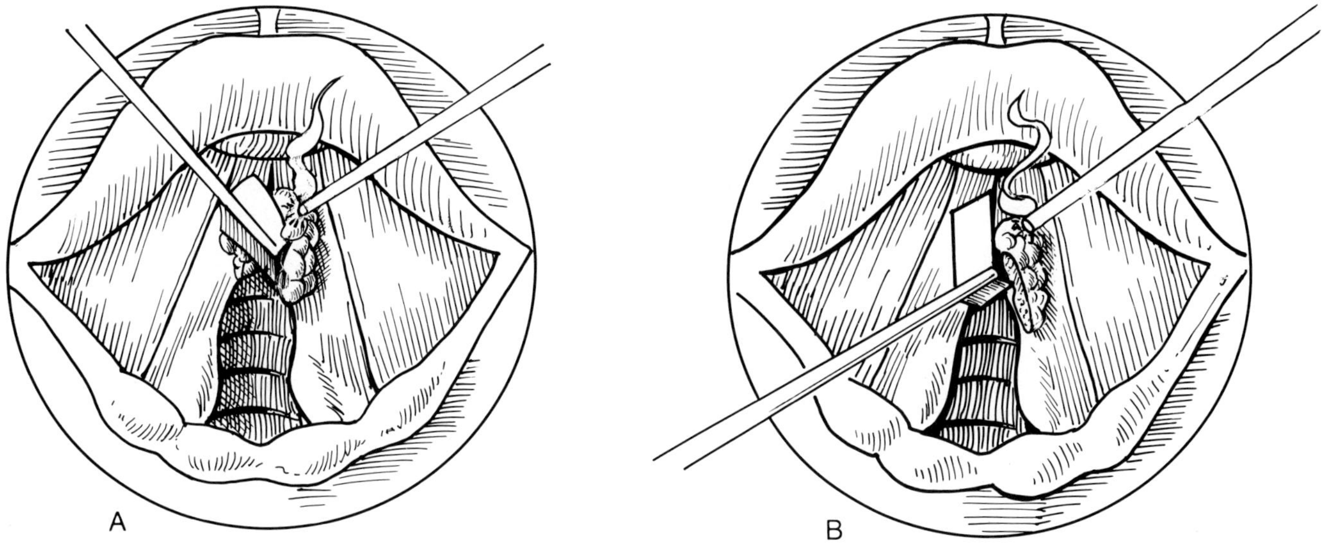

A B

• **FIGURE 23-5.**

A, Vaporization of a laryngeal papilloma. *B*, Vaporization with a commissure retractor to protect the opposite side.

LARYNGEAL WEBS

Indications

The anatomic location and type of laryngeal webs are variable. Laryngeal webs can occur at the supraglottic, glottic, or subglottic level, may be thick or thin, and may be anterior or posterior. In addition, the webs may be congenital or acquired; the latter is often a result of intubation trauma.

Anesthetic considerations

Suspension microlaryngoscopy under general anesthesia is used. Venturi jet ventilation, apneic ventilation, or intubation with a laser-resistant endotracheal tube may be used. Because an endotracheal tube may obstruct the operative field, Venturi jet and apneic techniques may be the better approaches for treating laryngeal webs.

Procedure

- Thin laryngeal webs may be divided by either CO_2 laser or scissors and generally have a good response, regardless of the technique employed (Fig. 23–6*A*).

- Thick anterior webs are treated with a modification of the microtrapdoor flap approach. The CO_2 laser is used on a minimum thermal coagulation setting with 5 to 8 watts of power, 0.01- to 0.05-second pulse duration. With the smallest spot size possible (250 μm), a cut is made along the line of one vocal fold up to the anterior commissure (Fig. 23–6*B*).

- The web is then reflected toward the surgeon, and the mucosa and substance of the web itself are vaporized, preserving the superficial superior mucosa intact (Fig. 23–6*C* and *D*).

- The mucosa is then replaced to cover the raw surface of the vocal fold. Generally, the mucosa heals in place with minimal reformation of a web (Fig. 23–6*E* and *F*).

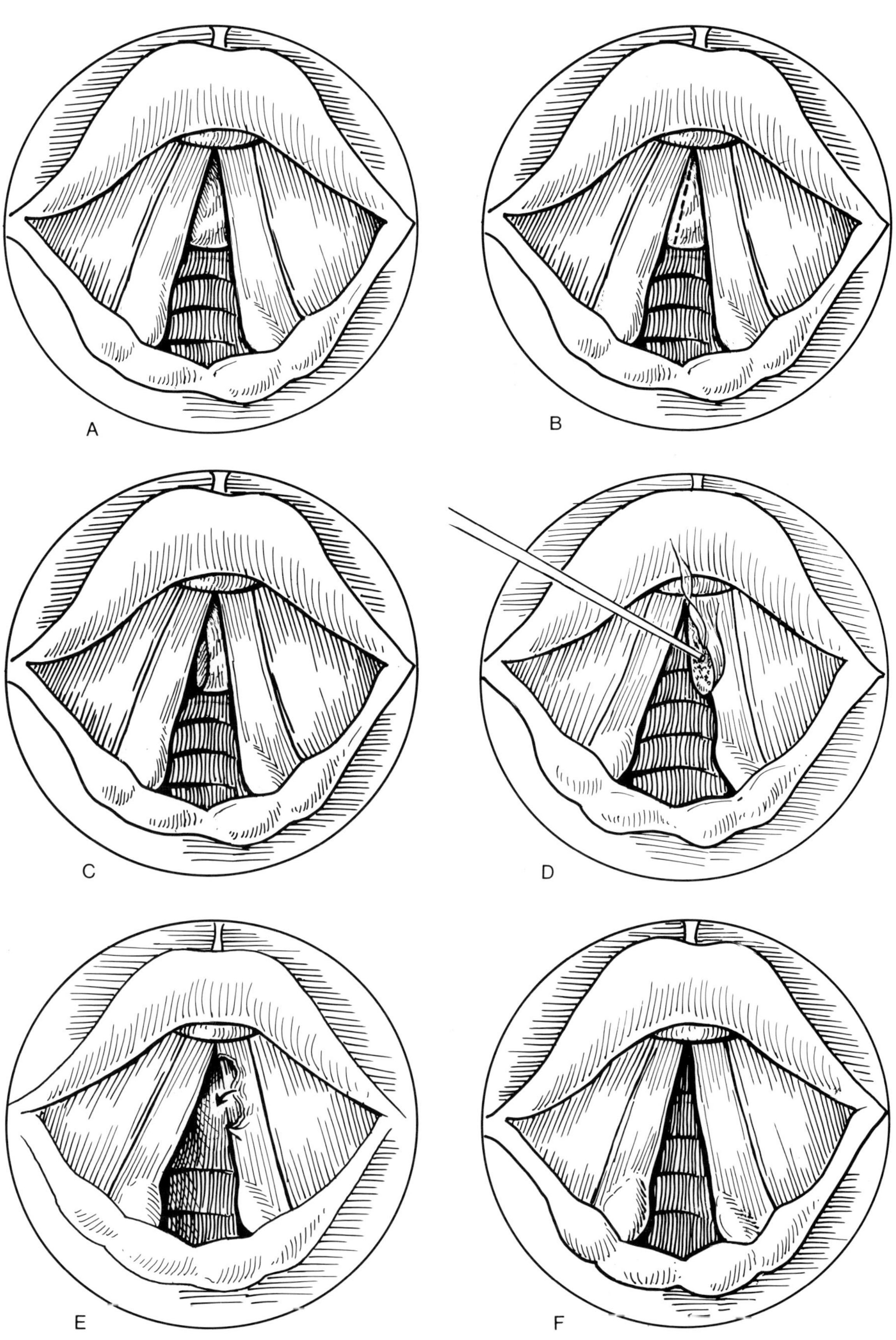

• FIGURE 23-6.

A, Division of thin laryngeal webs. *B*, Thick anterior webs require a modified version of the microtrapdoor flap approach. *C* and *D*, The mucosa and web are vaporized, preserving the superficial superior mucosa intact. *E* and *F*, The mucosa is then replaced to cover the raw area of the vocal fold. Healing occurs with minimal web reformation.

Illustration continued on following page

• Treatment of a posterior glottic web is slightly more involved but also uses a microtrapdoor flap. Posterior glottic webs are often thick and overlie the posterior lamina of the cricoid. A microtrapdoor flap is elevated, preserving the mucosa over the lumen (Fig. 23–6*G* through *J*).

• Once the flap has been elevated, the substance of the scar in the web is ablated using the CO_2 laser (Fig. 23–6*K* and *L*).

• Finally, the edges of the mucosa are incised and allowed to redrape over the raw surface that has been created (Fig. 23–6*M* and *N*).

Postoperative care

See General Principles of Postoperative Care.

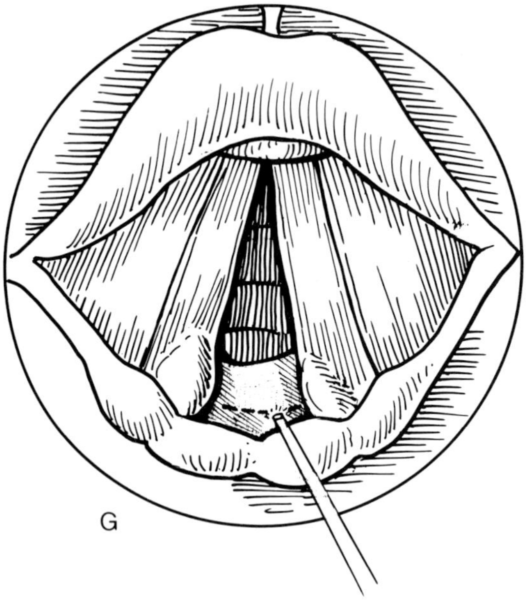

G

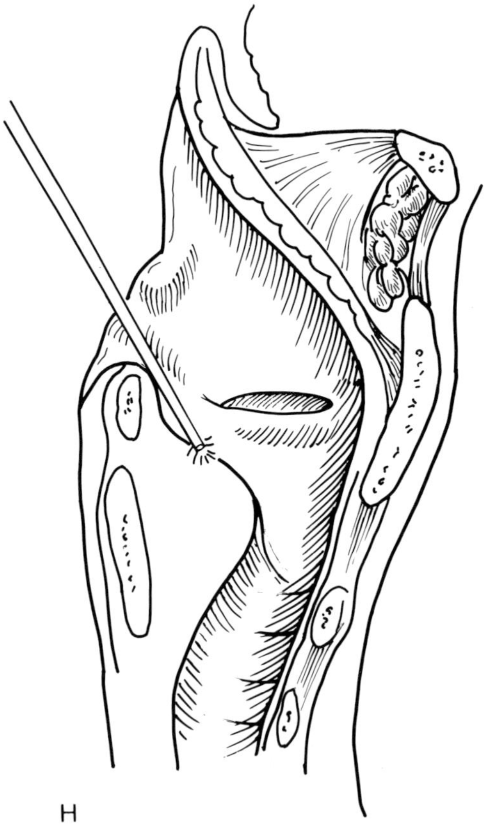

H

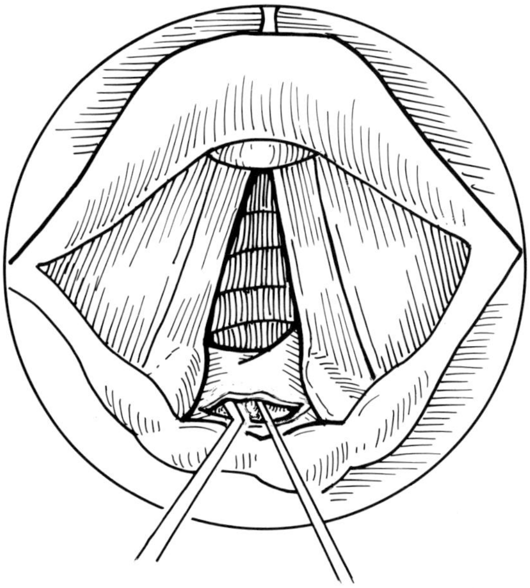

• **FIGURE 23–6.** *(continued)*

G through *J*, Use of a microtrapdoor flap to remove a posterior glottic web. The flap is elevated, preserving the mucosa over the lumen.

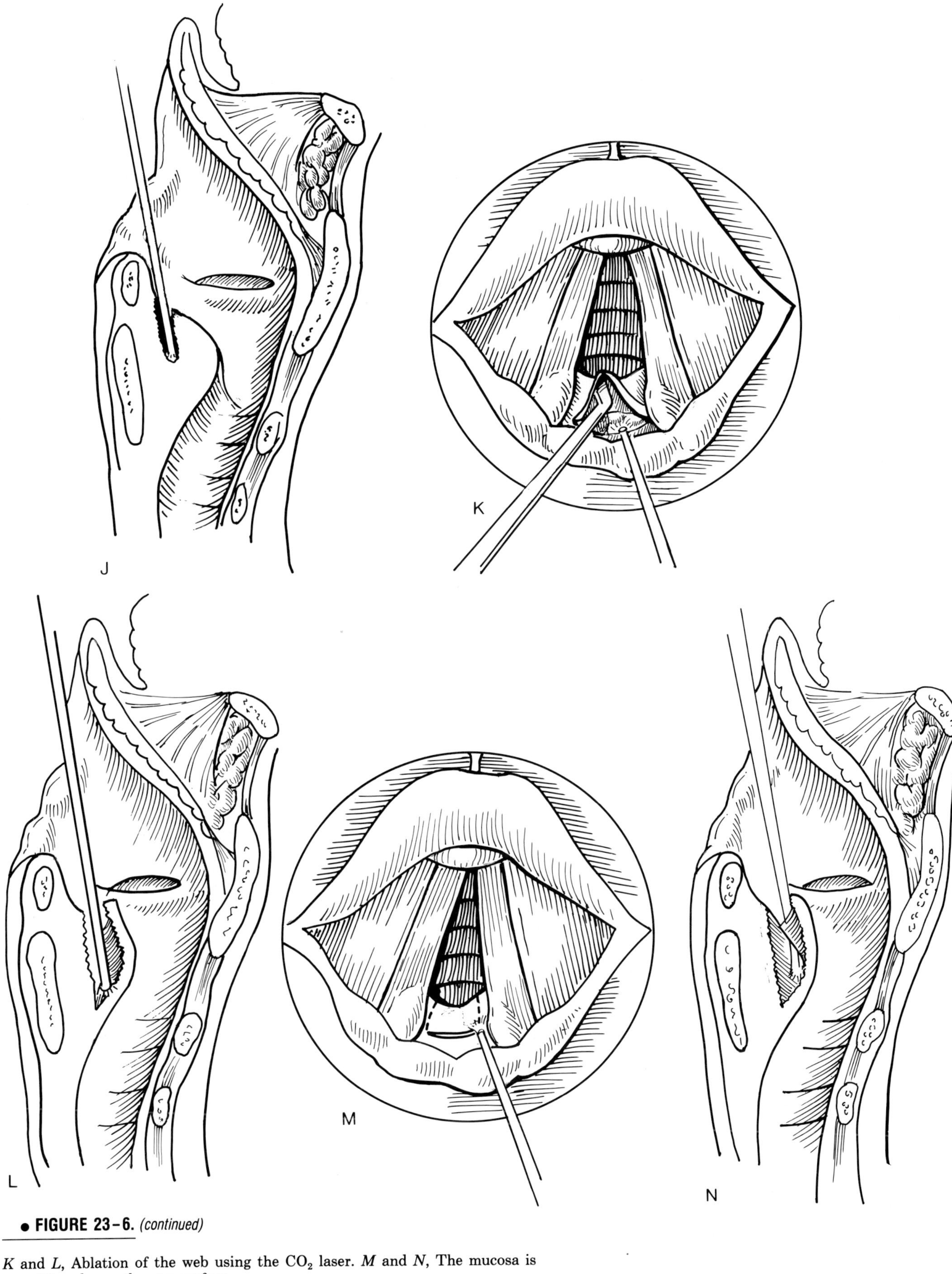

● **FIGURE 23–6.** *(continued)*

K and *L*, Ablation of the web using the CO_2 laser. *M* and *N*, The mucosa is repositioned over the raw surface.

VOCAL CORD NODULES

Indications

Vocal cord nodules rarely require surgical intervention in children. Most nodules resolve as the vocal abuse patterns are eliminated. If vocal nodules are to be surgically removed, cold steel excision techniques or excision with a microspot micromanipulator should be used.

Anesthetic considerations

Suspension microlaryngoscopy under general anesthesia should be used. Venturi jet ventilation or apneic ventilation gives good exposure without obstruction of the target by an endotracheal tube.

Procedure

LASER TECHNIQUE

- The CO_2 laser is used at the smallest spot size. Five to 8 watts of power with a pulse duration of 0.01 to 0.05 second are employed.

- The beam is not directed to have an impact over the center of the nodule; rather, the edge of the beam is used to shave away the nodule. An operative platform is used as a backstop to prevent beam spread distal to the vocal cord. Large spot sizes with the micromanipulator should be avoided, because lateral thermal damage may cause scarring to the underlying vocalis muscle (Fig. 23–7*A* and *B*).

NONLASER TECHNIQUE

- The nodule is grasped on the free edge using microsurgical forceps. Care should be taken not to include the underlying lamina. Tension is applied to stretch the nodule medially, and a pair of scissors is used to remove only the nodule. This should result in a smooth, free edge of the vocal cord without damage to underlying structures and without a depression in the cord. Direct removal with scissors is preferred to the older technique of cup forceps stripping, because the scissors affords a more precise removal with conservation of normal mucosa (Fig. 23–7*C*).

Postoperative care

Voice rest is encouraged. Postoperatively, speech therapy is continued in an attempt to prevent a recurrence of the vocal abuse patterns, which is usually the cause of these nodules.

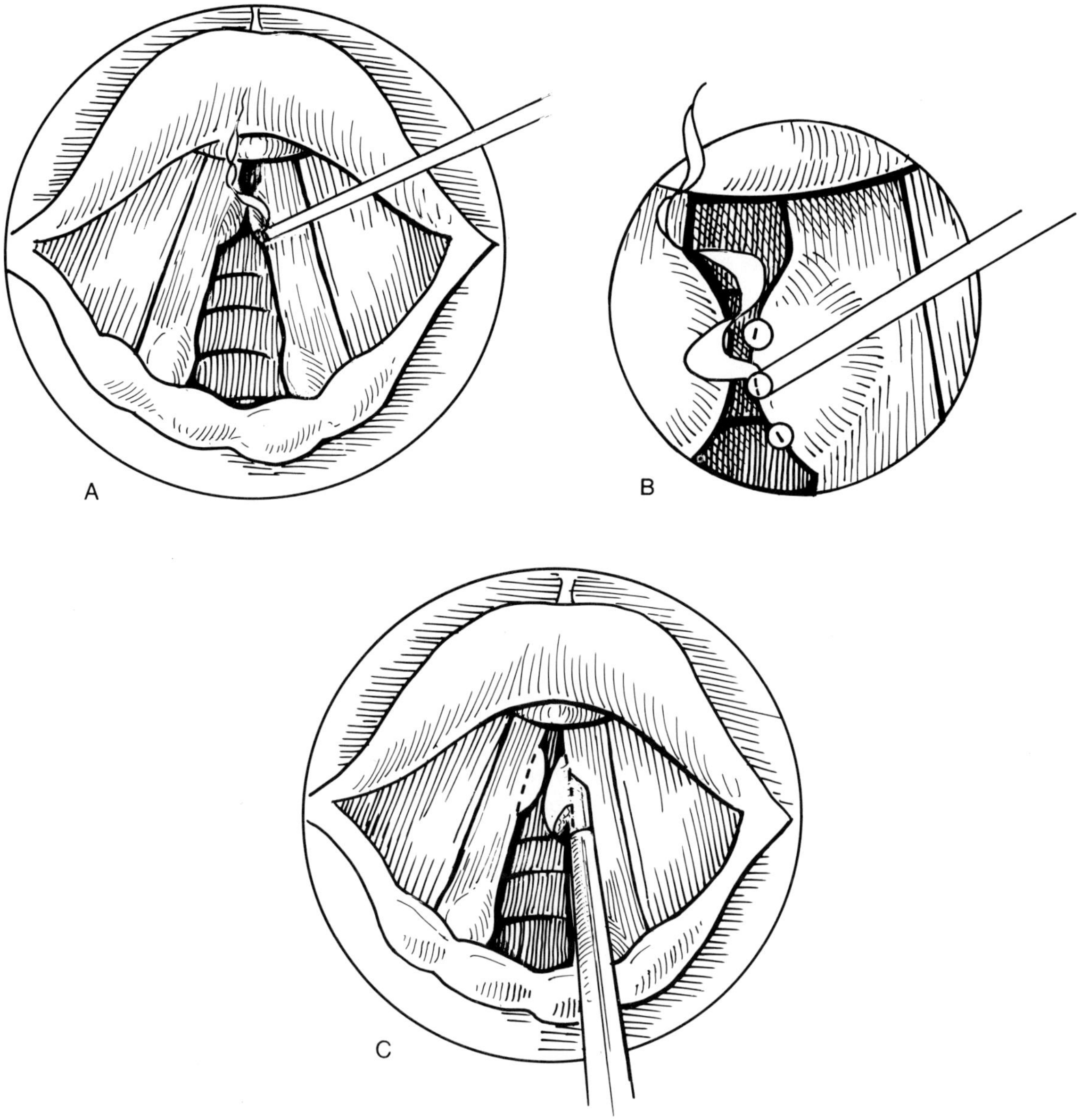

• **FIGURE 23-7.**

A and *B*, Removal of a vocal cord nodule with the CO_2 laser. *C*, Direct scissors removal of a vocal cord nodule.

REINKE'S EDEMA AND VOCAL CORD POLYPS

Indications

Reinke's edema and vocal cord polyps are uncommon in children, but when they occur and cause distortion in the voice, it is often of concern to the parents. Early or soft polyps may resolve spontaneously. Surgical intervention is indicated for polyps of documented chronicity or for polyps that are pedunculated, hemorrhagic, or fusiform.

Anesthetic considerations

Suspension microlaryngoscopy under general anesthesia should be used. Venturi jet ventilation or apneic ventilation gives good exposure without obstruction of the target by an endotracheal tube.

Procedure

- A series of spots outlining the proposed incision on the superior lateral surface of the true vocal fold is made with the CO_2 laser (Fig. 23–8*A*). These proposed incision marks are then connected, ablating the mucosa down to the level of the edema (Fig. 23–8*B*). The laser is often helpful in this part of the procedure because the true vocal fold is often inflamed, and the laser provides good hemostasis and improved visualization. (This incision may also be made with a microsurgical knife or scissors, but the resultant bleeding often obscures the proper tissue planes.)
- A blunt probe is then used to elevate the medial surface of the mucosa, identifying the edema or organized fibrous exudate (Fig. 23–8*C*).
- The edema is suctioned away with a microsuction or may be ablated using the CO_2 laser (Fig. 23–8*D*).

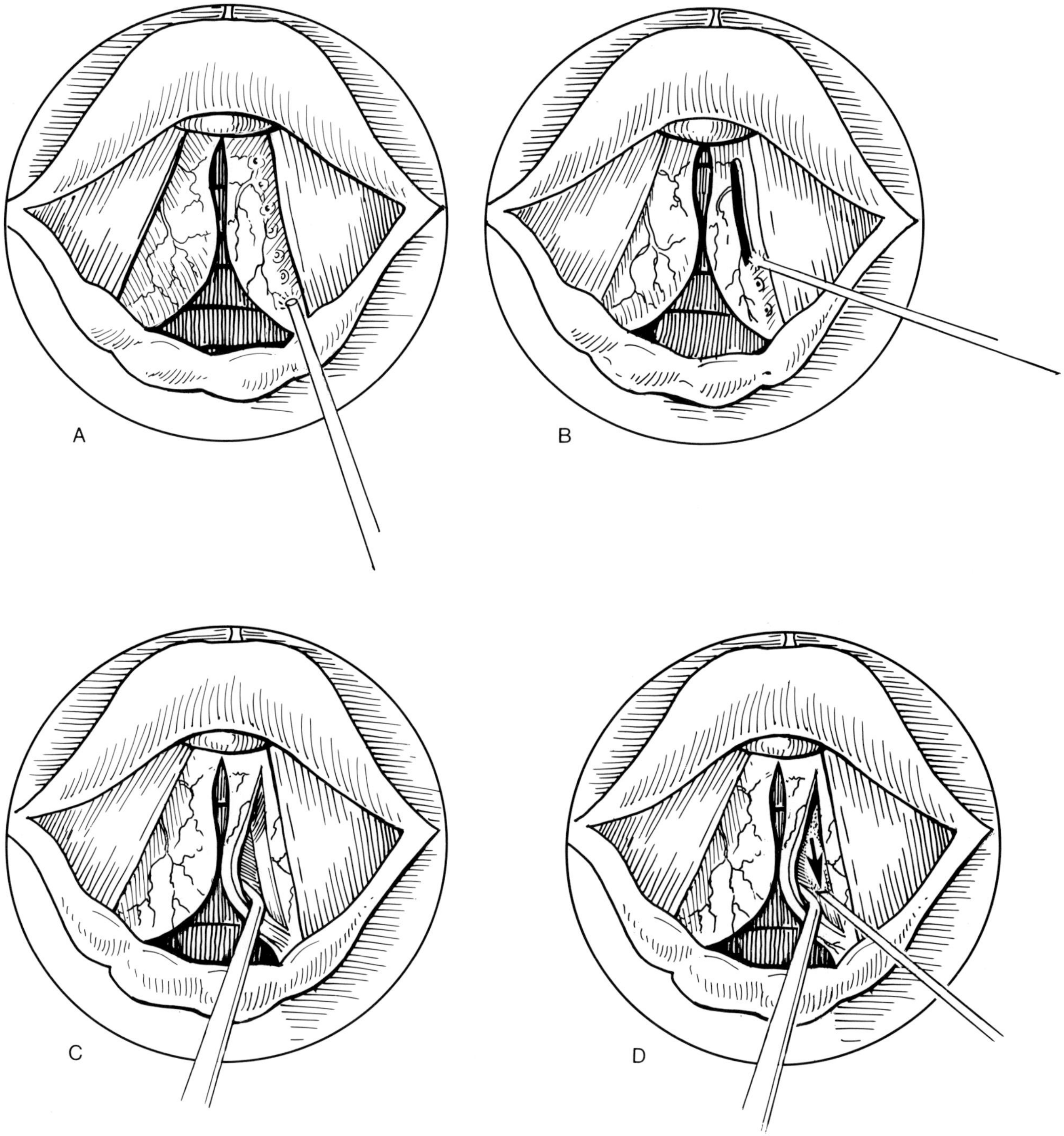

• **FIGURE 23-8.**

Incision marks are outlined (*A*), then connected (*B*) with the CO_2 laser, ablating the mucosa down to the level of the edema. A blunt probe elevates the medial surface of the mucosa (*C*), so that the edema can be removed (*D*) by microsuction or use of the CO_2 laser.

Illustration continued on page 505

- Once the edema has been removed, the excess mucosa is then trimmed using the laser or scissors, and the mucosa is allowed to fall back into position superiorly (Fig. 23–8*E* and *F*). The CO_2 laser on milliwatt power settings may then be used to weld or anneal the mucosa.

- Pedunculated vocal polyps are removed by grasping the polyp with a cup forceps and retracting medially. The CO_2 laser is then used to vaporize along the base (Fig. 23–8*G* and *H*). Care should be taken to apply the beam such that the majority of the beam diameter is directed to the polyp, and the edge of the beam is used to shave the polyp in line with the remainder of the vocal cord. Creating a depression on the vocal cord should be avoided whenever possible. Occasionally, pedunculated polyps are accompanied by a large feeding vessel, and this is carefully coagulated along its length with the laser before it is transected at the base of the polyp.

- Hemorrhagic polyps are most often capillary and rarely have large vessels within them. Hemorrhagic polyps are best dealt with by complete vaporization or ablation with the CO_2 laser. This laser affords generally good hemostasis for capillary-sized vessels. In order to effect coagulation with the CO_2 laser, powers of 5 to 8 watts are used with 0.2- to 0.5-second pulse duration to allow time for the heat diffusion into tissue to coagulate the vessels. Char should be removed as it is encountered, because this may lead to unwanted deeper thermal coagulation.

Postoperative care

See General Principles of Postoperative Care.

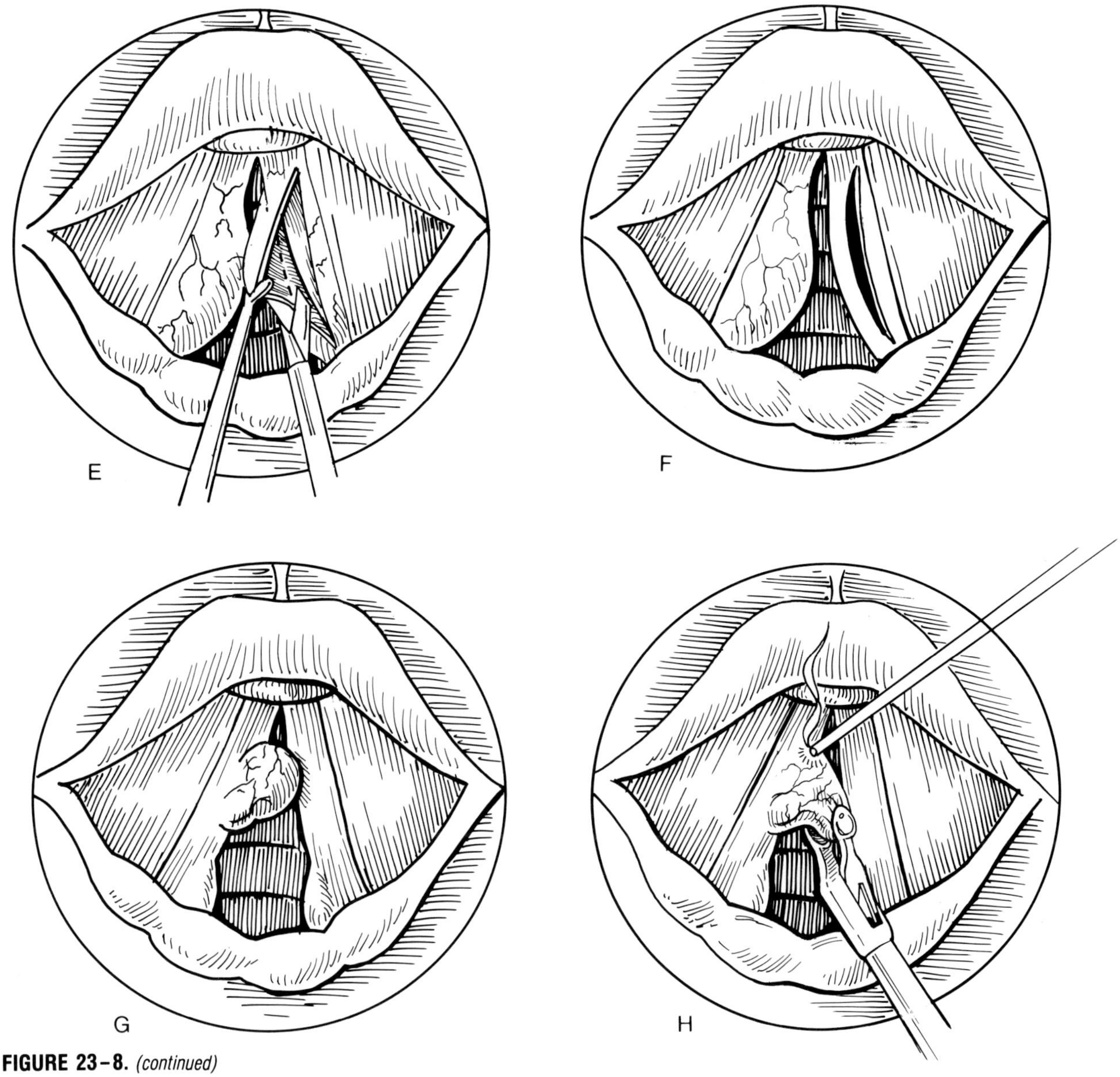

• **FIGURE 23-8.** *(continued)*

E and *F*, Excess mucosa is trimmed and repositioned. A pedunculated vocal polyp (G) is removed using the cup forceps and the CO_2 laser (*H*).

LARYNGEAL AND SUBGLOTTIC HEMANGIOMAS

Indications

Pediatric hemangiomas are typically subglottic whereas adult hemangiomas are usually glottic or supraglottic. Pediatric hemangiomas are generally capillary hemangiomas, whereas adult hemangiomas are often mixed capillary or cavernous hemangiomas. Capillary hemangiomas are typically able to be treated with the CO_2 laser, whereas cavernous hemangiomas may require a laser capable of deeper thermal coagulation (e.g., the argon, KTP, or Nd:YAG laser). Both types of hemangiomas are treated with suspension microlaryngoscopy with high magnification. Once the type of hemangioma has been determined, the appropriate laser may then be brought into the field.

Anesthetic considerations

For most laryngeal and subglottic hemangiomas, Venturi jet ventilation or apneic ventilation must be employed to give adequate exposure. An endotracheal tube would obstruct visualization of the subglottic region. As most of these patients had a prior tracheostomy to establish an airway, the tracheostomy tube is changed to a metal tracheostomy tube to remove any flammable material from the airway. In addition, the presence of an established airway allows the surgeon to proceed in a cautious, serially progressive manner.

Procedure

- Typical power levels for the CO_2 laser for ablation of a capillary hemangioma are 5 to 8 watts of power and 0.2- to 0.5-second pulse duration. The microspot micromanipulator is used to reach the subglottis because of the lack of parallax. The spot size is slightly defocused to give a larger spot than 250 μm in order to obtain wider thermal coagulation. Because the depth and the extent of the hemangioma are generally not able to be determined from an endoscopic evaluation, endoscopic removal of hemangiomas is limited to removing 2 to 3 mm of tissue at a time. This can be compared with chopping off the top of an iceberg and waiting for the iceberg to float back to the top to chop again. Several procedures may be required, but by minimizing the aggressiveness of the approach, potential complications (e.g., scar or damage to supporting cartilage) are also minimized (Fig. 23–9).

- Mixed cavernous and capillary hemangiomas are best treated with a laser with a slightly deeper thermal effect. In this case the argon, KTP, or Nd:YAG laser is used to coagulate the hemangioma. Care is taken to avoid deep thermal effect, because, as previously mentioned, the depth and extent of the hemangioma are not known. Coagulation is established to the depth of the optical penetration depth for the appropriate laser. Six to 10 weeks are then allowed to elapse to allow slough of the necrotic tissue and fibrosis and contracture to enlarge the airway.

- Adjunctive measures in the treatment of subglottic hemangiomas include use of systemic steroids or triamcinolone (Kenalog) injection into the bed of the hemangioma.

Postoperative care

See General Principles of Postoperative Care.

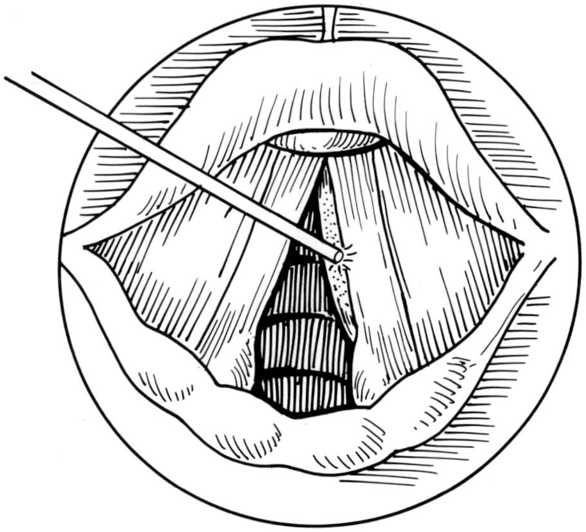

• **FIGURE 23-9.**

Removal of a subglottic hemangioma with a CO_2 laser.

SUBGLOTTIC STENOSIS

Indications

The characterization of the scar in subglottic stenosis determines the type of approach used. Subglottic stenosis may be either thin or thick and may be circumferential or involve only a segmented part of the subglottis.

Anesthetic considerations

Suspension microsubglottoscopy with the appropriate subglottiscope is employed. In general, Venturi jet ventilation or apneic ventilation is used to give exposure, unless the patient has an indwelling tracheostomy tube to establish an airway. In this case, the tracheostomy tube must be changed to a metal trachesotomy tube to ensure that there is no flammable material in the airway.

Procedure

- The CO_2 laser is generally used in an ablation mode with 5 to 8 watts of power, 0.01- to 0.05-second pulse duration, and 250-μm spot size, to minimize thermal coagulation.
- Thin subglottic webs may be incised radially. In this technique, incisions are made in the web in each of three or four quadrants, preserving bridges of mucosa between the laser incisions. The area is allowed to heal and contract, and procedures may be repeated at 6- to 8-week intervals.
- Dilatation after radial incision may be of some benefit because it may compress and break the scar adhesions. However, dilatation is being performed against a fixed obstruction (i.e., the cricoid ring).
- Thick subglottic stenosis is difficult to treat by almost any method but is amenable occasionally to serial radial incision or to serial microtrapdoor flap excision of scar (Fig. 23–10*A1* and *A2*). Serial radial incision is carried out in a manner similar to the previous technique.
- Serial microtrapdoor flap excision is performed by the excision of scar in a microtrapdoor fashion in quadrant sections over a period of time. The microtrapdoor flaps are elevated in small segments (i.e., from 12 o'clock to 3 or 4 o'clock). The mucosa is incised (Fig. 23–10*B*).
- The mucosa is elevated and maintained, while the deep scar tissue is ablated using the CO_2 laser. Care must be taken not to expose cartilage (Fig. 23–10*C*).
- The mucosa is then incised along the edge, leaving the mucosa attached to the inferior side as a flap (Fig. 23–10*D*).
- The mucosa is allowed to adhere to the area of scar ablation and provides mucosa coverage for approximately one half of the surface area due to shrinkage of the mucosa flap during the procedure. Although this procedure is technically difficult, the free edge of the flap may be welded into position with the defocused laser (Fig. 23–10*E*).

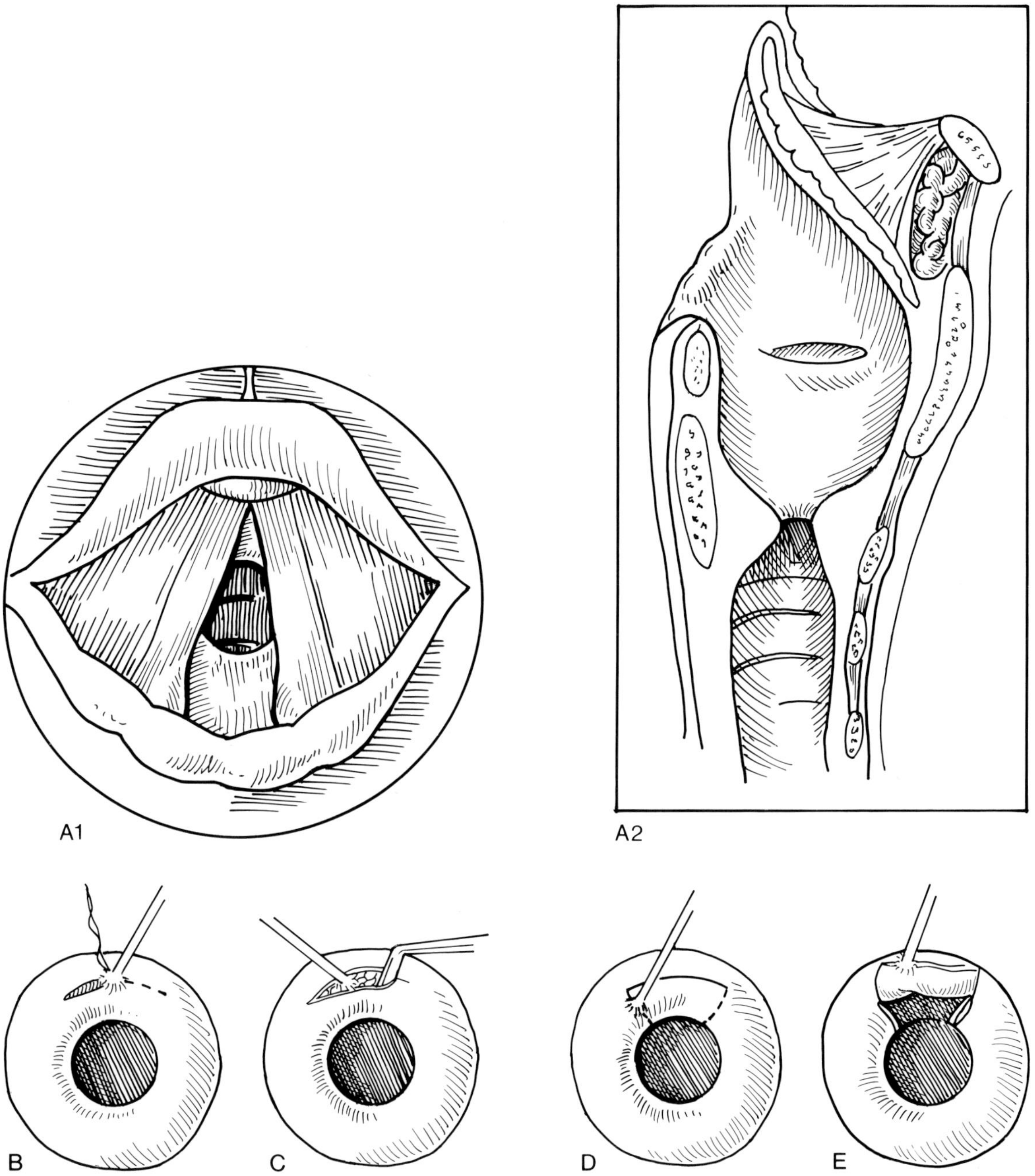

• FIGURE 23-10.

A1 and *A2*, Thick subglottic stenosis. *B* through *E*, A serial microtrapdoor flap excision of the subglottic stenosis. The mucosa is incised (*B*), then elevated while deep scar tissue is ablated with the CO_2 laser (*C*). The mucosa is then incised along the edge (*D*) and allowed to adhere to the area of scar ablation. The free edge of the flap may be welded into position with the defocused laser (*E*).

Illustration continued on page 511

- The scar tissue is excised, and serial procedures are repeated over 6- to 8-week intervals (Fig. 23–10*F*). Even in cases in which serial microtrapdoor flaps are unable to provide an adequate airway, it generally results in a much larger mucosa-covered lumen that improves the success of subsequent laryngotracheoplasty.

Postoperative care

See General Principles of Postoperative Care.

TRACHEAL STENOSIS

Indications

When tracheal stenosis is distal to the subglottis, a bronchoscope must be used to obtain exposure. If the lumen is large enough (7.5-mm absolute diameter or larger), a CO_2 laser ventilating bronchoscope may be used. For lumens that are smaller, a smaller bronchoscope may be used with a laser that may be transmitted through an optical fiber.

Anesthetic considerations

General anesthesia through the side port of the bronchoscope is employed. The humidifier circuit is not connected in the anesthesia machine to minimize vapor buildup on the internal optics.

Procedure

- For both thick and thin tracheal scars the CO_2 laser may be used in a fashion similar to that employed in the laser excision of subglottic stenosis (see earlier). The spot size with a 250-mm bronchoscope is approximately 300 μm and is appropriate for use in this area. With larger bronchoscopes, the spot size is appropriately larger due to the defocusing effect caused by the length of the bronchoscope.

- Stenosis in a small lumen that would not allow the admission of a CO_2 laser ventilating bronchoscope may be treated with a standard ventilating bronchoscope and the KTP, argon, or Nd:YAG laser. Appropriate modifications to protect the surgeon's eyes (appropriate filters) or glasses should be used. The laser may be directed down an optical fiber that is placed down the side port of these bronchoscopes. In general, depending on which laser is available (e.g., argon, KTP, or Nd:YAG), the laser with the shallower thermal effect is preferred. In addition, the smallest fiber available is used. The guideline for the general technique of excision of scar with these lasers is to use power densities that are high enough and pulse durations that are short enough to effect vaporization with minimal thermal coagulation. The scar tissue is generally treated in a radial incision and dilatation manner, because it is exceedingly difficult to attempt to raise a microtrapdoor flap with these fibers. The success of treatment of tracheal stenosis with these other lasers has been only fair to date.

Postoperative care

See General Principles of Postoperative Care.

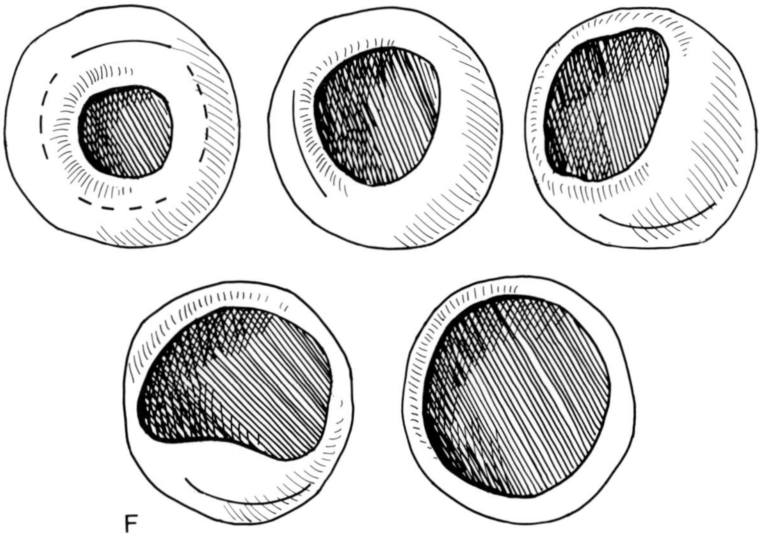

• **FIGURE 23-10.** *(continued)*

F, Scar tissue is excised, and serial procedures are repeated at 6- to 8-week intervals.

TRACHEAL GRANULATION

Indications

Granulation tissue of the trachea may occur in several sites. Commonly, it may occur at the superior edge of the tracheostomy tube stoma, at the tip of the tracheostomy tube on the anterior tracheal wall, or near the carina due to vigorous suctioning. Granulation tissue may also occur at the location of the tip of indwelling endotracheal tubes in patients who have had orotracheal intubation for some time. In general, the CO_2 laser is the laser of choice for the excision of this granulation tissue; however, the argon, KTP, or Nd:YAG laser may also be used.

Anesthetic considerations

General anesthesia is employed through the side port of the ventilating bronchoscope. The humidification circuit is not connected.

Procedure

- The CO_2 laser is used on airways that may be larger than 7.5 mm in absolute diameter (because this is the smallest commercially available CO_2 ventilating bronchoscope at present). Once the granulation tissue is identified, the CO_2 laser is used in a vaporization mode with a moderate coagulation effect (5 to 8 watts of power, 0.05- to 0.2-second pulse duration). The granulation tissue is vaporized to its base, taking care not to extend the vaporization to the cartilage of the tracheal rings.

- If the CO_2 laser is not available or the tracheal lumen is too small, the argon, KTP, or Nd:YAG laser may be used through the ventilating bronchoscope. The technique here is very similar to that used for subglottic stenosis in that the fiber is passed through the side channel of the ventilating bronchoscope and is brought to bear on the granulation tissue. Owing to the deep thermal coagulation effect of these lasers, the technique is to coagulate the granulation tissue and then to use the tip of the bronchoscope to gently remove the granulation tissue from the tracheal wall (Fig. 23–11*A* and *B*). Experience with each of the different wavelengths provides the surgeon with the skill to recognize the depth of coagulation with each of these lasers. Repeat endoscopy several days later is required occasionally for suction removal of the eschar.

Postoperative care

See General Principles of Postoperative Care.

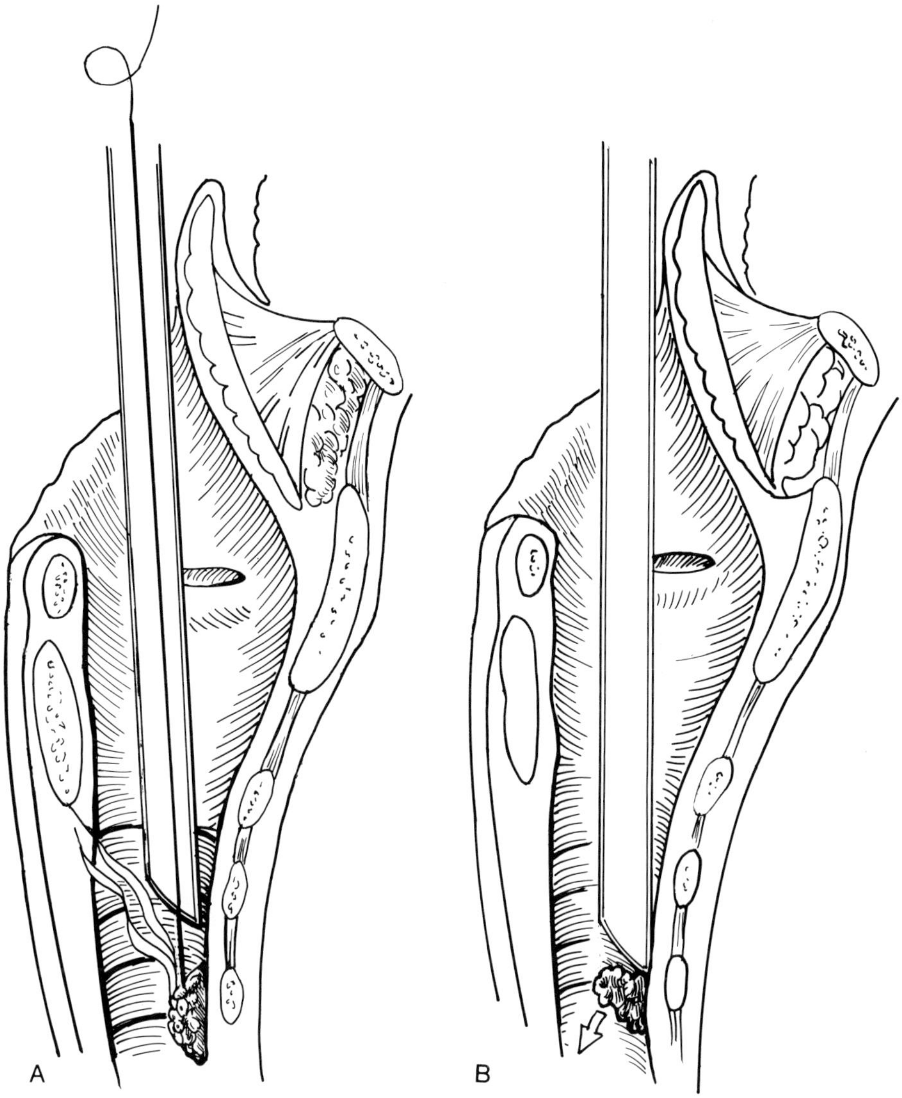

• **FIGURE 23-11.**

A and *B*, Removal of granulation tissue from the tracheal wall using the laser through the ventilating bronchoscope.

BIBLIOGRAPHY

Benjamin B and Croxson G: Vocal cord granulomas. Ann Otol Rhinol Laryngol 94:538–541, 1985.

Booth JB and Birck HG: Operative treatment and postoperative management of saccular cyst and laryngocele. Arch Otolaryngol Head Neck Surg 107:500–502, 1981.

Boulnois JL: Photophysical processes in recent medical laser developments: A review. Lasers Med Sci 1:47–66, 1986.

DeSanto LW: Laryngocele, laryngeal mucocele, large saccules, and laryngeal saccular cysts: A developmental spectrum. Laryngoscope 84:1291–1296, 1974.

Harris DM and Werkhaven JA: Biophysics and applications of medical lasers. *In* Myers EN and Bluestone CD (eds): Advances in Otolaryngology—Head and Neck Surgery, Vol 3. Chicago, Year Book Medical Publishers, 1989, pp 91–123.

Holinger LD, Barnes DR, Smid LJ et al: Laryngocele and saccular cysts. Ann Otol Rhinol Laryngol 87:675–685, 1978.

Jako GJ: Laser surgery of the vocal cords. Laryngoscope 82:2204–2216, 1972.

McKenzie AL and Karruth JAS: Lasers in surgery and medicine. Phys Med Biol 29:619–641, 1984.

Mizono G and Dedo HH: Subglottic hemangiomas in infants: Treatment with CO_2 laser. Laryngoscope 94:638–641, 1984.

Monday LA, Cornut G, Bouchayer M et al: Epidermoid cysts of the vocal cords. Ann Otol Rhinol Laryngol 92:124–127, 1983.

Ossoff RH, Toriumi DM, and Duncavage JA: The use of the laser in head and neck surgery. *In* Myers EN, Bluestone CD, Brackman DE, and Krause CJ (eds): Advances in Otolaryngology—Head and Neck Surgery, Vol 1. Chicago, Year Book Medical Publishers, 1987, pp 217–240.

Sheppard L, Werkhaven J, Mickelson S et al: The effect of steroids or tissue precooling on edema and tissue thermal coagulation after CO_2 laser impact. Lasers Surg Med 12:137–141, 1992.

Strong MS and Vaughn CW: Vocal cord nodules and polyps—the role of surgical treatment. Laryngoscope 81:911–923, 1971.

Strong MS, Vaughn CW, Healy GB et al: Recurrent respiratory papillomatosis: Management with the CO_2 laser. Ann Otol Rhinol Laryngol 85:508–516, 1976.

Vaughn CW: Use of the carbon dioxide laser in the endoscopic management of organic laryngeal disease. Otolaryngol Clin North Am 16:849–864, 1983.

chapter

24

Congenital Malformations of the Neck

MARK A. RICHARDSON, M.D.

THYROGLOSSAL CYST

A thyroglossal cyst generally presents as a firm cystic mass near the midline, just below the level of the hyoid bone. The mass may be located superiorly, laterally, or inferiorly, and it may be draining if the patient had a previous infection or prior incision and drainage.

Thyroglossal cysts are thought to be an abnormality of thyroid formation and can exist anywhere from the base of the tongue to the level of the thyroid gland.

Indications

- Enlargement of the mass
- Infection
- Diagnosis of a mass present in the anterior of the neck

Anesthetic considerations

General endotracheal anesthesia is used. The tube should be taped to the upper lip to allow the surgeon access to the mouth.

Preparation

A preoperative evaluation should consist of a thyroid scan or ultrasonography of the thyroid to identify normal tissue to rule out association of a lingual thyroid with the thyroglossal cyst. If a lingual thyroid is identified and it is the only source of thyroid hormone production, thyroxine levels should be obtained preoperatively.

Procedure

SPECIAL INSTRUMENTS: LARYNGEAL SCISSORS

The hypoglossal nerve and the superior laryngeal nerve should be avoided. The fistula itself should not be dissected free from the surrounding tissue; instead, a core of tissue along with the middle third of the hyoid bone should be excised.

OPERATIVE PROCEDURE

The patient's neck is extended by placing a roll underneath the shoulders, and the anterior part of the neck is prepared and draped to the level of the lower lip using sterile technique.

An incision is created overlying the mass to permit an approach to the hyoid bone. The incision is carried through the skin and subcutaneous tissue to the level of the anterior strap muscles, and the anterior strap muscles are retracted laterally to expose the cystic lesion or inflammatory mass (Fig. 24–1).

The cyst is carefully dissected free from the surrounding soft tissue and pedicled to the middle third of the hyoid bone.

Muscular attachments to the hyoid bone are carefully eliminated with the use of the Bovie coagulator so that the hyoid bone can be visualized at its junction between the middle and lateral thirds (Fig. 24–2).

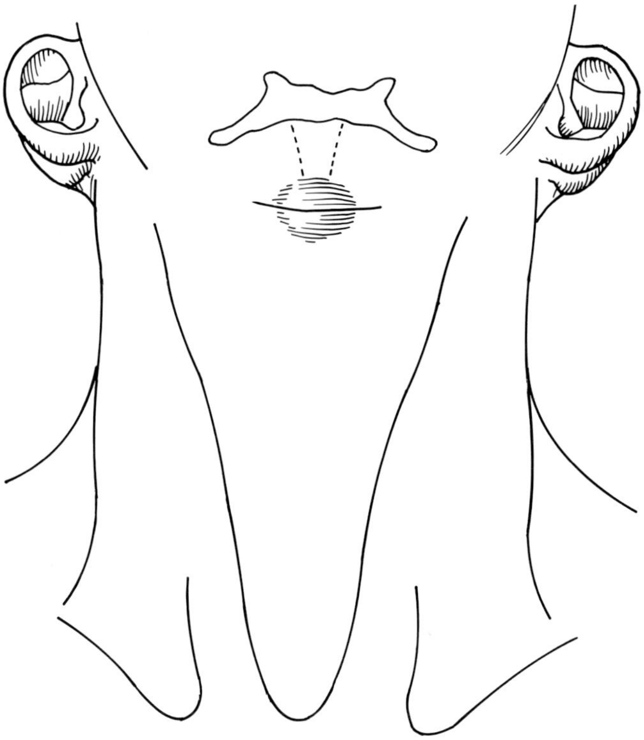

• FIGURE 24-1.

Incision site for removal of a thyroglossal cyst. (Redrawn from Peters GE: Excision of thyroglossal duct. *In* Johns ME, Price JC, and Mattox DE: Atlas of Head and Neck Surgery, Vol 1. St. Louis, Mosby-Year Book, 1990, p. 365.)

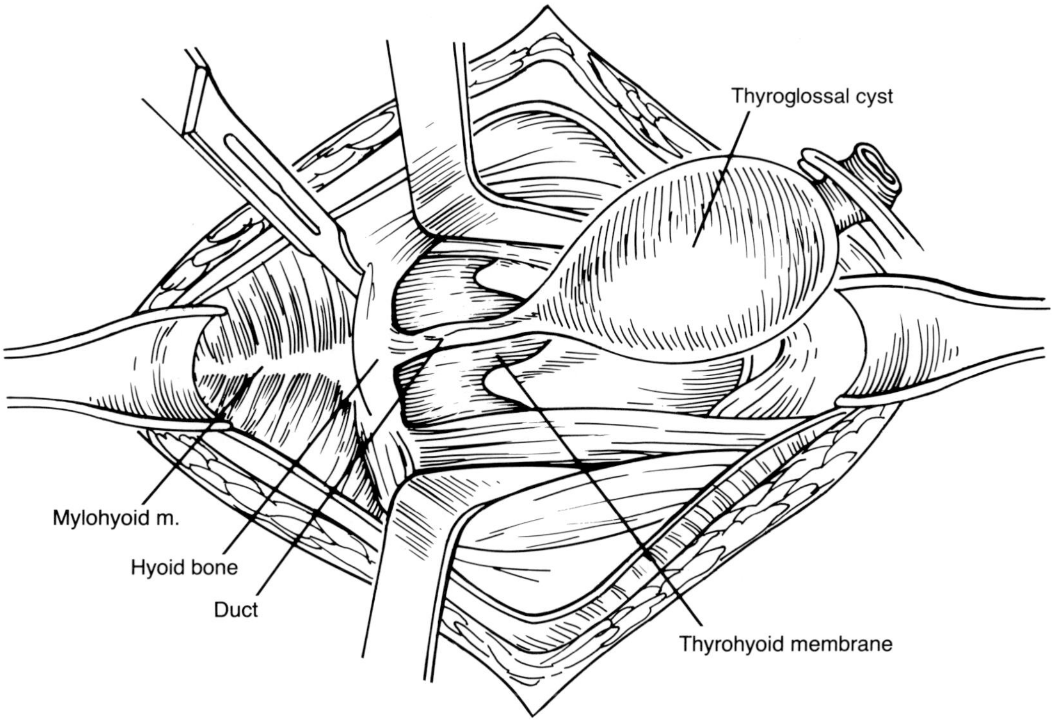

• FIGURE 24-2.

An incision is made along the superior border of the hyoid bone. (Redrawn from Loré JM: Atlas of Head and Neck Surgery, 3rd ed. Philadelphia, WB Saunders, 1988, p. 675.)

The laryngeal scissors are then used to resect the middle third of the hyoid bone and the cyst. An Allis clamp is used to put traction on the cyst and hyoid (Fig. 24–3).

At this point, using the nondominant hand and after double-gloving, the surgeon places a finger into the oral cavity and palpates the vallecula and the base of the tongue.

With an assistant holding the cyst and the hyoid bone, a core of muscular tissue with its apex at the base of the tongue is carefully excised. (It is not generally necessary to penetrate the mucosa [Fig. 24–4].)

Bleeding is controlled using the Bovie coagulator. Prior to removal of the surgeon's finger from the oral cavity, a suture of 3-0 chromic is used to close the muscles in the deep space. Further closure of dead space is accomplished using interrupted sutures of 3-0 chromic after adequate hemostasis has been obtained.

The strap muscles are replaced in their anatomic position, and a drain (generally a $\frac{1}{4}''$ Penrose drain) is placed into the wound prior to skin closure.

The skin is closed using 4-0 Vicryl sutures in the subcutaneous and subcuticular layers. A compressive dressing is applied, and the patient is awakened in the usual fashion.

Postoperative care

A drain is placed for 1 day postoperatively and a compressive dressing is applied. Patients may eat if they choose to do so, but discomfort is common and may prevent eating a normal diet for 24 to 48 hours.

CYSTIC HYGROMA

A soft, doughy mass usually presents at birth 50% of the time and is present by 3 years of age 80% of the time. There is an equal incidence among males and females.

Cystic hygroma and lymphangioma represent a spectrum of lymphatic malformations and are thought to arise from a common congenital blockage or arrest of normal development of the primordial lymph channels.

Both lesions are characterized by a heterogeneous collection of endothelially lined, thin-walled lymphatic cysts and channels that can vary in size from a few millimeters to more than 20 cm.

A widely accepted classification by Landing and Farber[1] categorizes these lesions according to the size of their vascular spaces:

- Lymphangiomas simplex consist of a capillary-like lymphatic vasculature.
- Cavernous lymphangiomas consist of dilated lymphatic channels with one or several endothelial layers (with or without an adventitial layer).
- Cystic hygromas or cystic lymphangiomas have large multiloculated cysts.

A cystic hygroma may increase rapidly in size owing to infection or trauma and, if in a suprahyoid location, may cause respiratory distress or feeding difficulties.

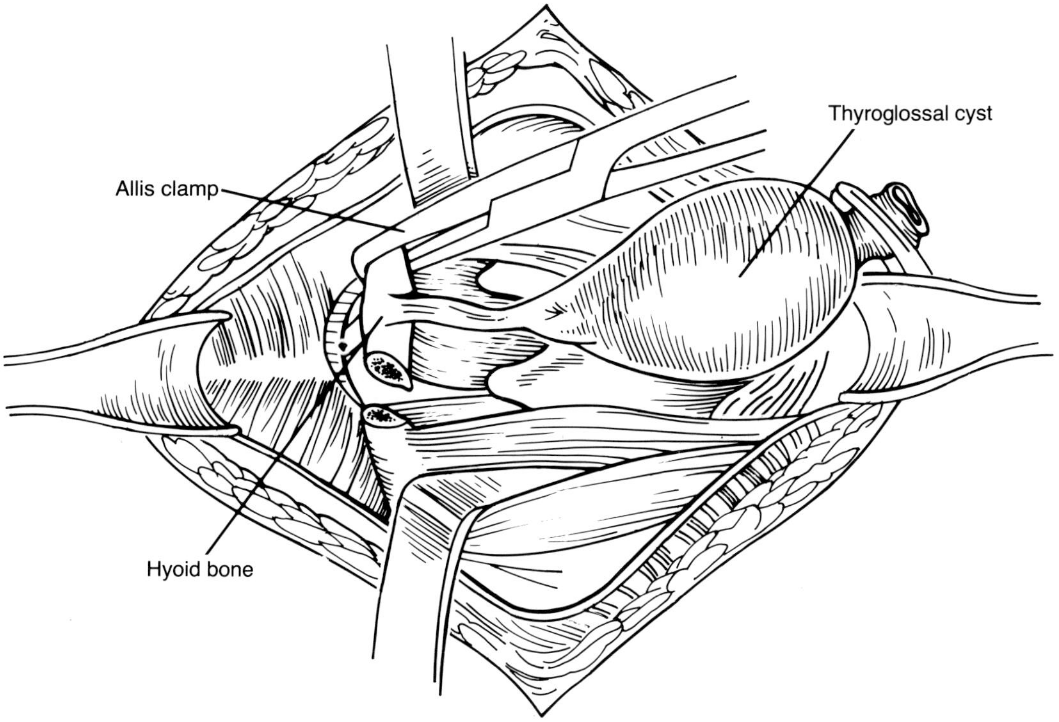

• FIGURE 24-3.

The hyoid bone is sectioned at each side with laryngeal scissors. (Redrawn from Loré JM: Atlas of Head and Neck Surgery, 3rd ed. Philadelphia, WB Saunders, 1988, p. 677.)

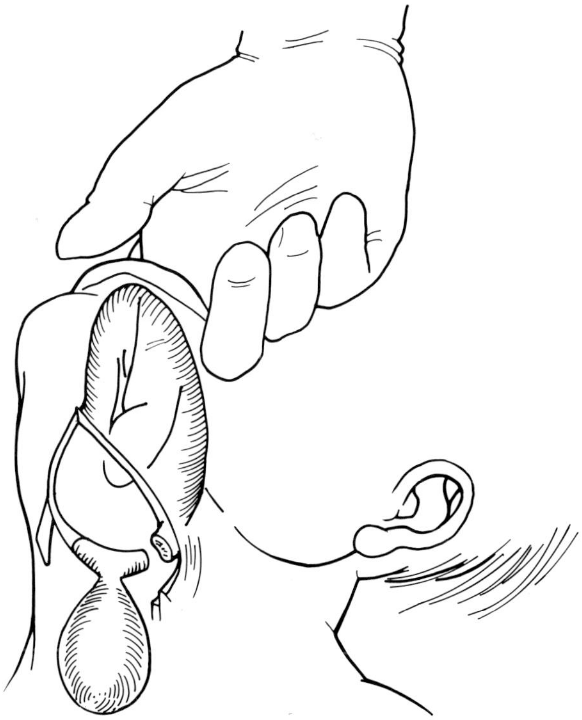

• FIGURE 24-4.

A finger is used to elevate a core of muscular tissue. (Redrawn from Rankow RM: An Atlas of Surgery of Face, Mouth and Neck. Philadelphia, WB Saunders, 1968, p. 207.)

Indications

- Nonregression
- Enlargement
- Pain
- Infection
- Airway or respiratory distress

Anesthetic considerations

Special instrumentation includes the use of a nerve stimulator. The anesthesiologist should not use paralyzing agents.

Preparation

Multiple site involvement in suprahyoid locations worsens the prognosis for one-stage uncomplicated removal. Timing for surgery should be based on the appearance of complications, or an elective excision should be performed when appropriate for the surgeon and the patient.

A preoperative evaluation should include a computed tomography (CT) or magnetic resonance imaging (MRI) scan. The addition of contrast to the CT examination is helpful to determine the vascular nature of the tumor. A preoperative work-up should also include a complete blood count (CBC) and a blood typing and cross-match.

Antibiotic prophylaxis that generally covers oral organisms should be administered prior to surgery. The patient's neck is generally extended and the head is rotated.

Procedure

- An attempt is made to remove the entire tumor and to preserve all normal and vital structures in a one-stage operation. The cystic hygroma is removed from the parotid anterior superior neck node chain and submandibular areas.

- An incision is planned to provide access for protection of nerves that run within the area to be dissected and to allow complete access to the tumor. The incision is created through the skin and subcutaneous tissues through the level of the platysma.

- A skin flap is elevated over the parotid gland and sternomastoid muscle using the Shaw knife (a Teflon-coated blade that uses heat but not electrical stimulation). The facial nerve is identified and dissected from the stylomastoid foramen in the usual fashion, with separation of the parotid from the cartridge of the ear and use of a neural stimulator to identify the facial nerve trunk.

- If a superficial parotidectomy is done, all branches of the facial nerve are dissected free; however, only the marginal branch and buccal branches are identified and dissected because of the extension of the tumor in this area.

• In a plane directed anterior to the sternomastoid muscle, the dissection is carried deep to the level of the vascular sheath, where the digastric muscle is identified directly lateral to the vascular sheath.

• The cystic hygroma often extends below the level of the digastric muscle; however, at this point, branches of the external carotid artery and the hypoglossal nerve are encountered and must be preserved.

• Once these structures have been identified, dissection proceeds from a lateral to a medial direction. The inferior limit of the tumor can be elevated superiorly to the residual specimen now based in the submandibular triangle.

• The facial artery where it enters the specimen is carefully identified, clamped, and suture-ligated. As the specimen is elevated along with the involved portion of submandibular gland, the glossopharyngeal nerve can be seen, and the lymphangioma is excised from the submandibular space.

• The dissection then proceeds anteriorly, with the marginal branch of the facial nerve elevated safely out of the way. The facial vein is ligated, and the gland and tumor are retracted inferiorly. The lesion's extension through the mylohyoid is carefully dissected free, again using the Shaw knife to eliminate any excessive bleeding. The submandibular duct is ligated using a right-angle clamp and a 3-0 chromic suture.

• The specimen is then passed from the field; the wound is copiously irrigated with saline; and the flaps are replaced in their anatomic position over a straight drainage using a $\frac{1}{4}''$ Penrose drain. A compressive dressing is applied after closure is obtained using subcuticular and subcutaneous stitches of 4-0 Vicryl. The patient is taken to the recovery room, where an evaluation of the facial nerve is undertaken.

Postoperative care

• Prolonged drainage is sometimes needed with a pressure dressing.

• If surgical extirpation has been done at a site where it is difficult to perform dressing changes, preoperative fitting of a Jobst dressing may be helpful to maintain pressure on clean dressings postoperatively.

• Owing to the interruption of lymphatics because of the congenital disorder, prolonged edema in superior or nearby structures (e.g., at the tongue, cheek, or lips) may occur.

• Antibiotics should be continued postoperatively.

Adjunctive treatments include the following:

• The laser, carbon dioxide to the intraoral involvement of the palate, tonsil, and mucosal surfaces.

• A partial glossectomy is done if the tongue is involved and is causing dentofacial abnormalities, airway distress, or difficulty with feeding.

• Antibiotics are administered intermittently for any swelling or bleeding that may occur.

FIRST BRANCHIAL CLEFT FISTULA

This cleft fistula is thought to represent a duplication of the external ear canal and is divided into types I and II by the classification of Work.[2]

It may present anywhere from anterior to the ear below the level of the tragus to the anterior cervical triangle, usually below the mandible. In some cases, the mass or fistula may be behind the ear. The cyst and fistula generally drain intermittently; however, a first branchial cleft cyst may also present as a simple mass without fistula formation or discharge. In some cases, abnormalities may be visualized in the external ear canal of the affected side.

Indications

- Surgical removal is indicated if there is drainage, swelling, or infection.

Anesthetic considerations

No paralysis can be induced because of the potential need for stimulation and identification of the facial nerve at the time of surgery.

Preparation

A CT scan should be performed, and the facial nerve injury should be discussed with the patient or parents. The patient's neck is extended and the head is rotated to the side opposite the fistula or first branchial cyst. The face and neck areas are draped in order to permit visualization of the eye and the corner of the mouth. A nerve integrity monitor can be placed for greater ease in identifying the facial nerve and its branches. Additional sterile drapings are applied to permit continued visualization of the face with a sterile field.

Procedure

During the surgery, the fistula may lead below the facial nerve to a cartilaginous tube that contains dermal elements. All must be excised. A superficial parotidectomy may be necessary to avoid injury to the nerve.

- A preauricular incision, extending behind the ear and incorporating the fistulous tract in the neck, is created. The flap is elevated in order to expose the parotid, and the fistulous tract is identified and dissected free from the surrounding tissue (Fig. 24–5*A*).

- As the dissection proceeds superiorly, identification of the facial nerve becomes mandatory. The facial nerve is identified in the standard fashion using the normal landmarks found in adults. In younger children, the nerve is located further laterally and, because the mastoid tip is not as well defined, the nerve can be approached sooner anatomically than might be expected (Fig. 24–5*B*).

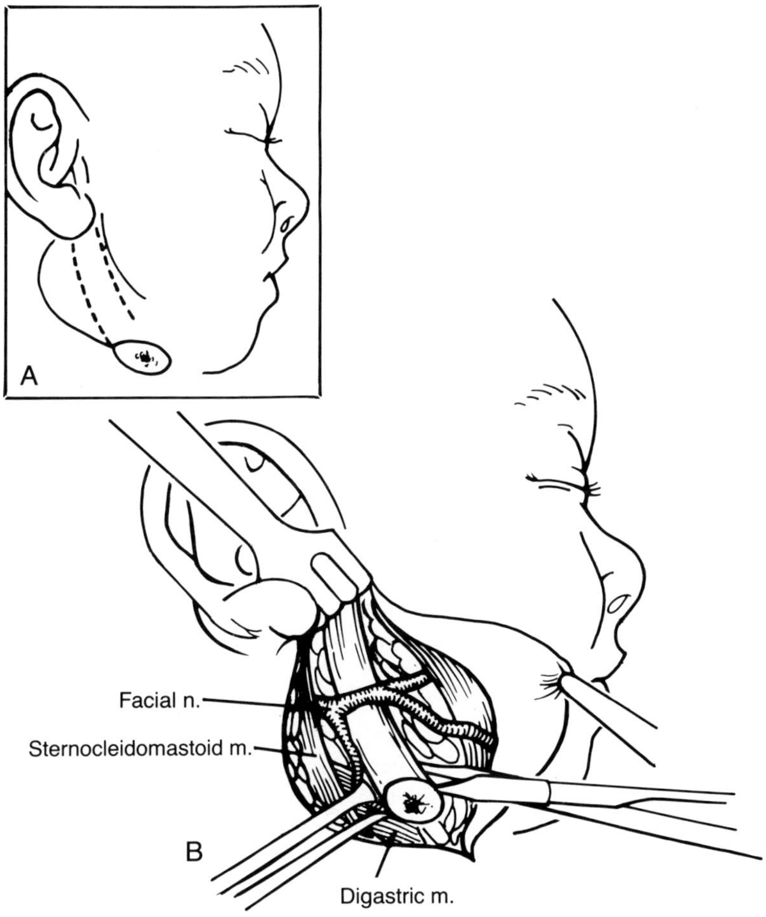

• FIGURE 24-5.

A, Incision site. *B*, Intraoperative view clearly showing the location of the facial nerve. (Redrawn from Orobello PW: Excision of first branchial cleft. *In* Johns ME, Price JC, and Mattox DE: Atlas of Head and Neck Surgery, Vol 1. St. Louis, Mosby-Year Book, 1990, p. 345.)

• After the facial nerve has been identified and the lower or marginal branch has been dissected free from the surrounding tissue, dissection along the fistulous area can be continued. The fistula usually passes medial to the facial nerve trunk and its branches, ending either directly in the external ear canal or within a duplicated cartilaginous structure next to the ear canal, which must be dissected free and excised. This excision, in some cases, leaves a small defect in the external canal that should be closed primarily.

• Copious irrigation of the wound is performed. A drain is placed, and the skin flaps are sutured in place using interrupted sutures of 4-0 Vicryl for the subcutaneous tissue and a fast-dissolving plain suture for the skin of the parotid incision.

In some cases, it may be necessary to do a complete superficial parotidectomy in order to identify and preserve all branches of the facial nerve if there is confusion with regard to their location. As the dissection proceeds deep to the facial nerve, superficial temporal vascular branches may be encountered and should be ligated.

• A compressive dressing is applied, and the patient is awakened and taken to the recovery room. The drain is generally left in place for 1 to 3 days, depending on the amount of drainage.

Postoperative care

• Postoperatively, a drain is placed through the face-lift type of incision.

SECOND AND THIRD BRANCHIAL CLEFT FISTULA

Branchial cleft abnormalities can exist as sinuses with no connection to the intraoral cavity, as fistulas that do connect, or as cysts that may connect to the skin or to the oral cavity. If the entity is familial, it can be associated with hearing loss, and an audiogram should be obtained preoperatively.

If the patient has draining sinuses or fistulas, it is probably advisable to perform the excision at an earlier age, when it can sometimes be done through a single incision. Because a pediatric patient's neck will elongate during growth, a stepladder incision is necessary in older children.

Second and third branchial cleft fistulas are differentiated by their course through the neck. The second cleft fistula traverses between the external and internal branches of the carotid artery and over the ninth cranial nerve. The third branchial fistula loops over the hypoglossal nerve, runs downward and medial to the carotid arteries, and pierces the thyrohyoid membrane near the pyriform sinus. The superior laryngeal nerve and hypoglossal nerve are sometimes encountered in the dissection.

The existence and pathway of a fourth branchial cleft is controversial, but such a cleft may be manifested by thyroiditis and a pit at the apex of the pyriform sinus. The exact tract is unknown, but excision of the thyroid and the pit seem necessary to cure these patients.

Indications

- A draining pit or fistula in the anterior triangle of the neck
- Infection within the fistulous tract
- A mass in the anterior cervical triangle

Preparation

- The endotracheal tube must be well secured because, in some cases, these fistulas may be bilateral, and some rotation of the head is necessary during the course of surgical dissection.
- No paralysis should be induced in case neurostimulators are required.
- Lacrimal probes should be present on the surgical set.
- The patient's neck is generally extended.
- The neck is draped from the clavicle to the chin.
- If the patient has an infection, antibiotics are given preoperatively.

Procedure

- A lacrimal probe is placed within the fistulous tract as far as it will easily pass, and an elliptical incision is made along skin tension lines surrounding the fistula.
- Using sharp dissection, the tract is pulled away from the surrounding tissue and is dissected free from the attaching muscle fibers.

- Using Ragnell retractors, exposure of the deepest part of the fistula tract is permitted unless the patient has an excessively long tract that would require a second or stepladder incision. This second, more cranially placed incision is created by passage of a hemostat along the dissected fistulous tract to its most distal point; a small skin incision is made, and the fistula is brought out through the skin incision. Dissection is continued further by sharp dissection, and a right-angle clamp is placed at the fistula's entrance to the mucosa (Fig. 24–6).

- A suture, generally a 3-0 chromic, is placed around the stump of the fistula and is tied when the fistula has been excised. Owing to the limited nature of the dissection, no drains are placed. The incisions are closed using subcutaneous and subcuticular Vicryl sutures. A light compressive dressing is applied. No special precautions are indicated or needed. The patient can usually be discharged on the same day, unless an extensive dissection has been performed.

Postoperative care

Postoperative care consists of a compressive dressing. Generally, if the dissection has gone smoothly, no drains are necessary because the dissection is limited.

TORTICOLLIS

Fibromatosis colli is thought to represent an injury to the sternomastoid muscle, incurred either in utero or during delivery. The deformity is usually noted at birth or within the first 10 days of life.

A firm mass becomes palpable in the muscle and progresses to a maximal size (e.g., 1 to 3 cm), generally within 1 month of its appearance. The head is usually tilted toward the side of the shortened muscle, and the chin rotates toward the opposite (normal) side.

If left untreated, the condition may cause developmental asymmetry of the face and ocular imbalance. Conservative management, which consists of range of motion exercises, is generally successful in resolving the problem; however, surgery may be necessary in rare cases.

Other evidence of injury should be looked for, such as a fracture of the clavicle or a cervical spine injury or abnormality.

Indications

- A mass within the body of the sternomastoid muscle that does not resolve with aggressive physical therapy

Anesthetic considerations

Surgical procedures are performed under general endotracheal anesthesia.

Preparation

- The patient's neck is extended, and the head is rotated away from the side of the torticollis to make the mass as prominent as possible.

- The neck is prepared from the clavicle to the chin.

• FIGURE 24-6.

A step-ladder incision is created by passing a hemostat along the dissected fistula tract. (Redrawn from Loré JM: An Atlas of Head and Neck Surgery, 3rd ed. Philadelphia, WB Saunders, 1988, p. 693.)

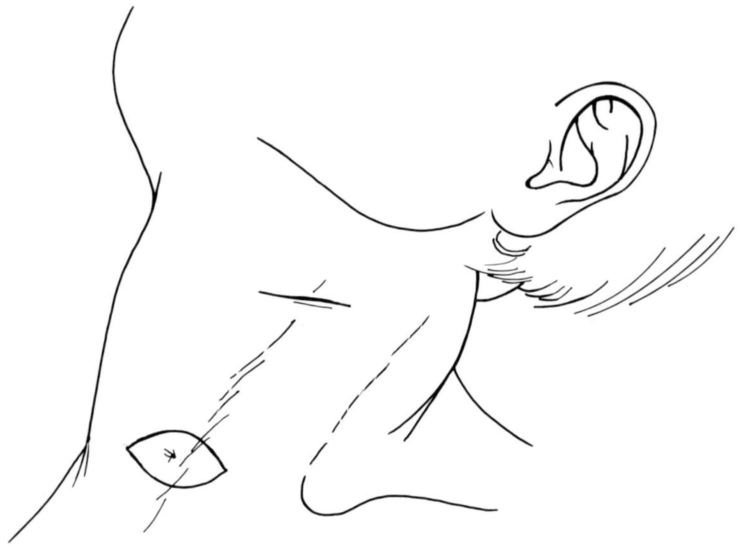

Procedure

- A horizontal incision is created over the mass and is carried through the skin's subcutaneous tissue. If appropriate, preservation of the greater auricular nerve is indicated.
- The mass can generally be separated from normal muscle fiber with preservation of the portion of the sternomastoid muscle that is not involved with the fibrosis. Preservation of the accessory branch to the sternomastoid muscle is also indicated.
- The incision is closed immediately in the standard fashion.

Postoperative care

- In the first day postoperatively, the patient performs range of motion exercises to maintain the release that has been surgically created.

REFERENCES

1. Landing BH and Farber S: Function of the cardiovascular system. *In* Atlas of Tumor Pathology. Washington, DC, Armed Forces Institute of Pathology, 1956.
2. Work WP: Newer concepts of first branchial cleft defects. Laryngoscope 82:1581–1593, 1972.

BIBLIOGRAPHY

Bill AH and Sumner DS: A unified concept of lymphangioma and cystic hygroma. Surg Gynecol Obstet 120:79–86, 1965.

Farrior JB and Santini H: Facial nerve identification in children. Otolaryngol Head Neck Surg 93:173–176, 1985.

Gonzales J, Ljung BM, Guerry T, and Schoenrock L: Congenital torticollis: Evaluation by fine-needle aspiration biopsy. Laryngoscope 99:651–654, 1989.

Hoffman MA and Schuster SR: Thyroglossal duct remnants in infants and children: Reevaluation of histopathology and methods for resection. Ann Otol Rhinol Laryngol 97:483–486, 1988.

Howie AJ and Proops DW: The definition of branchial cysts, sinuses and fistulae. Clin Otolaryngol 7:51–57, 1982.

Karmody CS: Developmental anomalies of the neck. *In* Bluestone CD and Stool SE (eds): Pediatric Otolaryngology, Vol II. Philadelphia, WB Saunders, 1983, pp 1386–1401.

Kennedy TL: Cystic hygroma-lymphangioma: A rare and still unclear entity. Laryngoscope 99(Suppl):1–10, 1989.

May J and D'Angelo AJ Jr.: The facial nerve and the branchial cleft surgical challenge. Laryngoscope 99:564–565, 1989.

Mickel RA and Calcaterra TC: Management of recurrent thyroglossal duct cysts. Arch Otolaryngol Head Neck Surg 109:34–36, 1983.

Mulliken JB and Young AE: Lymphatic malformations. *In* Vascular Birthmarks, Hemangiomas, and Malformations. Philadelphia, WB Saunders, 1988.

Ricciardelli EJ and Richardson MA: Cervicofacial cystic hygroma: Patterns of recurrence and management of the difficult case. Arch Otolaryngol Head Neck Surg 117:546–553, 1991.

Sedwick CE and Walsh JF: Branchial cysts and fistulas: A study of seventy-five cases relative to clinical aspects and treatment. Am J Surg 83:3–8, 1952.

Simpson RA: Lateral cervical cysts and fistulas. Laryngoscope 79:30–58, 1969.

Sistrunk WE: The surgical treatment of cysts of the thyroglossal tract. Ann Surg 71:121–124, 1920.

Tom LWC, Handler DS, Wetmore RF, and Potsic WP: The sternocleidomastoid tumor of infancy. Pediatr Otorhinolaryngol 13:245–255, 1987.

Tom LW, Rossiter JL, Sutton LN, et al: Torticollis in children. Otolaryngol Head Neck Surg 105:1–5, 1991.

chapter

25

Tumors of the Head and Neck

MICHAEL J. CUNNINGHAM, M.D.

PERCUTANEOUS NEEDLE BIOPSY

Percutaneous needle biopsy may be used in the evaluation of both cystic and solid childhood head and neck masses. A close working relationship between the surgeon and pathologist is essential for the technique to succeed. The principal role of percutaneous needle biopsy as a diagnostic tool is to determine whether the mass is benign or malignant. In the hands of an experienced cytopathologist, aspiration biopsy can also be highly accurate in predicting the specific type of tumor.

Sampling errors do occur, and a negative finding on a percutaneous needle biopsy should never be considered definitive when there is clinical suspicion of malignancy. A subsequent open surgical biopsy is necessary under such circumstances.

Indications

- Head and neck lesions in which a preliminary histopathologic diagnosis better selects or modifies future operative intervention
- The diagnosis of inflammatory or cystic lesions that may not require additional surgery
- The diagnosis of clinically unresectable lesions

Anesthetic considerations

In the older pediatric and adolescent population, needle biopsy of superficial cervical lesions can be performed under local anesthesia using 1 or 2% lidocaine and 1:100,000 epinephrine solution. General anesthesia is often used for infants and young children. The need for a concomitant endoscopic evaluation of the aerodigestive tract or the biopsy of deep cervical lesions under radiologic guidance may also require general anesthesia, regardless of age.

Preparation

- Percutaneous needle biopsy can be performed by either large-bore or fine-needle aspiration (FNA) technique.
- Large-bore needles provide core tissue fragments from which fixed sections for histopathologic examination can be obtained. The Vim-Silverman (12-gauge) needle (Fig. 25–1*A*) and the disposable Tru-Cut (14-gauge) biopsy needle (Fig. 25–1*B*) are used for such purposes.
- The FNA technique uses much smaller 22- to 25-gauge needles of $1\frac{1}{2}$ to $3\frac{1}{2}$ inches in length, depending on the depth of the lesion (Fig. 25–1*C*).
- Needles of 18- to 20-gauge diameter may be necessary for the aspiration of cystic lesions containing thick, mucoid material.
- The child is positioned and draped such that the proposed biopsy site is readily available to the surgeon, and the surrounding anatomic landmarks can be easily visualized (Fig. 25–2).

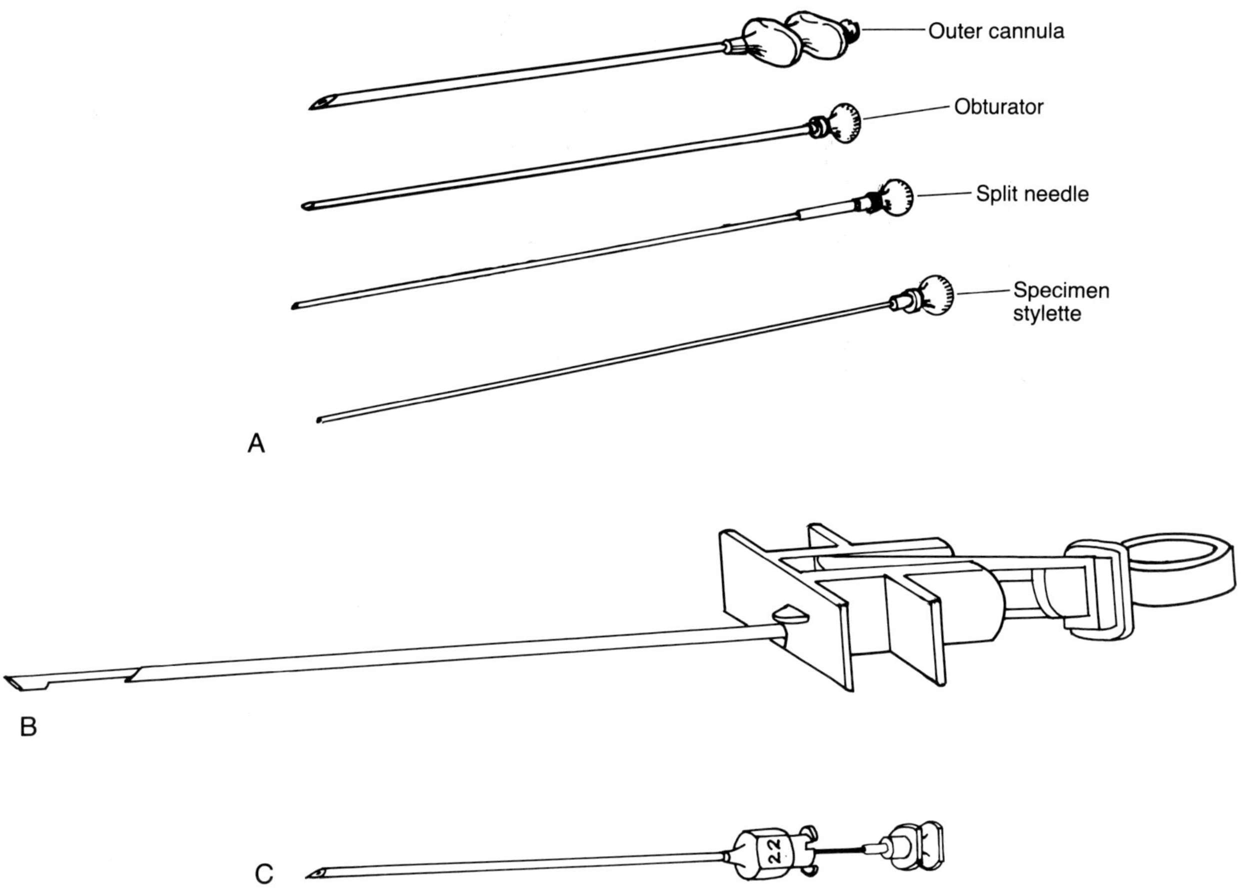

• **FIGURE 25-1.**

A, Vim-Silverman (12-gauge) needle. *B*, Tru-Cut biopsy needle. *C*, 22-gauge $3\frac{1}{2}''$ needle.

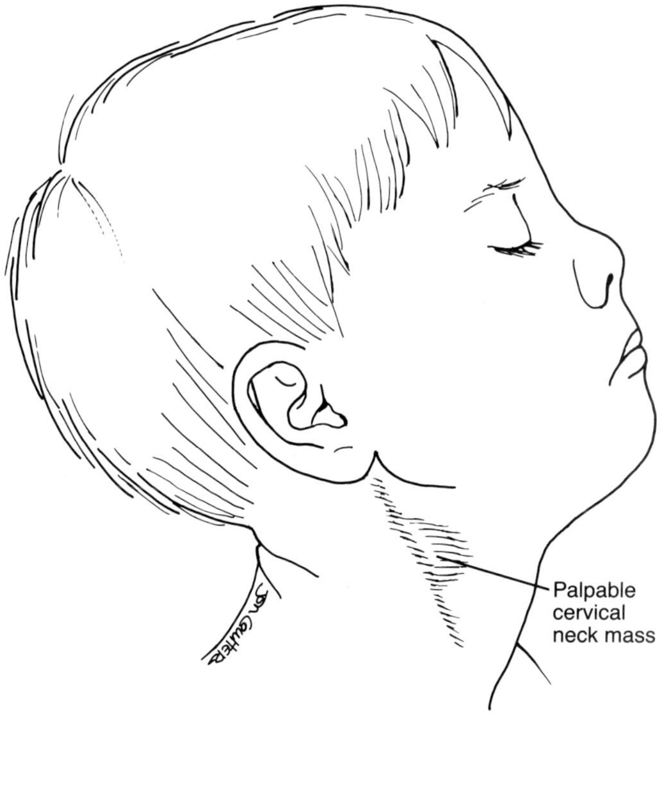

• **FIGURE 25-2.**

The patient is positioned so that the biopsy site is easily accessible to the surgeon.

Procedure

- If only local anesthesia is planned, the anesthetic solution is infiltrated into the skin over the planned biopsy tract; this step is not necessary when the procedure is being performed under general anesthesia.

- In the case of a superficial lesion, the mass is stabilized with the thumb and the index finger of the opposite hand (Fig. 25–3). In deep cervical lesions, either specific measurements for needle localization and depth placement should have been preoperatively calculated from radiologic studies, or the biopsy should be performed under radiologic guidance.

- In large-bore needle biopsy, a 1- to 2-mm skin incision is made with a No. 11 scalpel blade prior to needle insertion (Fig. 25–4). The biopsy technique does vary with the type of large-bore needle used; the Tru-Cut needle, for example, comes with its own specific instructions. In general, the needle is advanced into the mass using a smooth, rapid motion. At least two passes are recommended; the second biopsy attempt should be made through the same incision but at a different angle. The specimens obtained are expelled onto filter paper and placed into saline, formalin fixative, or another special medium, depending on the suspected pathology.

- In FNA technique, no skin incision is necessary. The needle chosen is attached to a 20-ml syringe and syringe holder. A constant vacuum is applied while the needle is passed at least twice at different angles into the mass (Fig. 25–5). The vacuum is then released slowly to avoid aspiration of material into the syringe. The needle is withdrawn. The syringe is separated from the needle, filled with air, and reattached. The material within the needle is then expelled onto glass slides, spread over a small area, and quickly air-dried. Ideally, such slides are passed immediately to the pathologist. In the absence of a readily available pathology consultation, such slides can be immediately fixed by placement in 95% alcohol solution. Lymph node aspirates should additionally be placed into saline or special cell culture media for lymphocyte marker analysis.

- Pressure is immediately applied to the biopsy site. After an FNA procedure, a plastic adhesive bandage dressing usually suffices. A small pressure dressing may be necessary after a large-bore needle biopsy.

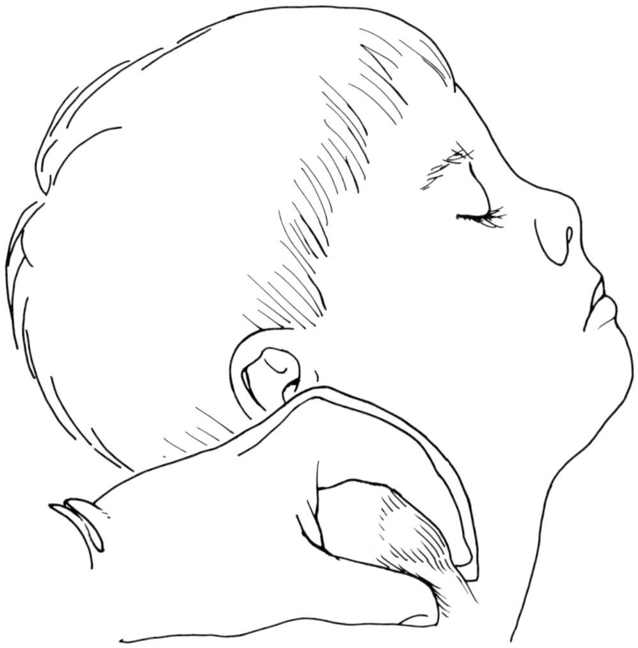

• FIGURE 25–3.

Superficial lesions can be stabilized with the thumb and index finger.

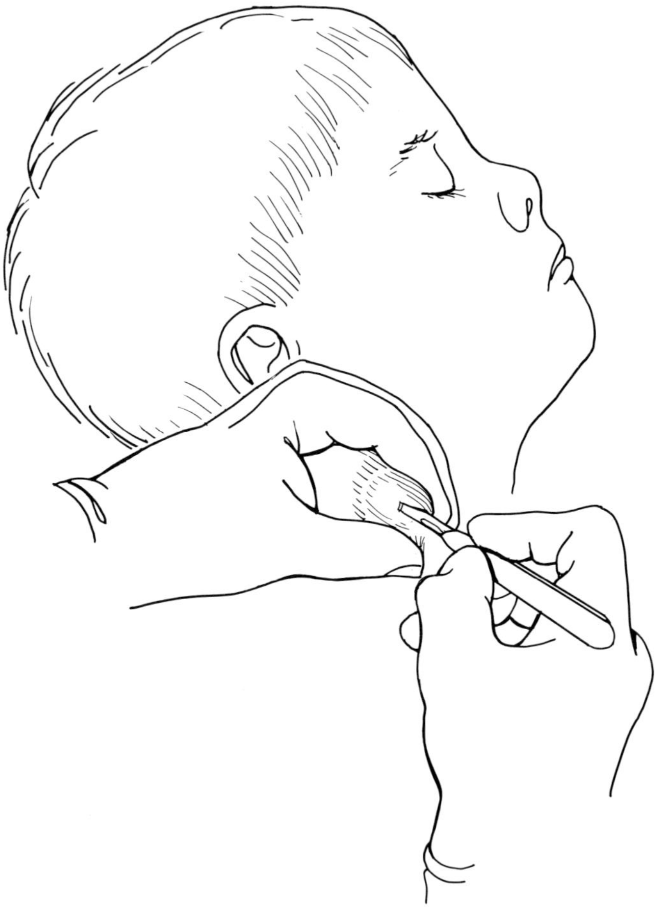

• FIGURE 25-4.

A large-bore needle biopsy requires that a 1- to 2-mm skin incision be made prior to needle insertion.

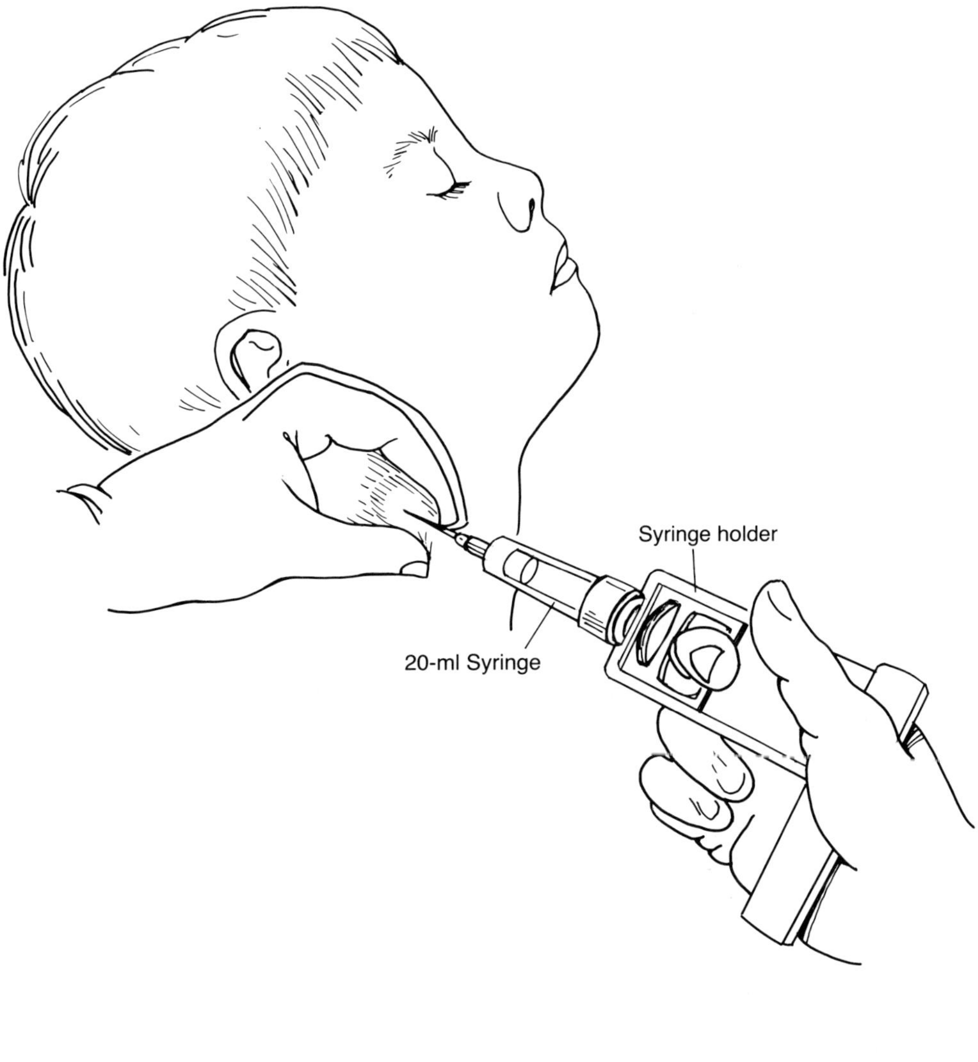

• FIGURE 25-5.

Fine-needle aspiration technique is shown.

Postoperative care

- The potential dissemination of malignancy from mechanical trauma is a major concern in large-bore needle biopsy. This implantation problem has theoretically been eliminated by the FNA technique.
- Bleeding with hematoma formation is a potential complication, particularly in the biopsy of vascular masses or in patients with underlying clotting defects. This risk has been reduced by using the FNA technique.
- There are additional site-specific risks, such as pneumothorax in the biopsy of supraclavicular masses.

CERVICAL LYMPH NODE BIOPSY

In adults, open lymph node biopsy is strongly contraindicated due to the high likelihood of metastatic carcinoma. Cervical nodal biopsy is much more frequently performed in children and adolescents due to the relatively higher incidence of chronic inflammatory or infectious disorders and lymphomatous malignancies in this age group. Excisional biopsy is favored. Incisional biopsy is reserved for clinically unresectable lesions.

Specific characteristics of a cervical neck mass in the pediatric population suggest the need for a thorough diagnostic evaluation, including endoscopic examination of the aerodigestive tract and a potential biopsy. The anatomic patterns of cervical lymph node drainage are an aid in locating primary aerodigestive tract lesions that otherwise might be undetected. Details of these drainage patterns are not covered in this chapter. In brief, the preauricular parotid nodes relate to the parotid gland, scalp, and periorbital tissues; the jugulodigastric nodes relate to the tonsil, gingivae, pharynx, mouth, and larynx; the submental nodes relate to the lips and anterior of the mouth; the submandibular nodes relate to the buccal mucosa, anterior of the mouth, and submandibular gland; the spinal accessory nodes relate to the posterior scalp and nasopharynx; and the lower cervical chain relates to the thyroid, upper esophagus, and infraclavicular structures.

Indications

A firm cervical neck mass with any of the following characteristics:

- Greater than 3 mm in diameter
- A history of rapid or progressive noninflammatory growth
- Fixation to underlying tissues or overlying skin ulceration
- A supraclavicular location
- Clinical presentation suggestive of malignancy

Anesthetic considerations

The procedure is performed under general anesthesia.

Preparation

- Preoperative consideration should be given to performing solely a diagnostic nodal biopsy as opposed to a biopsy with frozen-section histopathologic assessment and the possibility of cervical neck dissection.
- A preoperative pathology consultation is also important in suspected lymphoma cases.
- The child is positioned and draped such that the mass and the surrounding anatomic landmarks can be easily visualized.

Procedure

• The incision is outlined in a cervical skin crease near the mass (Fig. 25–6). Infiltration of the incision with 1% lidocaine with 1:100,000 epinephrine solution provides hemostasis.

• The skin, subcutaneous tissues, and platysma muscle are transected down to the level of the superficial layer of the deep cervical fascia (Fig. 25–7). Knowledge of the regional anatomy is necessary.

• The mass should be carefully delineated before being removed (Fig. 25–8). If feasible, the entire mass or the largest of multiple masses should be removed to maximize the chances of obtaining a successful histopathologic diagnosis. Frozen-section examination is requested when appropriate. Microbiology specimens should also be sent routinely for examination.

• After irrigation and hemostasis, the placement of a small Penrose drain may be necessary when extensive or deep dissection was required. Closure is performed in two layers using interrupted absorbable sutures for platysma muscle and subcutaneous tissue approximation and either interrupted or a single subcuticular nylon suture in the skin (Fig. 25–9). The application of a pressure dressing completes the procedure.

Postoperative care

• Hemorrhage with secondary hematoma or seroma formation reflects inadequate hemostasis or drainage.

• Additional postoperative sequelae relate to the specific biopsy site. Particular care is necessary in the vicinity of the tail of the parotid or the submandibular triangle, and in the posterior triangle of the neck, to avoid potential injury to the facial nerve and spinal accessory nerve, respectively.

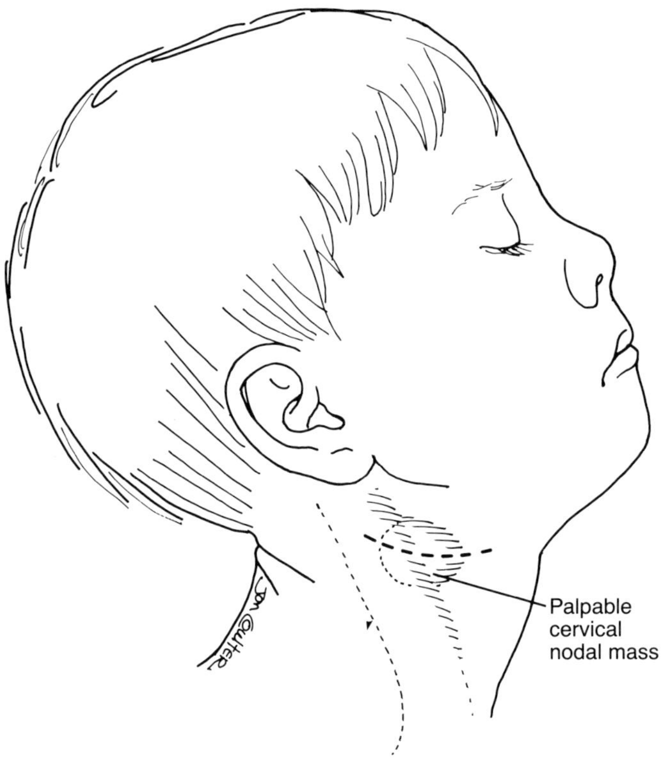

• FIGURE 25–6.

The incision is outlined in a cervical skin crease.

• FIGURE 25-7.

The mass beneath the superficial layer of the deep cervical fascia.

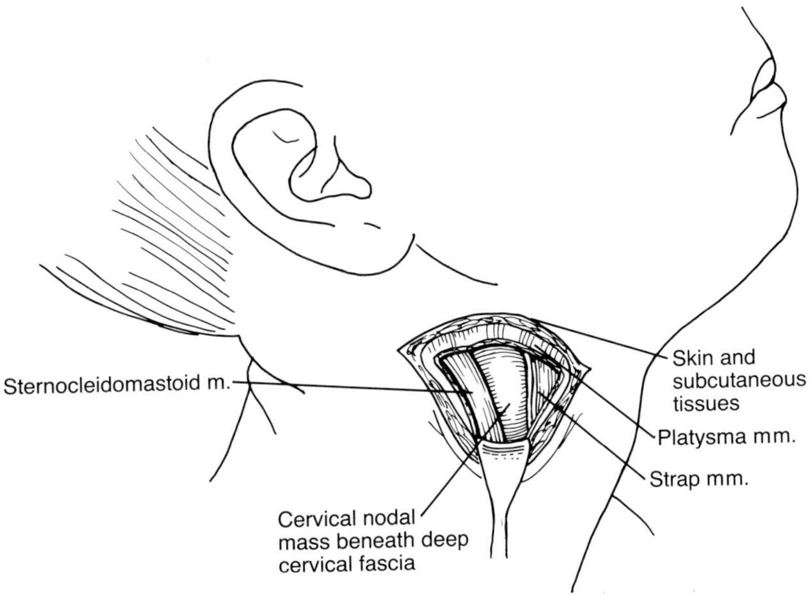

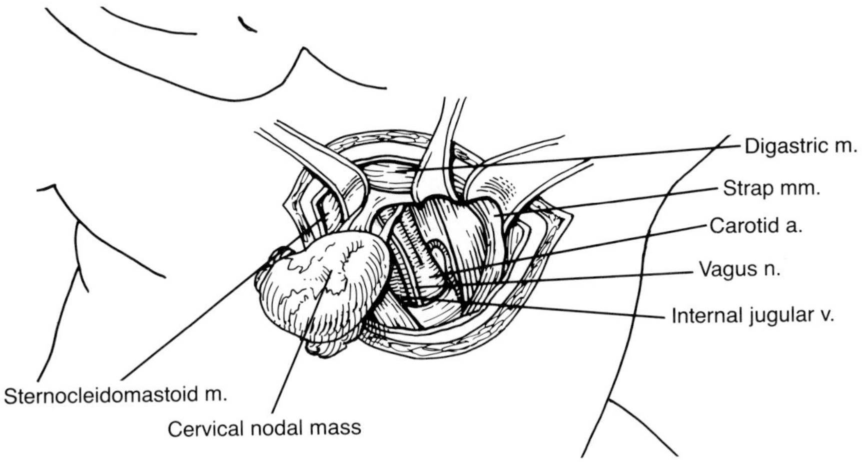

• FIGURE 25-8.

Removal of the cervical nodal mass.

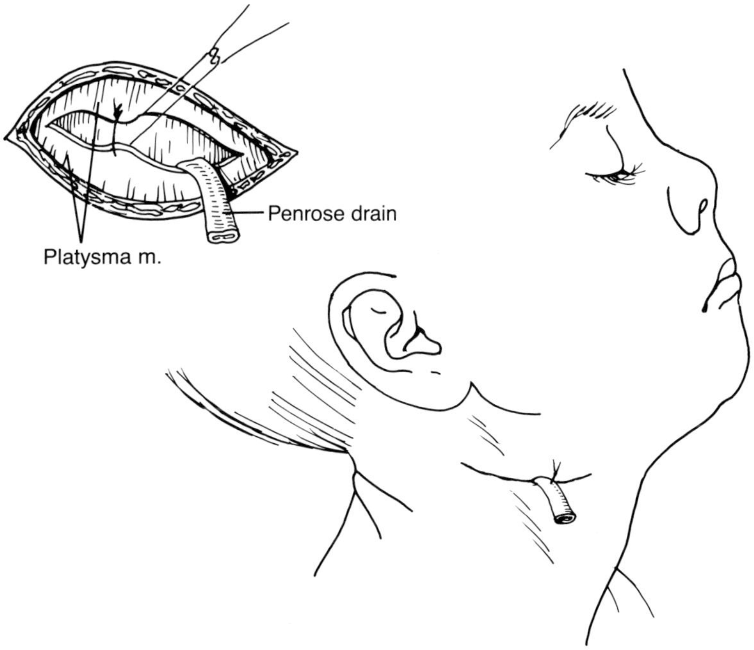

• FIGURE 25-9.

The incision is closed after placement of a small Penrose drain.

SUPERFICIAL AND TOTAL PAROTIDECTOMY

During childhood, the parotid glands and paraparotid lymph nodes are subject to various infectious and inflammatory and neoplastic conditions that can produce a solid mass in the parotid region. In contrast to the softer and often clinically apparent vasoformative and congenital cystic lesions, many of the chronic inflammatory processes present as indolent, firm masses indistinguishable from common benign and malignant pediatric parotid neoplasms. Laboratory evaluation, including serologic studies, skin tests, and various radiologic imaging techniques (e.g., contrast sialography, ultrasound, computed tomography, and magnetic resonance imaging), may suggest but typically cannot confirm the specific underlying disease process.

FNA biopsy has a limited role in the diagnosis of solid parotid lesions in the pediatric population. If the child's age necessitates general anesthesia for the performance of needle biopsy, the more detailed histopathologic examination afforded by excisional biopsy is appropriate. More important, the definitive treatment of many of the inflammatory as well as neoplastic causes of solid parotid masses in children is surgical excision. Excisional biopsy, by means of superficial parotidectomy, proves to be therapeutic as well as diagnostic in such cases.

As in adults, neither incisional biopsy nor the isolated enucleation of parotid lesions is recommended. Total parotidectomy rarely proves necessary in the pediatric population.

Indications

- Solid parotid mass of unknown or uncertain etiology
- Chronic recurrent parotitis
- First and second branchial system anomalies
- Vasoformative lesions

Anesthetic considerations

The procedure is performed under general anesthesia.

Preparation

- Informed consent regarding the risk of facial nerve injury is an absolute necessity.

- The child is positioned supine with the head turned toward the uninvolved side. The operative field is draped with sterile, transparent plastic sheeting to provide exposure of the entire face on the involved side, including the corners of the eye and mouth (Fig. 25–10). This allows for the intraoperative assessment of facial nerve function.

• FIGURE 25-10.

The patient is positioned so that facial nerve function can be assessed.

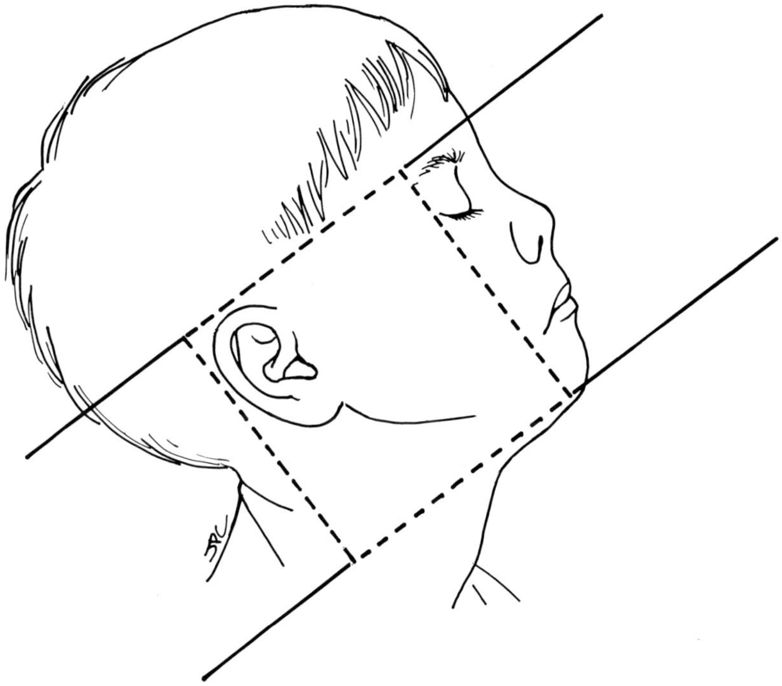

Procedure

- Typically in older children and adolescents, an S-shaped incision is used (Fig. 25–11*A*). This incision begins in the preauricular crease and extends in curvilinear fashion within a natural skin crease, approximately two fingerbreadths below the angle of the jaw. A Y-shaped incision with a retroauricular extension is an alternative approach (Fig. 25–11*B*). In the infant or very young child, the use of a single, curved incision, beginning 1.5 to 2 cm below the mandible and extending posterosuperiorly over the mastoid prominence reportedly protects the superficially located facial nerve trunk in this age group (Fig. 25–11*C*).
- Infiltration of the planned incision with 1% lidocaine and 1:100,000 epinephrine solution provides local hemostasis.

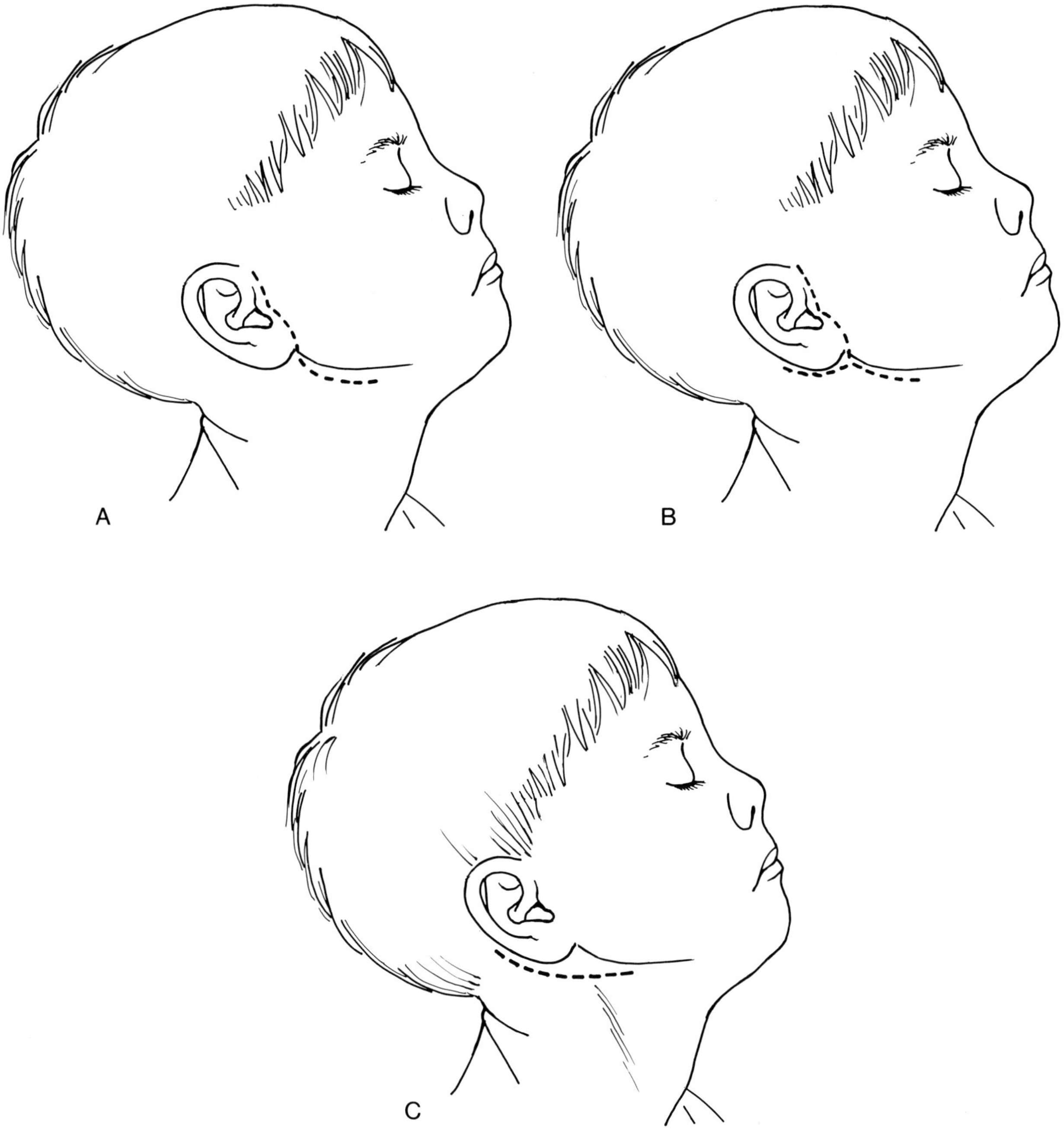

• **FIGURE 25-11.**

A, An S-shaped incision is used for older children and adolescents. *B*, A Y-shaped incision with a retroauricular extension. *C*, A single curved incision of potential use in infants or small children.

• An anterior skin flap is elevated. The plane of dissection is deep to the subcutaneous tissues and superficial to the investing fascia of the parotid gland. This dissection ends at the parotid gland's anterior border in order to avoid inadvertent transection of small facial nerve branches emerging from the gland over the masseter muscle (Fig. 25–12).

• Flap dissection is also carried in a posteroinferior direction in the subplatysmal plane until the anterior border of the sternocleidomastoid muscle is clearly identified (see Fig. 25–12). Care is particularly necessary in infants and young children because limited posterior development of the parotid gland may result in exposure of a large portion of the facial nerve (Fig. 25–13). In older children, the tail of the parotid gland often needs to be separated from the sternocleidomastoid muscle. Both the greater auricular nerve and the posterior facial (retromandibular) vein are typically encountered and need to be sacrificed for gland retraction and exposure.

• Using both superior traction on the earlobe and anterior traction on the parotid gland, blunt dissection along the tragal cartilage and adjacent mastoid bone allows separation of the small fibrous septa that attach the posterior border of the parotid gland to these structures (Fig. 25–14). The goal of progressive medial dissection in this fashion is to identify the main trunk of the facial nerve as it emerges from the stylomastoid foramen. In older children and adolescents, the location of the facial nerve can be anticipated approximately halfway between the tip of the mastoid process and a triangular extension of the cartilaginous external ear canal, the so-called pointer. Immediately before the facial nerve, the temporoparotid fascia often arises from the tympanomastoid fissure as a firm band extending into the parotid gland. Conservative use of the nerve stimulator during this portion of the procedure helps to distinguish fascia from nerve. Hemostasis is crucial for visualization purposes; bipolar cauterization in a moist field is advocated to decrease the likelihood of cautery-induced neural damage.

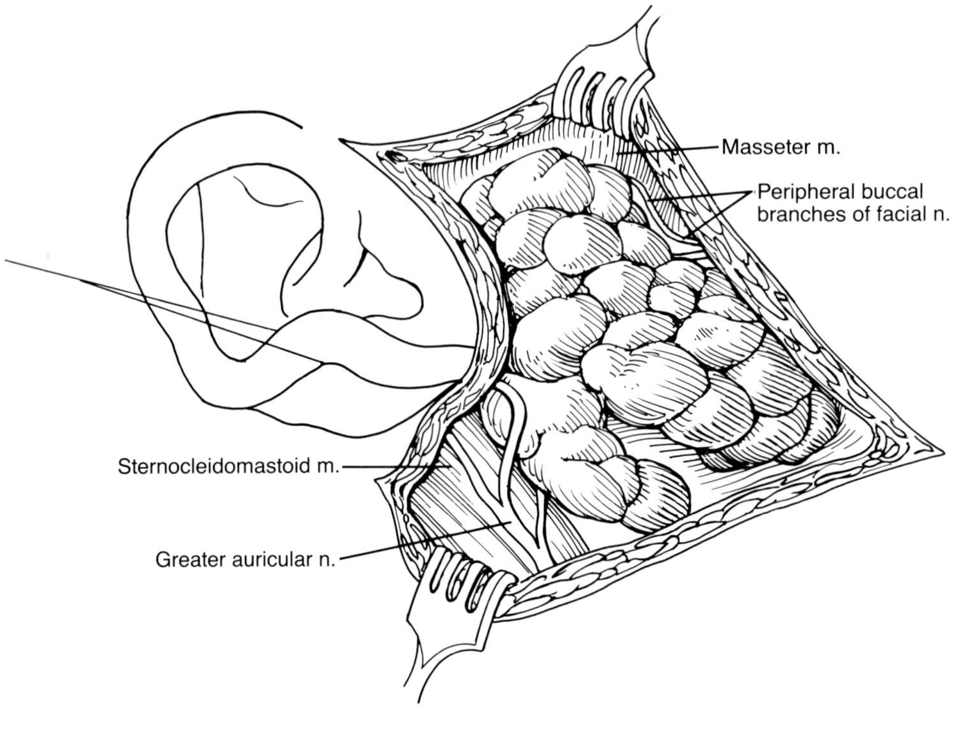

• FIGURE 25–12.

Elevation of the anterior flap.

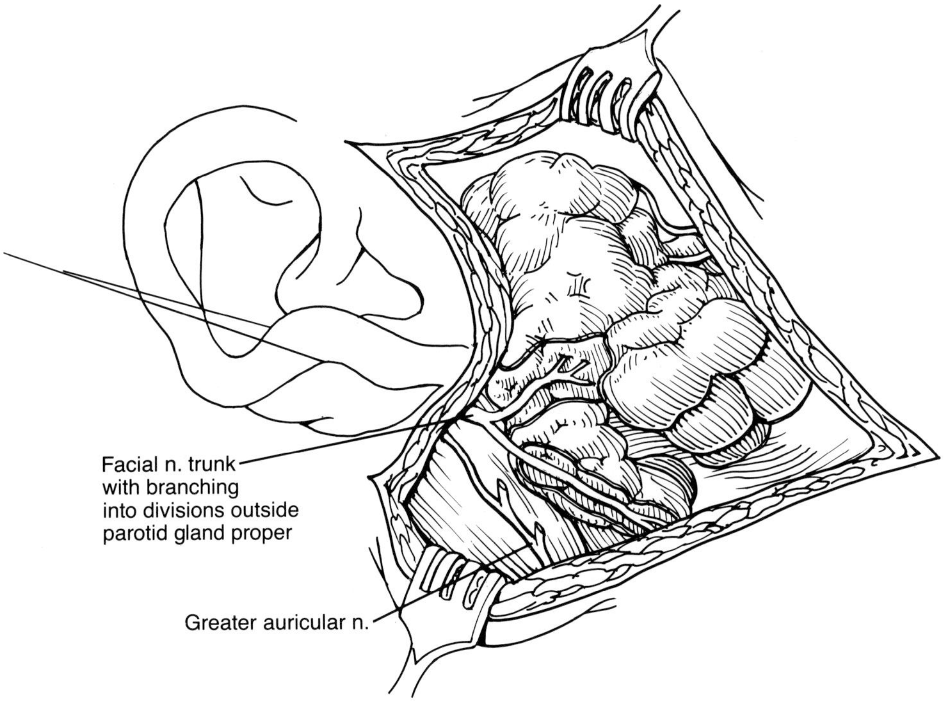

• FIGURE 25-13.

A large portion of the facial nerve may be exposed in younger children due to limited parotid gland development. (Modified from Welch KJ, Randolph JC [eds]: Pediatric Surgery, Vol. I. Chicago, Year Book Medical Publishers, 1986, p 500.)

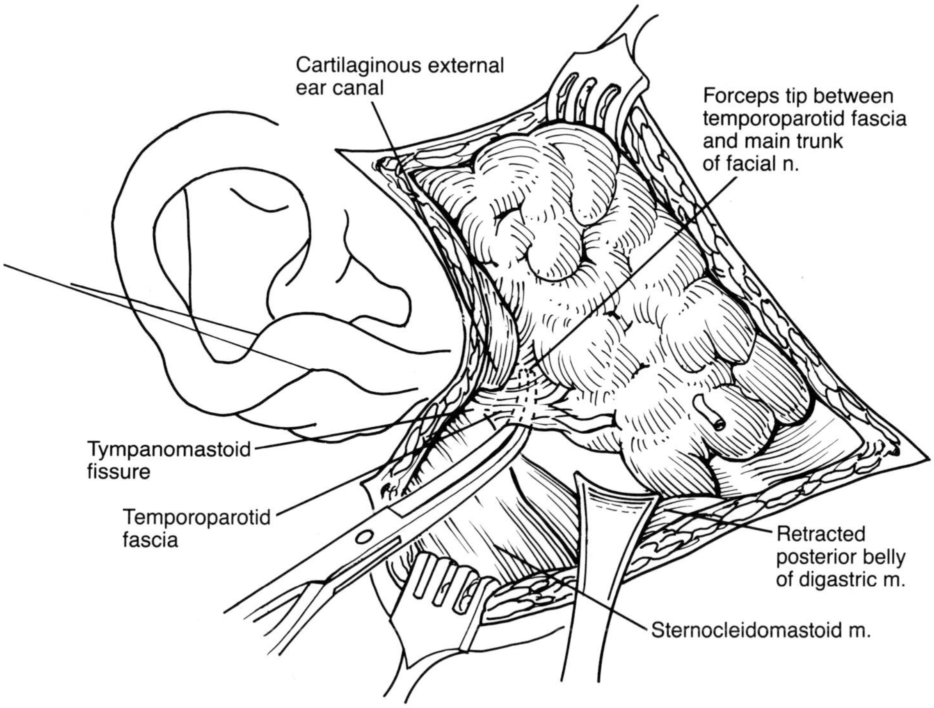

• FIGURE 25-14.

Separation of the small fibrous septa in this manner allows the main trunk of the facial nerve to be identified. (Modified from Welch KJ, Randolph JC [eds]: Pediatric Surgery, Vol. I. Chicago, Year Book Medical Publishers, 1986, p 500.)

- In infants and young children, limited mastoid development results in less well-defined bony landmarks for facial nerve identification (Fig. 25–15). In addition, some of the inflammatory conditions necessitating parotidectomy in children pathologically involve the external auditory canal, creating scarring in this region and placing the main trunk of the facial nerve in further jeopardy. An alternative method of finding the facial nerve in such circumstances is to follow the anterior border of the sternocleidomastoid muscle superiorly to its temporal bone insertion and to locate the posterior belly of the digastric muscle just deep to this insertion site. Using blunt dissection and working anteriorly, the facial nerve trunk can typically be found within the triangle formed by these two muscles and the cartilaginous ear canal (Fig. 25–16).

- In revision surgical procedures with extensive cervical scarring, an alternative approach is to use the retroauricular extension of a Y-shaped skin incision (see Fig. 25–11*B*). A limited mastoidectomy is then performed to provide access to the facial nerve in the descending portion of the fallopian canal prior to its skull base exit.

- Once the main trunk of the facial nerve is clearly identified, it is followed anteriorly to the pes anserinus. In adolescents and older children, this requires dissection into the parotid gland. In infants, the pes may actually be in the retromandibular region outside of the parotid gland proper (see Fig. 25–13).

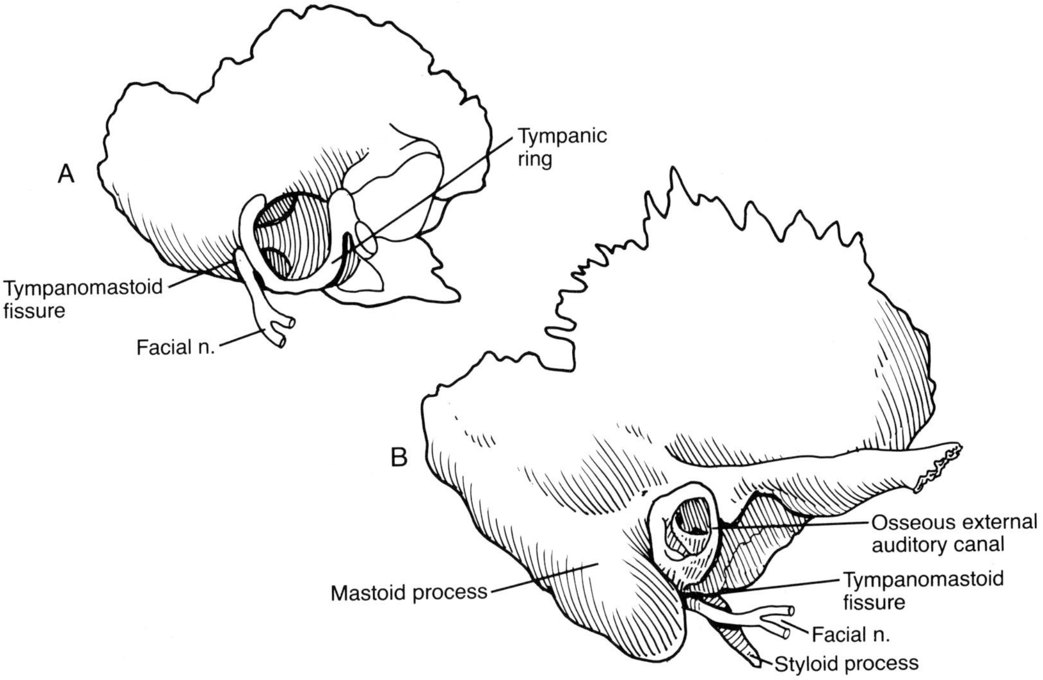

• FIGURE 25-15.

A, Newborn temporal bone. *B*, Adult temporal bone. (Modified from Montgomery WW: Surgery of the Upper Respiratory System, Vol. II. Philadelphia, Lea & Febiger, 1989, Fig. 3-11.)

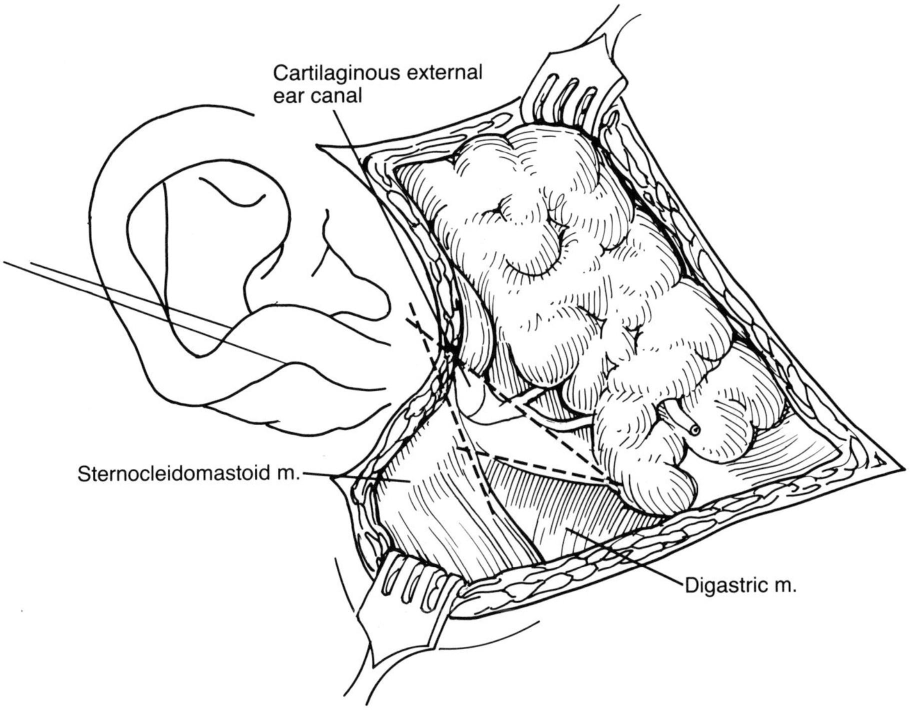

• FIGURE 25-16.

The triangle formed by the sternocleidomastoid muscle, the digastric muscle, and the cartilaginous ear canal. (Modified from Montgomery WW: Surgery of the Upper Respiratory System, Vol. II. Philadelphia, Lea & Febiger, 1989, p 254.)

• A plane of cleavage through the parotid gland is developed as proximal to distal dissection of both the upper zygomaticotemporal and lower cervicofacial divisions of the facial nerve is performed (Fig. 25–17). Branches of the posterior facial (retromandibular) vein require ligation during this portion of the procedure, as does the parotid duct if identified and transected. Once the temporal, zygomatic, buccal, and mandibular branches of the facial nerve have been completely followed to the point of turning deeply toward the facial musculature, the remaining portions of the parotid gland can be separated from the investing fascia (Fig. 25–18). This completely mobilizes the superficial lobe of the parotid gland. The so-called deep lobe of the parotid gland is the glandular tissue that remains undisturbed under the preserved facial nerve.

• A superficial parotidectomy is adequate treatment for virtually all superficially located parotid masses and allows the complete operative dissection of first and second congenital branchial anomalies. A total parotidectomy may prove necessary if the mass in question is located within the deep lobe, or if the pathology involves the entire gland, as is the case in some vasoformative lesions and chronic inflammatory processes. In such circumstances, the main trunk and individual branches of the facial nerve can be retracted gently with rubber vascular loops to allow access to the underlying parotid tissue (Fig. 25–19). The deep parotid tissue is separated from the underlying facial musculature, temporomandibular joint, and mandible. Ligation of the deeply adjacent external carotid and branching maxillary and superficial temporal arteries may be necessary. Deep parotid lobe dissection also universally exposes the parotid duct.

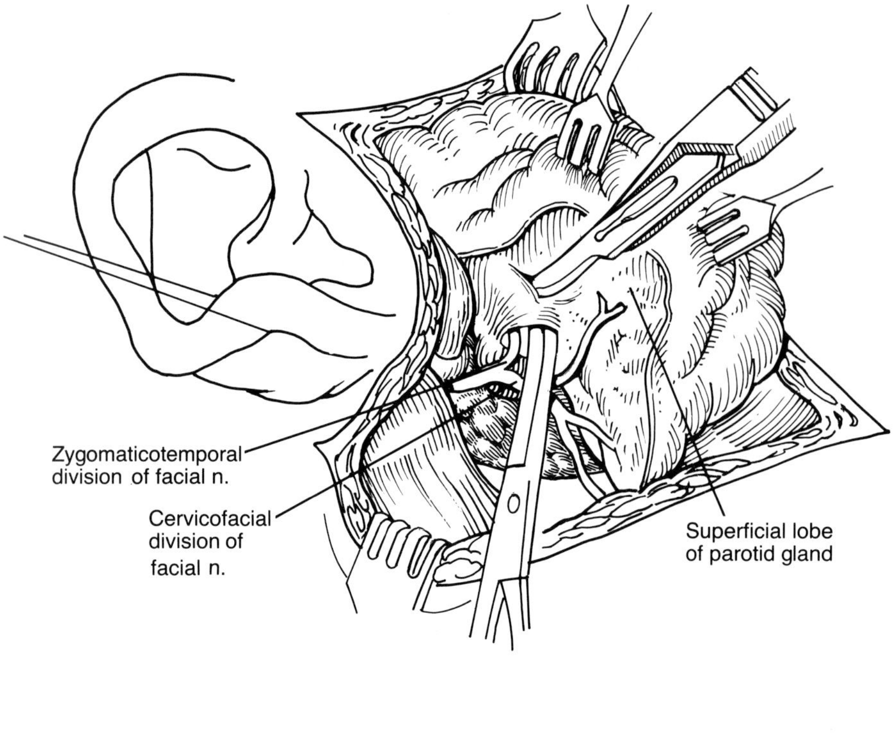

• FIGURE 25–17.

Development of a plane of cleavage through the parotid gland. (Modified from Welch KJ, Randolph JC [eds]: Pediatric Surgery, Vol. I. Chicago, Year Book Medical Publishers, 1986, p 500.)

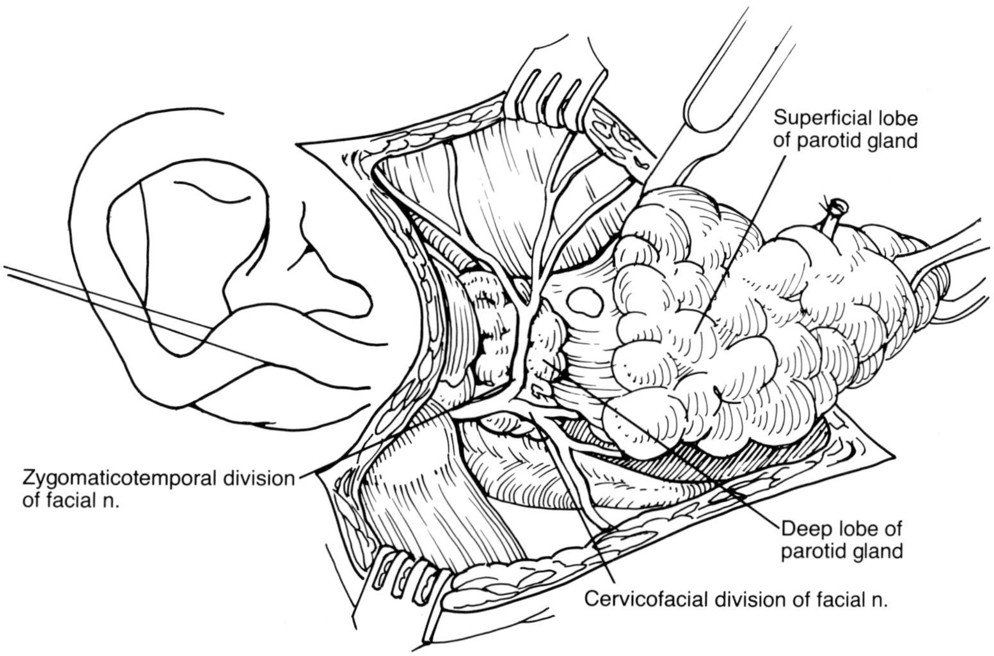

• FIGURE 25-18.

The remaining portions of the parotid gland are separated from the investing fascia, completely mobilizing the superficial lobe of the parotid gland. (Modified from Montgomery WW: Surgery of the Upper Respiratory System, Vol. II. Philadelphia, Lea & Febiger, 1989, p 256.)

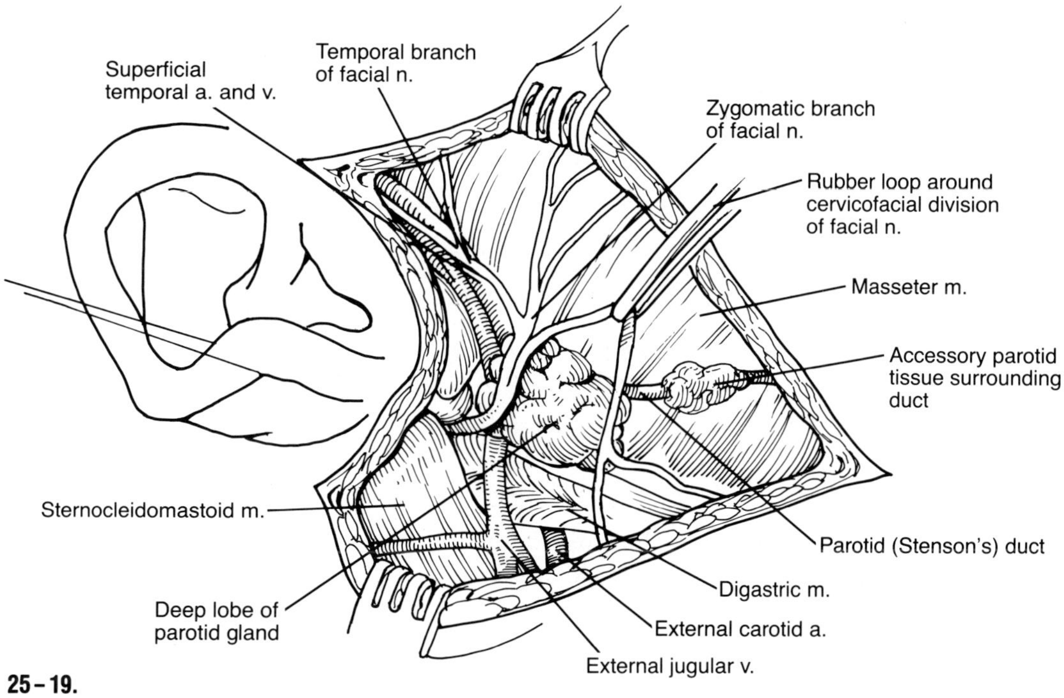

• FIGURE 25-19.

Retraction of the facial nerve with vascular loops allows access to parotid tissue. (Modified from Montgomery WW: Surgery of the Upper Respiratory System, Vol. II. Philadelphia, Lea & Febiger, 1989, pp 255 and 258; and from Loré JM: An Atlas of Head and Neck Surgery. Philadelphia, WB Saunders, 1988, p 717.)

- Invasion of the facial nerve is extremely infrequent in pediatric parotid malignancies. In the rare case of a resectable undifferentiated or sarcomatous malignancy, total parotidectomy with facial nerve resection is performed en bloc in conjunction with a neck dissection and perhaps a partial mandibulectomy. The proximal aspect of the facial nerve is typically identified within the vertical segment of the fallopian canal; the peripheral facial nerve branches are likewise identified and tagged (Fig. 25–20). Frozen-section histopathology is used to determine healthy neural margins. Immediate reconstruction by free autogenous nerve grafting is advocated using either the sural nerve or the greater auricular nerve from the opposite side of the neck; the harvesting of the former allows a two-team approach. Microanastamotic technique increases the likelihood of graft success.

- When the facial nerve has been preserved in parotid surgery, the main trunk, divisions, and individual branches of the nerve should be stimulated prior to wound closure to determine neural integrity. If the facial muscles do not twitch briskly with stimulation, the nerve must be inspected along its course for possible disruption. A transected nerve should be repaired immediately. An anatomically intact nerve may have been injured by stretching or compression.

- Following hemostasis and irrigation, suction drainage is recommended. A Jackson-Pratt drain is appropriate in older children and adolescents. In infants and young children, a Brent butterfly drain using a large test tube for vacuum purposes works well. The drain typically leaves the skin through a separate stab incision (Fig. 25–21).

- Closure is performed in two layers using interrupted absorbable sutures subcutaneously and either nylon or absorbable sutures in an interrupted or running fashion in the skin. The application of a pressure dressing completes the procedure.

Postoperative care

- Facial paresis may be observed on the side of the operation for days or even weeks postoperatively, depending on the extent of nerve mobilization. If gentle retraction was performed and no significant branches of the facial nerve have been severed, complete recovery is the rule.

- Gustatory sweating (Frey's syndrome) occurs secondary to the regrowth of parasympathetic motor fibers from the auriculotemporal nerve, which preoperatively innervated the parotid gland, into the skin. Efferent impulses that had induced salivation now stimulate the cutaneous sweat glands.

- Hypoesthesia of the earlobe is commonly present for up to several months. Permanent hypoesthesia can occur if the greater auricular nerve has been sacrificed.

- Hemorrhage with secondary hematoma or seroma formation reflects inadequate hemostasis or drainage.

- Salivary fistula formation may occur if the parotid duct has not been identified and ligated prior to transection.

• FIGURE 25-20.

Facial nerve anastomosis.

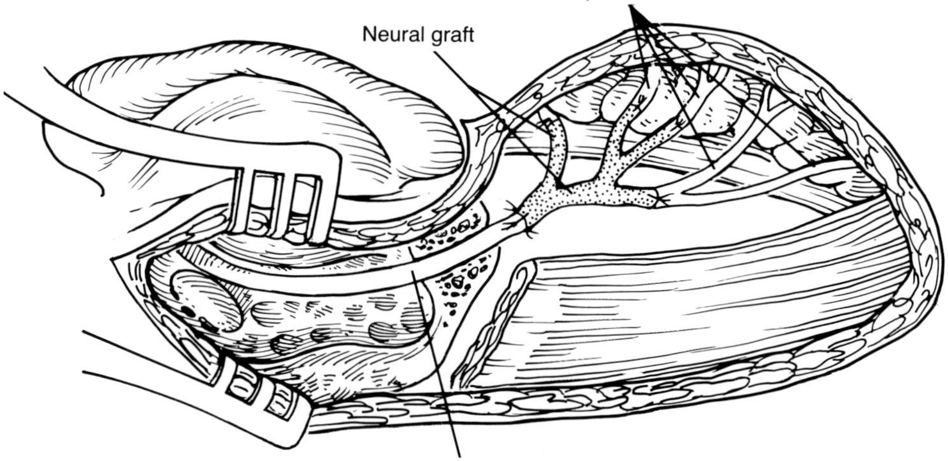

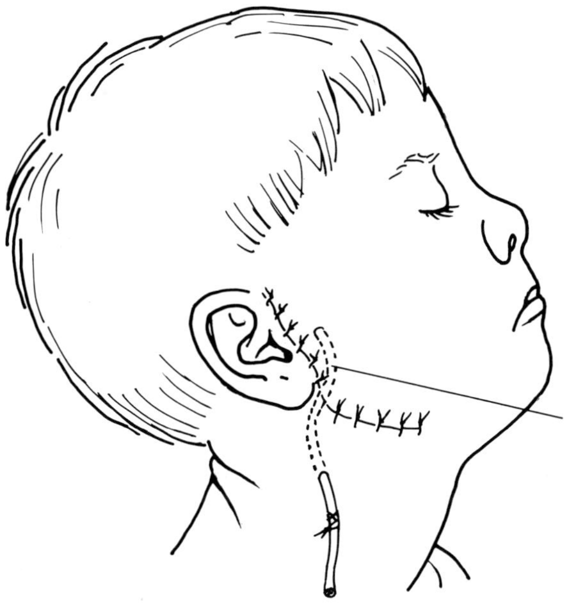

• FIGURE 25-21.

Placement of a drain through a separate stab incision.

SUBMANDIBULAR GLAND EXCISION

Submandibular gland neoplasms are extremely rare in the pediatric population. Vasoformative lesions, especially lymphangiomas, can arise within the submandibular triangle. The inflammatory processes that afflict the paraparotid lymph nodes can likewise involve the submandibular lymph nodes. The submandibular gland itself is also susceptible to a higher rate of stone formation (sialolithiasis) and secondary inflammation (sialoadenitis). Overall, excision of the submandibular gland in children is infrequently necessary.

Indications

- Chronic sialoadenitis with or without sialolithiasis
- A persistent, firm, submandibular mass of unknown or uncertain etiology
- Elective removal in an attempt to decrease salivary secretions in children with excessive drooling secondary to cerebral palsy and other neuromuscular disorders

Anesthetic considerations

The procedure is performed under general anesthesia.

Preparation

- Informed consent regarding the risk of marginal mandibular nerve injury is necessary.
- The child is positioned supine with the head turned toward the uninvolved side. The operative field is draped with sterile transparent plastic sheeting to provide exposure of the corner of the mouth on the involved side (Fig. 25–22). This allows for the intraoperative assessment of marginal mandibular nerve function.

Procedure

- A horizontal skin incision is made in a neck crease two fingerbreadths inferior and parallel to the angle and body of the mandible (Fig. 25–23).
- Infiltration of the incision with 1% lidocaine and 1:100,000 epinephrine solution provides local hemostasis.
- The skin, subcutaneous tissues and platysma muscle are divided down to the investing fascia of the submandibular gland. The mylohyoid muscle anteriorly, the sternocleidomastoid muscle posteriorly, and the digastric muscle inferiorly are exposed (Fig. 25–24).

• FIGURE 25-22.

Plastic sheeting is positioned to expose the corner of the mouth on the involved side.

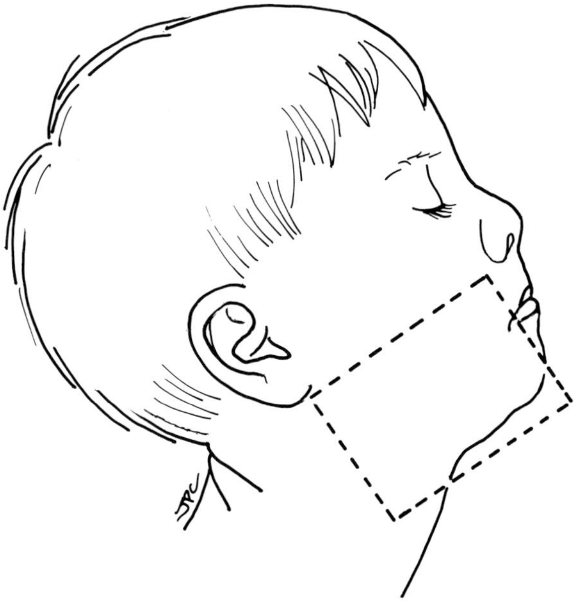

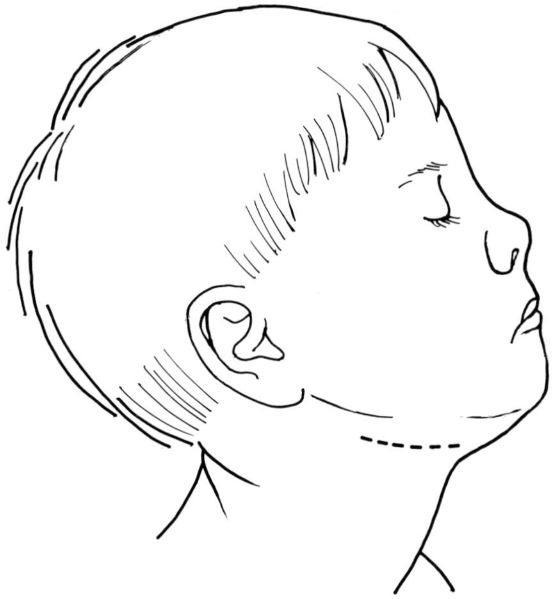

• FIGURE 25-23.

An incision is made in a neck crease.

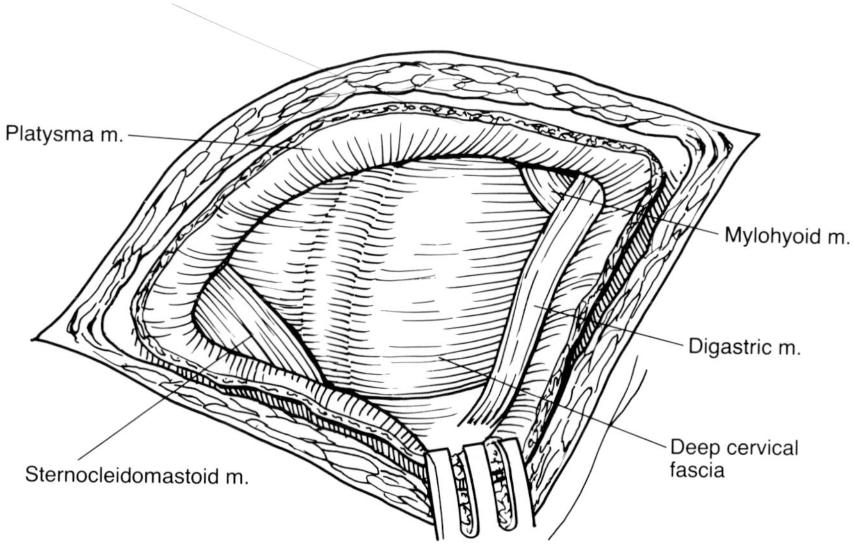

• FIGURE 25-24.

Exposure of the mylohyoid, sternocleidomastoid, and digastric muscles. (Modified from Montgomery WW: Surgery of the Upper Respiratory System, Vol. II. Philadelphia, Lea & Febiger, 1989, p 263.)

• The fascia over the submandibular gland is divided at its inferior aspect and elevated toward the mandible. The anterior facial vein is sought because this vein is usually crossed by the marginal mandibular branch of the facial nerve; ligation and elevation of this vessel with the fascia help to shield the marginal mandibular nerve from injury (Fig. 25–25). Direct identification with the use of a nerve stimulator is the best way to protect and preserve the nerve during elevation of the fascia.

• The mobilization of the submandibular gland is begun along its inferior aspect. The plane between the intermediate tendon of the digastric muscle and the submandibular gland is opened (Fig. 25–26). The hypoglossal nerve will be encountered deeply in the digastric triangle. The external maxillary (facial) artery enters the posterior aspect of the submandibular gland; this vessel is double-ligated before transection. Branches of the posterior facial (retromandibular) vein also require careful ligation.

• Anterior retraction of the mylohyoid muscle and gentle downward traction on the submandibular gland allow identification of the lingual nerve, its attached submandibular ganglion, and the submandibular (Wharton's) duct (Fig. 25–27). The duct is ligated and divided. The efferent fibers arising from the ganglion to the submandibular gland are also divided, freeing the lingual nerve from the gland. The submandibular gland is now completely mobilized by blunt dissection. The superior end of the external maxillary (facial) artery, if not previously ligated, will need to be identified and secured.

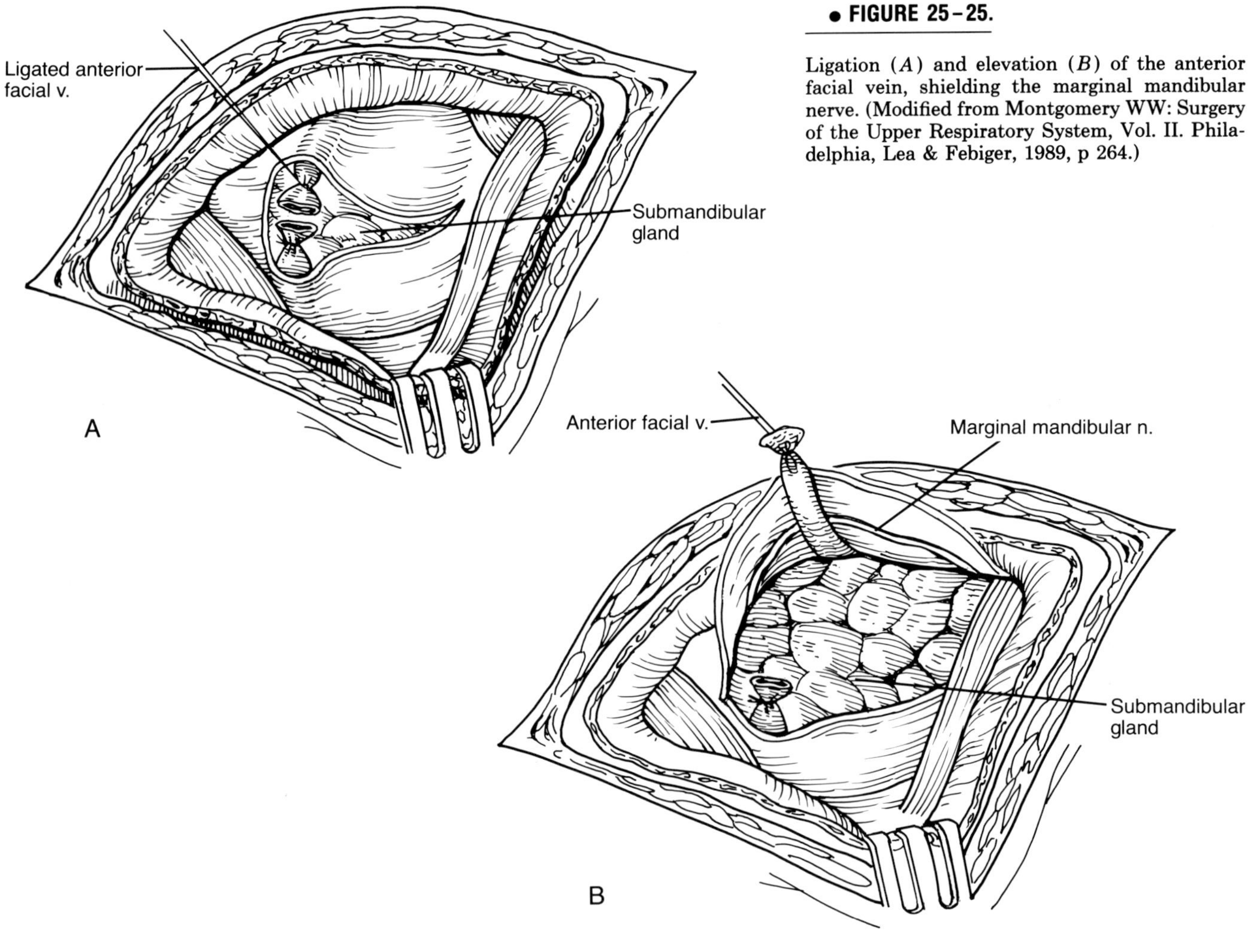

• FIGURE 25–25.

Ligation (*A*) and elevation (*B*) of the anterior facial vein, shielding the marginal mandibular nerve. (Modified from Montgomery WW: Surgery of the Upper Respiratory System, Vol. II. Philadelphia, Lea & Febiger, 1989, p 264.)

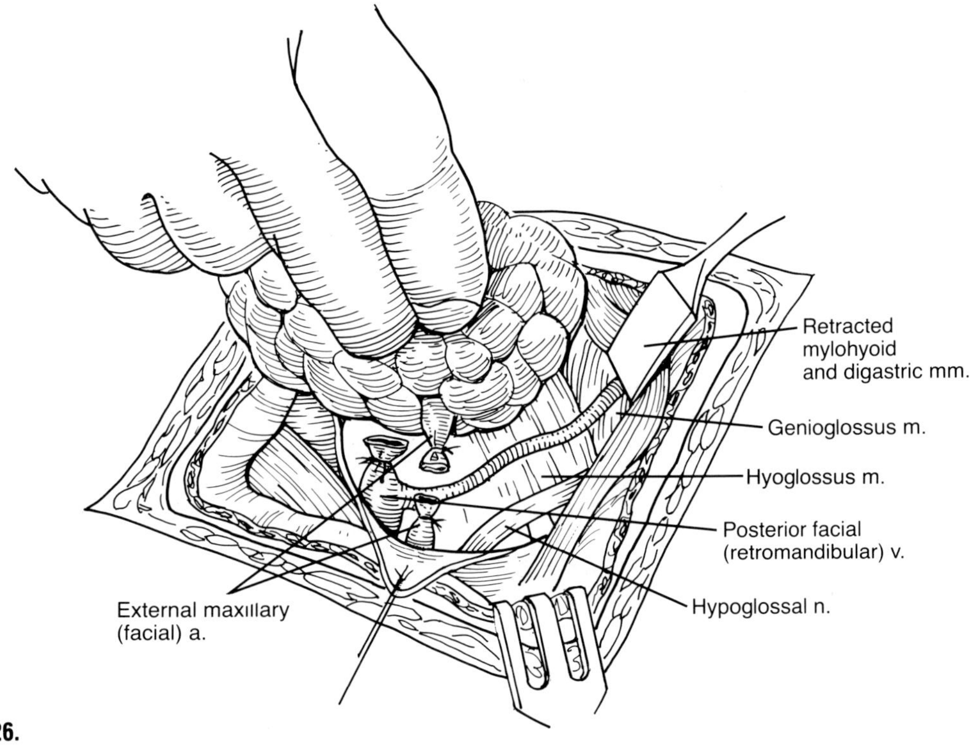

• **FIGURE 25-26.**

Exposure of the hypoglossal nerve. (Modified from Montgomery WW: Surgery of the Upper Respiratory System, Vol. II. Philadelphia, Lea & Febiger, 1989, p 269.)

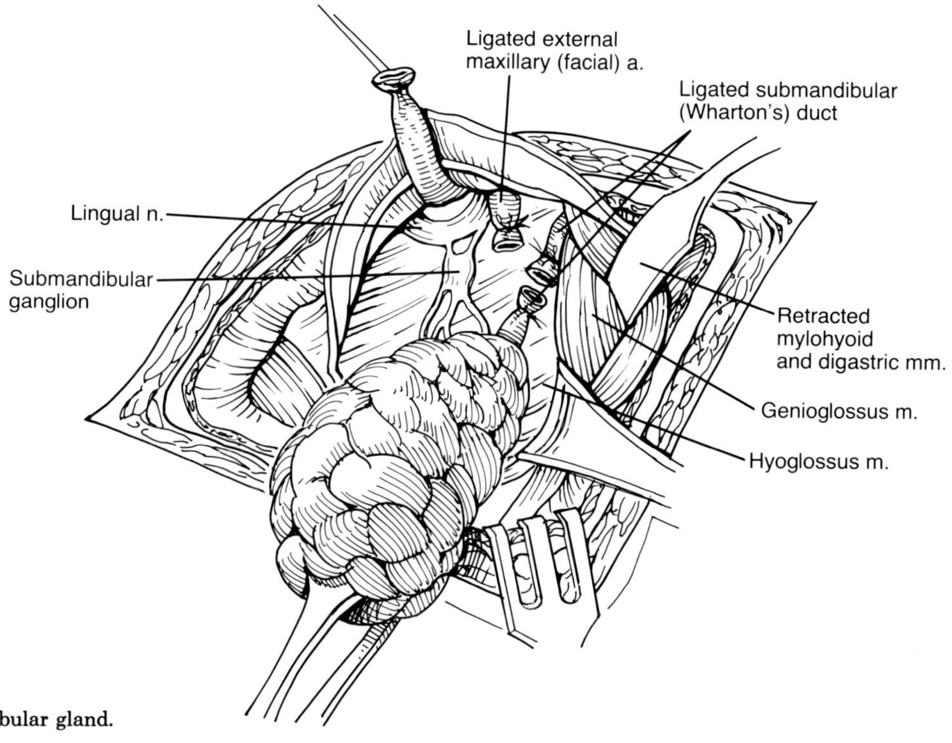

• **FIGURE 25-27.**

Complete mobilization of the submandibular gland.

• Upon removal of the specimen, the submandibular triangle is carefully explored (Fig. 25–28). The marginal mandibular nerve, if previously identified, should be stimulated to determine neural integrity.

• Following hemostasis and irrigation, a Penrose drain is placed. This drain leaves the skin through the operative incision (Fig. 25–29). Closure is performed in two layers using interrupted absorbable sutures for platysma muscle and subcutaneous tissue approximation and either interrupted or a single subcuticular nylon suture in the skin. The application of a pressure dressing completes the procedure.

Postoperative care

• Paresis or paralysis of the lower lip may occur secondary to injury to the marginal mandibular branch of the facial nerve. If the anatomic integrity of the nerve was operatively preserved, complete recovery is the rule.

• Because the platysma muscle aids in depressing the lower lip, there may be transient unilateral lip weakness secondary to its intraoperative division.

• Hemorrhage with secondary hematoma or seroma formation reflects inadequate hemostasis or drainage.

• Hypoglossal or lingual nerve injury is infrequent if these structures are properly identified intraoperatively.

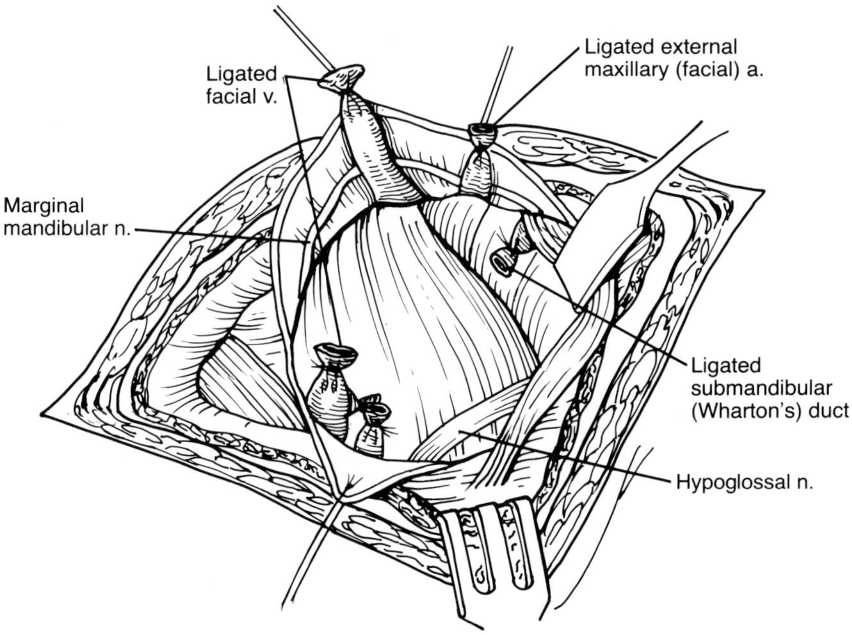

• FIGURE 25–28.

The submandibular triangle after gland removal. (Modified from Montgomery WW: Surgery of the Upper Respiratory System, Vol. II. Philadelphia, Lea & Febiger, 1989, p 269.)

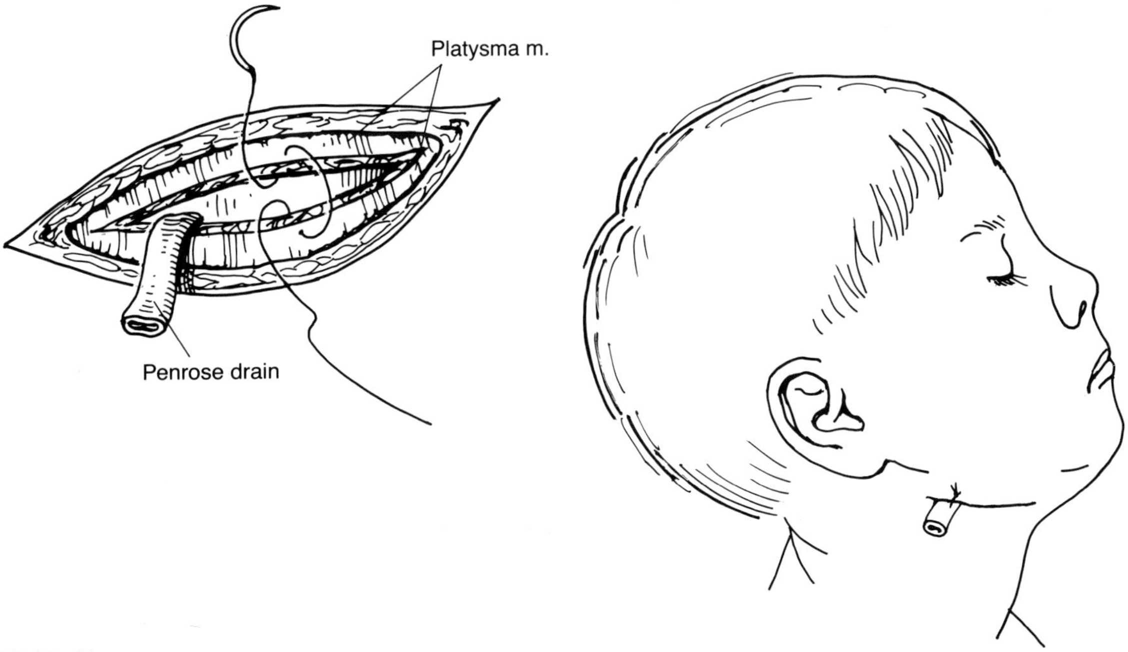

• FIGURE 25–29.

Insertion of a Penrose drain and closure. (Modified from Montgomery WW: Surgery of the Upper Respiratory System, Vol. II. Philadelphia, Lea & Febiger, 1989, p 269.)

TRANSCERVICAL RANULA EXCISION

A ranula is a retention cyst of the sublingual gland. Simple ranulas are true retention cysts of salivary gland origin that are localized to the floor of the mouth. The cervical or plunging ranula is a mucous extravasation pseudocyst that arises as a result of the escape of mucus through a ruptured sublingual duct. Such ranulas may extend through the gap between the posterior edge of the mylohyoid muscle and the anterior edge of the hyoglossus muscle into the superior cervical neck. The presence of a cystic floor-of-mouth swelling on the same side as a cystic swelling in the submandibular triangle region is suggestive of the diagnosis. Computed tomography or magnetic resonance imaging can distinguish a ranula from a cystic hygroma.

Indications

- Cervical (plunging) ranula

Anesthetic considerations

The procedure is performed under general anesthesia.

Preparation

Informed consent regarding the risk of marginal mandibular nerve injury is necessary.

Procedure

- The surgical approach described for submandibular gland resection is also used to treat this lesion. The submandibular duct passes through the same muscle cleft through which the ranula typically extends. The submandibular duct empties into the floor of the mouth medial to the sublingual gland; it provides a direct pathway to the site of ranula origin (Fig. 25–30).

- The anatomic proximity of these glandular structures often dictates the removal of the submandibular gland with ligation of its duct to allow complete removal of the plunging ranula cyst. The cervical approach provides greater exposure and protection of the lingual nerve than is possible transorally (Fig. 25–31).

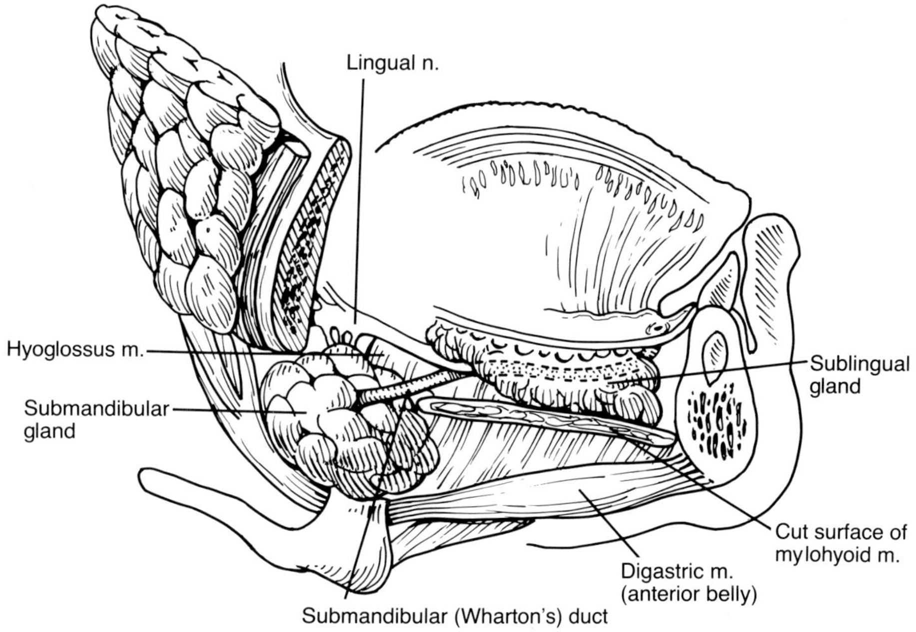

• FIGURE 25-30.

Sublingual gland showing the site of ranula origins.

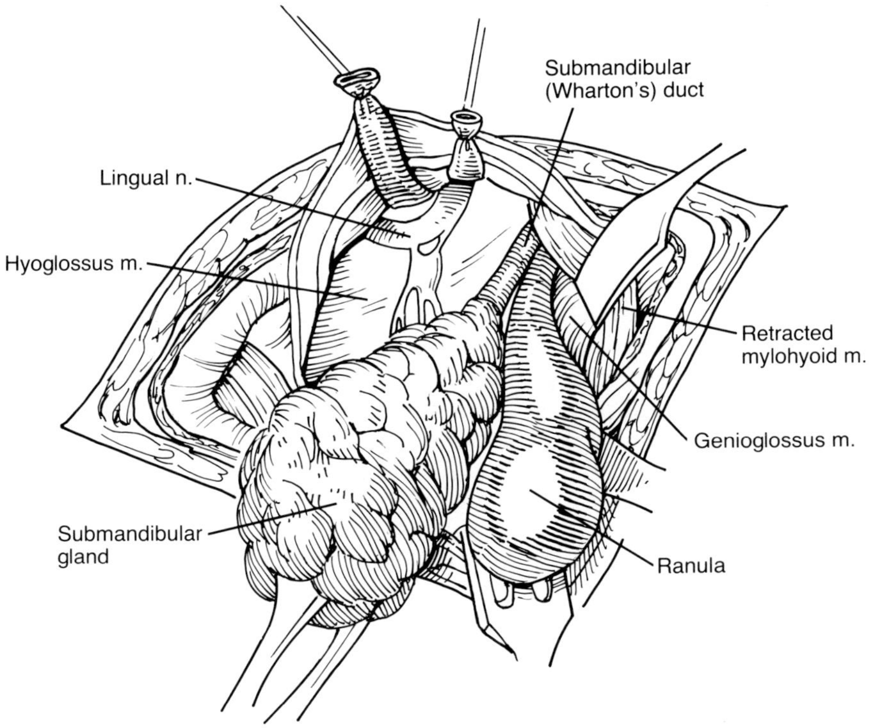

• FIGURE 25-31.

Note the well-exposed lingual nerve in the cervical approach.

• Gloved intraoral palpation on the ipsilateral floor of the mouth will help to deflect the sublingual gland into the operative field (Fig. 25–32). Complete removal of the sublingual gland is necessary.

• Cervical wound closure is performed as described in the previous section. If disruption of the floor-of-mouth mucosa occurs, closure by interrupted absorbable sutures is recommended. If removal of the submandibular gland is not planned and the submandibular duct is transected, the proximal end of the duct must be brought out through the floor-of-mouth mucosa for salivary drainage (Fig. 25–33).

Postoperative care

• The same postoperative sequelae described for submandibular gland excision can occur following the transcervical excision of a ranula. A ranula may recur if the sublingual gland is not operatively removed.

• Submandibular sialoadenitis may occur if the submandibular gland is left in place and the submandibular duct was injured intraoperatively.

THYROIDECTOMY

Thyroid surgery is not frequently performed in the pediatric age group. The common indications are a solitary thyroid mass and hyperthyroidism (Graves' disease) refractory to medical treatment.

A solitary thyroid mass in a child may represent a number of variable conditions, including thyroiditis, abscess, cyst, colloid nodule, hemiagenesis, ectopic thyroid, benign adenoma, and malignant tumors. Factors that raise suspicion for the diagnosis of malignancy include large size or rapid growth of the nodule, fixation to surrounding structures, the accompanying presence of vocal cord paralysis, associated enlarged cervical lymph nodes, a history of previous exposure to radiation therapy, or familial predisposition.

From a laboratory standpoint, the determination of serum T4, T3, thyroid-stimulating hormone (TSH), antithyroglobulin antibodies (ATA), and antimicrosomal antibodies (AMA) is necessary for the complete evaluation of the individual patient but is rarely of diagnostic help in the work-up of solitary nodules. The exception is an elevated serum calcitonin level indicative of medullary thyroid cancer.

Ultrasound examination is useful in evaluating the size, position, and multiplicity of thyroid lesions and in determining their cystic or solid character. Thyroid scanning, using ^{99}Tc or ^{123}I, complements ultrasonography, particularly in the evaluation of solitary childhood thyroid nodules. Thyroid cancer frequently appears as a cold nodule on the thyroid scan; rarely, warm or hot, nonsuppressible nodules have proved to be malignant.

FNA biopsy with cytopathologic evaluation is a valuable tool in the diagnostic work-up of thyroid nodules given the high specificity and the ease and safety of the technique in experienced hands. Positive FNA results can help to select the appropriate thyroid surgical procedure.

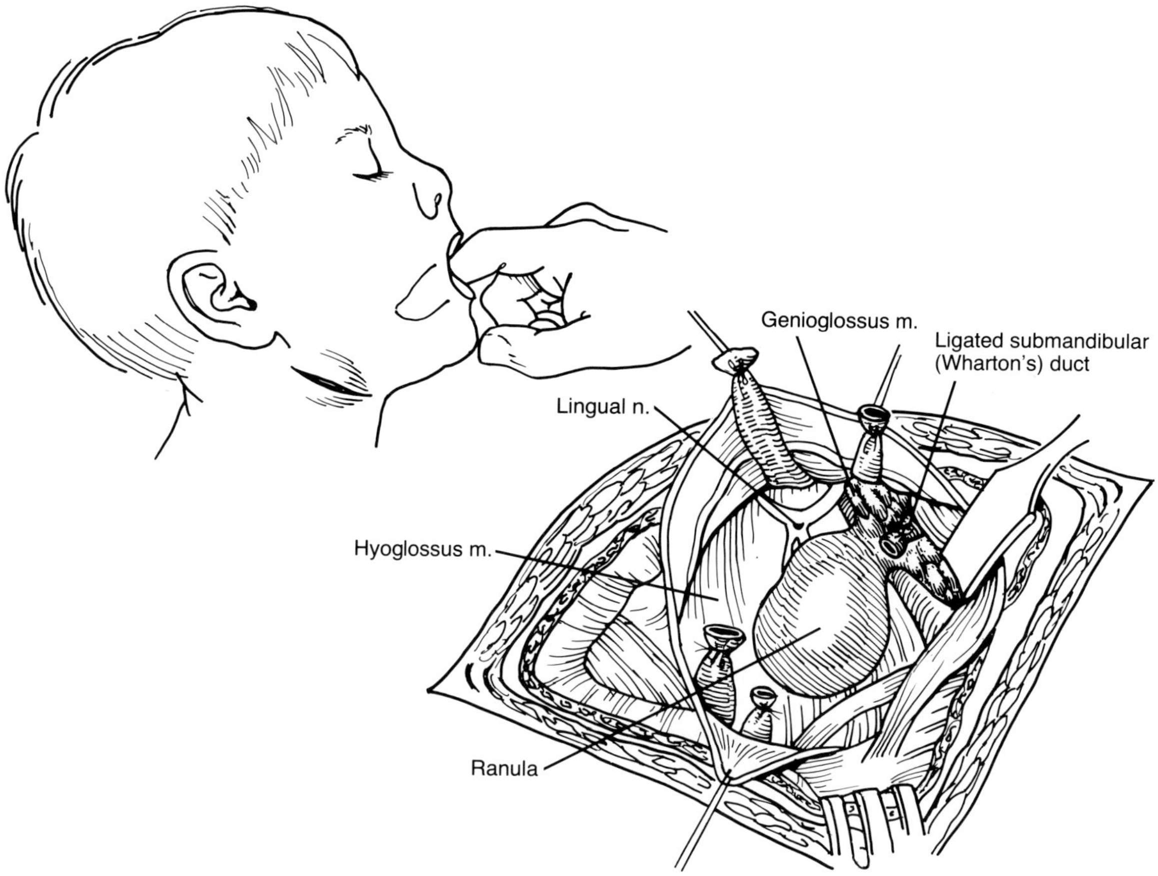

• FIGURE 25-32.

Gloved intraoral palpation displaces the ranula and sublingual gland into the operative field.

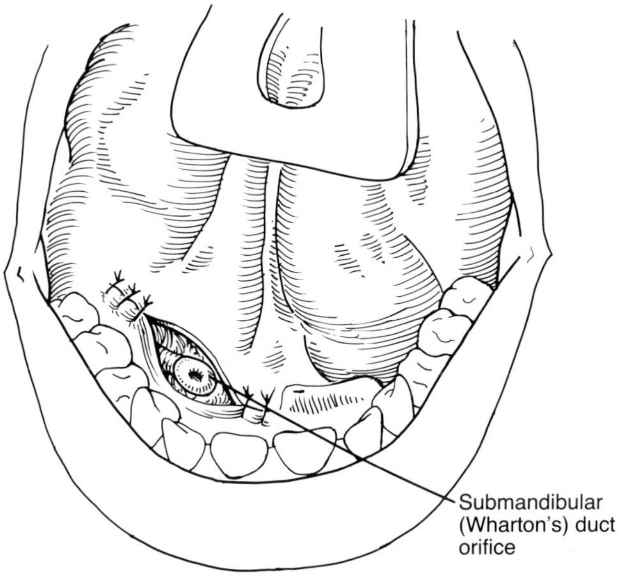

• FIGURE 25-33.

The proximal end of Wharton's duct is brought out through the floor of the mouth.

In many children with a solitary thyroid nodule, it is not possible to determine preoperatively whether the lesion is benign or malignant. Open surgical biopsy by means of total thyroid lobectomy (hemithyroidectomy) is advocated in such cases, with definitive surgery dictated by intraoperative frozen-section tissue diagnosis.

Indications

- Solitary thyroid nodule (especially a "cold" nodule or a "warm/hot" nodule that does not regress with thyroid hormone therapy)
- Hyperthyroidism (Graves' disease) refractory to medical therapy

Anesthetic considerations

The procedure is performed under general anesthesia.

Preparation

- A preoperative evaluation of vocal cord mobility is an absolute necessity. From a diagnostic standpoint, the presence of impaired vocal cord mobility is a clinical criterion that suggests the presence of a malignancy. In the case of frank vocal cord paralysis, it may be important in dictating the surgical course. In the presence of normal cord function, informed consent regarding the risk of recurrent laryngeal nerve injury is necessary.
- Children with hyperthyroidism should be rendered euthyroid prior to operative intervention. Propylthiouracil and methimazole are common antithyroid medications; propranolol is also used perioperatively at some centers. Preoperative treatment with iodine or Lugol's solution is also advocated to reduce thyroid vascularity.
- The child is positioned supine with the neck in full extension (Fig. 25–34).

Procedure

- A transverse collar incision is outlined in the lower neck. The exact position of the incision must take into account the relationship between the palpable portions of the laryngeal skeleton, the sternum, and the thyroid gland. The thyroid isthmus is situated immediately inferior to the cricoid cartilage. A natural skin crease is chosen within 1 to 2 cm of this level (Fig. 25–35). In young patients, the laryngeal structures may not be obviously palpable and may be at a considerably more cephalad level relative to the sternal notch than anticipated (Fig. 25–36).
- Infiltration of the planned incision with 1% lidocaine with 1:100,000 epinephrine solution provides hemostasis.

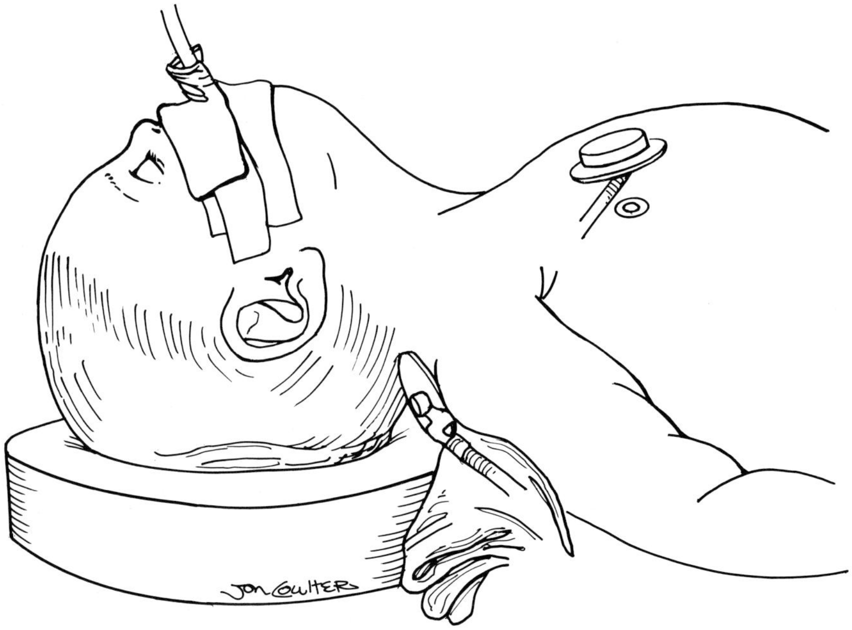

• FIGURE 25-34.

Thyroidectomy operative position.

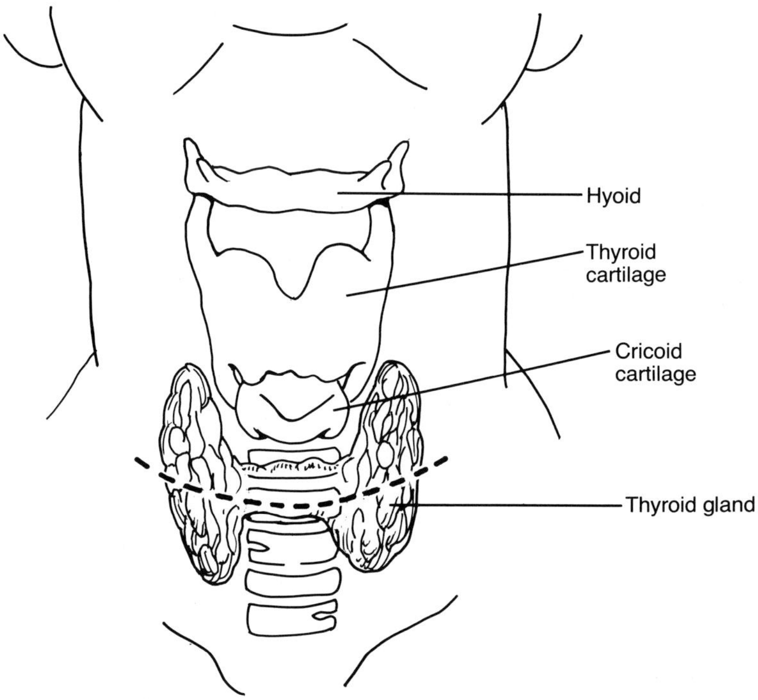

• FIGURE 25-35.

Standard incision site.

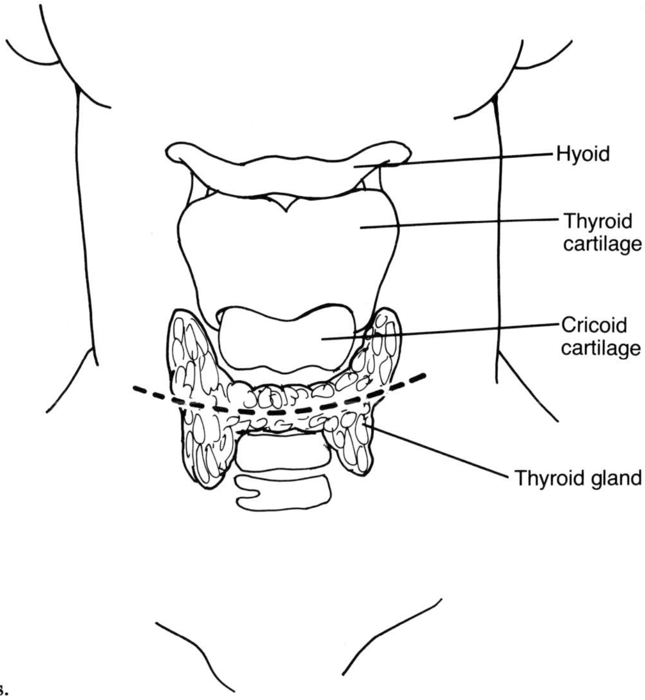

• FIGURE 25-36.

Incision site for younger patients.

• The skin, subcutaneous tissues, and platysma muscle are transected. The anterior borders of the sternocleidomastoid muscle serve as the lateral margins (Fig. 25–37). The incision should be long enough to allow adequate vertical exposure from the hyoid bone to the sternal notch.

• A superior flap is elevated in the subplatysmal plane to the level of the hyoid bone, and an inferior flap is elevated to the level of the sternal notch (Fig. 25–38).

• The midline raphe between the strap muscles is incised, and the sternohyoid and sternothyroid muscles are separated from one another and from the underlying thyroid gland (Fig. 25–39). Division of the strap muscles is infrequently necessary in the pediatric population; when required for operative exposure, the muscles should be divided high in the neck above the level of the cricoid cartilage to preserve ansa cervicalis innervation.

• Once the strap musculature is separated or divided, the sternocleidomastoid muscle on the side of the lesion is retracted so that the carotid sheath structures can be identified (Fig. 25–40). The thyroid lobe is retracted medially, and blunt dissection is carefully performed in the superior thoracic inlet just caudal to the inferior thyroid pole to identify the recurrent laryngeal nerve (RLN). When searching for the RLN, it is preferable to first identify the inferior thyroid artery. The nerve typically passes under this vessel but can cross superficial to it (Fig. 25–41).

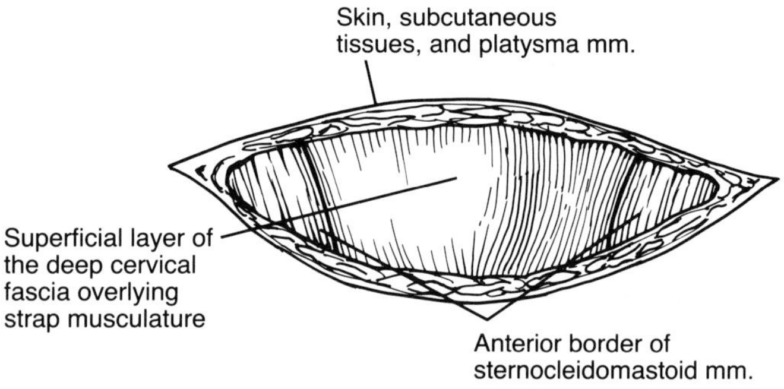

• FIGURE 25–37.

Transection of the skin, subcutaneous tissues, and platysma muscle. (Modified from Loré JM: An Atlas of Head and Neck Surgery, 3rd ed. Philadelphia, WB Saunders, 1988, p 759.)

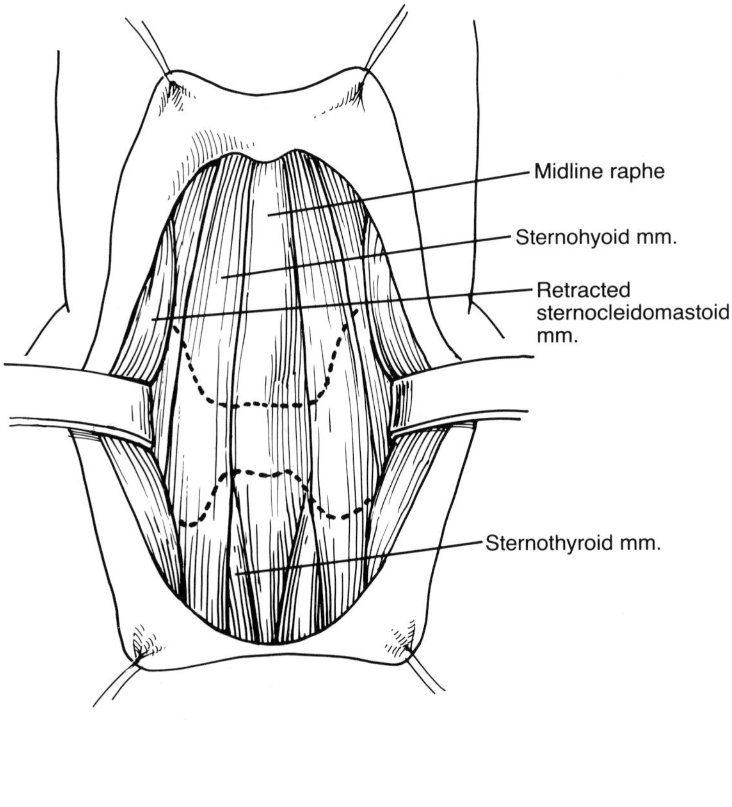

• FIGURE 25–38.

Elevation of the superior and inferior flaps. (Modified from Silver CE: Atlas of Head and Neck Surgery, p 263. New York, Churchill Livingstone, 1986.)

• FIGURE 25-39.

Retraction of the strap muscles.

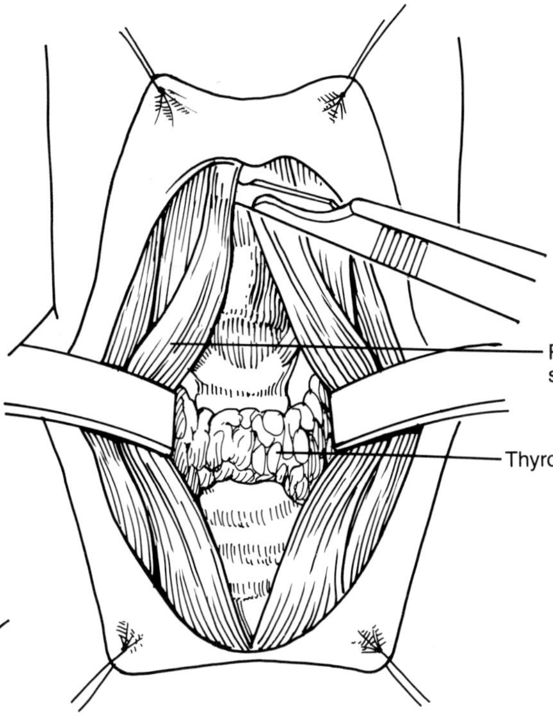

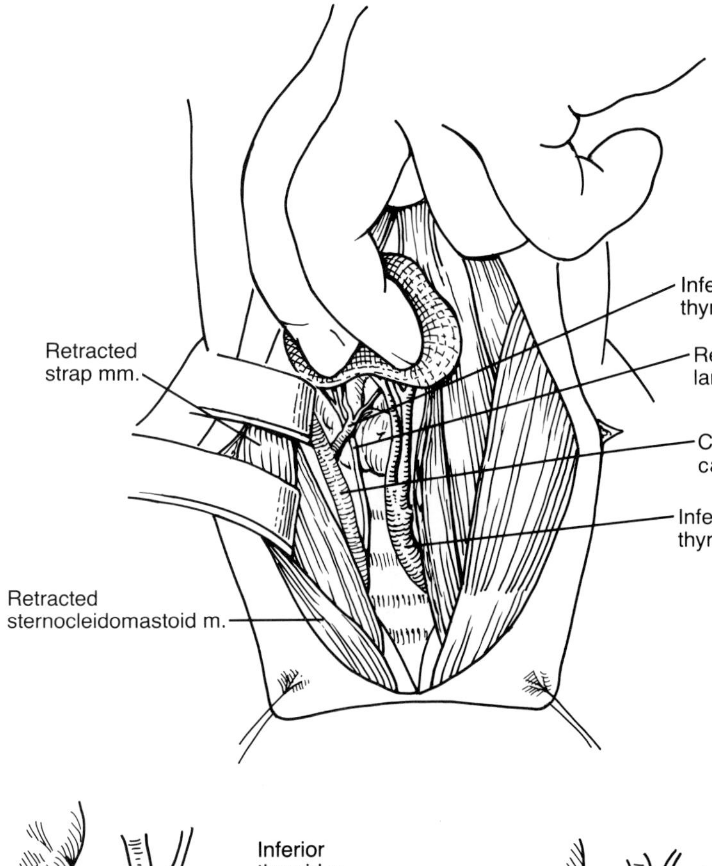

• FIGURE 25-40.

Retraction of the sternocleidomastoid muscle for carotid sheath exposure.

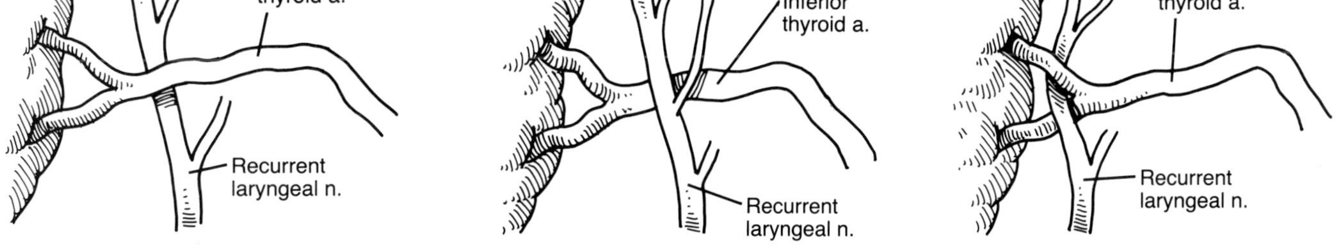

• FIGURE 25-41.

Possible positional relationships of the inferior thyroid artery and the recurrent laryngeal nerve. (Modified from Silver CE: Atlas of Head and Neck Surgery, p 261. New York, Churchill Livingstone, 1986.)

• The right RLN normally recurs beneath the right subclavian artery; the left RLN recurs beneath the aortic arch (Fig. 25–42*A*). Both recurrent nerves ascend toward the larynx in the tracheoesophageal groove. The left nerve ascends in a straight longitudinal direction parallel to the lateral border of the trachea. The right nerve follows a shorter course, approaching the larynx at a right angle, coursing medially as it ascends. Both nerves pass posterior to the thyroid lobes as they approach the cricoid cartilage. A nonrecurrent right RLN can arise horizontally off the vagus nerve in about 1% of individuals (Fig. 25–42*B*); a nonrecurrent left RLN is rare.

• Once the RLN is identified inferiorly, dissection proceeds cephalad. The inferior and middle thyroid veins on the side of the lesion will need to be ligated and divided for adequate gland mobilization (Fig. 25–43). Main truncal ligation of the inferior thyroid artery should be avoided to preserve the blood supply to the parathyroid glands; smaller, medial branches of this artery may be ligated on the capsule of the thyroid.

• The superior pole of the thyroid lobe is next mobilized by transection of the superior vascular pedicle (Fig. 25–44). Care must be taken during this portion of the procedure to avoid damage to the external branch of the superior laryngeal nerve. This nerve can sometimes be identified between the superior pole vessels and the laryngeal structures. If the plane of superior pole dissection continues bluntly along the presenting portion of the cricothyroid muscle, the likelihood of superior laryngeal nerve (SLN) injury is small. Ligation without clamping of the superior pole vessels may further decrease the likelihood of SLN injury.

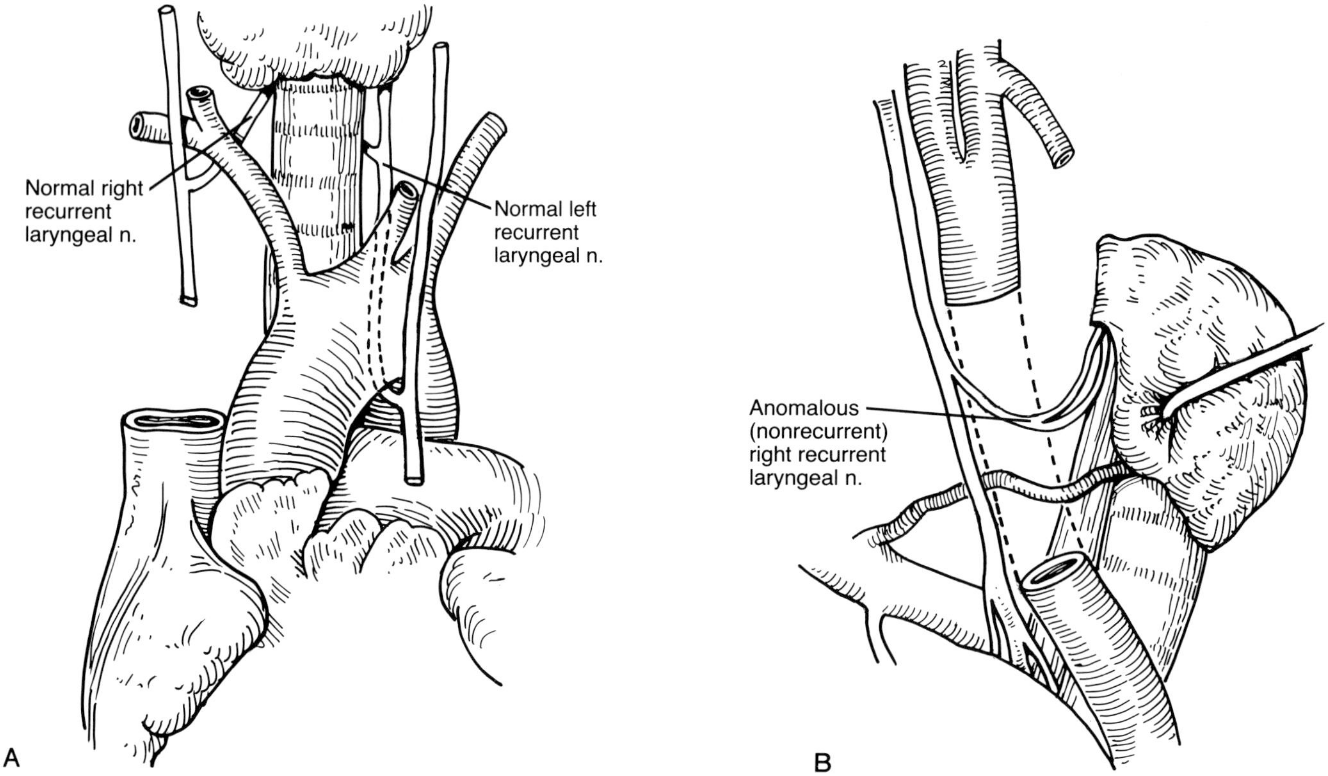

• FIGURE 25–42.

A, Normal right and left recurrent laryngeal nerves. *B*, Anomalous (nonrecurrent) right recurrent laryngeal nerve. (Modified from Silver CE: Atlas of Head and Neck Surgery. New York, Churchill Livingstone, 1986, pp 260–261.)

• FIGURE 25–43.

Ligation and division of the inferior and middle thyroid veins. (Modified from Silver CE: Atlas of Head and Neck Surgery. New York, Churchill Livingstone, 1986, p 265.)

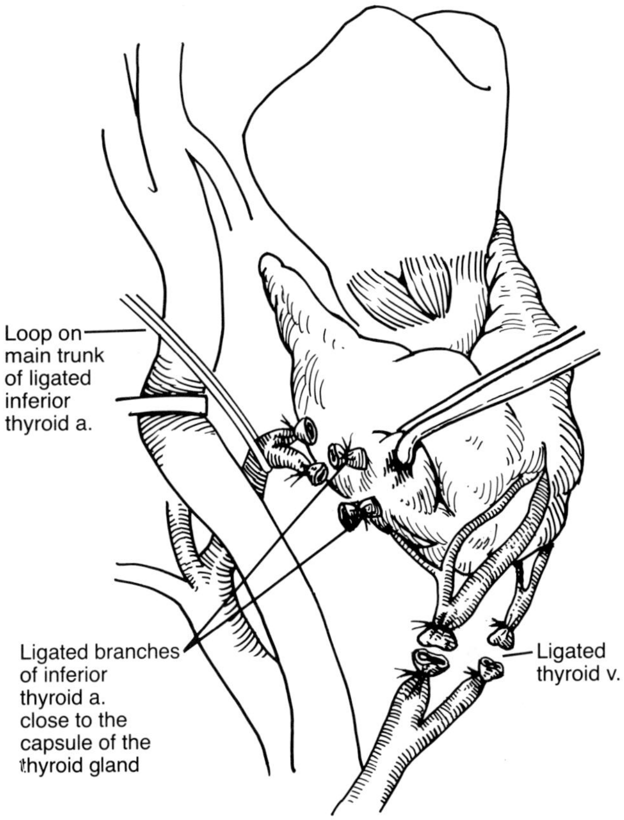

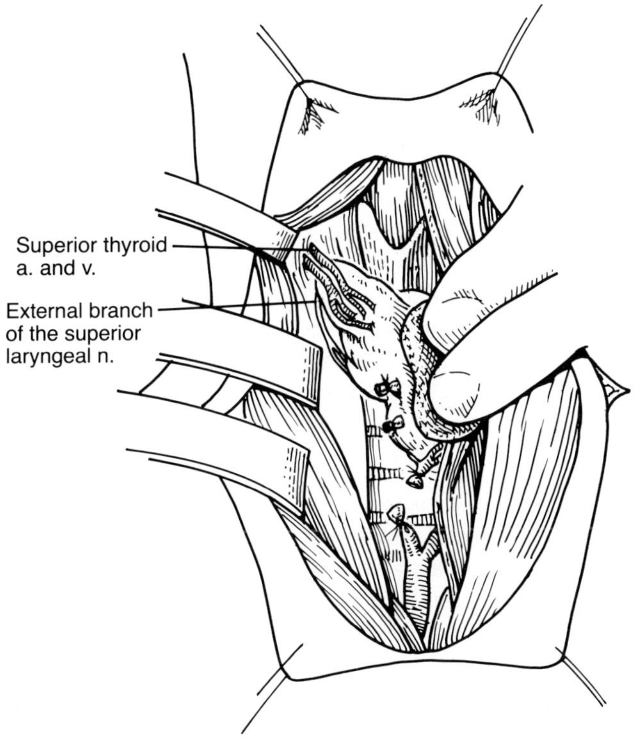

• FIGURE 25–44.

Transection of the superior vascular pedicle.

• Following transection of the superior vascular pedicle, the superior pole of the thyroid lobe is reflected inferiorly. The thyroid lobe now remains firmly attached by the lateral or posterior (Berry's) suspensory ligament (Fig. 25–45). This ligament extends bilaterally from the cricoid cartilage and first tracheal ring to the posteromedial aspect of each thyroid lobe. It is an extremely important structure because the RLN typically passes immediately deep to this ligament. Variations exist, however, and must be anticipated. Once the RLN has been clearly identified, the suspensory ligament is transected. A portion of thyroid tissue may also extend deep to this ligament and must be carefully removed.

• Once the suspensory ligament is transected, the remaining thyroid lobe separates easily from the surface of the trachea. Dissection proceeds medially until the entire isthmus has been elevated. The isthmus is transected at its junction with the contralateral lobe (Fig. 25–46).

• This completes a total thyroid lobectomy (hemithyroidectomy). If the indication for surgical intervention is a thyroid mass of unknown etiology, or if confirmation of needle biopsy findings is sought, a frozen-section examination of the hemithyroidectomy specimen is performed. Pathologic findings may dictate the further performance of a total or near-total thyroidectomy procedure.

• If the diagnosis of thyroid carcinoma (typically papillary or papillary follicular) is pathologically established, the decision needs to be made about whether to consider the hemithyroidectomy as the definitive procedure, taking a chance of a recurrence in the contralateral lobe, or to immediately perform a (near-) total thyroidectomy with its greater risk for permanent hypoparathyroidism and obvious need for lifelong thyroid hormone replacement. Near-total thyroidectomy allows for postoperative radionuclide scanning for the future detection of both local recurrence and metastases and enhances the efficacy of ^{131}I therapy, if needed.

• During removal of the contralateral lobe, the identical technique previously described for the ipsilateral lobe with exposure of the RLN is used. Identification and preservation of parathyroid tissue is crucial. In an effort to preserve contralateral parathyroid tissue, some surgeons advocate the performance of a so-called subtotal or near-total thyroidectomy technique. A small portion of the contralateral thyroid lobe is left in situ with its adjacent parathyroid gland(s); the inferior thyroid artery is also not ligated, in order to preserve the blood supply to these glands (Fig. 25–47).

• The concept of near-total thyroidectomy is controversial because of the possible future need, due to disease recurrence, to remove the small wedge of thyroid tissue left behind. There is a much greater risk to the RLN and residual parathyroid glands under such circumstances. There also appears to be little correlation between thyroid function and the amount of residual thyroid tissue. These problems have led many authors to consider the procedure of choice to be total thyroidectomy with identification and, if need be, reimplantation of the parathyroid glands.

• When more advanced thyroid cancer (as evidenced by the infiltration of surrounding tissues or cervical and systemic metastases) is present, total thyroidectomy with paratracheal lymph node removal is imperative. The accompanying performance of modified neck dissection depends on the specific thyroid malignancy and is not universally performed in children, even in the presence of cervical metastases.

• Following either hemithyroidectomy or (near-) total thyroidectomy, the operative site is carefully reinspected for the presence of parathyroid glands and for the integrity of the RLN and SLN. Following hemostasis and irrigation, a Penrose drain is placed and the strap muscles are loosely approximated in the midline.

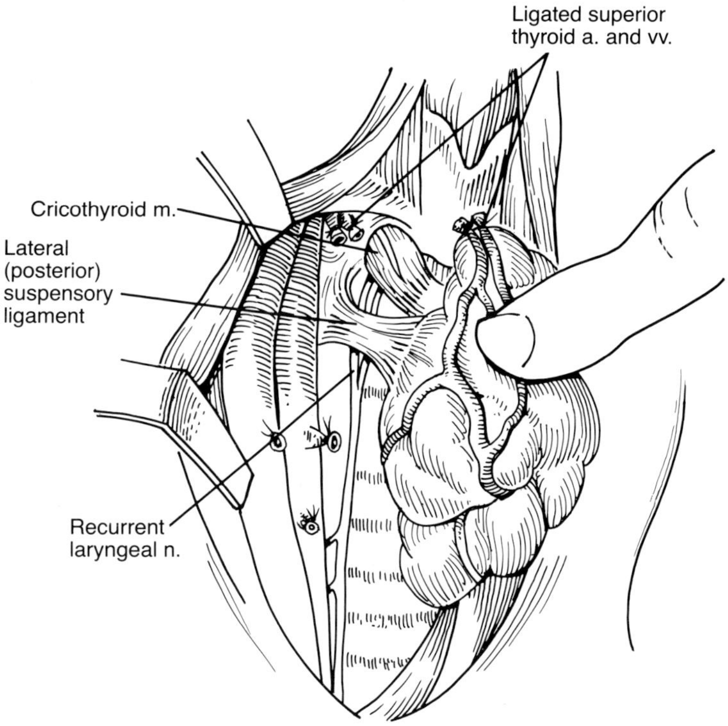

• FIGURE 25-45.

Lateral (posterior) suspensory ligament before transection. (Modified from Loré JM: An Atlas of Head and Neck Surgery, 3rd ed. Philadelphia, WB Saunders, 1988, p 775.)

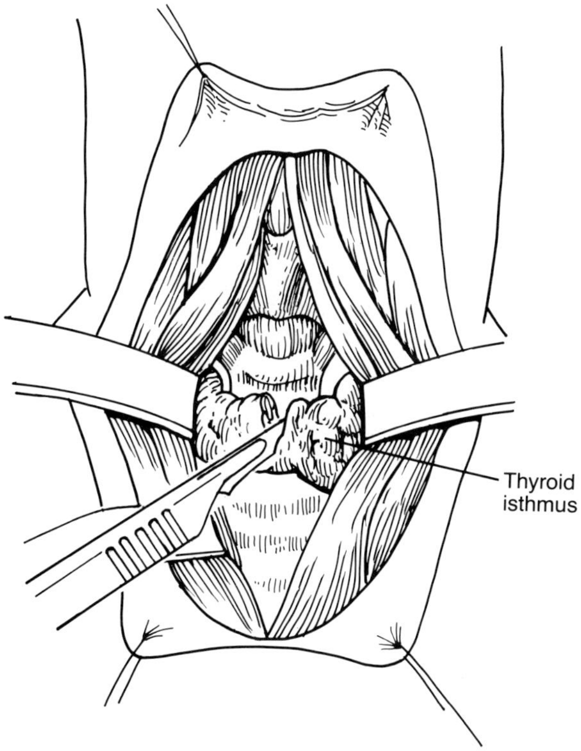

• FIGURE 25-46.

Transection of the thyroid isthmus.

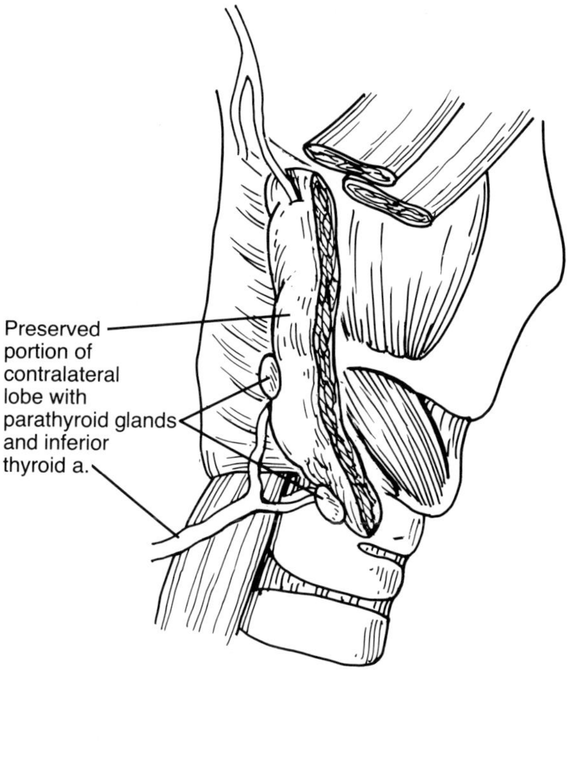

• FIGURE 25-47.

Remaining contralateral thyroid lobe and parathyroid glands after near-total thyroidectomy. (Modified from Silver CE: Atlas of Head and Neck Surgery. New York, Churchill Livingstone, 1986, p 271.)

• Closure is performed in two layers, using interrupted absorbable sutures to approximate platysma muscle and subcutaneous tissues and either interrupted or a single subcuticular nylon suture for skin (Fig. 25–48). The application of a pressure dressing completes the procedure.

Postoperative care

• Injury to either the RLNs or the external branch of the SLNs may occur. RLN injury typically results in an immobile vocal cord in a midline or paramedian position. SLN injury results in a bowed vocal cord. Both neural injuries adversely affect the voice; the former may also predispose to aspiration or airway obstruction.

• Hemorrhage with hematoma or seroma formation reflects inadequate hemostasis or drainage.

• Airway obstruction immediately following thyroid surgery may result either from hematoma formation with tracheal compression or from bilateral RLN injury during total thyroidectomy. In the event of acute postoperative airway obstruction, the dressing should be removed immediately for inspection of the neck. If no hematoma is found and airway intervention is not immediately necessary, a flexible laryngoscopic examination of the true vocal cords is indicated. The documentation of cord paralysis not anticipated from the intraoperative procedure dictates re-exploration to assess RLN integrity.

• Hypoparathyroidism with hypocalcemia may result from direct injury or resection of the parathyroid glands or their devascularization by ligation of the inferior thyroid artery(s).

• Hypothyroidism is an expected result following total thyroidectomy and also occurs frequently following near-total thyroidectomy procedures. Long-term thyroid hormone replacement is anticipated under such circumstances.

• The occurrence of a "thyroid storm" has been reported intraoperatively during total thyroidectomy in the treatment of hyperthyroidism (Graves' disease). As noted earlier, the likelihood of this complication is decreased by preoperatively rendering the patient euthyroid and by perioperatively using propranolol therapy.

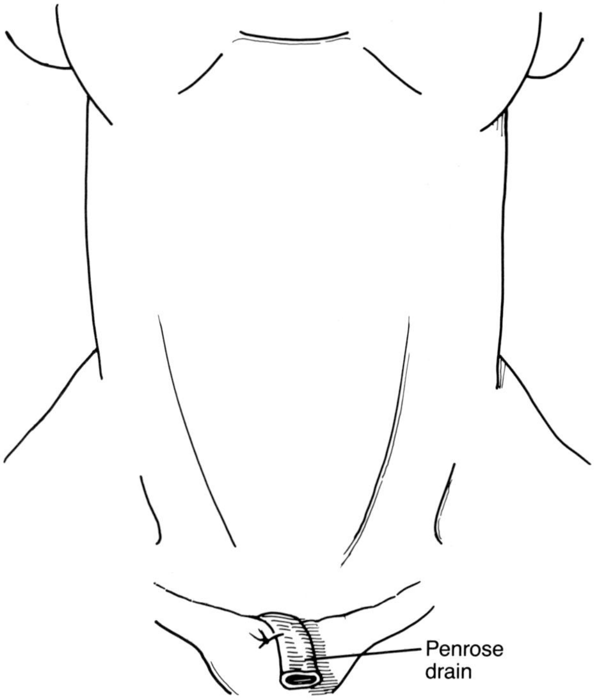

• FIGURE 25-48.

Penrose drain insertion and closure.

BIBLIOGRAPHY

Bryarly RC, Shockley WW, and Stucker FJ: The method and management of thyroid surgery in the pediatric patient. Laryngoscope 95:1025–1028, 1985.

Busby DR: Otolaryngologic surgery. *In* Manual of Ambulatory Surgery. Kassity KJ, McKittrick JE, Preston FW (eds): New York, Springer-Verlag, 1982, pp 40–43.

Camacho AE, Goodman ML, and Eavey RD: Pathologic correlation of the unknown solid parotid mass in children. Otolaryngol Head Neck Surg 101:566–571, 1989.

Ching T, Warden MJ, and Fefferman RA: Thyroid surgery in children and teenagers. Arch Otolaryngol Head Neck Surg 103:544–546, 1977.

Crysdale WS, Mendelsohn JD, and Conley S: Ranulas — mucoceles of the oral cavity: Experience in 26 children. Laryngoscope 98:296–298, 1988.

DeKeyser LFM and Van Herle AJ: Differentiated thyroid cancer in children. Head Neck Surg 8:100–114, 1985.

Farrior JB and Santini H: Facial nerve identification in children. Otolaryngol Head Neck Surg 93:173–176, 1985.

Jafek BW and Sasaki CT: Submandibular gland excision. *In* Loré JM: An Atlas of Head and Neck Surgery. New York, Grune & Stratton, 1983, pp 241–245.

Knight PJ, Mulne AF, and Vassy LE: When is a lymph node biopsy indicated in children with enlarged peripheral nodes? Pediatrics 69:391–396, 1982.

Knight PJ and Reiner CB: Superficial lumps in children: What, when, and why? Pediatrics 72:147–153, 1983.

Loré JM Jr: Endocrine surgery. *In* Loré JM: An Atlas of Head and Neck Surgery. Philadelphia, WB Saunders, 1988, pp 726–783.

Loré JM Jr: Excision of ranula. *In* Loré JM: An Atlas of Head and Neck Surgery. Philadelphia, WB Saunders, 1988, pp 618–619.

Loré JM Jr: The parotid salivary glands. *In* Loré JM: An Atlas of Head and Neck Surgery. Philadelphia, WB Saunders, 1988, pp 708–725.

Loré JM Jr: Resection of the submandibular salivary gland for benign disease. *In* Loré JM: An Atlas of Head and Neck Surgery. Philadelphia, WB Saunders, 1988, pp 708–725.

Luna MA, Batsakis JG, and El-Naggar AK: Salivary gland tumors in children. Ann Otol Rhinol Laryngol 100:869–871, 1991.

Matt BH and Crockett DM: Plunging ranula in an infant. Otolaryngol Head Neck Surg 99:330–333, 1988.

May M and D'Angelo AJ Jr: The facial nerve and the branchial cleft: Surgical challenge. Laryngoscope 99:564–565, 1989.

Mobley DL, Wakely PE, and Frable MAS: Fine-needle aspiration biopsy: Application to pediatric head and neck masses. Laryngoscope 101:469–472, 1991.

Montgomery WW: Surgery of the salivary glands. *In* Surgery of the Upper Respiratory System, Vol. II Philadelphia, Lea & Febiger, 1989, pp 225–269.

Myers EN and Cunningham MJ: Tumors of the neck. *In* Bluestone CD and Stool SE (eds): Pediatric Otolaryngology, Vol II. Philadelphia, WB Saunders, 1990, pp 1351–1356.

Reyes HM, Wright JK, and Rosenfield RL: Prevention of hypocalcemia in children due to parathyroid infarction after thyroidectomy. Surg Gynecol Obstetr 148:76–78, 1979.

Welch KJ. The salivary glands. *In* KJ Welch, JC Randolph, et al (eds) Pediatric Surgery, Vol I. Chicago, Yearbook Medical Publishers, 1986, pp 487–502.

Wesley JR, Buckingham BA, Gahr JA, et al: Surgical treatment of hyperthyroidism in children. Surg Gynecol Obstetr 145:343–346, 1977.

index

NOTE: Page numbers in *italics* refer to illustrations.

ISBN 0-7216-3711-6
90038
9 780721 637112